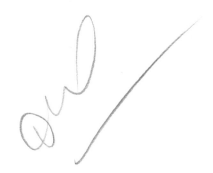

Clinical Emergency Radiology
Second Edition

This book is a highly visual guide to the radiographic and advanced imaging modalities – such as computed tomography and ultrasonography – that are frequently used by physicians during the treatment of emergency patients. Covering practices ranging from ultrasound at the point of care to the interpretation of CT scan results, this book contains more than 2,200 images, each with detailed captions and line art that highlight key findings. Within each section, particular attention is devoted to practical tricks of the trade and tips for avoiding common pitfalls. This book is a useful source for experienced clinicians, residents, mid-level providers, and medical students who want to maximize the diagnostic accuracy of each modality without losing valuable time.

J. Christian Fox received his undergraduate degree at University of California, Irvine, and his MD at Tufts Medical School. Since joining the UC Irvine faculty in 2001 as Chief of the Division of Emergency Ultrasound, he has directed the Ultrasound Fellowship. In 2010 he created a fully integrated four-year ultrasound curriculum at the School of Medicine. He is the editor of *Clinical Emergency Radiology* as well as *Atlas of Emergency Ultrasound*, and has authored over eighty articles on ultrasound.

Clinical Emergency Radiology
Second Edition

Edited by
J. Christian Fox
University of California, Irvine

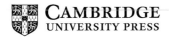
CAMBRIDGE
UNIVERSITY PRESS

CAMBRIDGE
UNIVERSITY PRESS

University Printing House, Cambridge CB2 8BS, United Kingdom

One Liberty Plaza, 20th Floor, New York, NY 10006, USA

477 Williamstown Road, Port Melbourne, VIC 3207, Australia

4843/24, 2nd Floor, Ansari Road, Daryaganj, Delhi – 110002, India

79 Anson Road, #06–04/06, Singapore 079906

Cambridge University Press is part of the University of Cambridge.

It furthers the University's mission by disseminating knowledge in the pursuit of education, learning, and research at the highest international levels of excellence.

www.cambridge.org
Information on this title: www.cambridge.org/9781107065796

First published 2008
Second edition 2017

Printed in the United Kingdom by Clays, St Ives plc

A catalog record for this publication is available from the British Library.

ISBN 978-1-107-06579-6 Hardback

Contents

Part IV—Magnetic Resonance Imaging

Contributors

Kenny Banh
University of California, San Francisco – Fresno

Gregory Hendey
University of California Los Angeles

Peter DeBlieux
Louisiana State University

Lisa Mills
University of California, Davis

Anthony J. Dean
University of Pennsylvania

Ross Kessler
University of Michigan

Eric Fox Silman
University of California, San Francisco

Olusola Balogun
University of Illinois, Chicago Christ Hospital

Natalie Kmetuk
University of Illinois, Chicago Christ Hospital

Christine Kulstad
University of Illinois, Chicago Christ Hospital

Kenneth T. Kwon
Mission Hospital, Mission Viejo, California

Lauren Pellman
University of Nevada, Las Vegas

Loren G. Yamamoto
University of Hawaii

Michael Peterson
University of California, Los Angeles

Seric S. Cusick
Hoag Hospital

Theodore Nielsen
FujiFilm SonoSite, Inc

William Scruggs
University of Hawaii

Laleh Gharahbaghian
Stanford University

Bret Nelson
Mount Sinai University

Eitan Dickman
Maimonides Medical Center

David Blehar
University of Massachussets

Romolo Gaspari
University of Massachussets

Chris Moore
Yale University

James Hwang
Scripps Memorial Hospital, La Jolla, California

Deepak Chandwani
University of California, Riverside

Daniel D. Price
Alameda County Medical Center, Highland Hospital

Sharon R. Wilson
University of California, Davis

Michael Lambert
University of Illinois, Chicago Christ Hospital

Viet Tran
Garden Grove Medical Center, California

Zareth Irwin
Legacy Emanuel Medical Center, Portland, Oregon

Paul R. Sierzenski
Christiana Care Health System, Delaware

Gillian Baty
University of New Mexico

Shane Arishenkoff
University of British Columbia

Tala Elia
Tufts University

JoAnne McDonough
Ellis Medicine, Schenectady, New York

Katrina Dean
University of California, Irvine

Anthony J. Weeks
Carolinas Medical Center, Charlotte, North Carolina

Resa E. Lewiss
University of Colorado

Tarina Kang
University of Southern California

Melissa Joseph
University of Southern California

Michael E. R. Habicht
Barton Memorial Hospital, South Lake Tahoe, California

Samantha Costantini
University of California, Irvine

Marlowe Majoewsky
University of Southern California

Stuart Swadron
University of Southern California

Monica Wattana
University of Texas, Houston

Tareg Bey
Saudi Arabia

Jonathan Patane
University of California, Irvine

Megan Osborn
University of California, Irvine

Nichole Meissner
Kaweah Delta Medical Center, Visalia, California

Matthew Dolich
University of California, Irvine

Swaminatha V. Gurudevan
Healthcare Partners Medical Group, Glendale, California

Reza Arsanjani
Cedars-Sinai Medical Center, Los Angeles, California

Kathleen Latouf
Canonsburg Hospital, Pennsylvania

Steve Nanini
University of Illinois, Chicago Christ Hospital

Martha Villalba
Jesse Brown Veterans Affairs Medical Center, Chicago, Illinois

Saud Siddiqui
George Washington Univeristy Hospital

Nilasha Ghosh
Northwestern University

Chanel Fischetti
Duke University

Andrew Berg
Northwestern University

Bharath Chakravarthy
University of California, Irvine

Joseph Dinglasan
St. Judes Hospital, Fullerton California

Asmita Patel
University of Illinois, Chicago Christ Hospital

Colleen Crowe
Medical College of Wisconsin

Brian Sayger
University of Illinois, Chicago Christ Hospital

Aaron Harries
Alameda County Medical Center, Highland Hospital

Andrew V. Bokarius
University of Chicago

Armando S. Garza
Orange Coast Memorial Medical Center, Fountain Valley, California

Bryan Sloane
University of California, Los Angeles

Mark Langdorf
University of California, Irvine

Lancelot Beier
Virginia Commonwealth University

Andrew Wong
University of California, Irvine

Kathryn J. Stevens
Stanford University

Shaun V. Mohan
Stanford University

Plain Radiography of the Upper Extremity in Adults

Kenny Banh and Gregory W. Hendey

Plain radiography remains the imaging study of choice for most applications in the upper extremity. Far and away the most common indication for plain radiography in the upper extremity is acute trauma. The shoulder, humerus, elbow, forearm, wrist, and hand are common radiographic series that are useful in diagnosing an acute fracture. Other imaging modalities such as CT, ultrasound, and MRI are not generally indicated in acute trauma but have an important role in diagnosing soft tissue pathology.

Another common indication for plain radiography of the upper extremity is the search for a foreign body in a wound. Plain films are an excellent modality for detecting common, dense foreign bodies in wounds, such as glass and rock, but they are much less sensitive in detecting plastic or organic materials (1). Other imaging modalities such as CT, ultrasound, and MRI are superior for detecting organic and plastic foreign bodies (2). The principles of using plain films for foreign body detection are similar regardless of the location in the body and are not discussed in further detail here.

In this chapter, discussion of the upper extremity is divided into three sections: 1) the shoulder, 2) the elbow and forearm, and 3) the wrist and hand. Within each section, the indications, diagnostic capabilities, and pitfalls are discussed, followed by images of important pathological findings.

The shoulder

Indications

The main indication for plain radiography of the shoulder is acute trauma. There are a number of acute injuries that may be discovered on plain radiography after acute trauma, including fractures of the clavicle, scapula, and humerus, as well as shoulder (glenohumeral) dislocation or acromioclavicular (AC) separation. Although many patients may present with subacute or chronic, nontraumatic pain, the utility of plain films in that setting is extremely low. For chronic, nontraumatic shoulder pain, plain films may reveal changes consistent with calcific tendonitis or degenerative arthritis, but it is not necessary to diagnose such conditions in the emergency setting.

Several studies have focused on whether all patients with shoulder dislocation require both prereduction and postreduction radiographs (3). Some support an approach of selective radiography, ordering prereduction films for first-

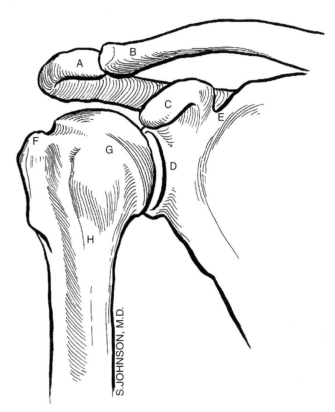

Anterior shoulder. A = acromion, B = clavicle, C = coracoid process, D = neck of scapula, E = scapular notch, F = greater tuberosity, G = anatomical neck, H = surgical neck

time dislocations and those with a blunt traumatic mechanism of injury, and postreduction films for those with a fracture-dislocation. It is also important to order radiographs whenever the physician is uncertain of joint position, whether dislocated or reduced. Therefore, it may be appropriate to manage a patient with a recurrent dislocation by an atraumatic mechanism without any radiographs when the physician is clinically certain of the dislocation and the reduction.

Diagnostic capabilities

In most settings, if the plain films do not reveal a pathological finding, no further imaging is necessary. MRI is an important modality in diagnosing ligamentous injury (e.g., rotator cuff tear), but it is rarely indicated in the emergency setting.

With the possible exception of the scapula, most fractures of the shoulder girdle are readily apparent on standard plain films, without the need for specialized views or advanced imaging. The shoulder is no exception to the general rule of plain films that at least two views are necessary for adequate evaluation. The two most common views in a shoulder series include the anteroposterior (AP) and the lateral, or "Y," scapula view. Other views that are sometimes helpful include the axillary and apical oblique views. The point of the additional views is to enhance the visualization of the glenoid and its articulation with the humeral head. These views may be particularly helpful in diagnosing a posterior shoulder dislocation or subtle glenoid fracture.

Another radiographic series that is sometimes used is the AC view with and without weights. Although the purpose of these views is to help the physician diagnose an AC separation, they are not recommended for the following reasons: 1) the views might occasionally distinguish a second-degree separation from a first-degree one, but that difference has little clinical relevance because both are treated conservatively, and 2) third-degree AC separations are usually obvious clinically and radiographically, without the need for weights or additional views.

Imaging pitfalls and limitations

Although most acute shoulder injuries may be adequately evaluated using a standard two-view shoulder series, posterior shoulder dislocation can be surprisingly subtle and is notoriously difficult to diagnose. When posterior dislocation is suspected based on the history, physical, or standard radiographic views, additional specialized views such as the axillary and apical oblique can be very helpful. Most radiographic views of the shoulder may be obtained even when the injured patient has limited mobility, but the axillary view does require some degree of abduction and may be difficult.

Clinical images

Following are examples of common and important findings in plain radiography of the shoulder:

1. Clavicle fracture (fx)
2. AC separation
3. Anterior shoulder dislocation
4. Posterior dislocation (AP)
5. Posterior dislocation (lateral scapula)
6. Luxatio erecta
7. Bankart fx
8. Hill–Sachs deformity
9. Humeral head fracture

The elbow and forearm

Indications

Similar to the shoulder, the most common use of elbow and forearm plain radiography is with acute trauma. There are numerous fractures and dislocations that can be easily visualized with plain films. Chronic pain in these areas is often secondary to subacute repetitive injuries of the soft tissue such as epicondylitis or bursitis. Many of these soft tissue diseases such as lateral "tennis elbow" and medial "golfer's elbow" epicondylitis are easily diagnosed on clinical exam and generally require no imaging at all. Plain films may reveal such soft tissue pathologies as foreign bodies and subcutaneous air.

No well-established clinical decision rules exist for imaging elbows and forearms in acute trauma. Patients with full range of flexion-extension and supination-pronation of the

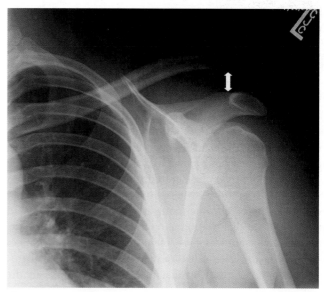

Figure 1.2. AC separation is commonly referred to as a "separated shoulder" and can be classified as grade 1 (AC ligament and coracoclavicular [CC] ligaments intact, radiographically normal), grade 2 (AC ligament disrupted, CC ligament intact), or grade 3 (both ligaments disrupted, resulting in a separation of the acromion and clavicle greater than half the width of the clavicle).

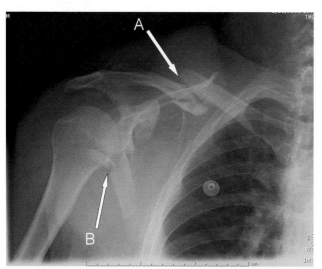

Figure 1.1. Clavicle fractures (A) are often described by location, with the clavicle divided into thirds: proximal, middle, or distal. Note the scapular fracture (B) as well.

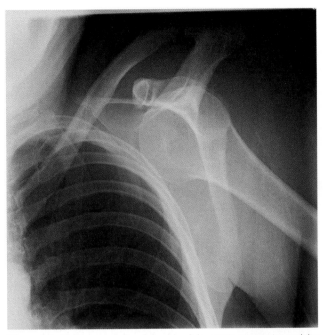

Figure 1.3. The large majority of shoulder dislocations are anterior, and the large majority of anterior dislocations are subcoracoid, as demonstrated in this AP view.

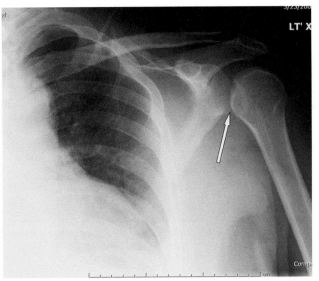

Figure 1.4. Posterior shoulder dislocation is uncommon and is difficult to diagnose on a single AP radiograph. Although it is not obvious in this single view, there are some hints that suggest posterior dislocation. The humeral head is abnormally rounded due to internal rotation (light bulb sign), and the normal overlap between the humeral head and glenoid is absent.

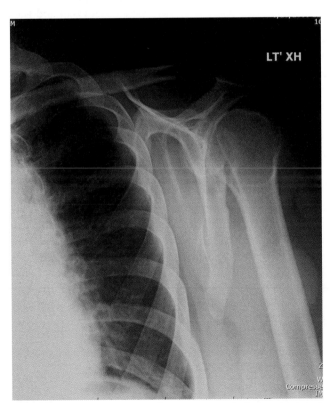

Figure 1.5. Posterior shoulder dislocation is clearly evident on this lateral scapula view, while it was much more subtle on the preceding AP view (see Fig. 1.4). This illustrates the importance of obtaining a second view such as the lateral scapula view or axillary view.

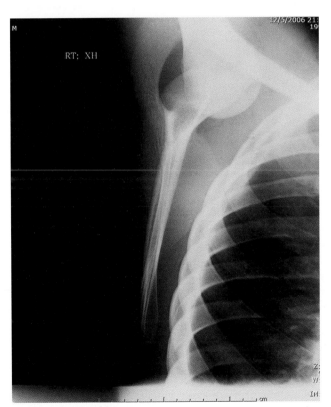

Figure 1.6. Luxatio erecta is the rarest of shoulder dislocations in which the humeral head is displaced inferiorly while the arm is in an abducted or overhead position.

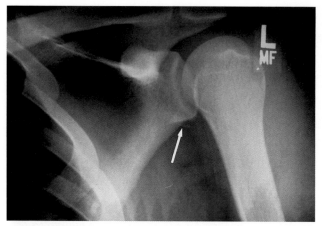

Figure 1.7. Although radiographically subtle, the Bankart fracture is a small avulsion of the inferior rim of the glenoid. The loss of the glenoid labrum destabilizes the glenohumeral joint and nearly ensures recurrent dislocations.

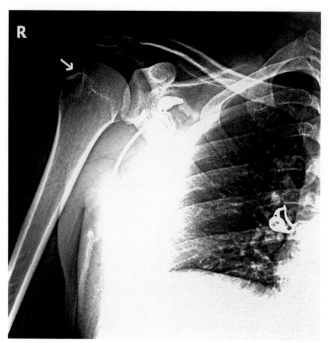

Figure 1.8. The Hill–Sachs deformity is a compression fracture of the superolateral aspect of the humeral head and is commonly noted in recurrent shoulder dislocations. It is believed to occur when the humeral head is resting against the inferior rim of the glenoid while dislocated.

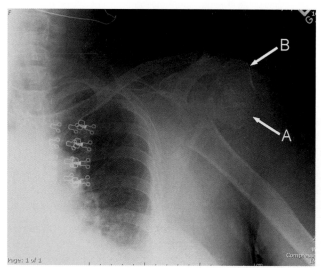

Figure 1.9. Humeral head fracture often occurs across the surgical neck (A) but may also occur at the anatomical neck (B).

elbow and no bony point tenderness rarely have a fracture, and they generally do not require imaging (4). Midshaft forearm fractures are usually clinically apparent, and deformity, swelling, and limited range of motion are all indications for obtaining radiographs. Some suggest ultrasonography may reduce the need for elbow radiography (5).

Diagnostic capabilities

In most cases, if no pathology is found in the plain films of the forearm or elbow, no further imaging is required. Although obvious fractures are easily visualized on plain film, some fractures leave more subtle findings. Radiographs of the elbow in particular may yield important indirect findings. The elbow joint is surrounded by two fat pads, an anterior one lying within the coronoid fossa and a slightly larger posterior fat pad located within the olecranon fossa. In normal circumstances, the posterior fat pad cannot be visualized on plain films, but a traumatic joint effusion may elevate the posterior fat pad enough to be visualized on a 90-degree lateral radiograph. The anterior fat pad is normally visualized as a thin stripe on lateral radiographs, but joint effusions may cause it to bulge out to form a "sail sign" (6). Traumatic joint effusions are sensitive signs of an intra-articular elbow fracture (7). In an adult with fat pads and no obvious fracture, an occult radial head fracture is the usual culprit.

Imaging pitfalls and limitations

The two standard views of the elbow are the AP view and the lateral view with the elbow flexed 90 degrees. The majority of fractures can be identified with these two views, but occasionally supplementary views may be obtained to identify certain parts of the elbow and forearm. The lateral and medial oblique views allow easier identification of their respective epicondylar fractures. The capitellum view is a cephalad-oriented lateral view that exposes the radial head and radiocapitellar articulation. The axial olecranon is shot with a supinated and flexed forearm and isolates the olecranon in a longitudinal plane.

Clinical images

Following are examples of common and important findings in plain radiography of the elbow and forearm:

10. Posterior fat pad
11. Radiocapitellar line
12. Elbow dislocation, posterior

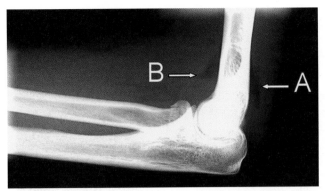

Figure 1.10. Subtle soft tissue findings such as this posterior fat pad (A) and sail sign (B) are markers for fractures that should not be dismissed.

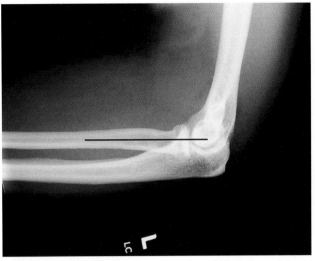

Figure 1.11. A radiocapitellar line is drawn through the radius and should bisect the capitellum regardless of the position of the elbow.

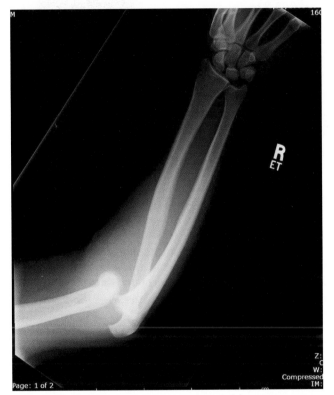

Figure 1.12. Elbow dislocation is a common joint dislocation, outnumbered only by shoulder and interphalangeal dislocations. Most elbow dislocations occur during hyperextension. The majority are posterior and are obvious clinically and radiographically.

13. Monteggia fracture
14. Galeazzi fracture (AP)
15. Galeazzi fracture (lateral)

The wrist and hand

Indications

As with the rest of the upper extremity, the major indication for imaging of the wrist and hand is with acute trauma. It is one of the most difficult areas to differentiate between soft

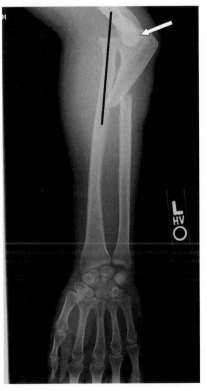

Figure 1.13. Monteggia fractures or dislocations are fractures of the proximal ulna with an anterior dislocation of the proximal radius. These injuries are usually caused by rotational forces, and the dislocation may not be obvious. Drawing a radiocapitellar line aids in diagnosis as it demonstrates the misalignment.

tissue and skeletal injury on history and physical examination alone. Imaging is necessary even with obvious fractures because the extent of the fracture, displacement, angulation, and articular involvement are important to determine if the patient needs closed reduction in the ED or immediate

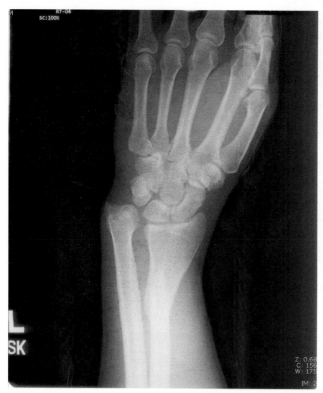

Figure 1.14. A Galeazzi fracture, or Piedmont fracture, is a fracture of the distal third of the radius with dislocation of the distal ulna from the carpal joints. This is the exact opposite of a Monteggia fracture and is also caused by rotational forces in the forearm, although more distal.

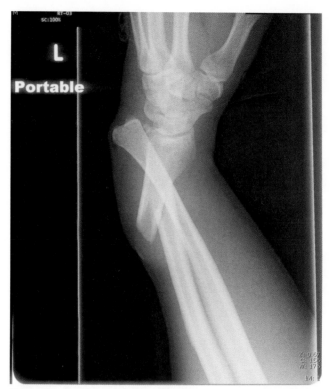

Figure 1.15. Often mistaken for a simple distal radius fracture on AP radiograph, the dislocation is clearly evident on a lateral forearm or wrist.

orthopedic referral for possible open reduction and surgical fixation.

There are still settings where imaging of the hand and wrist is not indicated. Carpal tunnel disease and rheumatologic and gouty disorders are chronic diseases that usually do not involve acute trauma and can be diagnosed based on a good history and physical exam alone.

Diagnostic capabilities

Besides searching for acute bony fractures and dislocations, plain films can reveal other important pathology. With high-pressure injection injuries to the hand, subcutaneous air is a marker for significant soft tissue injury and is often an indication for surgical exploration. Many carpal dislocations and ligamentous injuries are readily visualized on radiographs of the wrist and hand. Perilunate and lunate dislocations usually result from hyperextension of the wrist and fall on an outstretched hand (FOOSH) injury. They may be poorly localized on physical exam and films, and a good neurovascular exam, especially of the median nerve, is indicated.

Imaging pitfalls and limitations

Because of the size and number of bones, complete radiographic sets of hand and wrist films are often acquired.

The minimum standard views of the hand and wrist involve a posterior-anterior, lateral, and pronated oblique. This third view helps assess angulated metacarpal fractures that would normally superimpose on a true lateral. Accessory views of the hand such as the supination oblique or ball catcher's view can help view fractures at the base of the ring and little finger, while a Brewerton view allows better visualization of the metacarpal bases. The wrist accessory films include a scaphoid view, a carpal tunnel view that looks at the hook of the hamate and trapezium ridge, and a supination oblique view that isolates the pisiform. These accessory films should be ordered whenever there is localized tenderness or swelling in these areas.

Unlike the proximal upper extremity, fractures in the wrist and hand may not always be readily apparent on plain films. Scaphoid fractures often result from a FOOSH injury. About 10% to 20% of scaphoid fractures have normal radiographs on initial presentation to the ED (8). Therefore, it is extremely important not to disregard these clinical signs of scaphoid fracture: "anatomical snuff box" tenderness, pain with supination against resistance, and pain with axial compression of the thumb. These signs merit immobilization of the wrist in a thumb spica splint and follow-up in one to two weeks.

More advanced imaging modalities of the wrist and hand such as CT, MRI, and high-resolution ultrasound are much more sensitive for identifying fractures, bone contusions, and ligamentous injury that would be missed

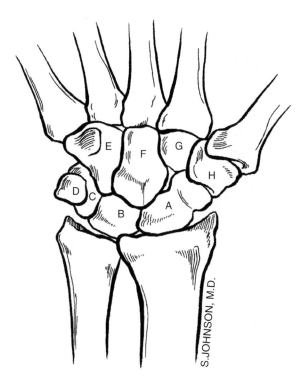

Bones of the wrist: palmar view. A = scaphoid, B = lunate, C = triquetrum, D = pisiform, E = hamate, F = capitate, G = trapezoid, H = trapezium

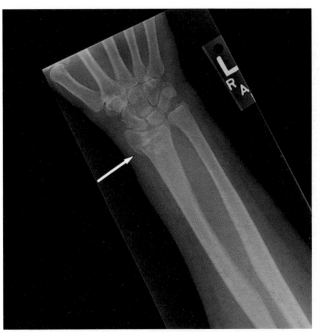

Figure 1.16. A Colles' fracture occurs at the distal metaphysis of the radius with dorsal displacement and radial length shortening. An extremely common injury pattern also seen in FOOSH injuries, the radial head is shortened, creating a disruption of the normally almost linear continuation of the radial and ulnar carpal surfaces.

on plain radiography (9). Whether advanced imaging is indicated in the emergency department may depend on local resources.

Clinical images

Following are examples of common and important findings in plain radiography of the wrist and hand:

16. Colles' fracture (AP)
17. Colles' fracture (lateral)
18. Smith's fracture (AP)
19. Smith's fracture (lateral)
20. Scaphoid fracture
21. Scapholunate dissociation
22. Lunate dislocation (AP)
23. Lunate dislocation (lateral)
24. Perilunate dislocation (AP)
25. Perilunate dislocation (lateral)
26. Boxer's fracture (AP)
27. Boxer's fracture (lateral)
28. Tuft fracture

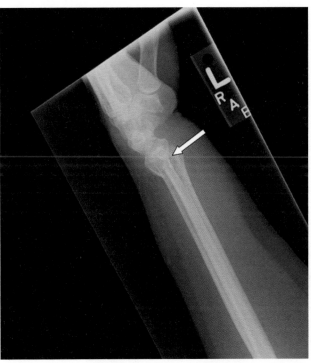

Figure 1.17. The dorsal displacement is evident on the lateral radiograph, and proper reduction is needed to restore this alignment.

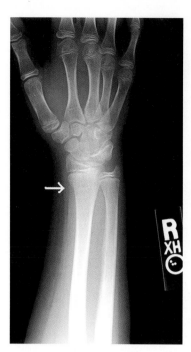

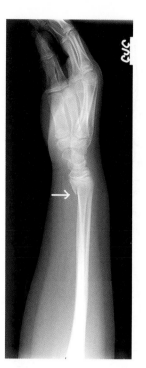

Figure 1.18. A Smith's fracture, also known as a reverse Colles' fracture, is a distal radius fracture with volar instead of dorsal displacement of the hand. Usually caused by direct blows to the dorsum of the hand, these fractures often need eventual surgical reduction.

Figure 1.19. Sometimes referred to as a "garden spade" deformity, the lateral view differentiates this type of fracture from the more common Colles' fracture.

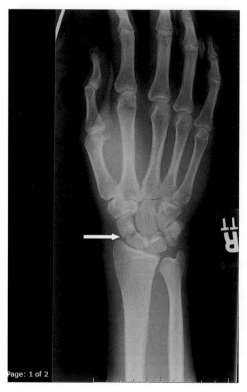

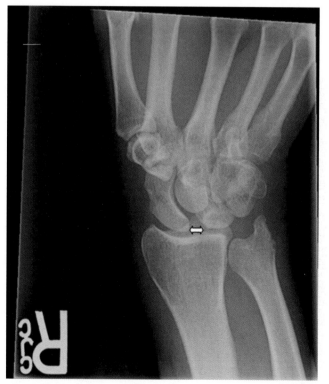

Figure 1.20. Because of the size and number of hand and wrist bones, many subtle fractures are missed on cursory views of plain radiographs. All AP hand views should be checked for smooth carpal arches formed by the distal and proximal bones of the wrist. Evidence of avascular necrosis in scaphoid fractures occurs in the proximal body of the fracture because the blood supply of the scaphoid comes distally from a branch of the radial artery. The arrow denotes a scaphoid fracture.

Figure 1.21. A tight relationship between adjacent carpal bones and the distal radius and ulna should be observed as well. The loss of this alignment or widening of the space, as seen here between the scaphoid and lunate bones, is a sign of joint disruption from fracture, dislocation, or joint instability. A widening of greater than 4 mm is abnormal and known as the "Terry-Thomas sign" or rotary subluxation of the scaphoid. The scaphoid rotates away and has a "signet ring" appearance at times.

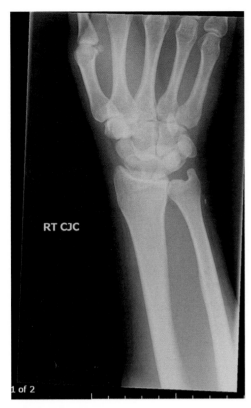

Figure 1.22. Lunate dislocations are the most common dislocations of the wrist and often occur from FOOSH injuries. They are significant injuries involving a volar displacement and angulation of the lunate bone. Notice how the carpal arches are no longer clearly seen.

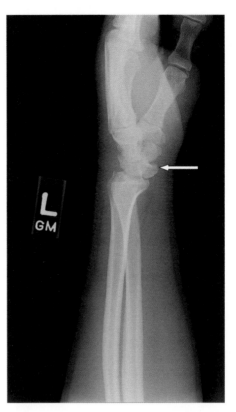

Figure 1.23. The lateral view shows the obviously dislocated and tilted "spilled teacup" lunate. Observe how the capitate and other wrist bones are in relative alignment with the distal radius.

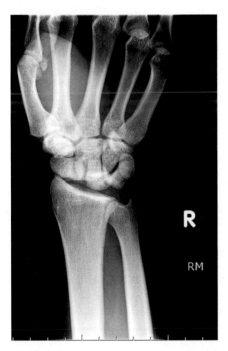

Figure 1.24. Perilunate dislocations are dorsal dislocations of the capitate and distal wrist bones. Once again, there is a loss of the carpal arcs with significant crowding and overlap of the proximal and distal carpal bones. Neurovascular exams for potential median nerve injuries are extremely important in these injuries.

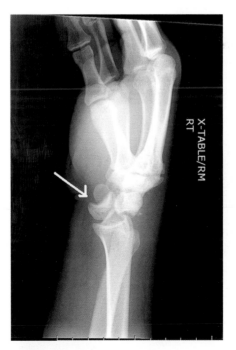

Figure 1.25. The lateral view of a perilunate dislocation shows the lunate in alignment with radial head. It is the distal capitate that is obviously displaced, in contrast to the lunate dislocation.

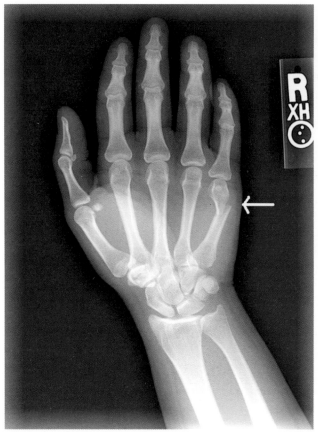

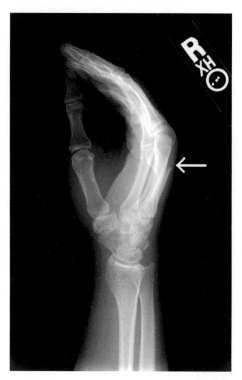

Figure 1.27. The lateral view reveals the degree of angulation. The amount of angulation that requires reduction or impairs function of the hand is controversial, but many believe greater than 30 degrees of angulation requires reduction (8).

Figure 1.26. Metacarpal neck fracture of the fifth metacarpal, commonly referred to as a boxer's fracture, typically occurs from a closed fist striking a hard object such as a mandible or wall.

References

1. Manthey DE, Storrow AB, Milbourn J, Wagner BJ: Ultrasound versus radiography in the detection of soft-tissue foreign bodies. *Ann Emerg Med* 1996;287–9.

2. Peterson JJ, Bancroft LW, Kransdorf MJ: Wooden foreign bodies: imaging appearance. *AJR Am J Roentgenol* 2002;**178**(3): 557–62.

3. Hendey G, Chally M, Stewart V: Selective radiography in 100 patients with suspected shoulder dislocation. *J Emerg Med* 2006;**31**(1):23–8.

4. Hawksworth CR, Freeland P: Inability to fully extend the injured elbow: an indicator of significant injury. *Arch Emerg Med* 1991; **8**:253.

5. Rabiner JE, Khine H, Avner JR, et al.: Accuracy of point-of-care ultrasonography for diagnosis of elbow fractures in children. *Ann Emerg Med* 2013;**61**(1):9–17.

6. Hall-Craggs MA, Shorvon PJ: Assessment of the radial head-capitellum view and the dorsal fat-pad sign in acute elbow trauma. *AJR Am J Roentgenol* 1985;**145**:607.

7. Murphy WA, Siegel MJ: Elbow fat pads with new signs and extended differential diagnosis. *Radiology* 1977;**124**:659.

8. Byrdie A, Raby N: Early MRI in the management of clinical scaphoid fracture. *Brit J Rad* 2003;**76**:296–300.

9. Waeckerle JF: A prospective study identifying the sensitivity of radiographic findings and the efficacy of clinical findings in carpal navicular fractures. *Ann Emerg Med* 1987;**16**:733.

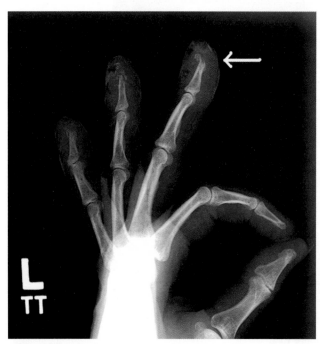

Figure 1.28. A crush injury to the distal phalanx often causes a tuft fracture. It is important to evaluate for open fractures, subungual hematomas, and concomitant nail bed injury.

Lower Extremity Plain Radiography

Anthony J. Medak, Tudor H. Hughes, and Stephen R. Hayden

Indications

Lower extremity injuries are common in ED and urgent care settings. As part of the workup of these patients, healthcare providers typically use some type of imaging modality. Plain radiography is frequently a starting point, as it is readily available, is inexpensive, and has few contraindications. In addition, plain radiography involves much lower levels of ionizing radiation than CT, for example. The medical literature has discussed at length the long-term risks and effects from ionizing radiation (1). As such, healthcare providers should give strong consideration to using additional plain radiograph views (gravity stress, weight bearing, etc.) rather than automatically opting for other modalities such as CT.

Plain radiography is useful in a number of clinical situations, including diagnosing fractures and dislocations and evaluating the end result after closed reductions performed in the ED. In addition, it is helpful in evaluating for radiopaque foreign bodies and assessing joint spaces for evidence of autoimmune or degenerative processes such as rheumatoid arthritis or avascular necrosis. Finally, plain films are also helpful in evaluating possible infections, including those involving the bone, as in osteomyelitis, or the adjacent soft tissues, as in necrotizing soft tissue infections.

Diagnostic capabilities

Lower extremity radiography is useful for diagnosing fractures and dislocations of the hip, knee, foot, and ankle, as well as demonstrating pathology of the femur, tibia, and fibula. Plain radiography is helpful in evaluating fractures of the lower extremity bones, as well as masses and malignancies, including pathological fractures. In some cases, these films will be supplemented with CT or MRI of the affected area to provide additional information. In addition to bony pathology, lower extremity radiography is helpful in assessing the soft tissues, as in the setting of joint effusions, inflammation of bursae, soft tissue calcifications, or soft tissue infections. Finally, plain radiography is also useful for visualizing radiopaque foreign bodies of the lower extremity.

When ordering radiographs of the lower extremity, one must give careful consideration to selecting the optimal views. Obtaining the proper radiographic views will significantly affect the utility of the study. For example, when looking for calcaneal pathology, it is advisable to obtain dedicated calcaneal views as opposed to imaging the entire foot, as this allows for better visualization of subtle pathology.

Imaging pitfalls and limitations

Information obtained from plain radiographs may be limited by several factors. Most notable is the quality of the technique employed. Penetration of the image and proper patient positioning are crucial to obtaining useful images. Improper positioning can mask findings of subtle hip, tibial plateau, or foot and ankle fractures.

Additionally, postoperative patients sometimes pose a challenge. If a patient has had prior surgeries or has an internal fixation device in place, interpretation of the films may be difficult. Also, plain radiography itself has inherent limitations, regardless of patient or technique. For example, many foreign bodies, including organic material, plastics, and some types of glass, are radiolucent and, therefore, not well visualized with plain radiography. Ultrasound and MRI are other imaging options in these cases.

Plain radiography is very good for evaluating most bony pathology; however, there are exceptions. In the case of osteomyelitis, for example, there is often a delay of 2 to 3 weeks between onset of symptoms (pain, fever, swelling) and onset of radiographic findings. As a result, plain radiography alone is relatively insensitive in diagnosing acute osteomyelitis (2). Other modalities, including MRI and bone scan, are often used in these cases.

Other limitations of plain radiography include failure to detect fractures with subtle radiographic findings, such as acetabular, tibial plateau, or midfoot (Lisfranc's) fractures. In many such instances, CT or MRI is necessary if clinical suspicion is high, even in the setting of negative plain films. It is well reported that, in patients with complex foot and ankle fractures, the sensitivity and negative predictive value of plain radiography alone are inadequate (3). In these cases, multidetector CT is the modality of choice. Another area where plain radiography alone yields insufficient anatomical detail is the proximal tibia. Many authors support supplemental imaging with CT to better delineate the anatomy and allow for preoperative planning and fracture management (4, 5).

Despite these limitations of lower extremity radiography, some simple measures may be taken to improve overall diagnostic accuracy. As noted previously, proper image penetration and patient positioning are imperative. Beyond this, the

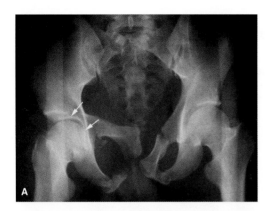

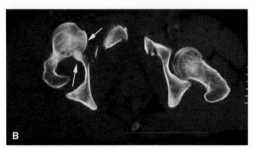

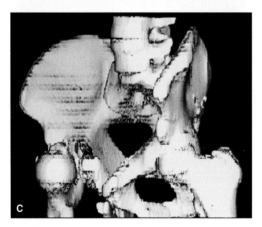

Figure 2.1. Anterior hip fracture-dislocation. The initial AP radiograph (A) shows the right leg to be externally rotated and the superior acetabulum to have a discontinuous margin due to an accompanying acetabular fracture. The CT scans, both axial (B) and 3D reconstructions (C), show the anterior dislocation of the femur, with both acetabular fracture and impaction fracture of the femoral head.

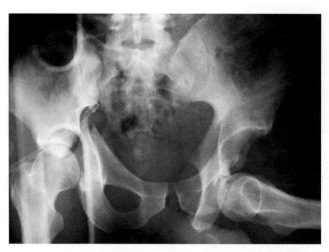

Figure 2.2. Open anterior fracture-dislocation of hip. An AP radiograph shows the left hip to be dislocated with the femoral head inferior, compatible with anterior dislocation. The leg is abducted and externally rotated, which is commonly the leg position that predisposes to anterior dislocation. In addition, note the acetabular fracture on the right.

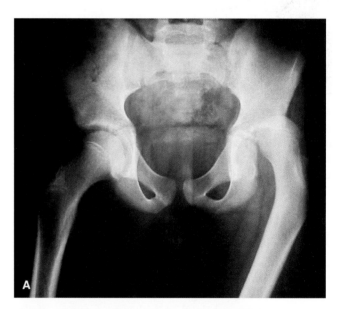

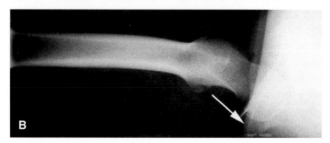

Figure 2.3. Posterior hip dislocation. AP (A) and lateral (B) radiographs of a 15-year-old male with a posterior left hip dislocation. Note the high position of the left femoral head on the AP view and the posterior position on the lateral view, which is projecting supine with the ischium (a posterior structure) at the bottom of the image (*arrow*).

use of stress imaging, whether it be weight bearing (to enhance Lisfranc injury) or gravity stress (to enhance ankle instability), can be very useful (6, 7). Stress views can reveal much more about the function of ligaments and as such are often superior and complementary to MRI.

Finally, as with any radiographic imaging, one must have sufficient knowledge of the normal anatomy to be able to recognize pathology. This includes the ability to distinguish normal variants from true pathology. For example, bipartite patella, presence of a growth plate, or sesamoid bone may all be mistaken for abnormalities if a basic understanding of normal anatomy is lacking.

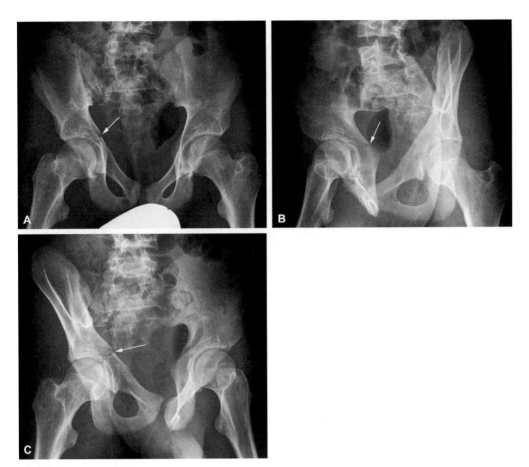

Figure 2.4. Acetabular fracture not well visualized on CT. This 19-year-old male sustained a horizontal fracture of the right acetabulum in a motor vehicle collision. The AP view (A) shows the fracture line over the medial acetabulum, and the Judet views (B, C), RPO (right posterior oblique), and LPO (left posterior oblique) show the involvement of the posterior column and anterior column, respectively (*arrows*). This fracture was very difficult to see on CT due to the fracture plane being the same as that of the axial CT images. This underscores the importance, in some cases, of multiple imaging modalities to properly characterize the injury.

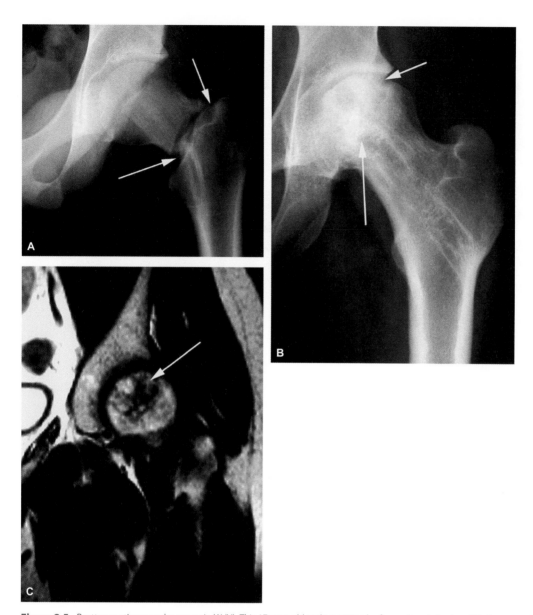

Figure 2.5. Posttraumatic avascular necrosis (AVN). This 17-year-old male sustained a femoral neck fracture (A). Four years later following decompression, the subsequent radiograph (B), as well as the coronal plane T1-weighted MRI (C), show sclerosis and lucencies on the radiograph (*arrows*) and well-defined margins of AVN on the MRI (*arrow*).

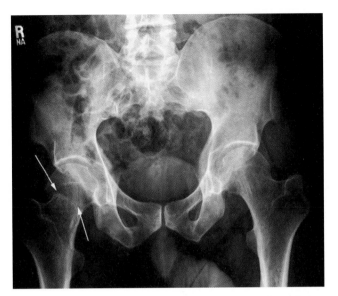

Figure 2.6. Impacted fracture of right femoral neck. An AP radiograph shows impaction of the lateral femoral neck as well as a band of sclerosis (*arrows*) in this 46-year-old male.

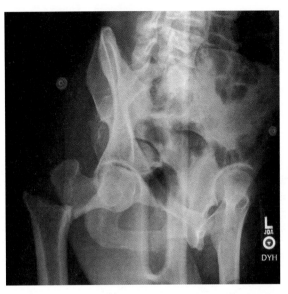

Figure 2.8. Horizontal intertrochanteric fracture. The left posterior oblique radiograph of the pelvis shows a relatively horizontal intertrochanteric fracture. Most fractures in this region are more oblique from superolateral to inferomedial.

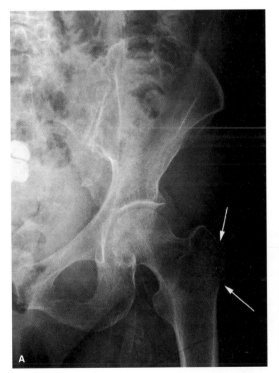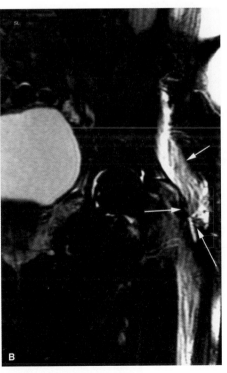

Figure 2.7. Greater trochanter fracture. This 68-year-old female sustained a greater trochanter fracture, difficult to appreciate with plain radiography (A). The subsequent coronal T2-weighted MRI (B) shows the edema in the greater trochanter and adjacent hip abductors (*arrows*). MRI is useful in the differentiation of surgical and nonsurgical management.

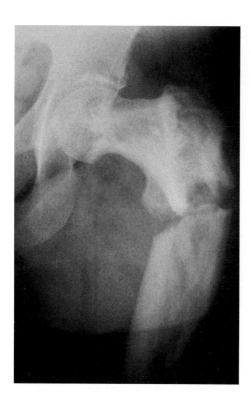

Figure 2.9. Pathological fracture of the left subtrochanteric femur. AP radiograph of the left hip in this 70-year-old male with Paget disease shows abnormal architecture of the proximal femur with a coarse trabecular pattern and cortical thickening typical of the sclerotic phase of this disease. A pathological fracture has occurred through the weakened abnormal bone.

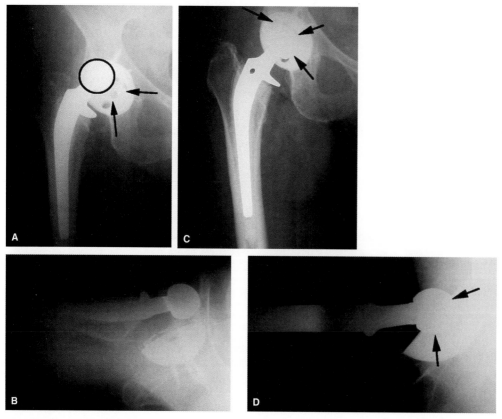

Figure 2.10. Dislocated total hip arthroplasty. AP and lateral views of the right hip with anterior dislocation (A, B) (the ring represents the femoral head) and following reduction (C, D). Note the femoral head must be concentric with the acetabulum on both views for it to be correctly located.

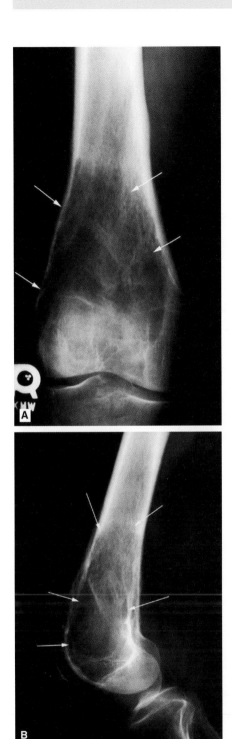

Figure 2.12. Subluxed patella. A bilateral Merchant view of the patellae shows the right patella to be laterally subluxed. Axial views of the patella are taken with the knees flexed 40 degrees and with the film either on the shins (Merchant projection) or on the thighs (Inferosuperior projection).

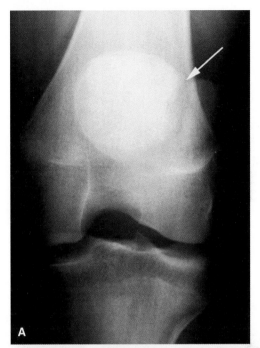

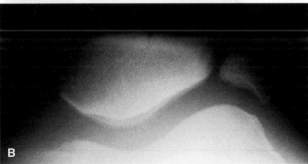

Figure 2.11. Giant cell tumor of bone involving the right distal femur. AP (A) and lateral (B) radiographs in a 37-year-old male show a lytic lesion involving the metaphysis and extending to the epiphysis (*arrows*). It has a mixed benign and aggressive appearance, with the lateral margin being well defined and the proximal margin more ill defined.

Figure 2.13. Bipartite patella. AP (A) and axial (B) views of the left knee in a 16-year-old male. Note that the accessory bone fragment is always superolateral. The margins are rounded and sclerotic, excluding an acute fracture.

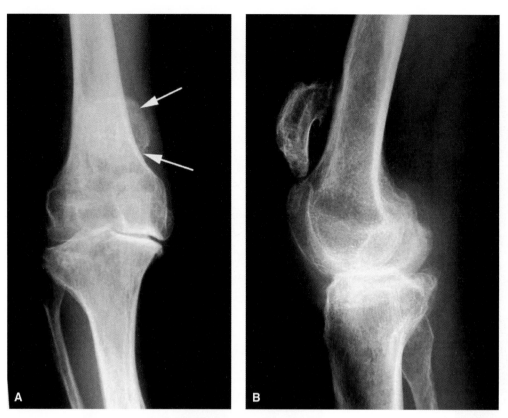

Figure 2.14. Patella alta. AP (A) and lateral (B) radiographs in a 55-year-old male show the patella to be in a higher location than is normal. The distance from the inferior articular surface of the patella to the tibial tubercle should be between 1.5 and 2 times the length of the articular surface of the patella.

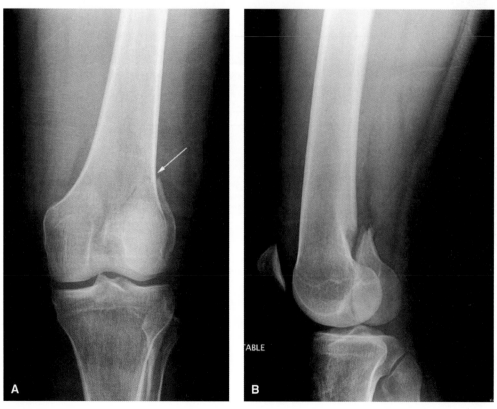

Figure 2.15. Femoral condyle fracture. AP (A) and lateral (B) radiographs of the left knee in a 37-year-old male show a coronal oblique fracture of the lateral femoral condyle. Sagittal plane condylar fractures are more common than coronal. Coronal fractures tend to occur on the lateral side and are called Hoffa fractures.

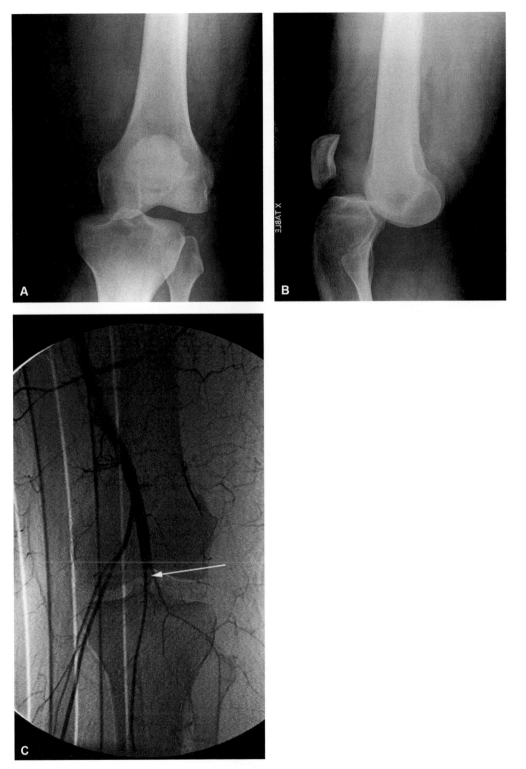

Figure 2.16. Knee dislocation. AP (A) and lateral (B) radiographs in a 77-year-old female show a knee dislocation. The subsequent postreduction angiogram (C) shows abrupt disruption of flow in the popliteal artery (*arrow*). Arterial injury is one of the major concerns in a patient with knee dislocation.

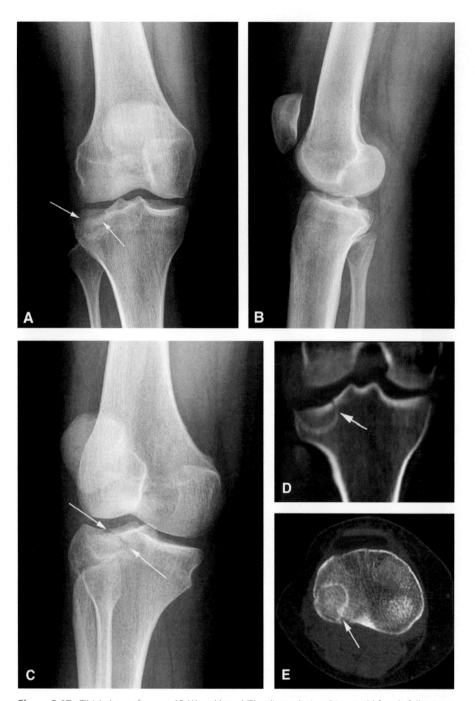

Figure 2.17. Tibial plateau fracture. AP (A) and lateral (B) radiographs in a 24-year-old female following trauma show irregularity of the lateral tibial plateau with a band of sclerosis between the subchondral bone plate and the epiphyseal scar (*arrows*). The oblique view (C) confirms this finding (*arrows*) and is often helpful in equivocal cases in the absence of CT. The CT images with coronal (D) and axial (E) reformations also confirm the impacted lateral tibial plateau fracture (*arrows*). CT is much more sensitive in detecting tibial plateau fractures than is plain radiography, and it is often used for preoperative planning and management decisions.

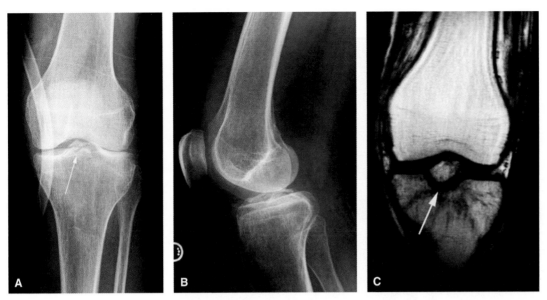

Figure 2.18. Tibial spine avulsion. AP (A) and lateral (B) radiographs in a 58-year-old male show avulsion of the tibial spines by the anterior cruciate ligament (*arrow*). The subsequent coronal T1-weighted MRI (C) confirms this finding (*arrow*). Due to the comparative strengths of ligaments and bones, this injury is more common in children, whereas ACL tears are more common in adults.

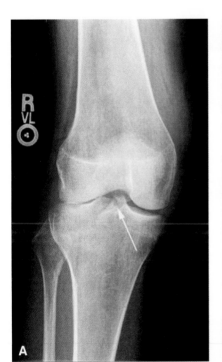

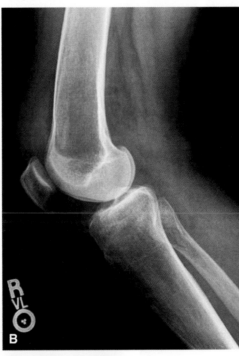

Figure 2.19. Knee lipohemarthrosis. AP (A) and lateral (B) radiographs in a 51-year-old female show a vertical split fracture of the lateral tibial plateau. In addition, the lateral recumbent view (C) shows a large joint effusion/hemarthrosis. The cross-table lateral view taken with a horizontal beam (C) shows a fat fluid level (lipohemarthrosis) within the knee (*arrows*). The fat is released from the bone marrow, confirming the intra-articular fracture. In some cases, this may be the only finding on plain radiography to suggest a fracture.

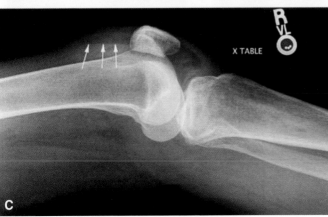

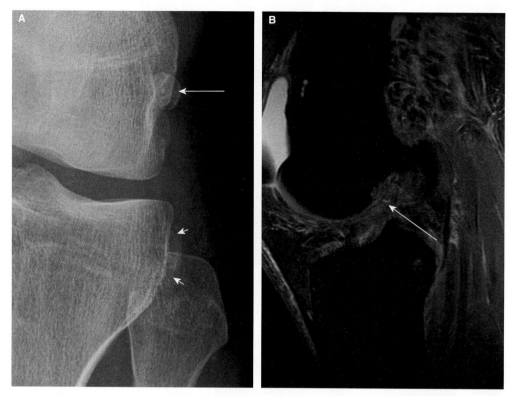

Figure 2.20. AP close-up radiograph of the lateral aspect of the left knee (A) in a 34-year-old man following trauma, shows a small bone fragment projecting over the lateral aspect of the proximal tibia and fibula (*arrowheads*). This represents a Segond fracture avulsion by the lateral capsular ligamentous complex and is a strong indicator of an ACL tear. The ACL injury (*arrow*) is shown in the accompanying sagittal proton density fat saturated MRI through the midline of the intercondylar notch of the same knee (B). Note that the rounded bone more superiorly overlying the lateral margin of the distal femur on the radiograph (*arrow*) is a normal variant, the fabella.

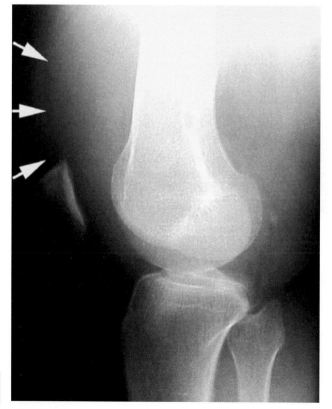

Figure 2.21. Large knee joint effusion. Lateral radiograph of the knee shows a bulging soft tissue density arising from the superior aspect of the patellofemoral joint due to an effusion. If the lateral knee radiograph is obtained flexed more than 30 degrees, an effusion may be pushed posteriorly so that it is no longer visible.

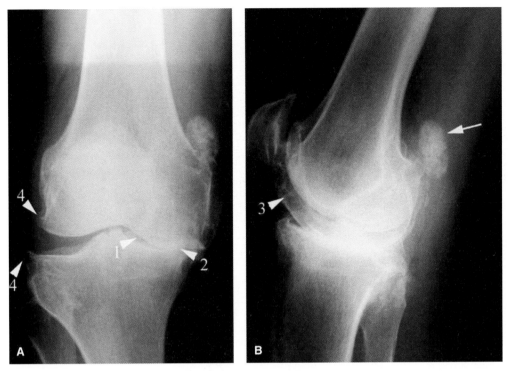

Figure 2.22. Osteoarthrosis of the knee. AP (A) and lateral (B) radiographs of the right knee in a 52-year-old male show the four cardinal signs of osteoarthrosis: 1) focal joint space narrowing, 2) subchondral sclerosis, 3) subchondral cysts, and 4) osteophytes. In addition, a large intra-articular body is seen in the popliteal recess (*arrow*).

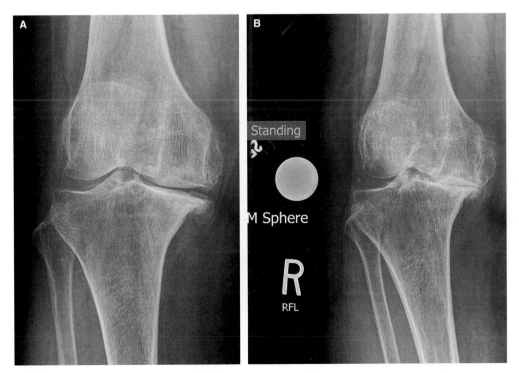

Figure 2.23. AP radiographs of the right knee in a 71-year-old female with severe osteoarthrosis. Although the non-weight-bearing view (A) shows severe medial compartment joint space narrowing, it is only with weight bearing (B) that the full extent of the accompanying genu varum deformity becomes apparent. This will likely affect the arthroplasty technique selected for definitive treatment.

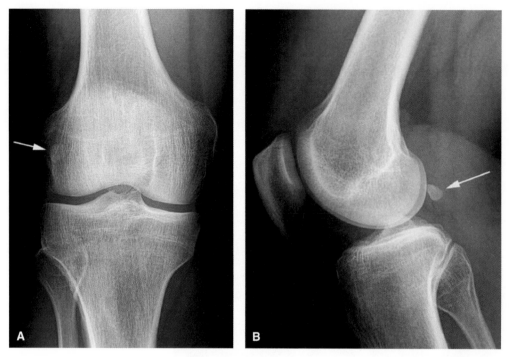

Figure 2.24. Fabella. AP (A) and lateral (B) radiographs of the knee of a 35-year-old male demonstrate a fabella, a sesamoid bone within the lateral head of the gastrocnemius muscle (*arrows*). The fabella is sometimes mistaken for an intra-articular ossified fragment. Note that the fabella is always lateral. In AP projection, the fabella is round. In the lateral view, the anterior margin should be flat or concave.

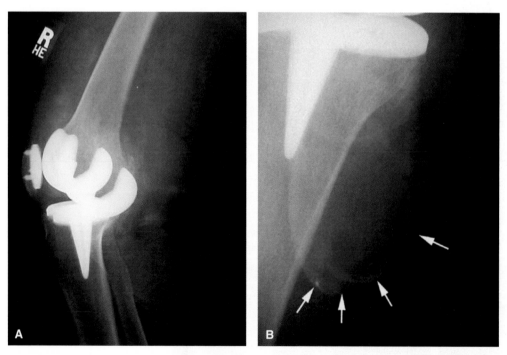

Figure 2.25. Metal synovitis of the knee. Lateral oblique radiograph (A), with coned down view (B), in a 69-year-old female who has extensive microfragmentation of a total knee arthroplasty. Metal has collected in the synovium, producing a synovitis.

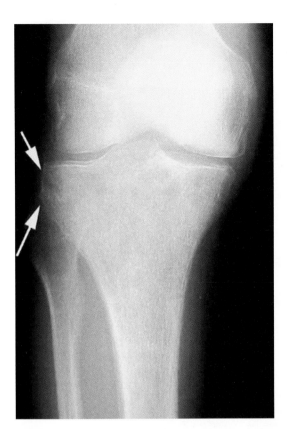

Figure 2.26. Acute osteomyelitis. AP radiograph of the proximal tibia shows an ill-defined lucency with periosteal reaction, compatible with an aggressive process – in this case, osteomyelitis.

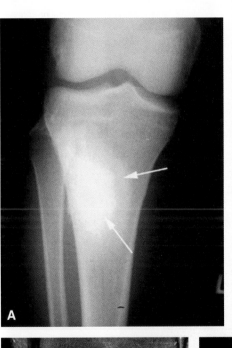

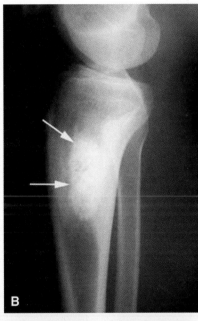

Figure 2.27. Osteosarcoma. AP (A) and lateral (B) radiographs of the right proximal tibia in a 16-year-old male show an ill-defined but dense area of sclerosis in the lateral proximal tibia. Coronal (C) and axial (D) T1-weighted MRI show low signal centrally, compatible with bone formation, and high signal peripherally, compatible with gadolinium uptake by growing tumor.

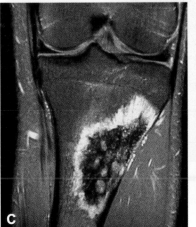

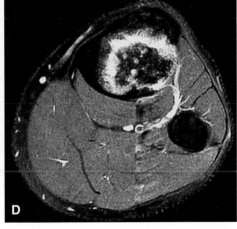

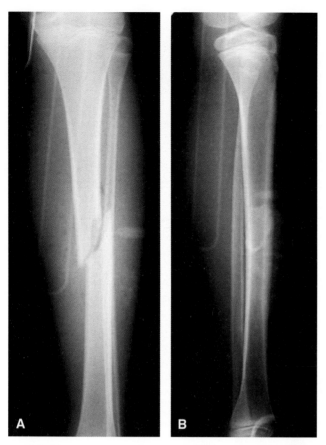

Figure 2.28. Tibial fracture. AP (A) and lateral (B) radiographs of a 16-year-old male following trauma. The AP view clearly shows the steep oblique fracture of the midtibial shaft. Note the difficulty of seeing the fracture on the lateral view, emphasizing the need for more than one view to assess trauma.

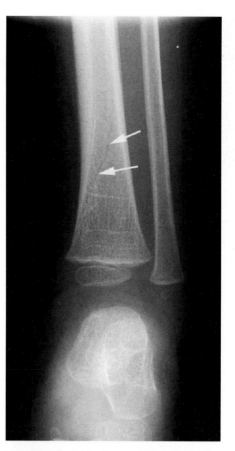

Figure 2.29. Toddler fracture. AP radiograph of a 22-month-old boy, whose leg became trapped beneath his mother while descending a slide, shows a spiral fracture of the distal tibia (*arrows*). These nondisplaced toddler fractures are often difficult to see on radiographs acutely.

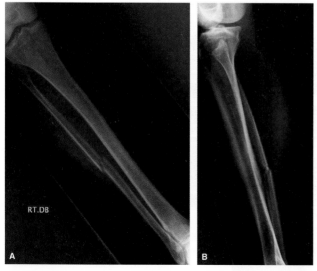

Figure 2.30. Fibular shaft fracture. AP (A) and lateral (B) radiographs of the tibia and fibula in a 45-year-old male following pedestrian versus auto accident. The fracture of the midshaft of the fibula has a butterfly fragment, which is strongly associated with direct trauma.

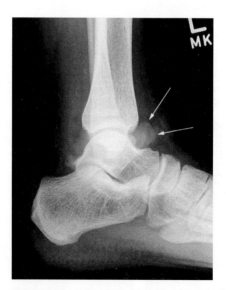

Figure 2.31. Ankle effusion. Lateral radiograph of the ankle in a 25-year-old male with chronic renal failure. Anterior to the ankle joint is a moderate-size effusion. When such a dense effusion is noted, presence of hemarthrosis must be considered.

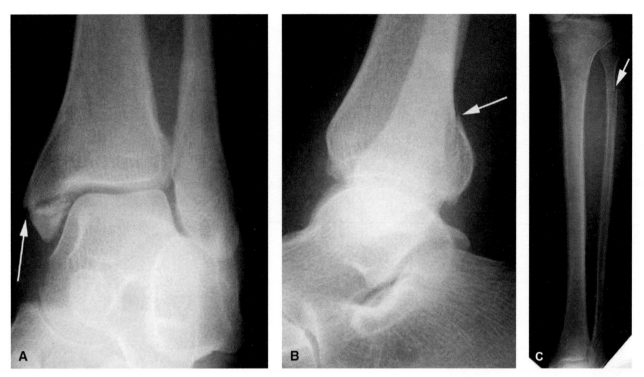

Figure 2.32. Maisonneuve fracture. Mortise (A) and lateral (B) projections of the left ankle in a 54-year-old male show a transverse fracture of medial malleolus (*arrow in Fig. 2.32A*), extending to involve the posterior malleolus (*arrow in Fig. 2.32B*). In this situation, especially if the distal tibiofibular space is widened, views of the proximal tibia and fibula (C) are recommended to look for a proximal Maisonneuve fracture of the fibula (*arrow in Fig. 2.32C*).

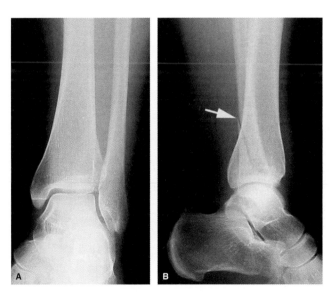

Figure 2.33. Lateral malleolus fracture. Mortise (A) and lateral (B) views of the left ankle show a fracture line passing from superoposterior to anteroinferior on the lateral view (*arrow*), which is difficult to see on the mortise view. This is a very common pattern of ankle fracture and emphasizes the need to look carefully at the lateral view.

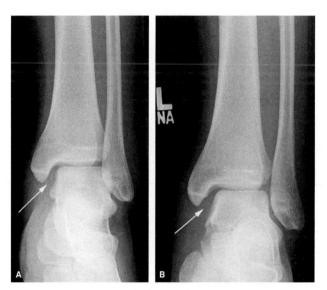

Figure 2.34. Wide medial and syndesmotic clear spaces. AP (A) and mortise (B) views of the left ankle in a 34-year-old male following a twisting injury. The ankle is incongruent, with the medial aspect of the joint wider than the superior joint space (*arrow*), indicating a medial ligament injury. In addition, the distal tibiofibular clear space is too wide. In this setting, views of the proximal fibula are recommended to evaluate for a Maisonneuve fracture (see Fig. 2.32).

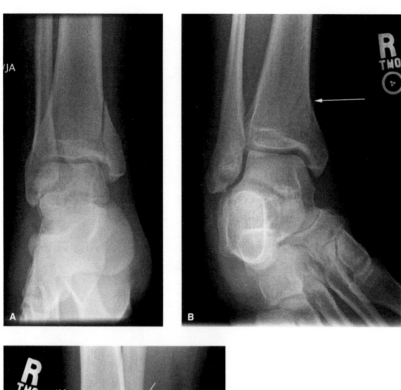

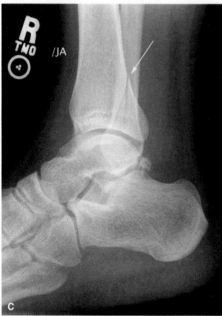

Figure 2.35. Medial and posterior malleolar fractures. AP (A), mortise (B), and lateral (C) views of the right ankle in an 18-year-old male show a medial malleolar fracture (*arrow in Fig. 2.35B*) that extends around to the posterior malleolus (*arrow in Fig. 2.35C*). Posterior malleolar fractures appear on the AP and mortise views as an inverted V–shaped lucent line. On the lateral view, it is important to discern whether the fracture is of the lateral malleolus or posterior malleolus.

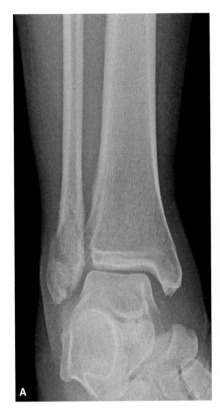
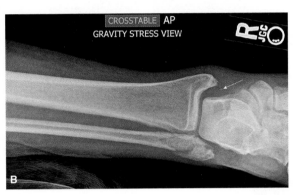

Figure 2.36. Frontal radiographs of the right ankle in a 48-year-old woman, without (A) and with (B) gravity stress. The stress views show widening of the medial mortise (*arrow*) compatible with a deltoid ligament injury. This upgrades the Lauge Hansen "supination external rotation" injury from a stable grade 2 to an unstable grade 4.

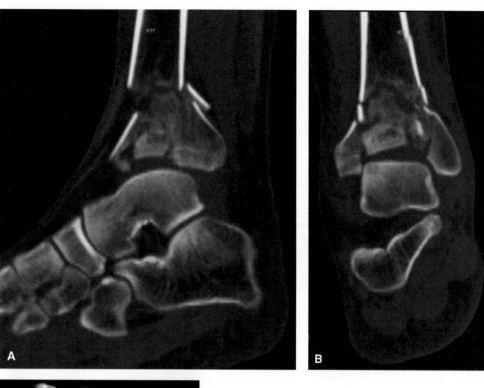

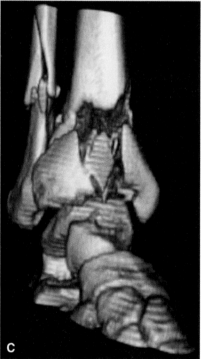

Figure 2.37. Tibial plafond fracture. Sagittal (A), coronal (B), and 3D reformations (C) of the distal tibia in a 35-year-old male following an all-terrain vehicle rollover accident. The tibial plafond is grossly comminuted, and the fractures have a vertical configuration compatible with a pilon-type fracture.

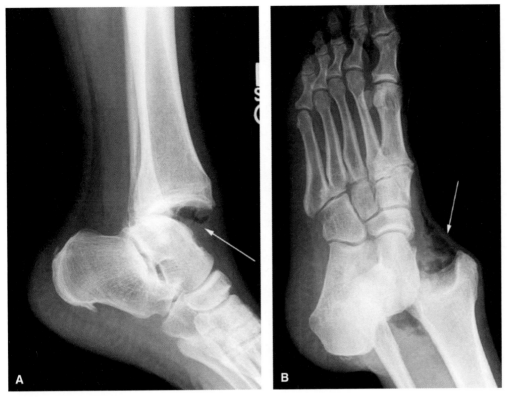

Figure 2.38. Ankle dislocation. Lateral (A) and oblique (B) radiographs of the left foot/ankle in a 59-year-old male show an open dislocation of the ankle, with gas seen within the joint (*arrows*).

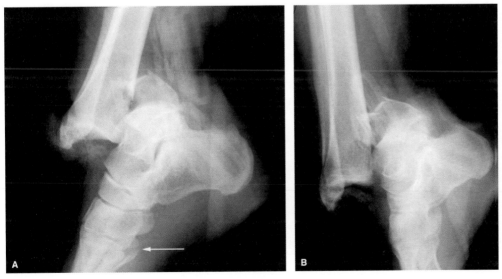

Figure 2.39. Ankle fracture-dislocation. Lateral (A) and oblique (B) radiographs of the right ankle show an ankle fracture-dislocation. On finding an obvious fracture such as this, it is important not to stop looking for the less obvious fracture, in this case, at the base of the fifth metatarsal (*arrow in Fig. 2.39A*).

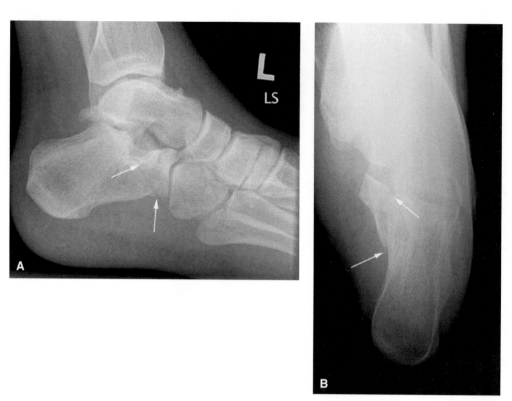

Figure 2.40. Calcaneal fracture. Lateral (A) and axial (Harris-Beath) radiographs (B) of the left heel in a 26-year-old male following a fall. The fracture of the anterior and medial calcaneus can be visualized on both views (*arrows*), with the axial view showing involvement at the base of the sustentaculum talus.

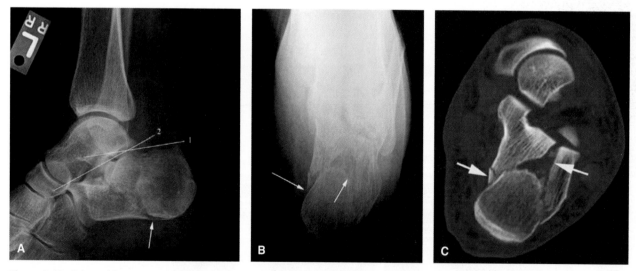

Figure 2.41. Calcaneal fracture. Lateral (A) and axial (Harris-Beath) radiographs (B) and coronal oblique CT (C) in a 44-year-old male with a calcaneal fracture following a fall. The lateral view is used to measure Boehler's angle. A line is drawn from the superior margin of the posterior tuberosity of the calcaneus, extending through the superior tip of the posterior facet (*line 1*), and another line from this latter point, extending through the superior tip of the anterior process (*line 2*). The angle made by the intersection of these lines should normally be between 20 and 40 degrees. When less than 20 degrees, this implies an intra-articular, impacted fracture. The axial view (B) and CT (C) clearly show the inverted Y configuration of the fractures that is a common pattern and the involvement of the posterior subtalar joint.

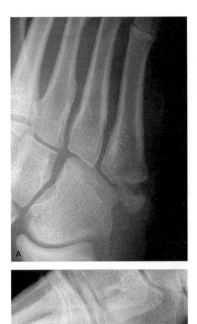

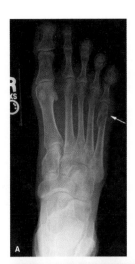

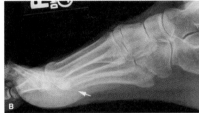

Figure 2.42. Avulsion fracture of base of fifth metatarsal. Oblique (A) and lateral (B) radiographs of the right foot in a skeletally immature patient show the transverse fracture superimposed on the open apophysis (*arrow*).

Figure 2.43. Dancer's fracture. PA (A) and lateral (B) radiographs of the right foot in a 46-year-old female show a spiral fracture of the distal shaft of the fifth metatarsal, known as a dancer's fracture (*arrows*).

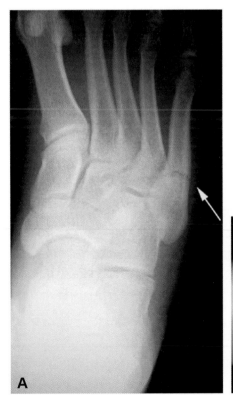

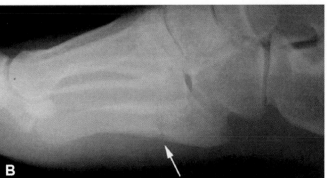

Figure 2.44. Jones fracture. PA (A) and lateral (B) radiographs of the right foot in a 33-year-old male show an extra-articular fracture of the proximal fifth metatarsal, known as a Jones fracture (*arrows*). Note that this fracture is distinctly different from the more common avulsion fracture of the fifth metatarsal tuberosity (see Fig. 2.42). Patients with the avulsion injury generally do well; however, the Jones fracture may result in nonunion and require surgical repair.

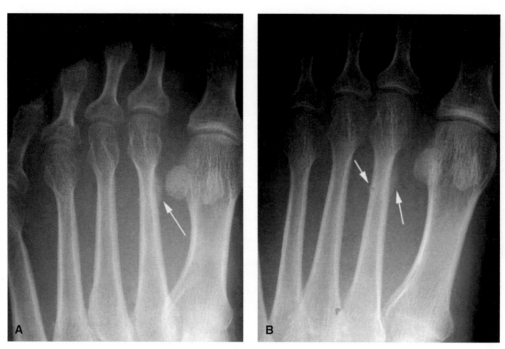

Figure 2.45. Metatarsal stress fracture. PA (A) and oblique coned down (B) radiographs of the left forefoot in a 48-year-old male show a fusiform periosteal reaction of the distal second metatarsal shaft/neck (*arrows*). This is typical of a stress fracture, if a fracture line can be seen, or may be called a stress reaction if the fracture line is not visualized. These may be very subtle and must be sought to be recognized.

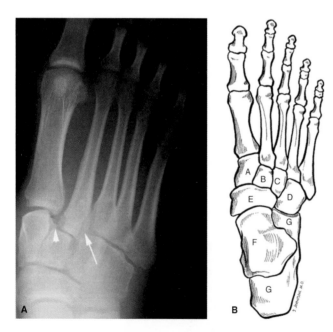

Figure 2.46. Lisfranc fracture subluxation. PA radiograph (A) of the right foot in a 23-year-old male shows malalignment at the medial tarsometatarsal joints (*arrowhead*) and a fracture at the base of the second metatarsal (*arrow*). As a rule, the medial side of the second metatarsal should always line up with the medial side of the middle cuneiform as illustrated (B).

Normal AP Right Foot: A = Medial cuneiform, B = Intermediate cuneiform, C = Lateral cuneiform, D = Cuboid, E = Navicular, F = Talus, G = Calcaneus

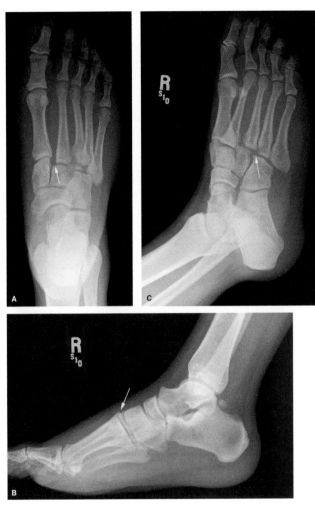

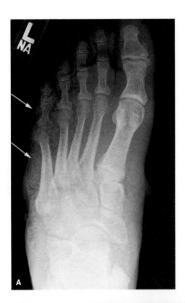

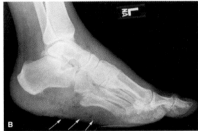

Figure 2.49. Soft tissue gas in an infected foot. PA (A) and lateral (B) radiographs of the left foot in a 65-year-old diabetic male show extensive gas within the soft tissues on the lateral side of the forefoot (*arrows*). A careful inspection of the bones for ill-defined erosion is needed to exclude osteomyelitis.

Figure 2.47. Lisfranc fracture subluxation. Three views of the foot of a 19-year-old male reveal another example of a Lisfranc fracture subluxation. PA view (A) demonstrates the lack of normal alignment between the medial margin of the second metatarsal with the medial margin of the middle cuneiform (*arrow*). Lateral projection (B) reveals a slight dorsal displacement of the metatarsals on the cuneiforms (*arrow*). Oblique view (C) illustrates the lack of normal alignment between the medial margin of the fourth metatarsal and the medial margin of the cuboid (contrast with illustration in Fig. 2.46B).

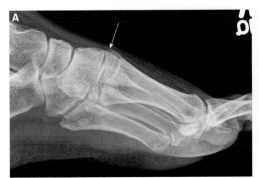

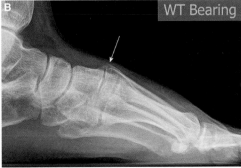

Figure 2.48. Lateral radiographs of the right foot in a 31-year-old woman with a chronic Lisfranc injury. Although a slight step is seen on the dorsal aspect of the middle cuneiform-second metatarsal joint, with the metatarsal displaced dorsally on the non-weight-bearing view (A), this becomes much more apparent and is accentuated by weight bearing (B), greatly aiding in this often difficult diagnosis (*arrows*).

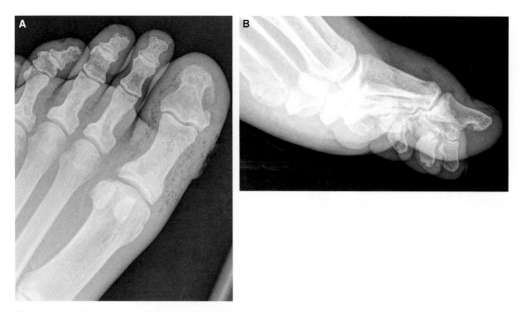

Figure 2.50. AP (A) and lateral (B) radiographs of the great toe in a 70-year-old man with diabetes and clinically dry gangrene of the great toe. The numerous small low densities represent soft tissue gas and are worrisome for gas gangrene, a more fulminant infection.

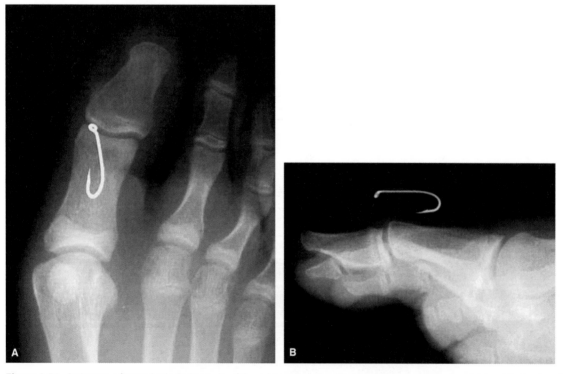

Figure 2.51. Radiopaque foreign body. Radiographs of the right great toe in a 13-year-old boy show a barbed fish hook in the dorsal soft tissues.

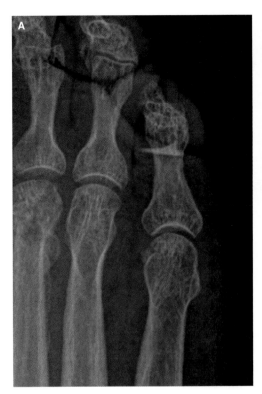
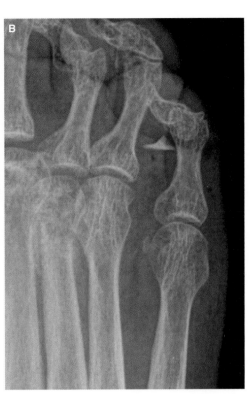

Figure 2.52. AP (A) and oblique (B) radiographs of the lateral forefoot in a 54-year-old man with diabetes. The sharp angular object of increased density adjacent to the fifth PIP joint is a shard of glass. There is accompanying gas in the soft tissue. Note how using two views of the affected area allows for localization of the glass to the plantar aspect of the foot.

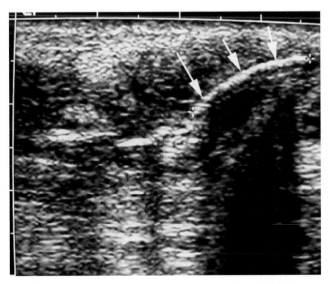

Figure 2.53. Radiolucent foreign body. Ultrasound of the dorsal soft tissues of the foot reveals a wooden (radiolucent, not visible on x-ray) foreign body between the markers (*arrows*). It is hyperechoic (bright) on ultrasound and casts an acoustic shadow because so much of the incident sound is reflected back by the body that little passes through to the deeper tissues.

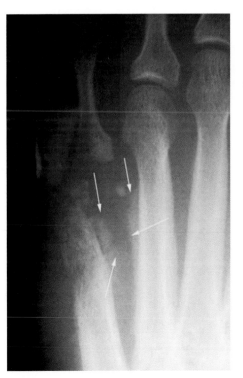

Figure 2.54. Osteomyelitis. Oblique coned down radiograph of the lateral forefoot in a 33-year-old male with diabetes shows extensive bony destruction of the fifth ray, centered at the metatarsal-phalangeal joint, and periosteal reactions (*arrows*) of the fourth and fifth metatarsal bones due to osteomyelitis.

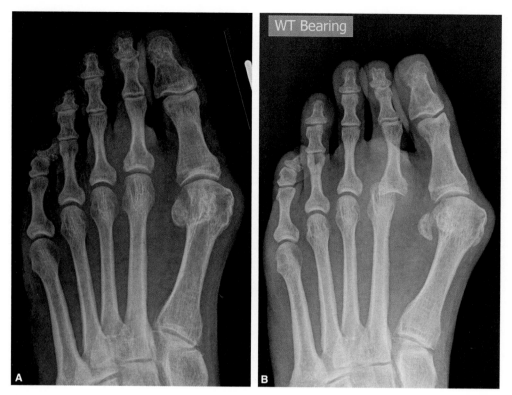

Figure 2.55. AP radiographs of the left foot of a 61-year-old female, without and with weight bearing. Although the non-weight-bearing view (A) shows the hallux valgus and first MTP joint osteoarthrosis, it is only with weight bearing (B) that the second MTP joint dislocation occurs and the degree of hallux valgus increases.

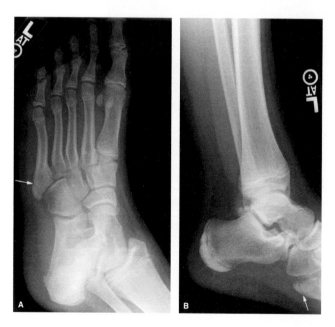

Figure 2.56. Open fifth metatarsal apophyseal growth plate. Oblique (A) and lateral (B) radiographs of the left foot in a skeletally immature patient show the orientation of the fifth metatarsal growth plate. Note how this mimics a fifth metatarsal avulsion fracture.

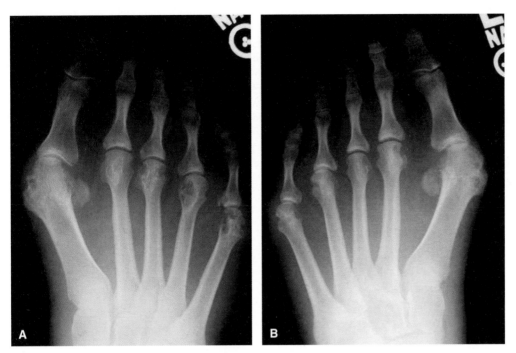

Figure 2.57. Rheumatoid arthritis. PA radiographs of both feet in a 43-year-old female show typical changes of rheumatoid arthritis. Note that the erosions of the metatarsal-phalangeal joints are symmetric.

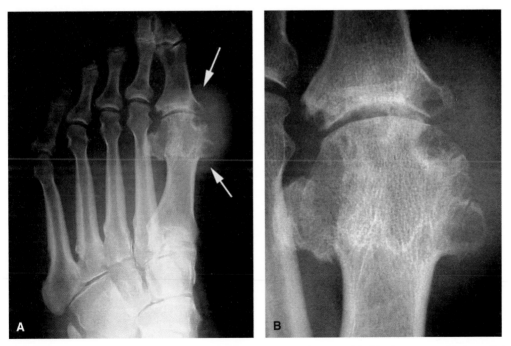

Figure 2.58. Gout. Oblique radiograph of the left foot (A) with a coned down view (B) of the first metatarsalphalangeal joint in a 53-year-old male with gout show eccentric soft tissue swelling (*arrows*) and well-defined erosions with overhanging edges but relative preservation of joint space.

References

1. Brenner DJ, Hall EJ: Computed tomography: an increasing source of radiation exposure. *N Engl J Med* 2007;**357**(**22**):2277–84.

2. Gold RH, Hawkins RA, Katz RD: Bacterial osteomyelitis: findings on plain radiography, CT, MR, and scintigraphy. *AJR Am J Roentgenol* 1991;**157**:365–70.

3. Haapamaki VV, Kiuru MJ, Koskinen SK: Ankle and foot injuries: analysis of MDCT findings. *AJR Am J Roentgenol* 2004;**183**(**3**): 615–22.

4. Mustonen AO, Koskinen SK, Kiuru MJ: Acute knee trauma: analysis of multidetector computed tomography findings and comparison with conventional radiography. *Acta Radiol* 2005;**46**(**8**):866–74.

5. Wicky S, Blaser PF, Blanc CH, et al.: Comparison between standard radiography and spiral CT with 3D reconstruction in the evaluation, classification and management of tibial plateau fractures. *Eur Radiol* 2000;**10**(**8**):1227–32.

6. Gupta RT, Wadhwa RP, Learch TJ, Herwick SM: Lisfranc injury: imaging findings for this important but often-missed diagnosis. *Curr Probl Diagn Radiol* 2008;**37**(**3**):115–26.

7. McConnell T, Creevy W, Tornetta III P: Stress examination of supination external rotation-type fibular fractures. *J Bone Joint Surg Am* 2004;**86-A**(**10**):2171–8.

Chest Radiograph

Peter DeBlieux and Lisa Mills

Indications

The chest radiograph (CXR) is the most commonly ordered plain film in emergency medicine and has correspondingly broad indications. It is ordered to evaluate patients with chest pain, breathing complaints, thorax trauma, fevers, and altered mental status. Patients who complain of chest pain have a broad differential diagnosis, and CXR is one of the first screening tests to be applied in chest pain complaints. This study is relevant when cardiac or pulmonary processes are suspected. CXR should be obtained when patients are suspected of having an occult infectious process, a fever, altered mental status, or hypotension. A screening CXR also helps initially evaluate patients for thoracic injury after thoracoabdominal trauma.

Diagnostic capabilities

CXR is useful to diagnose or identify primary cardiac and pulmonary pathology, abnormal pleural processes, thoracic aortic dilation, aspirated foreign bodies, and thoracic trauma. In cardiac disease, the CXR reveals pulmonary edema, moderate to large pericardial effusion, and cardiomegaly. CXR shows multiple primary pulmonary processes. It reveals infectious processes, such as lobar pneumonia, tuberculosis, atypical pneumonia, empyema, and lung abscess. Pulmonary processes such as pneumonitis, hyperaeration due to chronic obstructive pulmonary disease (COPD) and asthma, and lung masses are evident on CXR. Pleural processes such as pleural thickening, pneumothorax, hemothorax, and pleural effusions are also evident on CXR. CXR is the first radiologic screening test for thoracic aneurysm. The anteroposterior upright CXR shows 90% sensitivity for thoracic aneurysm, when any abnormality is considered a positive test (1). When aspirated foreign body is suspected, a CXR can reveal the location of radiopaque foreign bodies whether in the trachea, smaller airways, esophagus, or stomach.

In thoracic trauma, CXR evaluates for multiple bony and soft tissue injuries. CXR is the screening exam for thoracic aortic injury, pulmonary contusion, pneumothorax, hemothorax, and traumatic pericardial effusion. Skeletal injuries – including rib, scapular, clavicular, shoulder, and sternal fractures and dislocations – can be seen on CXR.

Imaging pitfalls and limitations

The most significant limitation of CXR is obtaining a limited number of studies. This is particularly true when only a supine film is obtained. In supine films, small collections of pleural fluid and small pneumothoraces are missed because these layer out along the lungs, rather than at the base or apex of the lung. The anteroposterior technique artificially enlarges the cardiomediastinal silhouette. Rib fractures, especially along the angle of the ribs, are difficult to see on a standard two-view chest series. Oblique views enhance the sensitivity of CXR for rib fractures. CXR identifies lung masses, pleural lesions, air-space disease, and hilar masses. However, CT better delineates the quality of these lesions.

Systematic approach to reading the CXR

A consistent approach to the CXR improves detection of pathology. The authors promote an alphabetical approach, A to F:

A = airway

B = bones

C = cardiomediastinum

D = diaphragms

E = everything else (pleura, soft tissue, visualized portions of the abdomen)

F = lung fields

See the normal posteroanterior (PA) and lateral CXR in Figure 3.1 for a demonstration of this technique.

Clinical images

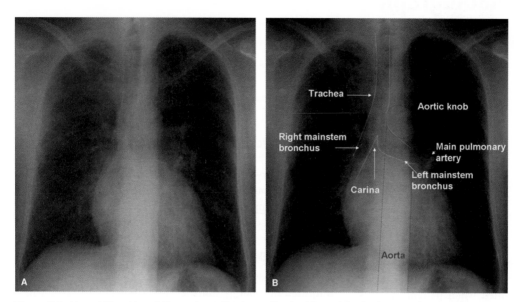

Figure 3.1. Normal PA and lateral. Airway: A good inspiratory film should reveal the diaphragm at the level of the eighth to tenth posterior ribs or the fifth to sixth anterior ribs. The trachea should be visible in the midline of the thoracic cavity equidistant between the clavicular heads. In the anteroposterior and posteroanterior views, the right paratracheal stripe is usually 2 to 3 mm wide, 5 mm being the upper limit of normal. On a lateral CXR, the posterior tracheal wall should be less than 4 mm wide. The trachea should smoothly divide at the carina with both major bronchi visible.

Bones: Examine the bones for lytic or blastic lesions, fractures, spinal alignment, and joint spaces. The thoracic spine should decrease in opacity (brightness) as it is followed inferiorly (caudally). An area of increased opacity suggests an overlying density in the lung. This is termed the "spine sign."

Cardiomediastinum: Examine the mediastinum for size and deviation. The trachea and aorta course down the middle of the thoracic cavity without significant deviation to either side. The aortic arch and knob should be visible. The widest diameter of the heart should be less than 50% of the widest diameter of the thoracic cavity, measured from the inner aspects of the ribs. Look for air lines to suggest pneumopericardium or pneumomediastinum. The aortic knob is the first "bump" of the mediastinum, lying in the left hemithorax. The left pulmonary artery is below the aortic knob separated by a small clear space called the "aortopulmonary window." The right pulmonary artery is usually hidden from visualization by the mediastinum. Behind the sternum, superior to the heart, is the anterior clear space. This should be the density of lung tissue. Soft tissue density suggests infiltrate or mass.

Diaphragms: Follow the mediastinum to the diaphragms. Follow the diaphragms, looking for a smooth course to the costophrenic angles and sharp costophrenic angles. Check for free air under the diaphragms. Both diaphragms should be seen in the lateral view, with the right diaphragm usually higher than the left, with a gastric bubble below.

Everything else: Follow the pleural lines from the costophrenic angles to the apex and around the mediastinum back to the diaphragms. Look for areas of thickening or separation from the chest wall. Check the visualized soft tissues for calcifications, mass effect, and air collections (subcutaneous emphysema). Examine the visualized portion of the abdomen.

Lung fields: The right lung is approximately 55% of the intrathoracic volume. The left lung is 45%. If these ratios change, consider hyperinflation or atelectasis in one hemithorax. Follow vascular patterns for signs of congestion or oligemia. Look for opacities and hyperlucent areas.

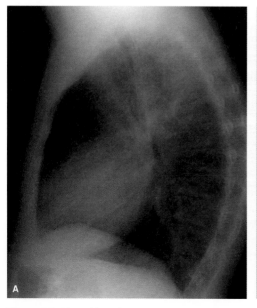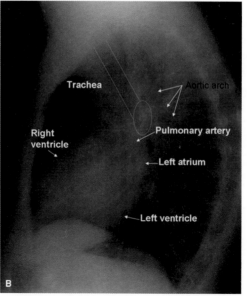

Figure 3.2. Normal lateral.

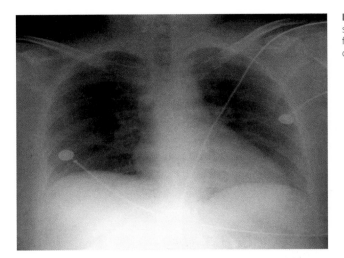

Figure 3.3. Normal supine. In the supine patient, the mediastinum is not stretched toward the feet by gravity. The result is crowding of the mediastinal features, giving the appearance of a larger mediastinum and larger transverse diameter of the cardiac silhouette.

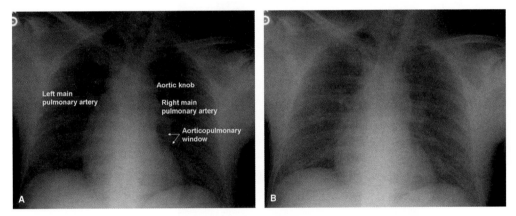

Figure 3.4. Normal anterosterior. This radiograph is usually taken as a portable study. The film cartridge is at the patient's back, and the patient is exposed from the front to the back. (This is the opposite of the PA, in which the patient faces the cartridge, and the back is exposed first.) The heart is artificially magnified, giving the appearance that the heart is larger than posterior structures. In addition, the structures in the thorax are more crowded as the patient remains seated. This causes vascular crowding. These inherent findings should be kept in mind when interpreting these films.

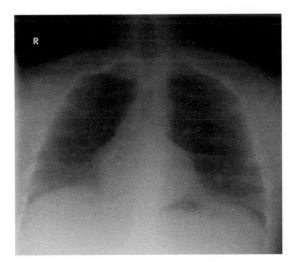

Figure 3.5. Normal apical. The apical view of the lungs focuses on the lung apices. The patient is positioned so the clavicles and ribs are moved away from the apices of the lung.

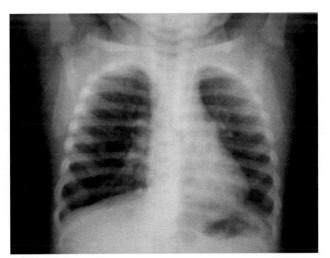

Figure 3.6. Normal infant. The normal infant has an enlarged cardiomediastinal silhouette due to the thymus extending into the thoracic cavity.

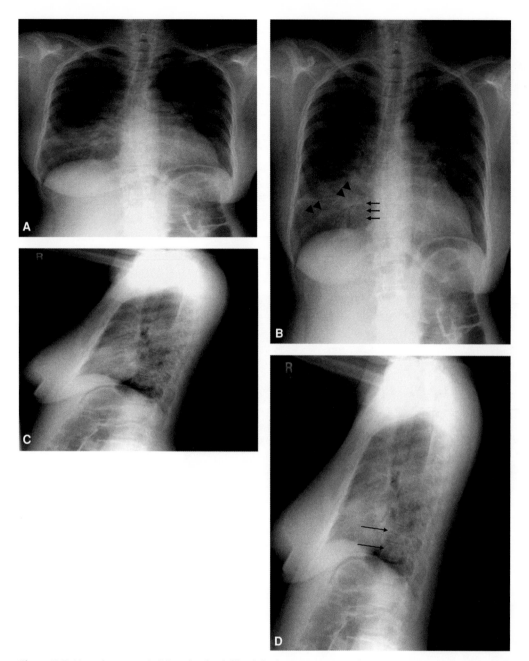

Figure 3.7. Normal pneumonia. When the alveoli fill with fluid, as in pneumonia, the contrast between tissue and air-filled alveoli is lost, creating opacity in the lung field. An area of focal density can correlate with pneumonia. However, opacities on CXR are nonspecific and should be correlated with the clinical picture.

Air-filled bronchi can contrast with the density of the fluid-filled alveoli, creating dark stripes through areas of opacity. This is an air bronchogram (B, *arrowheads*).

When opacity exists in the right middle lobe or left lingula, it obscures the cardiac margin. The adjacent diaphragm remains visible. This is called the "silhouette sign" (B, *arrows*) (2).

There is increased opacity of the last two thoracic vertebrae in the lung fields on this lateral radiograph. This is the "spine sign" (D, *arrows*).

Atelectasis and infiltrative processes such as pneumonia can usually be distinguished by examining the following features:

i. Volume: Atelectasis shows volume loss. Pneumonia shows normal or increased volume.

ii. Shifted structures: Atelectasis results in mediastinal and lung tissue shifting toward the side of the atelectasis. Pneumonia generally does not cause any shifting of structures.

iii. Shape: Atelectasis is usually a linear or wedge-shaped density with the apex pointed toward the hilum. Pneumonia is not linearly arranged and is not centered on the hilum.

iv. Air bronchograms can occur in both atelectasis and pneumonia.

v. Both infectious infiltrates and atelectasis respect anatomical divisions of the lung.

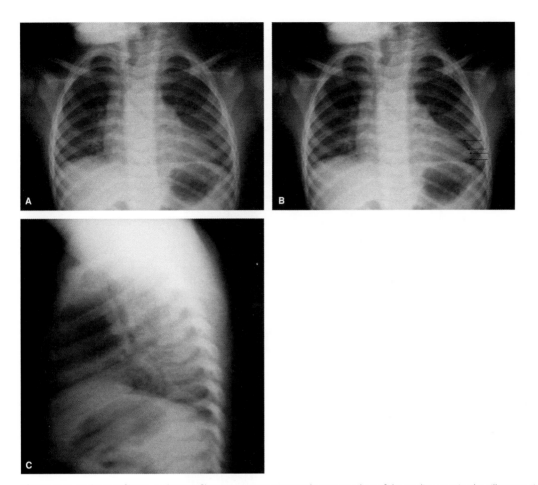

Figure 3.8. Pediatric infiltrate. Pediatric infiltrates are most commonly seen as a loss of the cardiac margin, the silhouette sign. This patient shows loss of the margin apex of the heart (B, *arrows*). This is best appreciated when the crisp margin of the right heart border is compared to the heart apex.

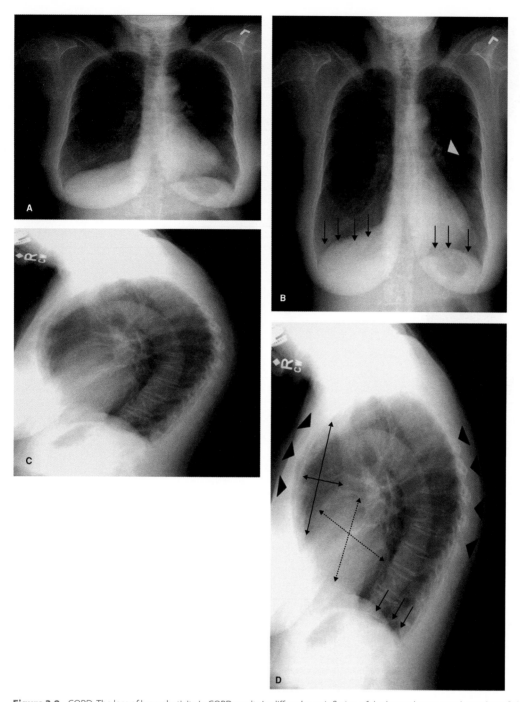

Figure 3.9. COPD. The loss of lung elasticity in COPD results in diffuse hyperinflation of the lungs that creates larger lung fields. The diaphragms flatten (B, *arrows*; D, *arrows*). There is increased AP diameter due to rounding of the sternum and thoracic spine, causing a barrel chest (D, *arrowheads*). The anterior clear (retrosternal) space is increased above the normal 1:2 ratio of anterior clear space (*solid double-headed arrows*) to heart (*dashed double-headed arrows*) (D). Bullae may be visible. In smokers, upper lung fields are more affected than lower. The left pulmonary trunk becomes visible as the heart is allowed to hang lower in the thoracic cavity (B, *arrowheads*).

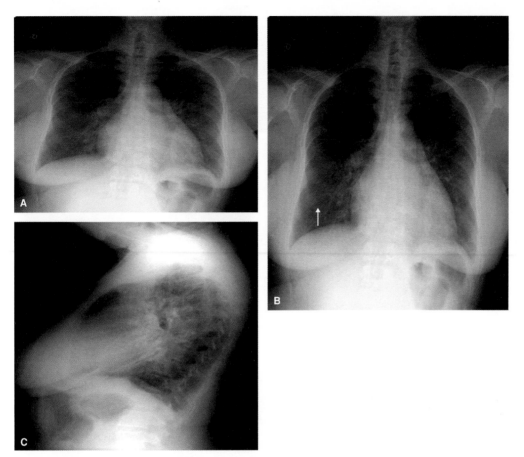

Figure 3.10. Pulmonary edema. In pulmonary edema, the interstitial pattern of increased fluid appears as a diffuse butterfly pattern of increased interstitial marking and soft, fluffy lesions (A). Kerley B lines are horizontal lines representing fluid-filled septae, extending away from the hila (B, *arrow*). They are less than 2 cm long and usually found in the lower lung zones. Effusions in the right horizontal fissure are common. Increased vascular marking may be present (A).

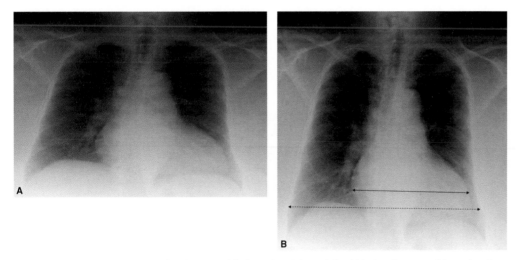

Figure 3.11. Cardiomegaly. The widest diameter of the heart (B, *solid arrow*) should be less than 50% of the widest diameter of the thoracic cavity (*dashed arrow*), measured from the inner aspects of the ribs.

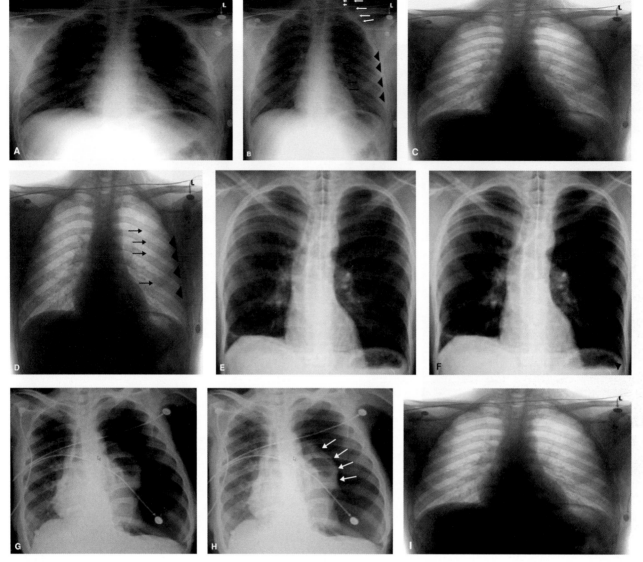

Figure 3.12. Pneumothorax. Air in the pleural space is seen as a black stripe without lung markings. Air will be located in the most elevated portion of the chest. In the upright patient, the air is lateral and superior (A). The line of a pneumothorax (B, *arrowheads*) can be confused with the scapular line (B, *black arrows*) and very subtle. An inverted color image can help distinguish these lines (C, D).

A small pneumothorax in the supine patient may be seen along the mediastinum. In the supine patient with a larger pneumothorax, the air may depress the diaphragm at the costophrenic angle, creating a "deep sulcus sign" (E and F, *arrowhead*). Subcutaneous air can be a clue to the presence of a pneumothorax (*white arrows*).

A tension pneumothorax pushes the mediastinum into the opposite hemithorax (G). The lung border is visible in the left chest (H, *white arrows*). The left hemithorax is hyperinflated. The mediastinum is shifted into the right chest (F–I).

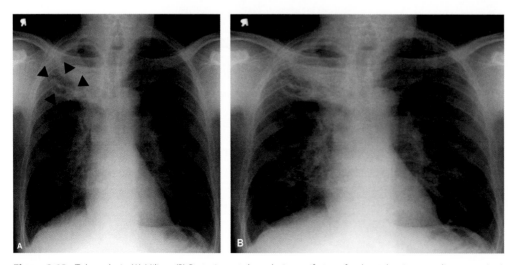

Figure 3.13. Tuberculosis. (A) Miliary. (B) Postprimary tuberculosis manifests as focal, patchy air-space disease, cavitations (A, *arrowheads*), fibrosis, pleural thickening, and calcification of lymph nodes. These changes are most often seen in the upper lobes and superior segments of the lower lobes.

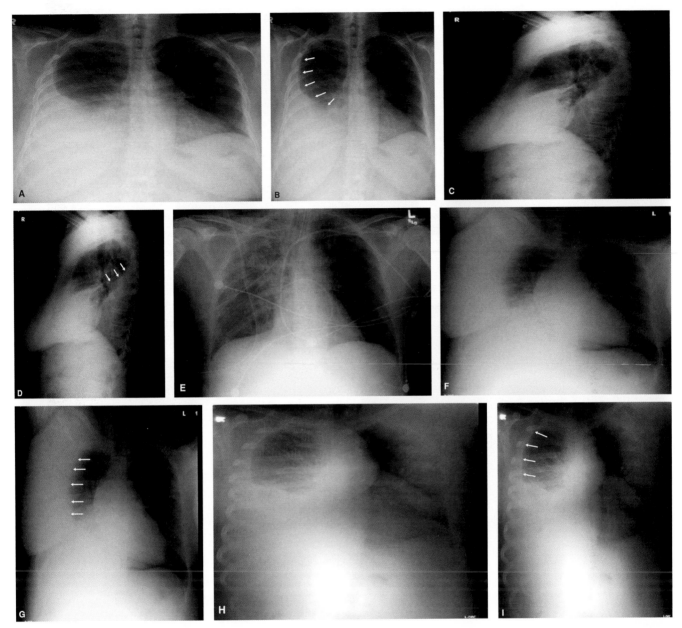

Figure 3.14. Pleural effusion/hemothorax. Pleural fluid creates increased density on CXR. A small amount of pleural fluid in the upright patient will cause blunting of costophrenic angle. The lateral view can be more sensitive for small amounts of fluid (C and D). Increasingly larger accumulations of fluid will track up the periphery of the lung, opacifying the encased lung tissue (B, *arrows*). In the supine patient, pleural fluid creates a generalized increased haziness to the entire affected hemithorax, without a focal area of opacification (E). Lateral decubitus.

   i. The decubitus film is taken with the patient lying on one side. A right decubitus film is taken with the patient lying on the right side (F), whereas the left decubitus film is taken with the patient lying on the left side. The decubitus position allows for fluid to shift when a pleural effusion is present to reveal underlying structures.

   ii. Classically, the decubitus film is taken with the affected side (side with the effusion) down. In this position, the pleural fluid shifts laterally (G, *arrows*), revealing the mediastinal structures.

   iii. With the affected side up, one can see the periphery of the affected hemithorax and loculated fluid (I). It is wise to have the decubitus taken with the affected side down and up, so the mediastinum and the lung periphery can be visualized with the free-flowing effusion.

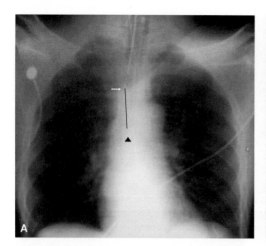
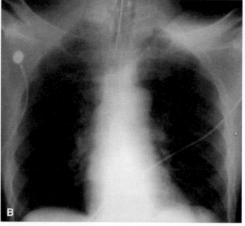

Figure 3.15. Intubation. The distal tip of the endotracheal tube (B, *arrow*) should be located 3 to 4 cm (B, *line*) above the carina (A, *arrowhead*).

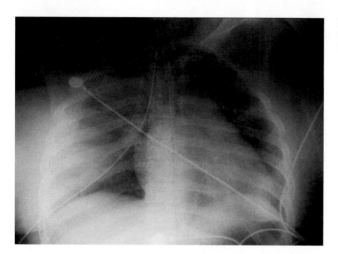

Figure 3.16. Chest tube. The chest tube can be visualized. Check for resolution of the attendant process after placement of the chest tube (e.g., resolution of the tension pneumothorax).

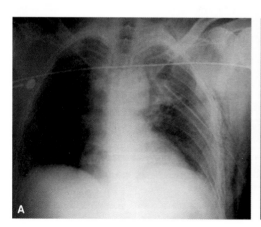
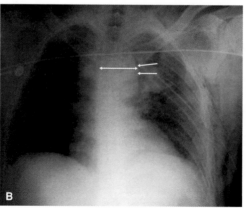

Figure 3.17. Wide cardiomediastinal silhouette. There are no strict measurements to define a "normal" cardiomediastinal silhouette. Cardiomediastinal silhouette widening is relative to the patient's body habitus, positioning, and clinical picture. It suggests a thoracic dilation from aneurysm or traumatic dissection.

Aortic dissection presents with a loss of the aortic knob (B, *arrows*). Look for a distinct aortic knob as an indicator that the widening may be secondary to positioning.

Whenever possible, assess the mediastinum in an upright view (B, *double arrow*).

Look for deviation of other mediastinal structures as an indicator that the aorta is enlarged and displacing adjacent tissue. An example is tracheal deviation into the right chest (A).

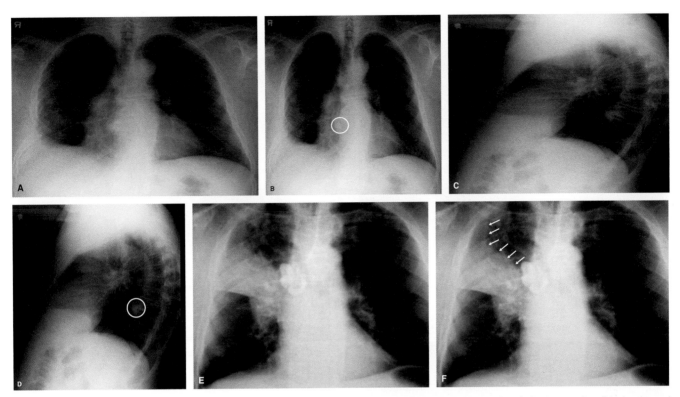

Figure 3.18. Mass and nodule. Localize the area on the lateral film compared to the PA view (A, C). Examine the mass for calcifications, quality of the border, and air-fluid levels to narrow the differential diagnosis.

Fifty percent of nodules that are less than 3 cm in diameter are malignant. The common etiologies of malignancy are bronchial adenoma, primary carcinoma, granuloma, hamartoma, and metastatic neoplasm. CXR is not the diagnostic modality to rule out malignancy.

When there is a mass adjacent to a fissure, the fissure may be S shaped (E, *arrows*). The proximal convexity is the distortion of the mass. The distal concavity reflects atelectasis distal to the mass. This is called the "S curve of golden" (E–F).

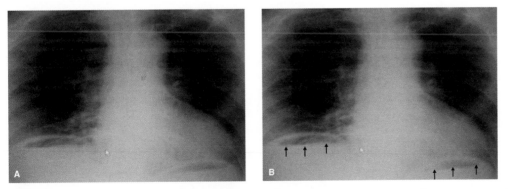

Figure 3.19. Free air. The CXR is used to assess for free intraperitoneal air. Free air in the peritoneal cavity appears as a black stripe between the dense tissue of the diaphragm and the underlying solid organ (spleen or liver) (B, *arrows*). The large, smooth surface area of the liver creates an ideal window for free air. Do not mistake the rounded, encapsulated stomach bubble for free air.

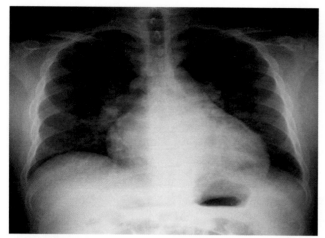

Figure 3.20. PCP. Presentations of PCP on CXR can appear highly variable, ranging from dense, multilobar infiltrates to apparently normal-appearing radiographs. Typically, CXR reveals a diffuse, hazy infiltrate involving all lung fields.

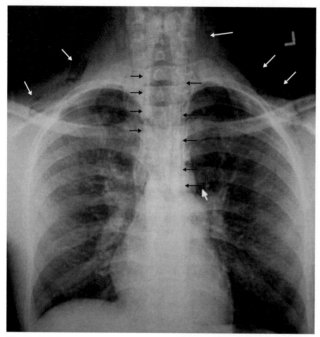

Figure 3.22. Pneumomediastinum. Air in the mediastinum (*black arrows*) appears as lucencies along the mediastinum that extend into the soft tissues of the neck (*white arrows*). The extension of the air into the neck distinguishes pneumomediastinum from pneumopericardium.

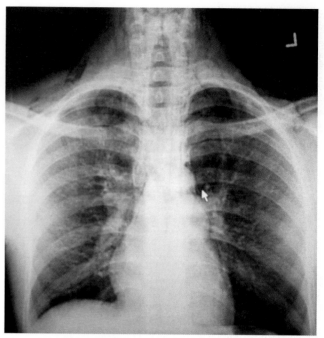

Figure 3.21. Subcutaneous emphysema. Air in the tissues around the thoracic cavity is seen as dark areas, often tracking linearly along tissue planes, interrupting the homogenously opaque appearance of normal soft tissue. Subcutaneous emphysema in the patient with penetrating thoracic trauma indicates communication of the intrathoracic cavity with the extrathoracic space and resultant pneumothorax.

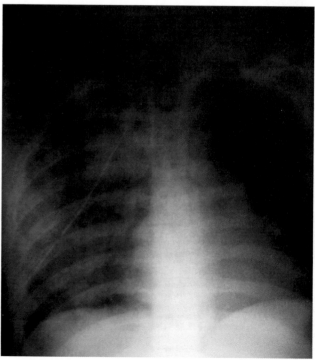

Figure 3.23. Pulmonary contusion. Pulmonary contusions appear as opacities on CXR that do not respect anatomical divisions of the lung. Seventy percent of lung contusions are visible within 1 to 2 hours following thoracic trauma. Thirty percent of contusions do not appear for 6 to 8 hours following trauma (3).

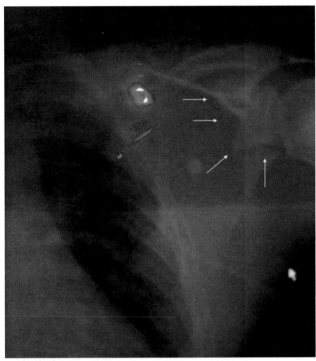

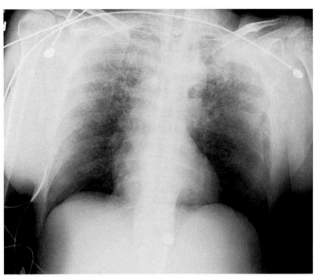

Figure 3.25. Rib fx. Assess for rib fractures by following the smooth lines of the ribs and watching for interruptions. A rib series is a more sensitive view for rib fractures; however, because the differentiation of rib fracture from contusion is not clinically significant, a rib series is rarely a necessary test. The important process to rule out when rib fractures are suspected is coincident pneumothorax and hemothorax. Acute rib fractures appear as irregularities interrupting the smooth lines of the ribs.

Figure 3.24. Scapular fracture. Scapular fractures are incidental, but clinically important, findings on the CXR of trauma patients. Forty-three percent of scapular fractures are missed on the supine film of a trauma patient (4).

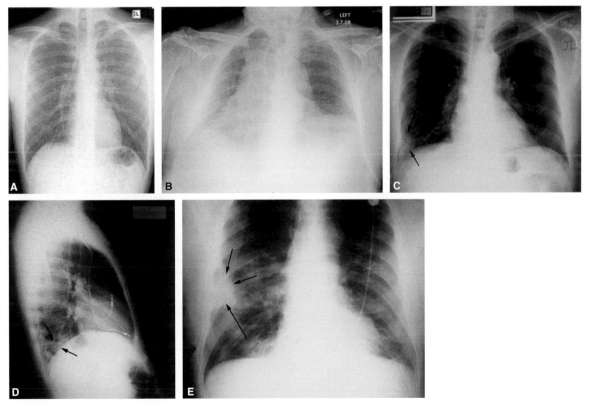

Figure 3.26. Pulmonary embolism. (A) The most common finding on CXR in pulmonary embolism is a normal CXR. Nonspecific CXR findings associated with pulmonary embolism are atelectasis, effusions, infiltrates, oligemia, and an upward shifted diaphragm. This CXR lacks these findings and is simply normal. Image courtesy of Michael Farner, MD. (B) Westermarkis sign is a dilation of pulmonary vascular proximal to the embolism and oligemia distal to the embolism. Note the absence of lung markings at the apices on this patient with massive bilateral PE. Image courtesy of Michael Farner, MD. (C) Hamptonis hump is a triangle-shaped opacity seen at the pleural with the apex pointed toward the hilum. It is often seen at the costophrenic angle on the PA view and behind the diaphragm on the lateral view. Image courtesy of Allen Cohen, MD. (D) Hamptons hump seen on PA and lateral views, courtesy of Anthony Dean, MD. (E) Hamptons hump outlined by arrows, courtesy of Anthony Dean, MD.

53

References

1. Klompas M: Does this patient have an acute thoracic aortic dissection? *JAMA* 2002;**287**:2262–72.

2. Felson B, Felson H: Localization of intrathoracic lesions by means of the postero-anterior roentgenogram: the silhouette sign. *Radiology* 1950;**55**:363.

3. Kirsh MM, Sloan H: *Blunt chest trauma*. Boston: Little, Brown and Company, 1977.

4. Harris RD, Harris JH Jr.: The prevalence and significance of missed scapular fractures in blunt chest trauma. *AJR Am J Roentgenol* 1988;**151**(4):747–50.

Plain Film Evaluation of the Abdomen

Anthony J. Dean and Ross Kessler

Indications

Although imaging of the abdomen is now largely performed utilizing CT, MRI, or ultrasound, plain film radiography can still be valuable in providing specific answers to urgent clinical questions regarding abdominal pain. In many cases, the more accurate and detailed information that advanced imaging modalities provide comes at the expense of delays and financial expenditures. In addition, because physicians in many locations still evaluate abdominal pain without rapid and easy access to advanced imaging, it is necessary to be familiar with significant plain film findings that might tailor the workup, direct supportive care, or mandate surgical interventions that preempt further imaging. The most common indication for abdominal plain film radiography is acute abdominal pain. Other indications, as dictated by clinical circumstances, might include vomiting, nonspecific abdominal complaints, history of trauma, or unexplained fever. Because abdominal plain films provide specific information about only a few diseases and give indirect or nonspecific clues about a much larger number, the decision to order abdominal films is subject to a variety of case- and practice-specific considerations. Case-specific factors include patient age, altered mental status, distracting injuries, medications (especially steroids and other immunosuppressive agents), and comorbid conditions (diabetes, other immunocompromising illnesses, or those predisposing to abdominal pathology).

Diagnostic capabilities

The normal plain film

An acute abdominal series (or "obstruction series") of the abdomen typically includes a supine view of the abdomen, an upright view of the abdomen, and an upright view of the chest. The supine abdominal "flat plate" view (also referred to as the "kidney-ureter-bladder," or KUB) can be used to identify many of the findings discussed below. This view of the abdomen is obtained with the patient lying supine and the x-ray beam directed vertically downward. It is useful in evaluating the overall bowel gas pattern and the presence of calcifications or soft tissue masses. The upright view of the abdomen is obtained with the patient standing or sitting and the x-ray beam directed horizontally. Alternatively, if the patient is unable to cooperate, a left lateral decubitus view can be obtained while the patient lies on her left side and the

x-ray beam is directed parallel to the floor. These views are essential in evaluating for free air and air-fluid levels within the bowel. Finally, an upright chest is obtained with the patient standing or sitting and the x-ray beam directed horizontally through the thorax. An upright chest is included in an abdominal series because the diaphragms may not be included in a large person's upright abdominal film and because common chest pathology such as basilar pneumonia or pleural effusions can be the etiology of abdominal symptoms.

In examining an abdominal plain film, it is often helpful to have a systematic approach. To recognize abnormal pathology, one must be familiar with normal radiographic findings. Under normal circumstances, bowel gas should invariably be present in the stomach, a few non-distended loops of small bowel, the colon, and the rectum. On an upright abdomen or chest radiograph, there is almost always an air-fluid level in the stomach, and a few small air-fluid levels may be seen in the small bowel. As the large bowel functions to remove fluid, there should be no air-fluid levels in the colon unless the patient has recently taken an enema. Small bowel is distinguished from large bowel by its more central location in the abdomen and by valvulae conniventes (also called plicae circulares), which traverse the entire width of the small bowel and are closely spaced. In contrast, the plicae semilunares of the colon are widely spaced and give rise to the characteristic haustral markings of that organ. Small bowel is normally less than 2.5 cm in diameter, the majority of colon less than 6 cm in diameter, and the cecum or sigmoid colon less than 9 cm in diameter. The risks of complications from obstruction (ischemia or perforation) significantly increase when the small bowel exceeds 5 cm and the cecum (the part of the colon most susceptible to perforation) exceeds 10 cm. Abnormal distribution or location of bowel gas (discussed below) may be a clue to a pathological process.

Between the lateral margin of the ascending and descending colon and the inner wall of the abdominal wall musculature (the transversalis fascia), a linear lucency created by the properitoneal fat can be seen. This should be checked for the following features: uniform radiodensity, well-defined margins, and symmetric thickness. Any retroperitoneal or peritoneal inflammation causing edema in this adipose layer will cause it to become relatively radiopaque, leading to loss of one or more of these radiographic features. In addition, the medial wall of the flank stripe should directly abut the adjacent bowel.

Evaluation of solid organs and soft tissue structures in the abdomen is limited because of their inherent radiographic density. The solid visceral organs (spleen, liver, and kidneys) should be evaluated for their location, size, external contour, and abnormal densities or radiolucencies. The outline of the kidneys and psoas muscles should be identified and compared side to side. These structures create a silhouette similar to the heart and diaphragm in the chest. The loss of this silhouette suggests an inflammatory process in that location. Abnormal collections of gas (discussed later in the chapter) or indirect evidence of a mass by displacement of bowel loops should be sought. Finally, the spine should be evaluated because a unilateral inflammatory process can cause local muscle spasm leading to scoliosis (concave) on the affected side.

Abnormal plain film findings and diagnosis

As noted, almost any abdominal complaint may be an indication for plain film radiography in certain circumstances. For that reason, it is more useful to think of the differential diagnoses for a particular patient and consider the ways that plain film may or may not be helpful in establishing or excluding those diagnoses. Thus, the following discussion is broken into diagnoses that are expected to give rise to fairly reliable findings on plain film; diagnoses for which nonspecific findings are common, but specific findings frequently unreliable; and diagnoses for which there are almost no indications for plain film. In almost all abdominal disease processes, plain film is insufficiently sensitive to exclude disease in situations where the pretest clinical suspicion is high. In such circumstances, further imaging with more advanced imaging modalities (usually CT) will be needed.

Indications for which plain films often give specific information
Perforated viscus

The most common cause of pneumoperitoneum is the rupture of an air-containing viscus. An upright chest or abdominal radiograph should include the diaphragms, which should be checked for abnormal subphrenic radiolucencies. Small volumes of free air tend to be crescent shaped and slit-like, in contrast to bowel gas, which usually has a rounder shape. The size of the radiolucent region is roughly proportional to the amount of free air. Free air is easier to recognize under the right hemi-diaphragm because of the soft tissue density of the liver in relation to air. Occasionally a small stomach bubble can be mistaken for free air, but it should be distinguishable by the presence of an air-fluid level on a true horizontal beam film. In addition, Chilaiditi's anomaly – loops of bowel interposed between the liver and the right diaphragm – can usually be identified by the presence of haustral colonic markings.

Patients who are unable to cooperate for an upright film can be placed in the left decubitus position, and the film should be inspected for a slit-like lucency between the liver and flank stripe. Free air is more difficult to detect in a supine KUB projection. Findings that have been described in this view include Rigler's sign (air outlining both sides of the bowel wall), the right upper quadrant sign (air outlining the liver), the falciform ligament sign (air outlining the falciform ligament), the "inverted V sign" (air outlining the umbilical "folds" or arteries in children or the inferior epigastric vessels in adults), and the football sign (a centrally located ovoid lucency).

For optimal horizontal beam projections, radiographic protocols call for the patient to be positioned (erect or decubitus) for at least 4 minutes prior to exposure of the film. Such conditions are seldom realized in the emergency department. Even under ideal conditions, small volumes of free air may not be evident on plain film, so if there is a high index of suspicion, a CT should be obtained.

Obstruction versus ileus

Mechanical bowel obstruction can be classified by location (large vs. small bowel), by cause, or by degree (complete vs. partial). Ileus may be localized or generalized. Both bowel obstruction and ileus are dynamic processes; therefore, findings will vary depending on when the radiographs are obtained as well as the cause and location of the pathologic process. The radiographic findings of generalized ileus and mechanical obstruction may overlap, but obstruction can be generally distinguished based on clinical features and, radiographically, by a disproportionate dilatation of small bowel compared to large bowel and by the absence of bowel gas distal to an obstruction. This is in contrast to an ileus that typically demonstrates a diffusely distended gas-filled GI tract, including the rectum. Another frequent, but not invariable, feature of obstruction is that air-fluid levels in adjacent loops of bowel on an upright film are characteristically at different levels ("step laddering" due to the hyperactive peristalsis seen in obstruction). In contrast, an ileus can demonstrate air-fluid levels throughout the small bowel and colon but typically does not demonstrate the "step laddering" appearance. This finding will be lost in advanced obstruction when the bowel develops a secondary ileus from the metabolic and mechanical insult of the obstruction.

The most common cause of generalized ileus is abdominal surgery, but in the ED it is more likely to be seen in the context of a severe abdominal (e.g., mesenteric ischemia), retroperitoneal (e.g., vascular catastrophe, ureteral colic), or systemic (e.g., sepsis, metabolic) illness. With generalized ileus, all parts of the abdominal gastrointestinal tract from the stomach to rectum are distended and filled with gas or fluid.

Localized ileus ("sentinel loop") is caused by a focal inflammatory process in the vicinity of one or more bowel loops that appear gas filled and distended. The location of the sentinel loop may offer a clue as to the cause but is not reliable. Classically, localized ileus in the right upper quadrant suggests cholecystitis; in the right lower quadrant, appendicitis; in the left upper quadrant, pancreatitis or peptic ulcer; and in the left lower quadrant, diverticulitis. It is important to remember that an early mechanical bowel obstruction may resemble a localized ileus, especially if the sentinel loops are located in the left upper quadrant.

Small bowel obstructions are most commonly caused by postoperative adhesions (accounting for >50%), hernias, neoplasia, and inflammatory bowel disease. Complete mechanical obstruction results in distended loops of bowel to a certain point, beyond which there is an abnormal paucity or absence of bowel gas. The bowel is usually distended with gas but can sometimes contain fluid and a paucity of gas, resulting in a failure to recognize the diagnosis. With careful inspection, the distended fluid-filled loops can usually be detected, with small bubbles of gas forming characteristic linear patterns between the valvulae conniventes (on both flat plate and upright films). This is described as the "string of pearls" sign. Partial bowel obstruction, most commonly caused by adhesions, allows some gas to pass the point of obstruction, and therefore gas may be visible in the colon beyond distended loops of small bowel. Generally, in a more distal small bowel obstruction, there will be a greater number of dilated bowel loops than in a proximal obstruction.

Large bowel obstruction results in dilatation of colon proximal to the obstruction and can be caused by neoplasia, volvulus, fecal impaction, inflammatory bowel disease, or intussusception. Pseudo-obstruction (Ogilvie's Syndrome) usually occurs in the elderly or chronically ill and is characterized by massive dilatation of the entire colon. Unlike a mechanical bowel obstruction, there is no obstructing lesion; it is instead caused by global loss of peristalsis. Distal large bowel obstruction, especially sigmoid (usually due to cancer or volvulus), may be confused with generalized ileus if the ileocecal valve is incompetent (allowing retrograde distension of the small bowel) but can usually be distinguished by absence of rectal gas. Partial obstruction allows the passage of some gas, so that its appearance may mimic that of localized ileus or early complete obstruction. Because the large bowel functions to reabsorb water, there are usually no air-fluid levels in a large bowel obstruction. The etiology of obstruction, with the exception of volvulus, is not usually apparent on plain film. Cecal volvulus tends to give rise to a loop of distended bowel in the form of a reversed "C" filling the left upper quadrant. Sigmoid volvulus typically reveals an inverted "U" or coffee bean arising from the left side of the pelvis and directed to the right upper quadrant. A barium enema study may demonstrate a loop of volvulated sigmoid colon tapering to a fine point, described as a bird's beak. Finally, toxic megacolon, a serious complication of inflammatory bowel disease, is characterized by marked dilatation of the colon (at least 6 cm in diameter of the transverse colon on supine radiograph) and submucosal bowel wall thickening, termed "thumbprinting."

Indications for which plain films often give nonspecific information but rarely give specific information

Solid organs

Splenic enlargement due to trauma or medical disease may be suggested by displacement of the splenic flexure, gastric bubble, or left kidney. An enlarged liver may be suggested by displacement of all bowel loops from the right upper quadrant to the iliac crest. Air in the biliary system presents as branching tube-like lucencies overlying the central region of the liver. This finding can be normal in the setting of an incompetent sphincter of Oddi or a surgical biliary-enteric anastamosis, or it may be pathologic, as seen in cholangitis from a gas-forming bacteria. Pneumobilia may also be associated with a gallstone ileus, in which a gallstone erodes through the wall of the bowel and creates a small bowel obstruction (with the offending radiolucent gallstone often impacted at the ileocecal valve). It is important to distinguish pneumobilia from portal venous gas, the latter presenting as thinner branching lucencies at the periphery of the liver, which can be an ominous sign of bowel ischemia.

Cholecystic mural calcification gives rise to the surgical finding of "porcelain gallbladder," which appears as a radiodense structure in the right upper quadrant. It is thought to occur in the setting of chronic gallbladder inflammation and was traditionally associated with a high incidence of gallbladder carcinoma, although recent reports have cast doubt on this association. Smaller lamellar calcifications or lucencies in the region of the gallbladder may be due to gallstones or emphysematous cholecystitis, respectively. Stippled pancreatic calcifications suggest recurrent or chronic pancreatitis. Their significance in the acute setting will need to be determined clinically. Other causes of right upper quadrant calcifications include echinococcal cysts, schistosomiasis, granulomatous diseases, and tumors (both benign and malignant). Occasionally, urinary retention overlooked on physical exam will be suggested by a large midline soft tissue mass arising from the pelvis.

Gastrointestinal tract pathology

Appendicitis can be suggested by a sentinel loop, loss of psoas or flank stripe shadows, scoliosis, the presence of an appendicolith, abnormal absence of gas in the ascending colon ("colon cut-off"), or the presence of a soft tissue mass (with or without abnormal gas collections in the case of perforation). Contiguous loops of bowel should be sought on the plain films to identify bowel wall thickening and pneumatosis intestinalis, although the absence of these findings does not rule them out. Diseases that may give rise to bowel wall thickening include inflammatory bowel disease, colitis, diverticulitis, and ischemia. Radiographically, the submucosal bowel wall edema leads to irregular narrowing of the bowel lumen with a characteristic "thumbprinting" appearance. Pneumatosis, best seen in profile, can be caused by necrosis of the bowel wall secondary to ischemia, severe mechanical obstruction that raises intraluminal pressure, or dissection of air from ruptured blebs in the setting of COPD. While mesenteric ischemia may give rise to pneumatosis and is a poor prognostic sign, in most cases it does not. However, plain films are usually indicated because other diagnoses identifiable on plain film may also be under active consideration in this clinical setting.

Abnormal fluid collections and soft tissue masses

Free peritoneal fluid may be identified by loss of the psoas or renal shadows, or displacement of the lateral walls of the ascending and descending colon from the flank stripes. The most common cause is ascites, but other causes, often suggested by the clinical context, include blood, urine, bile, succus entericus, and cerebrospinal fluid. Any soft tissue mass (e.g., splenomegaly, pseudocyst, renal tumor) may be suggested by abnormal displacement of the normal bowel gas pattern. Inflammatory processes (e.g., abscesses, acute pancreatitis) may also cause sentinel loops, colon cut-off, or extra-intestinal gas collections.

Retroperitoneal processes

Retroperitoneal inflammation or injury (e.g., due to acute pancreatitis, acute aortic aneurysm, or renal trauma) may give rise to loss of the normal kidney or psoas shadows. It may also cause thickening, increased radiodensity, or obscuration of the flank stripe because the fascial planes containing the properitoneal fat are continuous with the retroperitoneal compartments containing these organs. Retroperitoneal air can be caused by trauma, iatrogenic injury, or bowel perforation secondary to infection or inflammation (e.g., perforated diverticulitis). In contrast to pneumoperitoneum, retroperitoneal air appears as fixed, streaky lucencies that outline retroperitoneal structures, such as the psoas muscles, great vessels, or kidneys.

Other findings

A variety of abnormal radiodensities can be encountered on plain films. Most are due to abnormal calcifications within the soft tissues, although they can also be caused by foreign bodies, surgical clips, pills, or intramuscular injections. Most calcifications can be identified by examining their anatomical location and morphology. Vascular calcifications tend to have a railroad track appearance, representing calcification of the tubular walls, although the splenic and hepatic arteries can become remarkably tortuous. Aneurysms of any of these vessels can be seen on plain film if they have become calcified. In contrast to the delicate lamellar appearance of many gallstones, staghorn renal calculi have grotesque shapes. These and the diffuse stippling of nephrocalcinosis appear in characteristic locations.

The ureters run from the renal hilum crossing into the pelvic inlet medial to the sacroiliac joint. They cross the greater sciatic notch (visible on plain film) on the sidewalls of the pelvis before passing medially to the bladder. Ureteral stones tend to have an irregular radiodensity and outline in contrast to phleboliths, which usually have smooth, corticated margins and often a central lucency. Calculi originating from the kidney are often radiopaque and typically (80% to 85%) composed of combinations of calcium oxalate and calcium phosphate. The calculi then migrate from the kidney down the ureter to the bladder. Sizes can vary from <1 mm to >1 cm. More than 90% of urinary stones are radiopaque. (Uric acid and cystine stones are radiolucent.) Ureteral stones tend to become impacted at sites where the ureter is anatomically narrowed or compressed. Common sites include the ureteropelvic junction (where the renal pelvis or "infundibulum" tapers down into the proximal ureter), the pelvic brim (the ureter crosses the common iliac artery and vein and passes into the pelvis), and the ureterovesicular junction (UVJ) – the latter being narrowest and most common site of stone impaction. Stones that have passed through the UVJ can sometimes be seen in the bladder, but this is separate and distinct from a true bladder stone. The small size of most stones (<5 mm) makes them difficult to identify reliably on plain radiographs; therefore, noncontrast CT has become the modality of choice for the identification and measurement of ureteral calculi. However, with increasing concern among the public and healthcare providers about exposure to ionizing radiation from computed tomography, there has been renewed interest in the use of ultrasonography in the management of ureteral colic (discussed in detail in Chapter 18). Bladder stones are typically lamellar in appearance while fibroid calcifications tend to have a popcorn appearance and can become very large.

Skeletal structures are inspected for mineralization (focal or diffuse abnormalities), trabecular structure, compression, and fractures. Joints are inspected for alignment and evidence of degenerative or inflammatory processes.

Indications for which plain films are usually not indicated in the evaluation of the abdomen

Plain films are rarely indicated in the evaluation of gastrointestinal hemorrhage or gastroenteritis.

Imaging pitfalls and limitations

As noted, the most common pitfall is in using abdominal plain films to exclude a diagnosis for which there was high clinical suspicion. Plain films almost never definitively exclude the many diagnoses that they frequently rule in.

Clinical images

Normal plain films of the abdomen

The normal upright plain film of the abdomen shows a nonspecific bowel gas pattern with typical distribution and location of colonic gas from cecum to rectum. A loop of bowel is confirmed as large bowel (*white star*) by the presence of widely spaced haustral markings and its lateral location of descending colon. The gastric bubble is identified in the left upper quadrant (*white arrowhead*). The shadow of the liver can be seen (*white arrows*) medial to a clearly defined flank stripe. Black lines outline the psoas shadows. The kidney shadows are difficult to identify in this patient. There is mild scoliosis of the thoracolumbar spine. The sacrum, pelvis, hips, and articulations appear normal. The entire right diaphragm is not clearly seen, making this an inadequate series to rule out free air.

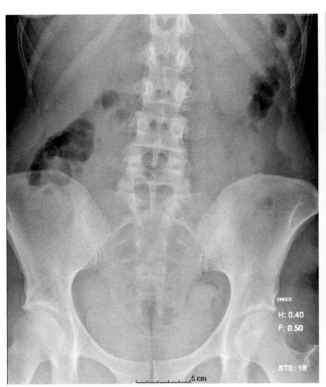

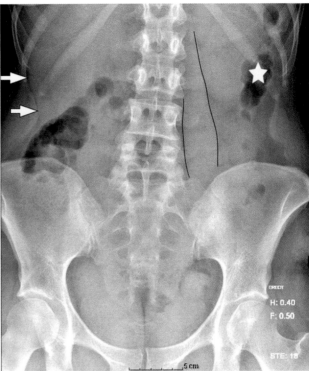

Figure 4.1A1 and 4.1A2. Normal upright abdomen.

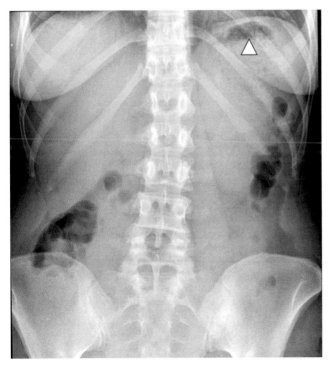

Figure 4.1B. Normal upright abdomen including diaphragms.

Free air

A patient with an expressive aphasia presents with weakness 17 days after an admission, in which the cause of anemia was identified as a peptic ulcer found via

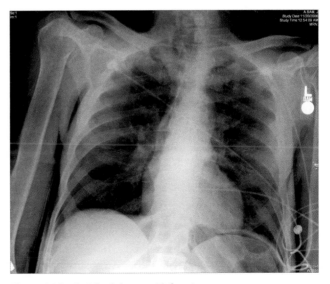

Figure 4.2A. Upright abdomen with free air.

esophagogastroduodenoscopy. Since discharge, the patient has been eating very little and not feeling well. He indicates mild abdominal pain and tenderness. There are no peritoneal signs. The initial chest film was done supine and did not reveal any abnormalities. Two hours later, an abdominal supine view was obtained with an upright chest view that showed free air under the left diaphragm (Fig. 4.2A). The free air on the supine view (Figs. 4.2B1 and 4.2B2) is not nearly so obvious, but the film demonstrates several of the recognized signs of free air (see the "Abnormal plain film

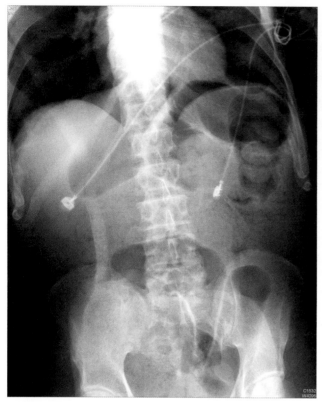

Figure 4.2B1. Supine abdomen with free air, no markings.

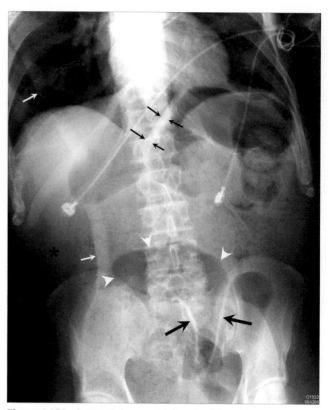

Figure 4.2B2. Supine abdomen with free air, with markings.

findings and diagnosis" section, earlier in this chapter). There is an inverted V sign (*large black arrows*), the suggestion of Rigler's sign (*small black arrows*), and the "football sign" (*white arrowheads*), and the lateral side of the ascending colon seems to be displaced from the flank stripe (*asterisk*). The prominent soft tissue density in the right flank is probably a skin fold because it can be seen continuing above the diaphragm (*small white arrows*). The patient was transfused for his hemoglobin of 5 and taken to the operating room.

Ileus

A 28-year-old presents with abdominal pain, nausea, vomiting, diarrhea, and fever for several days. He has a history of appendicitis. He has been passing flatus. An obstruction series shows a normal upright chest film. The supine and upright abdominal films are shown (Figs. 4.3A and B). Both films show gas through the small bowel (*above small white arrows*) and colon down to the rectum. In contrast to the usual findings on obstruction, in ileus, the loops of bowel on the upright do not show step laddering of their air-fluid levels (Fig. 4.3B2, *above white arrows*). This study demonstrates several normal soft tissue shadows, including bilateral well-demarcated flank stripes of homogeneous density (*between black arrows*), psoas shadows (Fig. 4.3A2, *white arrowheads*), and the liver margin (4.3B2, *white arrowheads*). The radiographic findings of ileus can be seen in gastroenteritis, as in this case.

Small bowel obstruction

A patient presents 2 days after takedown of a diverting colostomy. He has nausea, vomiting, and the absence of flatus. The flat plate (Figs. 4.4A1 and A2) shows multiple loops of small bowel with the valvulae conniventes traversing the small bowel. Occasional loops of colon are suggested by their by appearance and location (Fig. 4.4A2, *black arrows*). However, the upright film (Fig. 4.4B) reveals these also to be loops of small bowel. The upright film also shows marked step laddering of the air-fluid levels within single loops of bowel (Fig. 4.4B2, *pairs of white arrows on left and right sides*) and absence of colonic gas. This suggests vigorous peristalsis, consistent with early obstruction. A small gastric bubble above the soft tissue shadow of the stomach distended with fluid can be seen on the upright (Fig. 4.4B2, *white arrowheads*). Another case of small bowel obstruction is shown in Figures 4.4C (supine) and 4.4D (erect). The small bowel is distended with a striking paucity of gas in the colon. In addition, there is evidence of perforation with free air under the right hemidiaphragm (*white arrow*), suggestion of a Rigler's sign (*white arrowheads*), and extra-luminal subhepatic air (*black circle*).

Sentinel loop with appendicitis

A patient presents with 12 hours of anorexia, fever, and right lower quadrant pain. This film shows an appendicolith (*arrow*) and a loop of distended bowel (*asterisk*) with an air-fluid level.

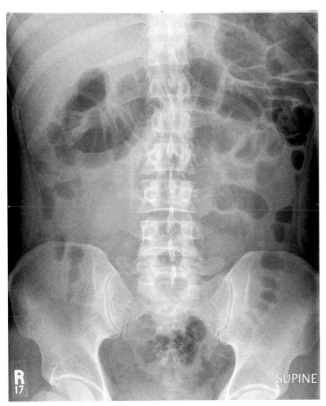

Figure 4.3A1. Supine ileus with no markings.

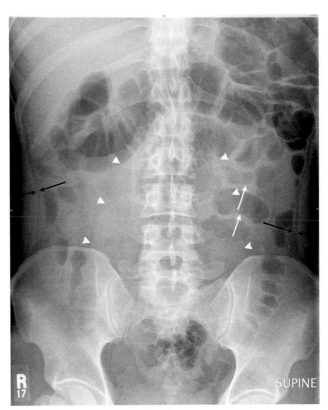

Figure 4.3A2. Supine ileus with markings.

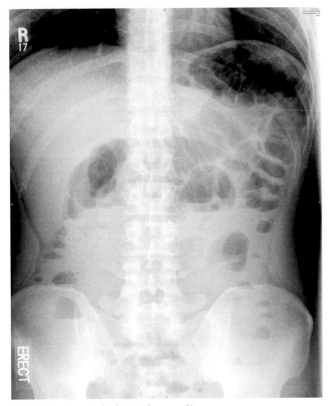

Figure 4.3B1. Upright ileus with no markings.

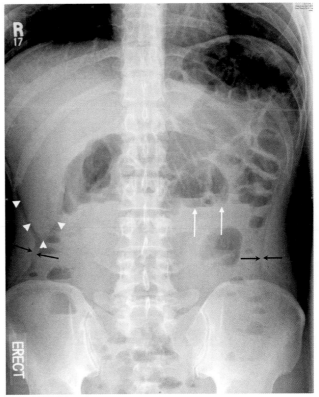

Figure 4.3B2. Upright ileus with markings.

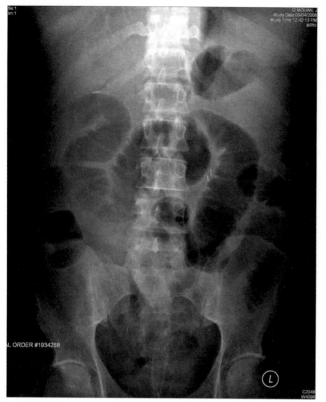

Figure 4.4A1. Supine view of obstruction without markings.

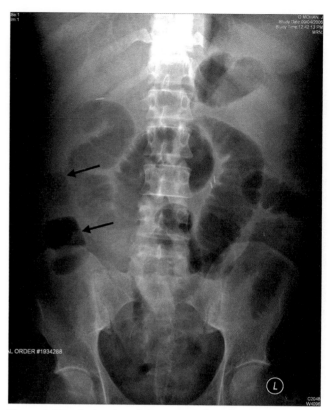

Figure 4.4A2. Supine view of obstruction with markings.

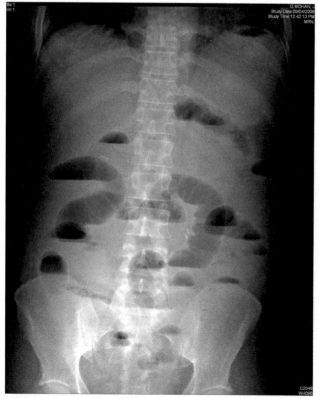

Figure 4.4B1. Upright view of obstruction without markings.

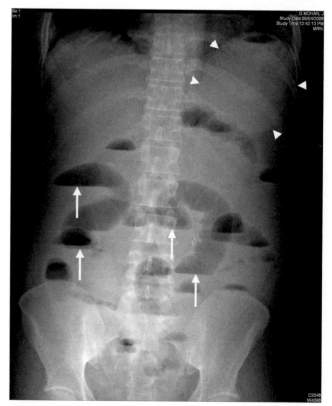

Figure 4.4B2. Upright view of obstruction with markings.

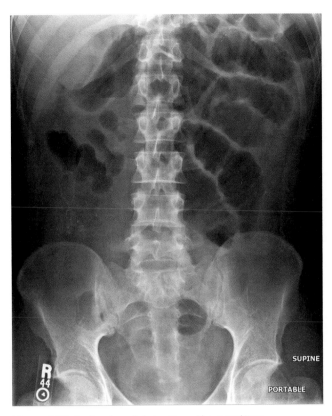

Figure 4.4C. Supine view of obstruction without markings.

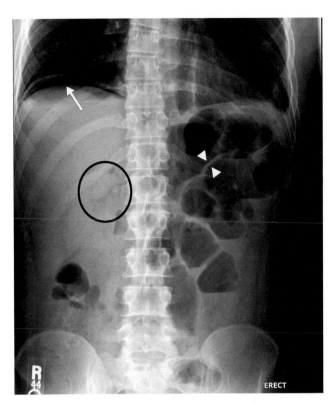

Figure 4.4D. Upright view of obstruction with free air with markings.

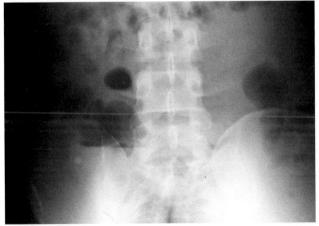

Figure 4.5A1. Sentinel loop without markings.

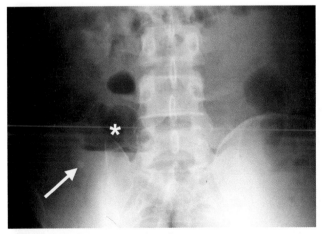

Figure 4.5A2. Sentinel loop with markings.

In this limited film, it is not possible to determine whether the loop is cecum or small bowel. There is a suggestion of scoliosis due to spasm of the right-sided lumbar muscles.

Cecal volvulus

A volvulus is a twisting of the intestines around the anchoring mesentery. Cecal volvulus typically occurs in younger patients than sigmoid volvulus, which is primarily a condition of the elderly. Cecal volvulus involves the cecum and a portion of the ascending colon and gives rise to a loop of distended bowel in the form of a reversed "C,"

filling the central abdomen and left upper quadrant. The white arrows outline the dilated cecal loop, which forms a "kidney bean" shape. Notice the thickened bowel wall of this loop (adjacent to left flank stripe), as well as the dilated loops of proximal small bowel.

Sigmoid volvulus

Sigmoid volvulus is more common than cecal volvulus. It occurs due to the loose mesenteric attachment of the sigmoid colon. Patients are usually elderly, have abdominal pain and distention, and have a history of decreased bowel

63

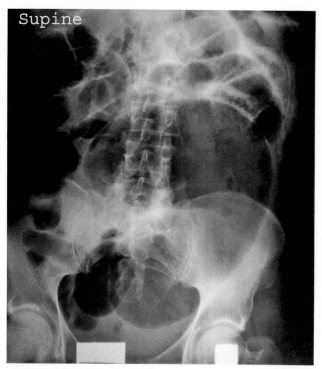

Figure 4.6A1. Cecal volvulus without markings.

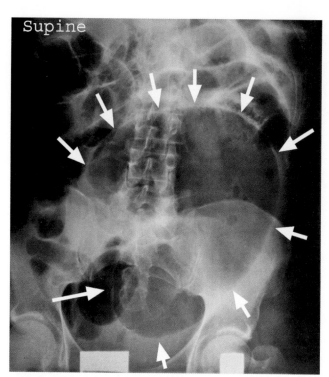

Figure 4.6A2. Cecal volvulus with markings.

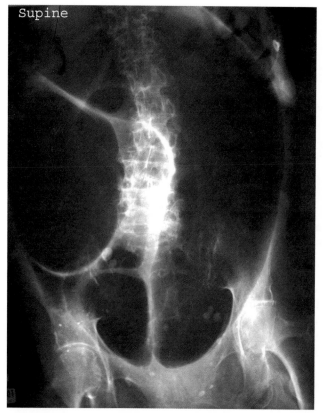

Figure 4.7A1. Sigmoid volvulus without markings.

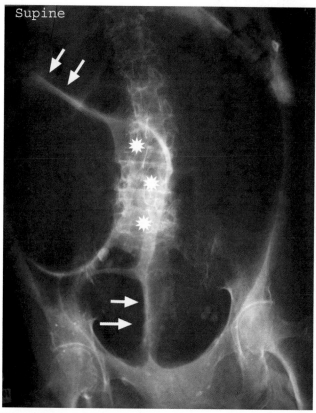

Figure 4.7A2. Sigmoid volvulus with markings.

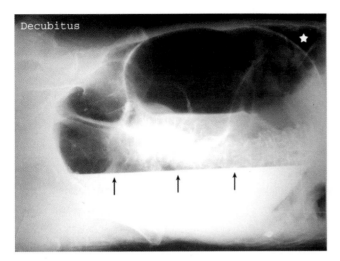

Figure 4.7B. Sigmoid volvulus decubitus view.

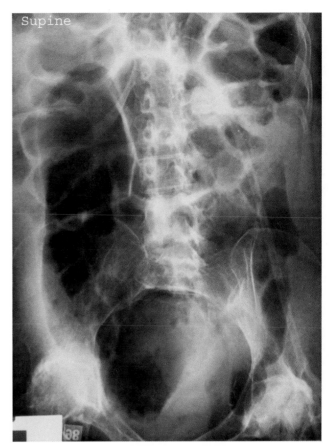

Figure 4.8A1. Large bowel obstruction without markings.

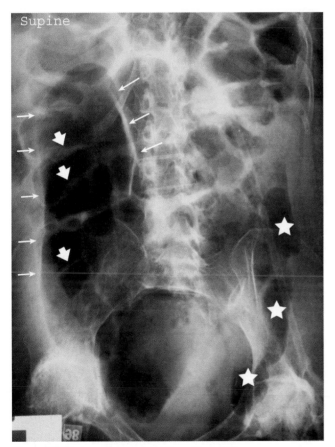

Figure 4.8A2. Large bowel obstruction with markings.

movements and absence of flatus. Supine and decubitus views show a massively dilated sigmoid colon forming an inverted "U" arising from the left side of the pelvis and directed to the right upper quadrant. In the pelvis, the twisted end(s) of the closed loop of bowel are often seen to taper down to a fine point, described as a "bird's beak" (not seen on these images). The adjacent walls of edematous

bowel and mesentery create the characteristic central "stripe" (*asterisks*). The haustral markings identify this as large bowel (*white arrows*). The decubitus view (Fig. 4.7B) demonstrates the air-fluid layer consistent with a closed-loop obstruction (*narrow black arrows*). Note the overlapping bowel (*white star*) that could be mistaken for free air. Many phleboliths with characteristic central lucencies are seen.

Large bowel obstruction

There is a dilated loop of ascending colon (*small white arrows*), and there is air in the descending and sigmoid colon (*white stars*), but none in the rectum. The markings of the superimposed small bowel can also be seen (*white arrows*), indicating an incompetent ileocecal valve. These findings are highly suspicious for an obstructing sigmoid carcinoma, which could be sought by CT with rectal contrast or proctoscopy. Colonic tumors are the most common cause of large bowel obstructions. Distal large bowel obstructions frequently present with relatively mild symptoms because most are gradually progressive and do not interrupt any of the metabolic functions of the GI tract (particularly water absorption, in contrast to small bowel obstruction). Radiographic findings on plain abdominal films are nonspecific. An upright or decubitus image may reveal air-fluid

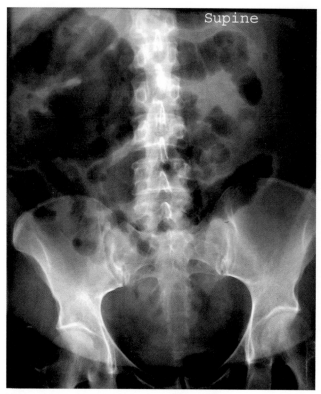

Figure 4.9A1. Toxic megacolon without markings.

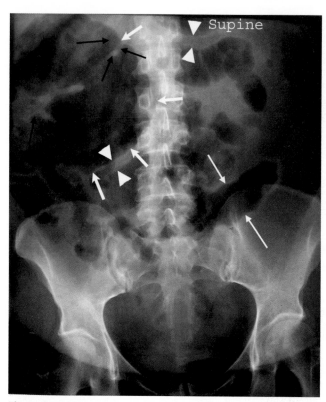

Figure 4.9A2. Toxic megacolon with markings.

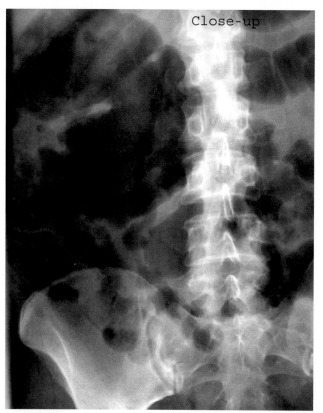

Figure 4.9B1. Toxic megacolon without markings close-up.

levels but would not identify the underlying cause of the obstruction.

Toxic megacolon

Toxic megacolon should be considered in patients with ulcerative colitis presenting with diarrhea, fever, abdominal pain, and distension. It is also seen in patients with Crohn's disease or other severe forms of colitis. It usually involves the entire large bowel, although the dilatation of the transverse colon is most striking on a supine radiograph. There is no consensus regarding a diagnostic colonic diameter for this condition; however, a diameter >6 cm is concerning, and one >10 cm puts the patient at high risk for perforation. The characteristic bowel wall pathology of ulcerative colitis consisting of areas of ulceration and intervening segments of inflammation and edema, with or without pseudopolyps, can be inferred from luminal irregularities known as "thumbprinting" (*black arrows*). The plain films in this case (Figs. 4.9A1 and A2) demonstrate a portion of the large bowel that is edematous and dilated (*large white arrows*). Other loops of bowel demonstrate effacement of normal bowel markings (*thin white arrows*) and marked thickening (*white arrowheads*). The close-up images (Figs. 4.9B1 and B2) show a large area of bowel edema, resembling a thumbprint smudge (*small white arrows*), as well as bowel wall crowding that forms a dense stripe (*star*). Crowding refers to the

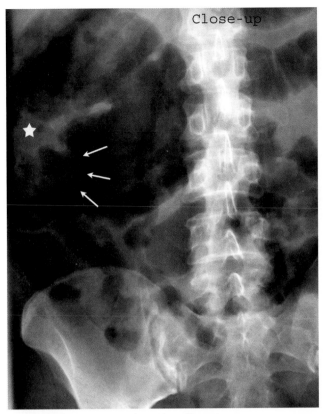

Figure 4.9B2. Toxic megacolon with markings close-up.

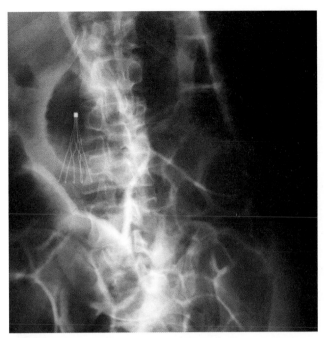

Figure 4.10A1. Pseudo-obstruction without markings.

appearance of adjacent thickened bowel folds in the setting of bowel wall edema.

Pseudo-obstruction (Ogilvie syndrome)

Pseudo-obstruction, also known as Ogilvie syndrome, is a mimic of large bowel obstruction. This condition is usually found among elderly patients and those with chronic illnesses, laxative abuse, or prolonged immobility, which results in markedly slowed colonic transit time that can progress to bowel atony. A portion of the intestine – most commonly, the lower colonic segment – is dilated and has mixed air and fecal contents without air-fluid levels. The films shown in Figures 4.10A1 and A2 are those of a patient who presented from a nursing home with fever and change in mental status. The patient had a benign abdominal exam without guarding or rebound but did have decreased bowel sounds. This single abdominal image demonstrates several findings: a number of dilated loops of large bowel (*asterisks*) and the lack of air-fluid layers or free air. A Greenfield filter (*arrow*) is incidentally noted. Although this single image is not diagnostic, the clinical presentation is suggestive of a pseudo-obstruction. Figure 4.10B shows the plain film of an elderly patient presenting with low back pain and a history of no bowel movements in 6 days. The image shows diffuse small and large bowel dilation and an apparent absence of gas in the rectum. However, CT revealed no obstruction, strictures, or masses, and the patient did well with nasogastric tube decompression, bowel rest, and gentle hydration. Pseudo-obstruction

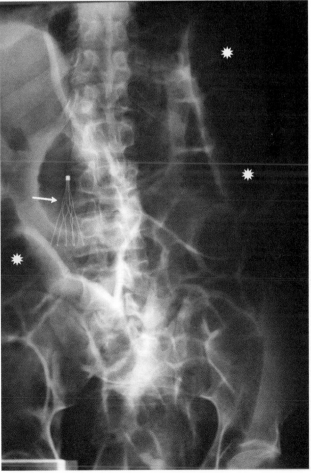

Figure 4.10A2. Pseudo-obstruction with markings.

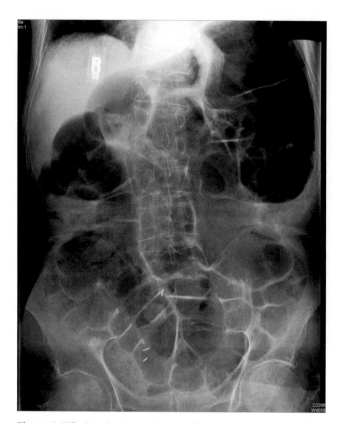

Figure 4.10B. Pseudo-obstruction second case.

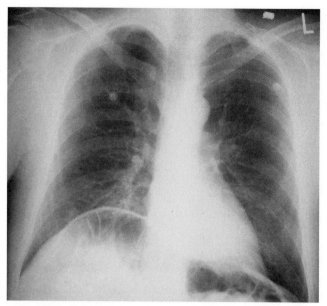

Figure 4.11. Chilaiditi finding.

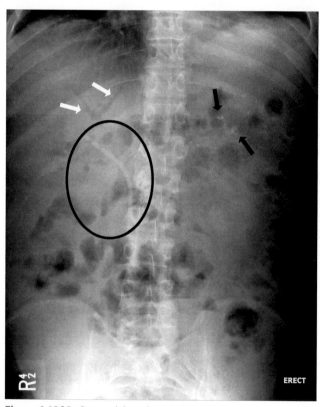

Figure 4.12A2. Pneumobilia with markings.

is a diagnosis of exclusion that can rarely be reached in the ED. Its consideration should prompt CT to exclude mechanical causes and a surgical consult.

Chilaiditi finding

Dimitrios Chilaiditi, a Greek radiologist first described loops of bowel seen between the liver and diaphragm in 1910. They

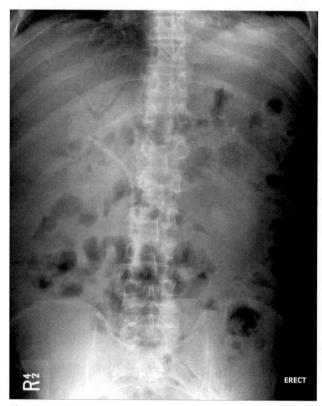

Figure 4.12A1. Pneumobilia without markings.

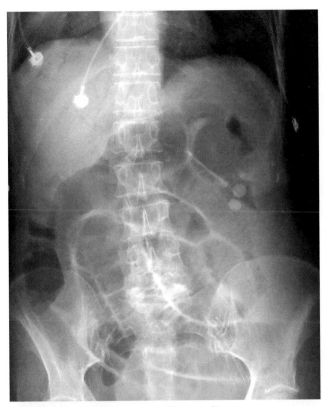

Figure 4.13A1. Portal venous gas without markings.

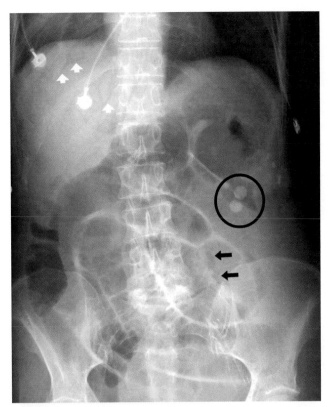

Figure 4.13A2. Portal venous gas with markings.

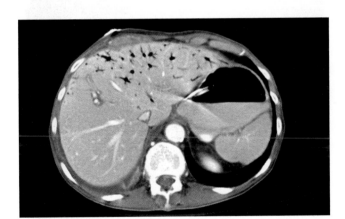

Figure 4.13B. Portal venous gas CT axial.

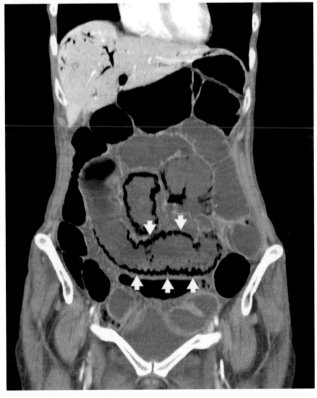

Figure 4.13C. Portal venous gas with obstruction CT coronal.

may give the impression of free air, but careful inspection reveals bowel markings as seen in this example. It is due to a small or absent bare area of the liver. Rarely, a patient's abdominal symptoms may be due to this condition, but in the vast majority it is chronic and of no clinical significance.

Pneumobilia

Air in the biliary system presents as branching tube-like lucencies overlying the central region of the liver. This finding can be benign in the setting of an incompetent sphincter of Oddi or a surgical biliary-enteric anastomosis, or pathologic, as seen in gallstone ileus or cholangitis from a gas-forming

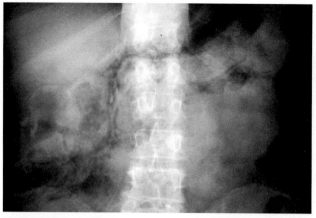

Figure 4.14A1. Pneumatosis without markings.

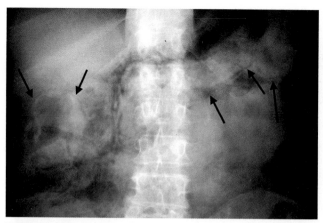

Figure 4.14A2. Pneumatosis with markings.

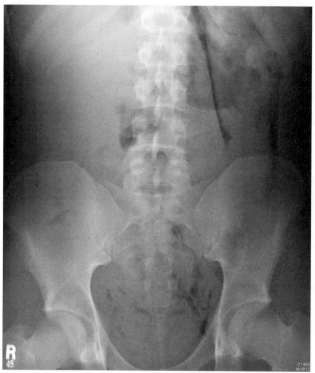

Figure 4.15A1. Retroperitoneal air without markings.

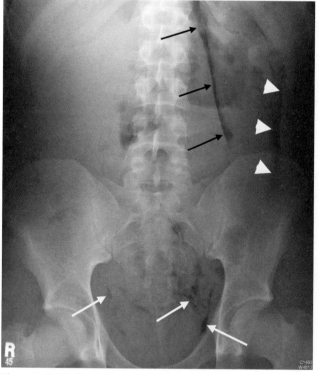

Figure 4.15A2. Retroperitoneal air with markings.

bacteria. The plain films in this case demonstrate pneumobilia (*white arrows*) in a patient with a recently placed biliary stent (*black ovoid*). In addition, small calcifications (*black arrows*) are seen within the pancreas, indicating the presence of chronic pancreatitis.

Portal venous gas

Portal venous gas is the accumulation of gas in the portal veins, presenting as thin branching lucencies at the periphery of the liver. This is in contrast to the central lucencies demonstrated in pneumobilia. Although traditionally considered an ominous finding of ischemic bowel, portal venous gas is increasingly

recognized in a variety of other conditions causing bowel distention, such as endoscopy with bowel insufflation or ileus. The plain films in this case demonstrate a small bowel obstruction with dilated loops of small bowel (Figs. 4.13A1 and A2). Portal venous gas is seen at the periphery of the liver (*white arrowheads*) and pneumatosis intestinalis is demonstrated within the walls of the small bowel (*black arrows*), both concerning for ischemia. Recently ingested radiopaque pills are incidentally seen en face within the stomach (*black circle*). The patient subsequently received a CT of the abdomen for further evaluation, which clearly demonstrates extensive portal venous gas within the liver (Fig. 4.13B). On the CT coronal

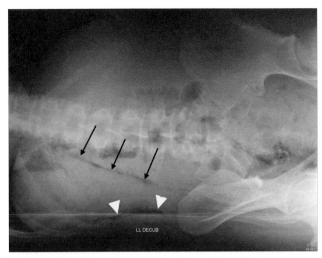

Figure 4.15B1. Retroperitoneal air decubitus without markings.

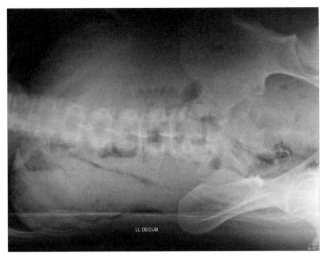

Figure 4.15B2. Retroperitoneal air decubitus with markings.

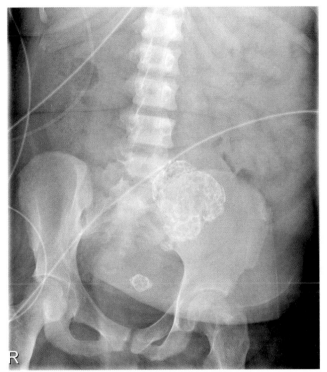

Figure 4.16A1. Uterine fibroids without markings.

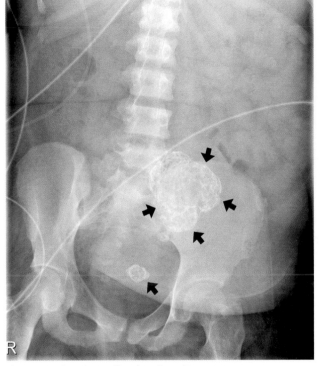

Figure 4.16A2. Uterine fibroids with markings.

image (Fig. 4.13C), there is marked dilatation of the small bowel with extensive pneumatosis intestinalis (*white arrowheads*) in keeping with an ischemic small bowel obstruction.

Pneumatosis intestinalis

A patient arrives from the nursing home, septic, with an acute abdomen. This plain film reveals multiple areas of pneumatosis (Fig. 4.14A2, *arrows*). At surgery, she was found to have ischemic and necrotic areas of bowel. Pneumatosis is usually an ominous sign because it indicates breakdown of the barrier between intestinal contents and the bloodstream. It can be caused by severe mechanical obstruction, ischemia,

inflammatory bowel disease, or, rarely, pulmonary sources such as ruptured blebs in the setting of COPD.

Retroperitoneal air

While demonstrating acrobatic tricks with a broom 45 minutes before presenting to the ED, a young, healthy patient landed on the point of the handle. He was complaining of severe rectal pain. The plain film (Fig. 4.15A2) shows areas of pelvic (*white arrows*) and lumbar (*black arrows*, also seen in Fig. 4.15B2) retroperitoneal air. Air is also seen in the left flank stripe (Figs. 4.15A2 and 4.15B2, *arrowheads*). Because of the bizarre mechanism and the patient's comfortable

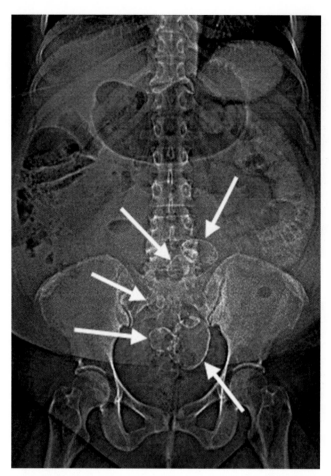

Figure 4.16B. Uterine fibroids CT scout view.

condition, the consulting surgeons expressed doubt as to the accuracy of the finding. To confirm it, and to exclude intra-peritoneal free air, a decubitus film (Figs. 4.15B1 and B2) was obtained. It demonstrates the same findings without migra-tion of the air. At surgery, the patient was found to have a rectal perforation extending into the extraperitoneal fascial planes of the pelvis.

Uterine fibroid calcifications

This supine image shows irregularly shaped clustered calcifi-cations (Figure 4.16A2, *black arrows*). Their dispersed loca-tion and the lack of smooth borders ("popcorn" appearance) differentiate them from bladder, ureteral, or renal stones. Uterine fibroids can often be palpated on examination of the lower abdomen, but many are not calcified. Their identity can easily be established by bedside ultrasonography. Figure 4.16B is a reconstructed abdominal CT scout film showing another case of multiple calcified fibroids extending out of the pelvis (*white arrows*).

Renal stone

The patient in Figures 4.17A and B presented with hematuria and left flank pain. She had had several previous episodes of "kidney infection," which were resolved with antibiotics. The supine abdominal film demonstrates a normal bowel gas pattern with an abnormal density in the left upper quad-rant (*long arrow*). The outline of the right kidney (*short arrows*) is seen, while that of the left is not, suggesting in the clinical context that inflammation of the kidney may be pre-sent, causing its margins to be obscured. The single CT image shows the calcific density located in the inferior pole of the left kidney without hydronephrosis (Fig. 4.17B2). Most renal stones do not cause hydronephrosis because they are too large to enter the ureter to obstruct it (although this one would be small enough to do so). Renal stones can become extremely large with bizarre shapes, leading to the term "stag-horn calculus" (see the next case). They should be suspected in patients with recurrent urinary tract infections, despite appropriate antibiotic therapy.

Staghorn calculus

This supine image demonstrates marked dilation of the right intrarenal collecting system (*star*) due to the presence of a large staghorn calculus. The location of the kidney is nor-mally just lateral to the psoas shadow. This image nicely demonstrates the left psoas shadow (*large arrows*), but the right psoas shadow is difficult to see, suggesting retroperito-neal edema or adjacent intraperitoneal fluid. The right side calcifications fill the collecting system. The midline calcifica-tion (*small arrows*) represents a horseshoe configuration of the kidney. Staghorn calculi are usually composed of struvite: a combination of magnesium (rendering them radiopaque), ammonium, and phosphate. They are classified as infected stones because they are associated with urea-splitting organ-isms, including Proteus, Pseudomonas, Providencia, Klebsiella, Staphylococci, and Mycoplasma.

Ureteral stone

Small densities along the tract of the ureter may represent a ureteral stone (Figure 4.19A2, *arrows*), which tend to have an irregular, angular, and non-uniformly radiodense appear-ance similar to the one in Fig. 4.19A2, in contrast to phlebo-liths (seen in Fig. 4.7A). Although there is some individual variation in the anatomy of the ureter, it is necessary to have an understanding of its typical course. This can be reviewed in standard anatomy texts but is easily appreciated from radio-graphs showing stents or intravenous pyelogram. The intravenous pyelogram in Figure 4.19B demonstrates contrast throughout a normal collecting system, outlining the course of the ureters (*white arrowheads*). No filling defects are identified to suggest the presence of a stone. Multiple calcified phleboliths in the pelvis are incidentally noted, which lie outside the collecting system (*black arrows*).

Plain radiography is not considered sufficient to exclude ureterolithiasis because most ureteral stones, although radiopaque, are too small to be identified on plain film or cannot be distinguished from other calcifications. Another case, demonstrating the difficulty of identifying ureteral

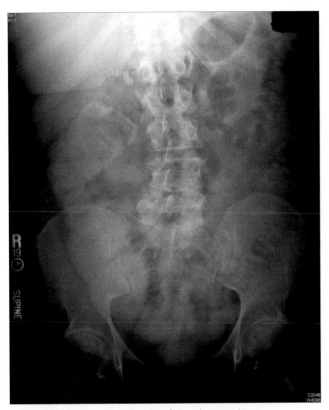

Figure 4.17A1. Renal calculus plain film without markings.

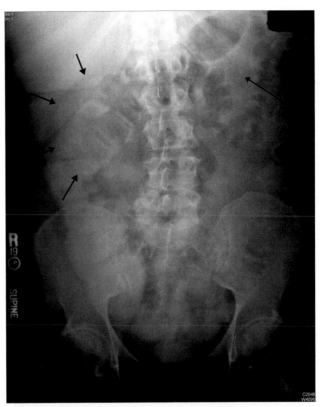

Figure 4.17A2. Renal calculus plain film with markings.

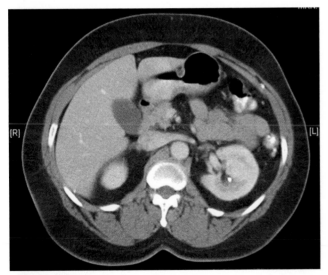

Figure 4.17B1. Renal calculus CT without markings.

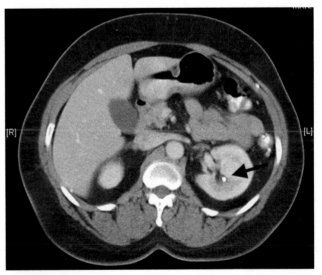

Figure 4.17B2. Renal calculus CT with markings.

stones on plain film, is shown in Figure 4.19C (*arrow*). This stone was not identified with certainty but was confirmed by CT (Fig. 4.19D). The combination of plain film, which reliably identifies larger stones (>5 mm) that are less likely to pass spontaneously, combined with ultrasound to identify hydronephrosis, is only slightly less accurate than CT. This alternative imaging approach is advocated by some as an alternative to CT, since it involves a much lower radiation exposure, the vast majority of small stones pass

spontaneously, and the initial management of all but the largest stones is expectant anyway.

Bladder stone

The rounded opaque structure located in the low pelvis is a bladder stone. This can be differentiated from contrast material in the bladder because there is no enhancement of the kidneys or ureters and the structure is small with well-delineated smooth margins.

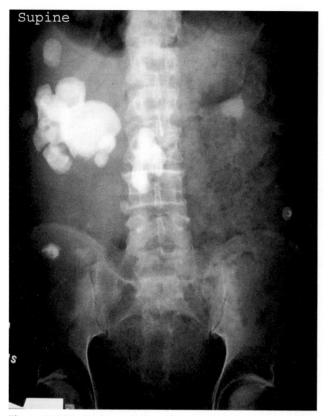

Figure 4.18A1. Staghorn calculus without markings.

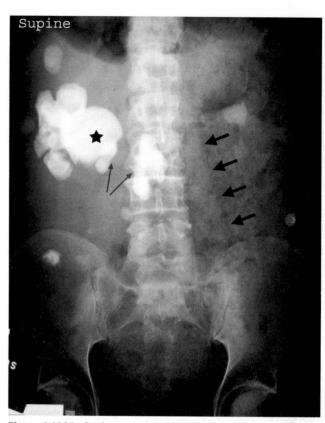

Figure 4.18A2. Staghorn calculus with markings.

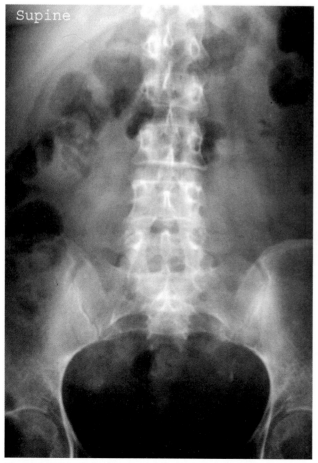

Figure 4.19A1. Ureteral stone plain film without markings.

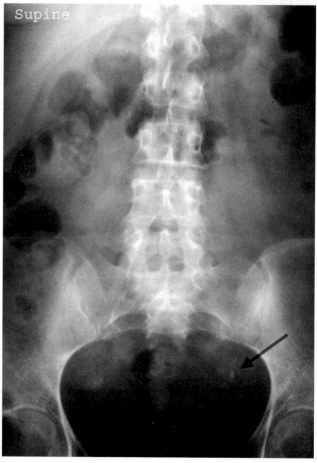

Figure 4.19A2. Ureteral stone plain film with markings.

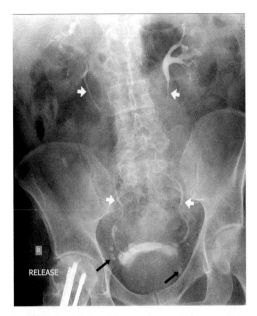

Figure 4.19B. Normal Intravenous pyelogram (IVP) demonstrating contrast in ureters.

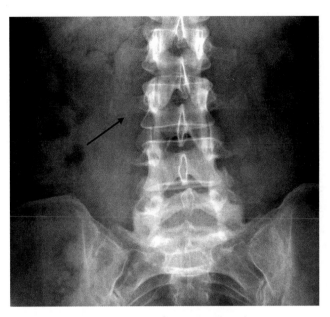

Figure 4.19C. Ureteral stone plain film case 2 with markings.

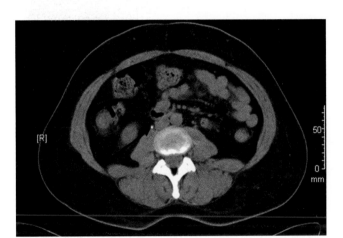

Figure 4.19D. Ureteral stone CT case 2 with markings.

Pancreatic calcifications

This image shows the characteristic stippling of pancreatic calcifications. They extend from the right upper quadrant, across the midline, to the left upper quadrant (*black arrows*). They reflect recurrent episodes of inflammation. The patient's complaints and clinical condition will determine the significance of this finding. See also Figure 4.12.

Porcelain gallbladder

The circular structure in the right upper quadrant is the calcified "shell" of the gallbladder. The close-up shows the presence of fine densities within the gallbladder as well (Fig. 4.22A2, *black circle*). A follow-up study and surgical consultation should be obtained because patients will often require cholecystectomy.

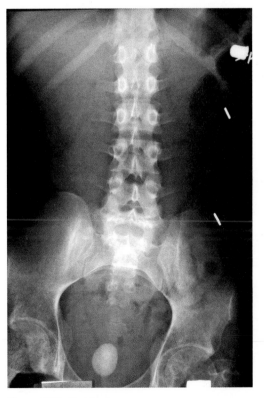

Figure 4.20. Bladder stone.

Vascular calcifications

Figures 4.23A and B show a large splenic artery aneurysm, which was an unexpected finding on the lumbosacral series obtained in a patient complaining of low back pain. The patient's symptoms did not seem to be related to the finding. Atherosclerotic calcifications are frequently seen on

75

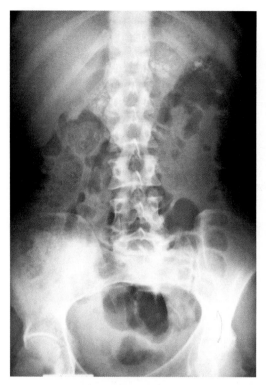

Figure 4.21A1. Pancreatic calcifications without markings.

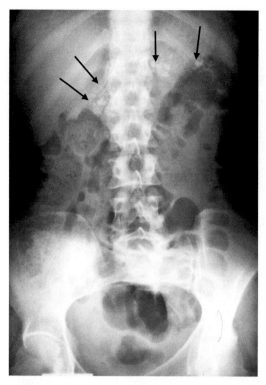

Figure 4.21A2. Pancreatic calcifications with markings.

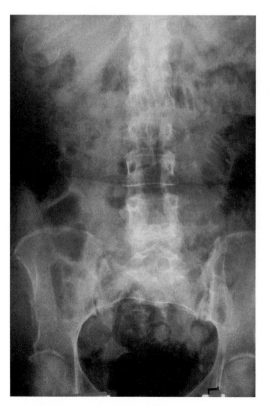

Figure 4.22A1. Porcelain gallbladder.

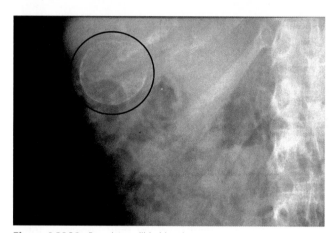

Figure 4.22A2. Porcelain gallbladder close-up.

abdominal films. Figure 4.23C shows the calcifications of a tortuous splenic artery (*white long arrow*) and the (normal) descending thoracic aorta (*white arrowheads*). Figure 4.23D demonstrates the rim-like calcification of a known abdominal aortic aneurysm (*black arrows*).

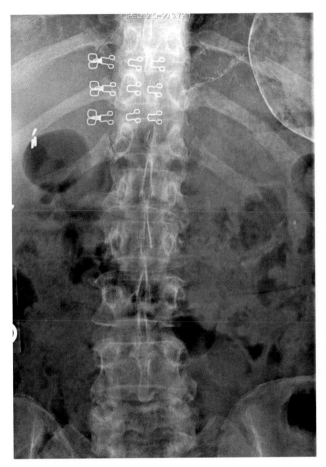

Figure 4.23A. Splenic artery aneurysm.

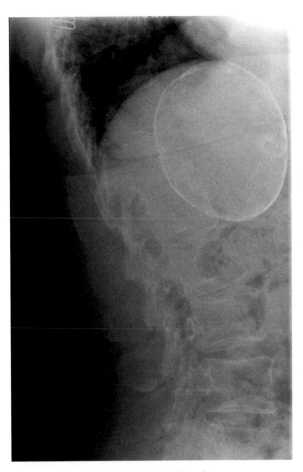

Figure 4.23B. Splenic artery aneurysm lateral view.

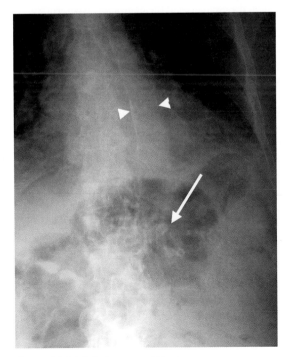

Figure 4.23C. Splenic artery calcifications.

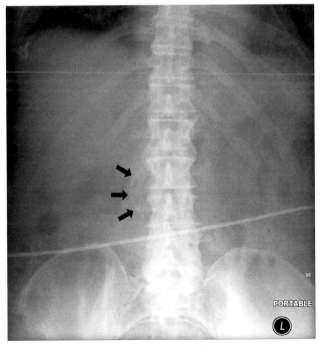

Figure 4.23D. Abdominal aortic aneurysm calcification.

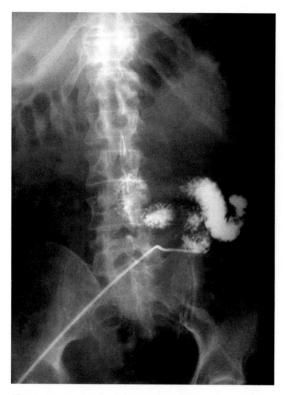

Figure 4.24A. Feeding tube replacement.

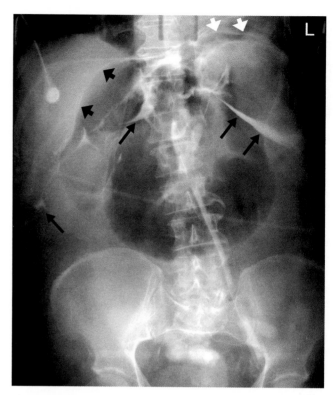

Figure 4.24B. Feeding tube extravasation.

Feeding tube replacement

Emergency physicians are frequently called on to replace feeding tubes. This procedure is usually followed by a contrast exam to confirm placement. Figure 4.24A shows a jejunostomy tube in the appropriate location: the dye can be seen outlining the characteristic multiple small jejunal mucosal folds. A contrast study done on another patient with recent placement of a gastrostomy tube (Fig. 4.24B) demonstrates intraperitoneal extravasation of contrast outside of the stomach (*black arrows*). Contrast is identified outlining the liver (*black arrowheads*). There is also contrast outlining the left hemidiaphragm (*white arrowheads*), with a moderate amount of subphrenic free air. A distended loop of bowel is seen in the mid-abdomen.

References

Ahn SH, Mayo-Smith WW, Murphy BL, et al.: Acute nontraumatic abdominal pain in adult patients: abdominal radiography compared with CT evaluation. *Radiology* 2002;**225**:159–64.

Anyanwu AC, Moalypour SM: Are abdominal radiographs still overutilised in the assessment of acute abdominal pain? A district general hospital audit. *J R Coll Surg Edinb* 1998;**43**:267–70.

Flak B, Rowley A: Acute abdomen: plain film utilization and analysis. *Can Assoc Radiol J* 1993;**44**(6):423–8.

Gupta K, Bhandari RK, Chander R: Comparative study of plain film abdomen and ultrasound in non-traumatic acute abdomen. *Ind J Radiol Imaging* 2005;**15**:109–15.

Kellow ZS, MacInnes M, Kurzencwyg D, et al.: The role of abdominal radiography in the evaluation of the nontrauma emergency patient. *Radiology* 2008;**248**:887–93.

Laméris W, van Randen A, Van Es HW, et al.: Imaging strategies for detection of urgent conditions in patients with acute abdominal pain: diagnostic accuracy study. *British Med J* 2009;**339**(7711):29–33.

MacKersie AB, Lane MJ, Gerhardt RT, et al.: Nontraumatic acute abdominal pain: unenhanced helical CT compared with three-view acute abdominal series. *Radiology* 2005;**237**:114–22.

Otero HJ, Ondategui-Parra S, Erturk SM, et al.: Imaging utilization in the management of appendicitis and its impact on hospital charges. *Emerg Radiol* 2008;**15**:23–8.

Rao PM, Rhea JT, Rao JA, Conn AK: Plain abdominal radiography in clinically suspected appendicitis: diagnostic yield, resource use, and comparison with CT. *Am J Emerg Med* 1999;**17**:325–8.

Stoker J, van Randen A, Lameris W, Boermeester MA: Imaging patients with acute abdominal pain. *Radiology* 2009;**253**(1):31–46.

van Randen A, Lameris W, Luitse, JSK, et al.: The role of plain radiographs in patients with acute abdominal pain at the ED. *Am J Emerg Med* 2011;**29**(6):582–9.

Plain Radiography of the C-spine

Chapter

5

Eric Fox Silman

Overview and capabilities

Cervical spine (C-spine) injury is a rare but important diagnosis in the ED. There are an estimated 11,000 new cases of spinal cord injury in the United States annually, nearly all of which are diagnosed in the ED. C-spine injury is present in 2% to 6% of all blunt trauma patients and may be present in up to one-third of those who present unconscious (1, 2). Because of the potentially devastating consequences of missed C-spine injury, ED providers must remain vigilant in evaluating patients at risk and must be experts in the area of appropriate diagnostic imaging for C-spine trauma.

Most C-spine injuries are the result of blunt trauma from motor vehicle collisions, falls, sports-related injuries, and assault. Decades of biomechanical studies have correlated injury patterns with mechanism of injury, but the details of these studies are beyond the scope of this chapter and will not be discussed. Important to recognize, however, are the regions and patterns of injury within the C-spine. One-third of C-spine fractures occur at C2, and about one-half between C5 and C6 (3). Noncontiguous injuries are common, especially in patients with severe mechanism of injury. In a large retrospective review, Nelson and colleagues found up to a 20% rate of noncontiguous C-spine fractures (4). The same study, and many others, found an increased incidence of C-spine fractures with increasing Injury Severity Score. The "stability" of C-spine fractures refers to the integrity of the spinal column overall following injury and the risk of a spinal cord injury. Stability is dependent on pre-existent conditions (i.e., rheumatoid or osteoarthritis) as well as degree of force and mechanism of injury. The most widely accepted classification of C-spine injury stability was described by Trafton (Table 5.1) (5).

Plain radiography of the C-spine was the traditional screening test of choice in patients with suspected C-spine injury. In recent years, much controversy has emerged regarding plain radiography versus CT scanning. This controversy and its supporting data and practice guidelines will be covered later in this chapter. Still, for certain patients and in many centers without easy access to CT, plain radiography remains the initial screening test of choice.

The standard C-spine radiographic study is a three-view series including anteroposterior (AP), lateral, and open-mouth odontoid views. An adequate AP film should clearly show all vertebrae from C3 to C7. The upper C-spine and occipitoatlantal joint are not reliably imaged on the AP film.

An adequate lateral film should show all levels from the cranium to the cervicothoracic junction, with the C7-T1 articulation of particular importance. In obese or muscular patients, soft tissue often obscures the C7-T1 junction. Downward traction on the arms or a "swimmer's view" with the arms raised may be obtained. The vertebral bodies, interbody spaces, transverse processes, articular masses with interfacet joints, laminae, and spinous processes should all be visible on the lateral view. The spinal ligamentous anatomy is not imaged by plain radiography; however, ligamentous integrity can be evaluated by following the four lines of lordosis on the lateral view. The open-mouth odontoid view should show the articulation of the lateral masses of C1 and C2 and the entire dens.

Flexion-extension (F/E) radiographs (Fig. 5.9) or fluoroscopic studies were traditionally used to reveal ligamentous instability in patients with no fracture on standard three-view radiographic series. Signs of instability on F/E imaging

Table 5.1: Cervical spine injuries and their relative stability (5)

Injury	Stability
Ruptured transverse ligament of C1	Least
Type II odontoid fracture	
Burst fracture with posterior ligamentous disruption (flexion teardrop fracture)	
Bilateral facet dislocation	
Burst fracture without posterior ligamentous disruption	
Hyperextension fracture-dislocation	
Compression fracture of C2 with anterior or posterior displacement (hangman fracture)	
Extension teardrop fracture	
Compression fracture of C1 with lateral displacement (Jefferson fracture)	
Unilateral facet dislocation	
Anterior subluxation	
Simple wedge compression fracture without posterior ligamentous disruption	
Pillar fracture	
Fracture of the posterior arch of C1	
Isolated spinous process fracture not involving the lamina (clay shoveler's fracture)	Most

Table 5.2: Canadian C-spine rule (9)

Any *high-risk* factor mandating radiography?[a]

  Age older than 65 years

  Paresthesias in extremities

  Dangerous mechanism

  Fall from more than 3 feet or five stairs

  Motor vehicle crash (MVC) with combined velocity >100 km/h (62 mph), rollover, or ejection

  Motorized recreational vehicle accident

  Bicycle collision

  Axial load to head (i.e., diving)

Any *low-risk* factor allowing safe assessment of range of motion?[a]

  Simple rear-end MVC

  Sitting position in ED

  Ambulatory at any time

  Delayed onset of midline cervical tenderness

Able to actively rotate head left and right 45 degrees?[a]

[a] Presence of *any* high-risk factor, absence of *all* low-risk factors, or *inability* to rotate head 45 degrees mandates radiography.

Table 5.3: NEXUS low-risk criteria[a] (11)

No midline C-spine tenderness

No evidence of intoxication

Normal level of alertness

No focal neurological deficit

No painful distracting injury

[a] *All* must be true to preclude radiography.

include >3.5 mm of horizontal displacement between adjacent disks, displaced apophyseal joints, widened disk spaces, loss of >30% of disk height, or presence of prevertebral hematoma, as evidenced by abnormal thickness or contour of the prevertebral soft tissues on lateral view (6). MRI has largely replaced F/E imaging to diagnose ligamentous injury, and F/E imaging has not been shown to add significant diagnostic information. F/E studies should *never* be performed on obtunded patients or those who have pain on range of motion. Oblique views allow visualization of intervertebral foraminae but have not been shown to add sensitivity over three-view series and should not be obtained in the ED (7).

Indications

Despite decades of research, there is still controversy regarding the indications for radiologic screening for C-spine injury in blunt trauma patients. In polytrauma patients with suspected multisystem injuries, there is little argument that C-spine imaging is mandatory. In obtunded patients with confirmed or suspected traumatic brain injury, imaging is similarly indicated. The controversy lies in the less-injured patient. Many of these patients have minor mechanisms of injury and can be clinically assessed for the need for radiographs. Most authorities agree that any patient with suspected C-spine injury who cannot be clinically cleared should be imaged. Plain radiographs of the C-spine have been the traditional screening test for fractures and ligamentous injuries. The American College of Radiology (ACR) gives plain radiography in patients who fail clinical clearance an appropriateness level of 6 out of 9, where 4–6 reflects imaging that "may be appropriate," and 7–9 reflects imaging that is "usually appropriate" (8).

Increasing concerns over cost and the risks of malignancy resulting from diagnostic medical radiation led to the development of two major decision instruments to aid clinicians in the decision to image patients at risk for C-spine injury. These rules assist physicians in clinically clearing the C-spine. The Canadian C-spine Rule (CCR) and the NEXUS Low-risk Criteria (NLC) are two decision rules designed to determine the need for C-spine imaging in alert, non-intoxicated patients presenting to the ED with neck injury.

The CCR (Table 5.2) is a three-step decision rule derived and validated in Canada (9). Step one is to assess for any high-risk factor that would immediately mandate imaging. Step two is to assess for any low-risk factor that will allow for active range-of-motion testing. Step three is to test active range of motion by asking patients to actively rotate their necks 45 degrees to both sides. Patients who can rotate their necks, regardless of pain, do not require imaging. In its derivation study, the rule was 100% sensitive and 42.5% specific for clinically important C-spine injuries (9). In addition, the four missed injuries in the study were categorized as not clinically significant. The rule was subsequently validated in a multicenter study that produced similar test characteristics as well as a 100% negative predictive value for clinically important C-spine injury (10).

The NLC proposed five low-risk criteria (Table 5.3), which allow clinical clearance of the cervical spine without radiography when all criteria are absent. The criteria were validated in a prospective study of 34,069 patients, in whom the sensitivity and specificity were 99% and 12.9%, respectively (11). Two of eight patients with missed injuries by the criteria had clinically significant injuries. Importantly, the NEXUS investigators defined a "painful distracting injury" as long bone fractures, visceral injury requiring surgical consultation, large lacerations, crush injuries, and large burns along with any injury that has "the potential to impair the patient's ability to appreciate other injuries."

It is important to note that patients excluded from the studies used to derive and validate the two decision rules included those with direct blows to the neck, those with penetrating trauma, and children under the age of 16 for the CCR. The NEXUS criteria have subsequently been validated in pediatric patients, mostly those older than 8 years old (12).

The two decision rules were compared directly in a prospective study of more than 8,000 patients in 2003 (13). The CCR and NLC showed sensitivities of 99.4% versus 90.7%, respectively. CCR would have missed one injury, whereas NEXUS would have missed 16. In terms of actual reduction in imaging, the CCR would have resulted in a 55.9% imaging rate versus 66.6% for the NLC. Despite these data, there is persistent controversy regarding bias and study design, which preclude conclusions about the superiority of either rule, and they both remain in widespread use. The NEXUS criteria are considered less cumbersome and may be used more widely.

Pitfalls in diagnosis

Pitfalls in the use of plain radiography for C-spine injury include its special issues in pediatric patients, its significant rate of inadequate imaging, and the ongoing controversy over its accuracy in diagnosing C-spine injury compared to CT scanning.

Plain radiography of the C-spine in pediatrics

Cervical spine injury in children is rare and occurs in 1% to 2% of severely traumatized children (14). Children are at increased risk of C-spine injury for several reasons. First, their relatively large head size creates increased forces on the C-spine in all directions during trauma. Their underdeveloped musculature offers less protection against injury, and the relatively horizontal orientation of their facet joints offer less resistance against translating forces. In addition, their incompletely ossified vertebrae and elastic intervertebral discs allow for more mobility and less resistance to deforming forces. Several congenital syndromes place children at higher risk of C-spine injury, the most common of which is Down's syndrome, which can results in atlanto-axial instability in up to 20% of patients.

Because children's tissues are more radiosensitive and relative doses of any radiologic study are higher than in adults, more thoughtful use of screening radiologic studies in children should be exercised. For this reason, clinical clearance should be attempted when appropriate.

The NEXUS criteria have been prospectively validated in a large study of more than 3,000 children, though few of these patients were younger than 8 years old (12). Thus, the NLC may be used to clear the C-spine of older children as it is used for adults. This statement is supported by the ACR in its latest appropriateness criteria (8). In a multicenter observational trial of more than 12,000 children younger than 3 years old, a separate clinical decision rule showed a negative predictive value of nearly 100% for children with a normal mental status

who were not involved in a motor vehicle collision (15). Taken together, these data suggest that radiographic evaluation is rarely indicated in children with normal mental status with an age-appropriate neurologic examination and a low-risk mechanism of injury, regardless of age.

There is little agreement by authorities in pediatrics, trauma, and radiology as to when CT should supplant plain radiography as the initial screening test in children. Therefore, in those children where radiographic evaluation is deemed necessary, the standard three-view C-spine series should be the starting point in all low-risk patients. Those with obvious polytrauma who are undergoing multiple other CT scans may be candidates for initial CT screening.

The final consideration in pediatric C-spine trauma is spinal cord injury without radiographic abnormality (SCIWORA). Initially described before the advent of MRI, SCIWORA was defined as objective signs of spinal cord injury in the presence of normal plain radiographs or CT (16). For all the reasons described above, the pediatric C-spine is more prone to soft tissue disruption, which can cause spinal cord injury in the absence of fracture. In more recent reports, MRI shows injury to soft tissue or spinal cord in up to two-thirds of cases (17, 18). Thus, many authorities recommend physicians abandon the term SCIWORA. Regardless of the term, in any child in whom pain radiographs or CT scans are normal and neurologic signs persist, MRI should be pursued.

Issues with inadequate imaging

A major pitfall of plain radiographs in patients with suspected C-spine injury is the risk of a missed injury. The most common reason for missed injury is inadequacy of the images due to a combination of radiographic technique and patient anatomic factors such as presence of a cervical collar, obesity, or decreased range of motion in the setting of pain or muscle spasm (19). Up to 72% of plain radiographs may provide inadequate imaging of the C-spine (20). In addition, plain films tend to miss fractures in certain areas such as the occiput to C3 and C6 to C7, which are often suboptimally visualized but are also common areas for fractures (21). Though the fractures missed by plain radiography tend to be those that do not require specific interventions (9, 11), there is still controversy that outcomes may suffer. However, there is less data to support this argument.

Controversy of plain radiographs versus CT

Major controversy remains as to whether plain radiography is adequately sensitive to be used as the primary screening modality for C-spine injury. Though the NEXUS study found that plain radiography failed to diagnose C-spine injury in 0.07% of all patients and 0.008% of those with unstable injuries (11), several subsequent controlled trials showed significantly better test characteristics for CT as the initial screening test. An often-cited meta-analysis of these trials showed a pooled sensitivity of 52% for plain radiography versus 98% for CT (22). The studies included in this review were significantly heterogenous and, in many cases, included only ICU admissions, patients with altered mental status, and on average a very ill cohort. This highlights the difference in study populations between the large plain radiography trials, which tend to enroll "all comers" to the ED with overall lower risk, compared with the trauma surgery studies, whose subjects tend to be more injured. Other reasoning for the move from plain radiography to CT-based screening includes increased efficiency and cost-effectiveness, both of which have been shown in various studies (23).

In the face of increasing data supporting CT-based screening for C-spine injury, the major trauma surgery authorities have moved to recommending CT as the initial screening test in blunt trauma patients. Citing increased sensitivity and cost-effectiveness, the Eastern Association for the Surgery of Trauma (EAST) practice-management guidelines as well as the Advanced Trauma Life Support (ATLS) guidelines have been updated in the past 5 years to recommend CT-based screening (24, 25).

Despite conflicting data and changing recommendations, it is clear that a risk-stratification tool is needed to determine the need for plain radiography versus CT screening for C-spine injuries. At some level of risk, CT may in fact be more sensitive and cost-effective. One group has attempted to define this level and has derived and internally validated a decision rule for determining which blunt trauma patients can be screened with plain radiography and which need CT. The Harborview Criteria (Table 5.4) were shown to identify patients at high (>5%) risk of cervical spine injury in whom CT-based screening is warranted (26). Using the six mechanistic and clinical criteria resulted in stratification of 14% of patients as high risk, in whom CT showed C-spine injury in 8.7%. The remaining 86% of patients were screened with the standard three-view C-spine radiography series, and only 0.2% had an injury. This study included several patients transferred to the trauma center with known fractures and has not been externally validated. Nonetheless, these data suggest that some degree of risk stratification may be useful in determining which of those patients who cannot be clinically cleared need plain radiography versus CT as their initial screening test.

Despite the ongoing controversy regarding cervical spine clearance and imaging, it is clear that the goals of every screening protocol should be to diagnose significant C-spine injury with accuracy while balancing cost-effectiveness and radiation dose. What is needed is a universal algorithm for cervical spine imaging in adult blunt trauma patients that risk-stratifies patients, provides a route to clinical clearance, and includes plain radiography screening for low-risk patients and CT screening for higher-risk patients. Such an algorithm has been proposed in several forms and is shown in Figure 5.1.

Clinical images

Table 5.4: Harborview criteria for patients at high (>5%) risk of cervical spine injury (26)

Injury

1. High-energy mechanism

    High speed (>35 mph) motor vehicle or motorcycle collision

    Motor vehicle collision with death at the scene

    Fall from height >10 feet

2. High-risk clinical parameter

    Significant head injury, including intracranial hemorrhage or persistent unconsciousness in the ED

    Neurologic signs or symptoms referable to the cervical spine

    Pelvic or multiple extremity fractures

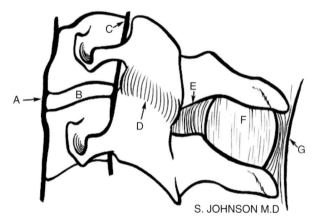

S. JOHNSON M.D

Figure 5.1. Suggested algorithm for cervical spine imaging in the emergency department.

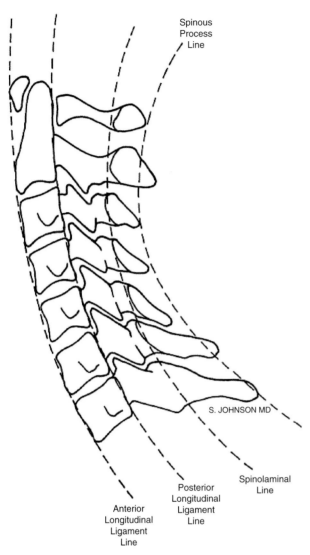

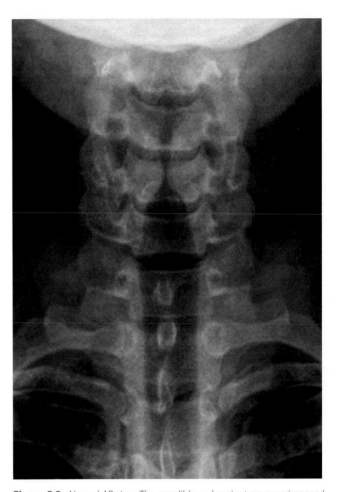

Figure 5.2. The four lines of lordosis. The anterior longitudinal ligament line, the posterior longitudinal ligament line, the spinolaminar line, and the posterior spinous line are each smooth and lordotic without disruption or angulation. Disruption of these imaginary lines should raise suspicion for ligamentous or bony injury.

Figure 5.3. Normal AP view. The mandible and occiput are superimposed over the first two cervical vertebrae; thus, an adequate film should clearly show the vertebral column from C3 to T1. There should be vertical and rotational symmetry of vertebral bodies, lateral masses, and spinous processes. Interbody and interspinous distance should be constant. Articular surfaces should be parallel to each other. "Step-offs" may indicate fractures, and isolated widened disc spaces can signify ligamentous disruption. Pathological rotation of cervical vertebrae, as in unilateral interfacetal dislocation, may manifest as deviation of spinous processes from normal vertical alignment. The trachea appears as a radiolucent air column that should lie in the midline.

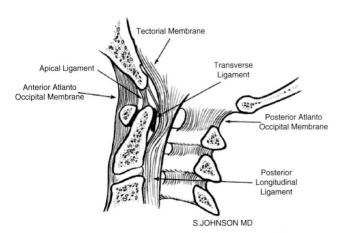

Figure 5.4. Ligamentous anatomy of the cervicocranium. The transverse atlantoaxial ligament, the alar ligaments, and the cruciate ligament stabilize the cervicocranial junction. The anterior longitudinal ligament arises from the tectorial membrane intracranially.

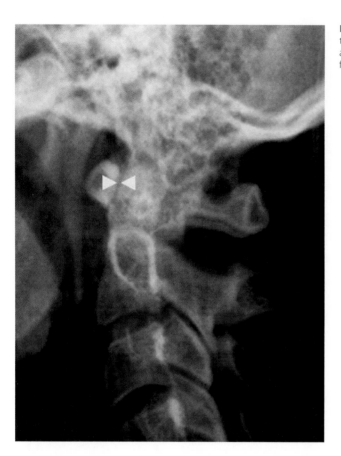

Figure 5.5. Normal atlantodens interval. The atlantodens interval is normally less than 3 mm in adults (small arrows). An atlantodens interval greater than 3 mm in adults or 5 mm in children suggests ligamentous injury or, more commonly, fracture of the arch of the atlas.

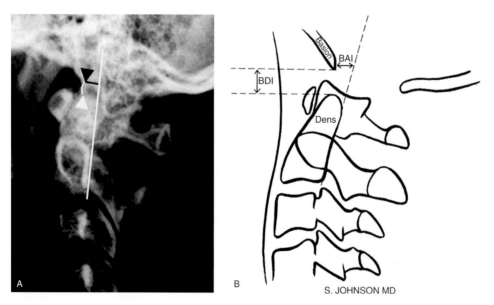

Figure 5.6. Normal occipitoatlantal (cervicocranial) articulation. A: The normal occipitoatlantal articulation. Both the basion-dental interval (BDI) and the basion-axial interval (BAI) assess the integrity of the cervicocranial junction; values of greater than 12 mm signify occipitoatlantal dissociation. The BDI (white bracket) is measured vertically from the basion to the tip of the dens. The BAI (*solid black line*) is measured from the basion horizontally to a line drawn vertically along the posterior cortex of the axis (*solid white line*).

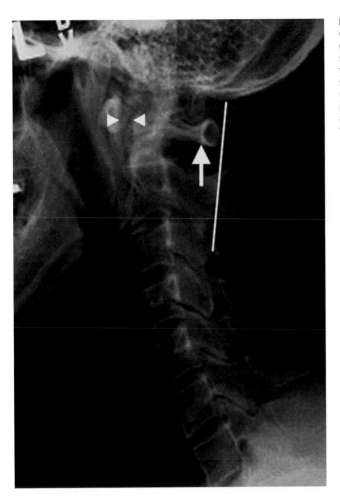

Figure 5.7. Atlantoaxial subluxation. Atlantoaxial subluxation most often results when C1 translates anteriorly on C2 due to an uncertain MOI with or without underlying degenerative pathology. The radiographic signs of atlantoaxial subluxation are a widened atlantodens interval (*small arrowheads*), usually greater than 3 mm in adults, and a posterior atlas arch that lies anterior to the spinolaminar line (*large arrow* and *solid line*). This condition is associated with rheumatoid arthritis, Down syndrome, Morquio syndrome, and Grisel syndrome in pediatric patients. This patient was diagnosed with ankylosing spondylitis shortly after this radiograph was obtained; note the "squared-off" appearance of the vertebral bodies.

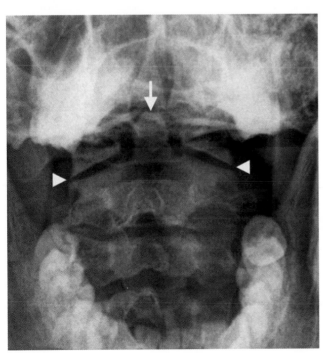

Figure 5.8. Normal open-mouth odontoid view. The dens and articulating surfaces of the lateral masses of C1 and C2 can be seen in their entirety. The dens should be equidistant from either arch of C1 and vertically aligned with the C2 spinous process. The lateral masses of C1 and C2 should articulate with less than 2 mm of lateral override (*small arrows*). It is important to note that two common masqueraders of odontoid fracture are failure of ossification of the base of the dens leading to persistent infantile odontoid and the radiographic shadow cast across the dens by either the occiput or the maxillary teeth.

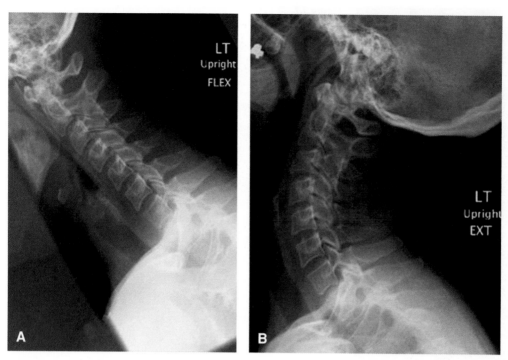

Figure 5.9. Normal flexion and extension view. The cervical spine is visualized from the occiput to C7; the anterior and posterior ligamentous lines are intact, as are the interbody distances; and there is no subluxation. Note that the smooth lordosis of the cervical spine is reduced or absent in flexion and exaggerated in extension. These views are useful in identifying anterior or posterior ligamentous injury, with resultant instability of the cervical vertebrae in extension and flexion, respectively. Inappropriate increases in the vertical distance between spinous processes or vertebral bodies can indicate the presence of anterior or posterior subluxation.

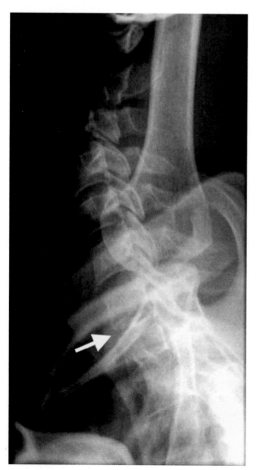

Figure 5.10. Normal Swimmer's view. If the standard lateral radiograph does not clearly show the entire cervical spine down to the C7-T1 junction and downward traction on the arms to lower the shoulders is either insufficient or contraindicated, the arm closest to the film may be raised and a Swimmer's view obtained. The adequate Swimmer's view reveals the C7-T1 junction (*arrow*), albeit often overlapping with the soft tissue and bones of the shoulder. Note the incidental appearance of a calcified annulus fibrosus (*arrowhead*) at the C6-C7 level; these can mimic avulsion fractures.

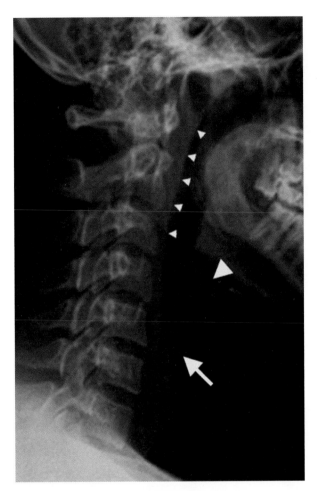

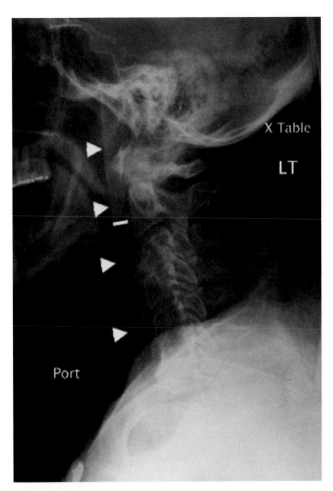

Figure 5.11. Normal prevertebral soft tissue. This lateral radiograph shows the normal width and contour of the prevertebral soft tissues (*small arrowheads*). The width of the prevertebral soft tissue should not exceed 6 mm anterior to the body of C2. Bulging or diffuse thickening is due to edema or hematoma and may signal underlying injury in an otherwise normal radiograph. Also seen in this view are the hyoid bone (*large arrowhead*) and epiglottis (*large arrow*).

Figure 5.12. Prevertebral soft tissue swelling. Prevertebral soft tissue swelling in conjunction with a fracture of the anterior arch of C1 is shown. Note the presence of a widened prevertebral space (*white line*) and the loss of the normal contour (*small arrowheads*). The thickness on lateral view should be no more than 6 mm at C2 and 22 mm at C6. Greater thickness is very specific but not adequately sensitive to identify a high percentage of occult fractures. Thus, a widened prevertebral soft tissue should raise the index suspicion of occult injury and mandate further imaging. The most common injuries associated with abnormal prevertebral soft tissue contour are occipitoatlantal dissociation, occipital condyle fracture, Jefferson burst fracture, odontoid fractures, C1 arch fracture, and traumatic rupture of the transverse atlantoaxial ligament.

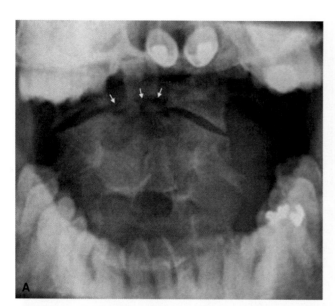
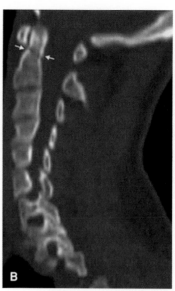

Figure 5.13. Type II odontoid fracture. The fracture line (small arrowheads) is present at the junction of the base of the odontoid process and the ring of C2, visible on plain film odontoid view (A) and CT (B). Type II fractures are the most common odontoid fracture and carry a 30% to 50% incidence of nonunion. Odontoid fractures result from diverse mechanisms of injury but require significant force. Type I fractures are uncommon and occur when the tip of the dens is avulsed at the insertion of the alar ligament. This fracture is stable. Type II and III fractures occur at the base of the dens and through the anterior axis body inferior to the dens, respectively. These fractures are unstable and can be associated with neurological deficits up to 10% of the time.

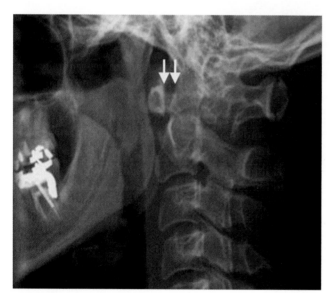

Figure 5.14. Increased atlantodens interval (ADI). The width of the predental space or ADI is normally less than 3 mm in adults and 5 mm in children. The ADI is determined by the stability of the dens in the anterior arch of the atlas, which is determined mostly by the integrity of the transverse ligament. Ligamentous injury is seen with hyperflexion, extreme lateral flexion, or vertical compression. Rupture of the transverse ligament is often seen with concomitant fracture, but in the absence of bony trauma, the ADI is the only indication of disruption. It should be noted that in patients with rheumatoid arthritis, the ADI may be pathologically widened.

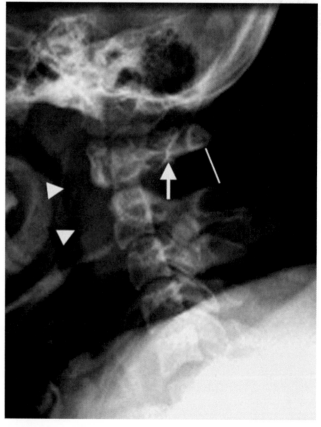

Figure 5.15. Isolated fracture of ring of C1. Isolated fracture of the C1 ring on the left side (*arrow*). Note the superior displacement of the vertebral ring, leading to an increased interspinous distance (*solid line*). There is also significant prevertebral soft tissue swelling and loss of contour (*arrowheads*).

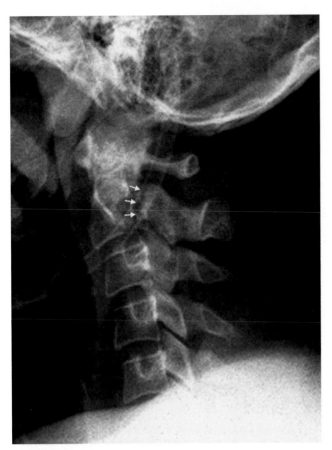

Figure 5.16. Traumatic spondylolisthesis of C2 (Hangman's fracture). Bilateral fracture of the pars interarticularis (not the "pedicles," which are poorly defined in the axis) of C2 results from extreme hyperextension, usually associated with MVC. Despite the relatively greater width of the spinal canal at this level, the Hangman's fracture is considered unstable because it is often associated with C2-C3 disc injury or C2-C3 interfacetal dislocation and resultant anterolisthesis.

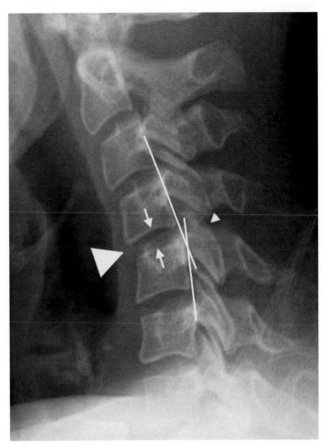

Figure 5.17. Anterior subluxation (AS). AS of "hyperflexion sprain" is a disruption of the posterior ligamentous complex resulting from hyperflexion, as in the flexion component of the "whiplash" injury associated with rapid deceleration in MVC. Although classic isolated AS is a purely ligamentous injury, AS can also be associated with facet joint dislocation, fractures, and spinal cord compression. Radiographically, AS presents as hyperkyphotic angulation (*solid lines*) at the level of injury, posterior "fanning" of the spinous processes, and anterior disc space narrowing in conjunction with posterior disc space widening (small arrows show overall disc space widening in this case). Variable amounts of facet joint displacement may be seen in more extensive cases. Anterior translation is usually less than 3 mm (*large arrowhead*), distinguishing pure AS from bilateral interfacetal dislocation, which presents as 50% or greater anterior translation of the vertebral body. In fact, subluxation (seen radiographically as incongruity of subjacent facets) is more common than frank dislocation.

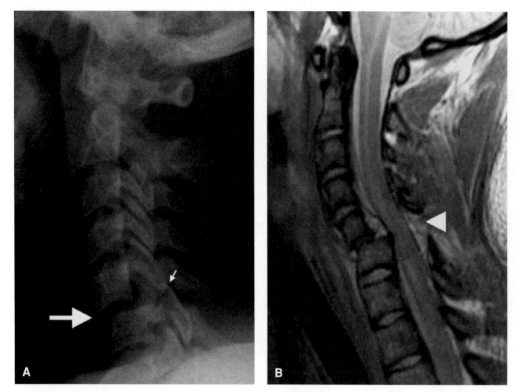

Figure 5.18. Anterior subluxation (AS) with perched facets. When flexion forces are significant, disruption of the posterior ligamentous complex can be accompanied by incomplete dislocation of the interfacetal joint leading to "perching" of the facets. A: Note AS of C5 on C6 with less than 50% overlap of vertebral bodies (*large arrow*) coupled with perching of the left articular facet (*small arrow*). B: MRI of the same patient, illustrating the potential for spinal cord injury when AS is coupled with facet joint dissociation. Note the complete disruption of the posterior ligamentous complex (*large arrowhead*).

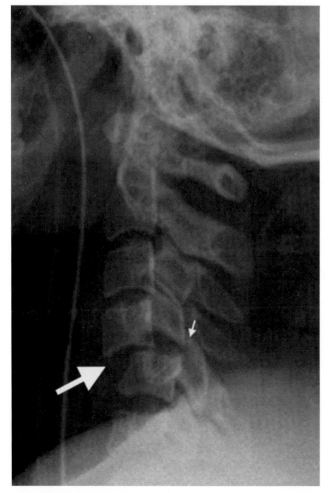

Figure 5.19. Bilateral interfacetal dislocation. Bilateral interfacetal dis- location occurs when extreme hyperflexion disrupts the entire posterior ligamentous complex. On lateral view, the superior facets come to rest anterior to their subjacent counterparts (referred to as "locked facets," *small arrow*), the superior vertebral body is subluxed anteriorly to an extent equal to or greater than 50% of its width (*large arrow*), and both soft tissue and bone are unstable. MRI is indicated to determine the degree of spinal canal encroachment and/or cord damage.

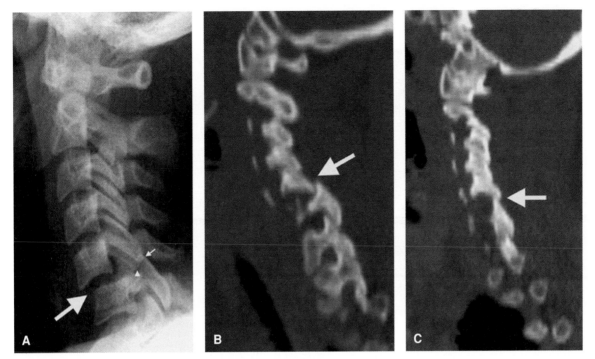

Figure 5.20. Anterior subluxation (AS) with perched and locked facets. This film shows AS of C5 on C6 with both perched and locket facets. A: AS of less than 50% vertebral body width is evident (*large arrow*), along with a perched left facet (*small arrow*) and locked right facet (*small arrowhead*). B and C: The reconstructed CT scans show the locked right facets and perched left facets, respectively.

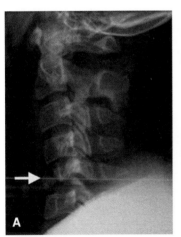

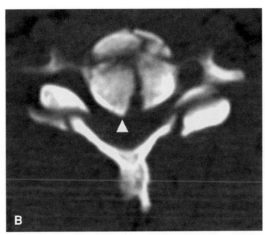

Figure 5.21. Burst fracture. A: Burst fracture of C5 on plain radiography (*large arrow*). Burst fractures result from an axial compressive force, usually a blow to the top of the head, and are characterized by lateral or AP displacement of fracture fragments (*arrowheads*) that may compress the spinal canal (B and C, showing CT and MRI of the same patient). Easily confused with simple wedge fractures due to the loss of vertebral height, burst fractures commonly have a vertical fracture line extending through the complete height of the vertebral body. These fractures are unstable.

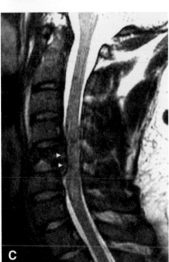

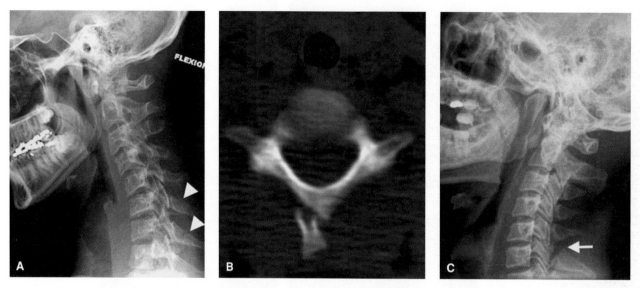

Figure 5.22. Clay shoveler's fracture. Clay shoveler's fracture of C6 and C7 (A, arrowheads) and C6 (B, *arrow*). C: CT of the patient in (B) showing the benign nature of the mildly displaced fractured spinous process. This simple avulsion fracture of the spinous process of a cervical vertebra occurs when the neck is forcefully flexed against the tensed posterior ligaments, a MOI often seen in football players and powerlifters. It occurs most often in C6 and C7 and is considered stable.

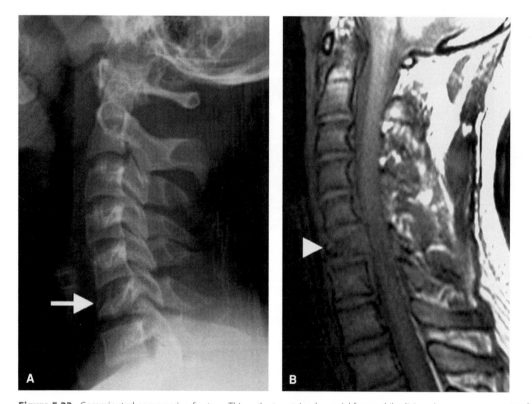

Figure 5.23. Comminuted compression fracture. This patient sustained an axial force while diving. A severe compression fracture of C6 (A), with greater than 70% loss of vertebral height anteriorly and retropulsion of fragments compressing the spinal cord (B). This patient exhibited a central cord syndrome.

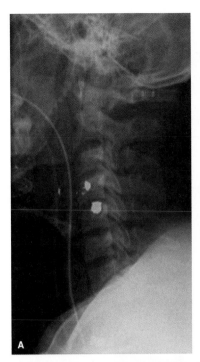

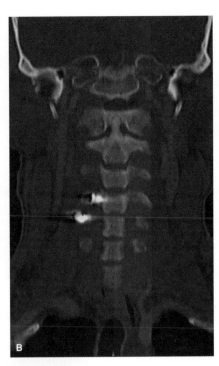

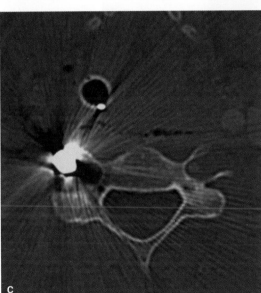

Figure 5.24. Gunshot wound to the neck. Plain films are helpful for initial localization of retained missile fragments, but CT provides more information about localization and involvement of bony and soft tissues. In this case, multiple bullet fragments are noted near C4 and C5 (A), but on CT (B and C) a large fragment is seen near the right transverse foramen of C5, dangerously close to the vertebral artery. Emphysema is noted in the soft tissues, a hallmark finding in cases of penetrating trauma.

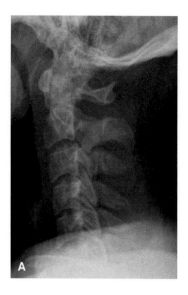

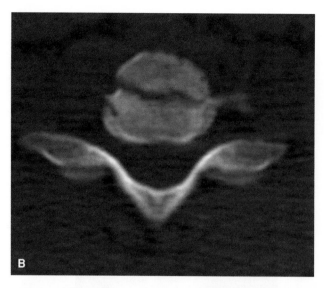

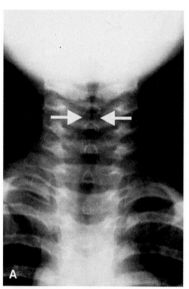

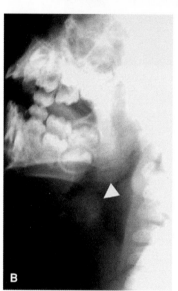

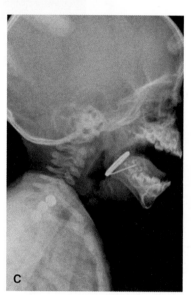

Figure 5.25. Importance of adequate films. A: An apparently normal lateral cervical radiograph. The cervical spine is well visualized only to the level of C5. CT reveals a significant fracture through the body of C6. This reinforces the concept of the necessity and utility of adequate views when performing C-spine radiography as well as the utility of CT for visualizing the entire cervical spine.

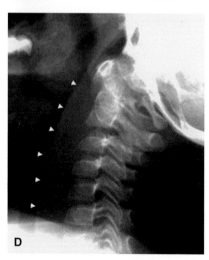

Figure 5.26. Use of plain radiography in nontraumatic conditions. Soft tissue radiography can be useful in identifying nontraumatic conditions in the neck, usually involving the airway and surrounding soft tissues. A: AP neck radiographs in croup display characteristic subglottic narrowing (large arrows), commonly referred to as "steeple sign." C: Epiglottitis produces an enlarged, edematous epiglottis (*large arrowhead*) visible on lateral radiographs. A radiopaque ingested foreign body at the level of the hypopharynx is clearly demonstrated on lateral views in (C). D: Markedly increased width of the prevertebral soft tissues (small arrowheads) on lateral radiograph in a patient with retropharyngeal abscess. Images courtesy of Dr. Kenneth Kwon.

References

1. Grossman MD, Reilly PM, Gillett T, et al.: National survey of the incidence of C-spine injury and approach to C-spine clearance in U.S. trauma centers. *J Trauma* 1999;**47**:684–91.

2. Greenbaum J, Walters N, Levy PD: An evidence-based approach to radiographic assessment of cervical spine injuries in the emergency department. *J Emerg Med* 2008;**68**(1):72–87.

3. Daffner RH, Sciulli RL, Rodriguez A, Protetch J: Imaging for evaluation of suspected C-spine trauma: a 2-year analysis. *Injury* 2006;**37**:652–8.

4. Nelson DW, Martin MJ, Martin ND, Beekley A: Evaluation of the risk of noncontiguous fractures of the spine in blunt trauma. *J Trauma Acute Care Surg* 2013;**75**(1):135–9.

5. Trafton PG: Spinal cord injuries. *Surg Clin North Am* 1982;**62**:61–72.

6. Bagley LJ: Imaging of spinal trauma. *Radiol Clin North Am* 2006;**44**:1–12.

7. Freemyer B, Knopp R, Piche J, et al.: Comparison of five-view and three-view C-spine series in the evaluation of patients with cervical trauma. *Ann Emerg Med* 1989;**18**(8):818–21.

8. American College of Radiology (ACR) Expert Panel on Musculoskeletal Imaging: *Suspected cervical spine trauma.* Reston, VA: ACR, 2012.

9. Stiell IG, Wells GA, Vandemheen KL, et al.: The Canadian C-spine Rule for radiography in alert and stable trauma patients. *JAMA* 2001;**286**(15):1841–8.

10. Stiell IG, Clement CM, Grimshaw J, et al.: Implementation of the Canadian C-spine Rule: prospective 12 centre cluster randomised trial. *BMJ* 2009;**339**:b41–6.

11. Hoffman JR, Mower WR, Wolfson AB, et al.: Validity of a set of clinical criteria to rule out injury to the cervical spine in patients with blunt trauma. National Emergency X-Radiography Utilization Study Group. *N Engl J Med* 2000;**343**(2):94–9.

12. Viccellio P, Simon H, Pressman BD, et al.: NEXUS group: a prospective multicenter study of cervical spine injury in children. *Pediatrics* 2001;**108**(2):E20.

13. Stiell IG, Clement CM, McKnight RD, et al.: The Canadian C-spine Rule versus the NEXUS Low-risk Criteria in patients with trauma. *N Engl J Med* 2003;**349**(26):2510–8.

14. Patel JC, Tepas JJ, Mollitt DL, Pieper P: Pediatric cervical spine injuries: defining the disease. *J Pediatr Surg* 2001;**36**(2):373.

15. Pieretti-Vanmarcke R, Velmahos GC, Nance ML, et al.: Clinical clearance of the cervical spine in blunt trauma patients younger than 3 years: a multi-center study of the American Association for the Surgery of Trauma. *J Trauma* 2009;**67**(3):543–9; discussion 549–50.

16. Pang D, Wilberger JE: Spinal cord injury without radiographic abnormalities in children. *J Neurosurg* 1982;**57**(1):114–29.

17. Yucesoy K, Yuksel KZ: SCIWORA in MRI era. *Clin Neurol Neurosurg* 2008;**110**(5):429.

18. Pang D: Spinal cord injury without radiographic abnormality in children, 2 decades later [review]. *Neurosurgery* 2004;**55**(6): 1325–42; discussion 1342–3.

19. Davis JW, Phreaner DL, Hoyt DB, Mackersie RC: The etiology of missed cervical spine injuries. *J Trauma* 1993;**34**(3):342–6.

20. Gale SC, Gracias VH, Reilly PM, Schwab CW: The inefficiency of plain radiography to evaluate the cervical spine after blunt trauma. *J Trauma* 2005; **59**:1121–5.

21. Woodring JH, Lee C: Limitations of cervical radiography in the evaluation of acute cervical trauma. *J Trauma* 1993;**34**:32–9.

22. Holmes JF, Akkinepalli R: Computed tomography versus plain radiography to screen for cervical spine injury: a meta-analysis. *J Trauma* 2005;**58**:902.

23. Blackmore CC, Ramsey SD, Mann FA, Deyo RA: Cervical spine screening with CT in trauma patients: a cost-effectiveness analysis. *Radiology* 1999;**212**:117–25.

24. Como J, Diaz J, Dunham C, et al.: Practice management guidelines for identifying cervical spine injuries following trauma: update from the Eastern Association for the Surgery of Trauma Practice Management Guidelines Committee. *J Trauma* 2009;**67**:651–9.

25. American College of Surgeons: *Advanced trauma life support student course manual*, 9th ed., 2012.

26. Hanson JA, Blackmore CC, Mann FA, Wilson, AJ: Cervical spine injury: a clinical decision rule to identify high-risk patients for helical CT screening. *Am J Roentgenol* 2000;**174**: 713–18.

Thoracic and Lumbar Spine

Olusola Balogun, Natalie Kmetuk, and Christine Kulstad

Radiographic evaluation of the pelvis and spine often begins with plain radiographs, most commonly ordered after a traumatic injury. Because of the limitations of plain films in these areas, discussed in more detail below, additional studies may be required. CT is performed to further delineate an injury noted on the radiograph or in cases where a high diagnostic concern exists. MRI may be necessary, especially in the thoracolumbar spine, to assess intervertebral disks, spinal nerves, and the spinal cord. Angiography can be a crucial study with severe fractures of the pelvis for the diagnosis and treatment of vascular injuries. Radiography of the thoracic and lumbar spine will be discussed separately from that of the pelvis.

Spine

Indications

Imaging of the thoracolumbar spine is often ordered after injury. Patients with pain or tenderness over the spine, high-risk injury mechanisms, known cervical spine fractures, palpable midline steps, and unreliable exams should be imaged (1, 2). Injury occurs less commonly in the thoracic spine because of its immobility and additional stability provided by the rib cage. Most fractures occur at the junction of the thoracic and lumbar spine.

Patients with nontraumatic back pain do not routinely need radiographs. Indications for plain films in these patients include those who have the acute onset of back pain and have major risk factors for cancer; spinal infection; or neurological deficits that are severe, progressive, or consistent with cauda equina syndrome (1). However, MRI is a better initial study in patients with neurological deficits or suspected infection.

Basic radiographs consist of an anteroposterior (AP) and a lateral view. Additional oblique views may be added to better visualize the neural foramina and facet joints. The beam can be centered at the thoracolumbar or lumbosacral junction to provide better visualization of these areas. The upper thoracic spine is difficult to evaluate on a lateral view because of the overlying shoulders, and a slightly rotated or a swimmer's view may be needed to visualize this area.

Diagnostic capabilities

Thoracolumbar radiology is capable of diagnosing fractures of the vertebral bodies, such as burst or compression fractures usually due to axial loading, or transverse fractures due to distraction injuries. More severe vertebral body fractures may extend into the posterior elements – pedicles, spinous processes, or lamina. Isolated fractures of the transverse processes can occur and have limited clinical significance except as a marker to evaluate for other significant injuries. Compression-burst fractures frequently have retropulsed fragments requiring CT or MRI for evaluation of spinal cord compromise. Ligamentous injuries can be identified by widening or rotation of the spinous processes or by dislocation of one vertebral body relative to another. Osteomyelitis, tumors, and Paget's disease can be visualized on plain radiography of the thoracolumbar spine.

Imaging pitfalls and limitations

In the thoracolumbar spine, a burst fracture may be mistaken for a less serious compression fracture (3, 4). Transverse and spinous process fractures can be hidden by overlying bowel gas or stool. A localized bulging of the paraspinal line should be recognized as an indication of a likely fracture of the thoracic spine with resulting hematoma. Computed tomography of the abdomen and pelvis, performed on many trauma patients, may be more accurate in diagnosing injuries of the thoracolumbar spine (5, 6). Fractures involving two of the three columns (anterior, middle, and posterior) of the thoracolumbar spine must be recognized as unstable.

Clinical images

On lateral projections, trace the alignment of the anterior and posterior borders of the vertebral bodies and the facet joints. These should form a smooth line. Trace the alignment of the superior and inferior borders of each vertebral body, checking for irregularities. Neighboring vertebral bodies should be the same height, and each body is roughly rectangular, not wedge shaped.

On an AP projection, vertebral bodies should gradually become taller and wider. Superior and inferior borders are smooth and clearly defined. Lateral borders have a smooth concave border. The normal paravertebral soft tissue line should be symmetric on either side of the spine and form a straight line. The distance between pedicles and spinous processes gradually increases throughout the lumbar spine. Alignment of vertebral bodies and spinous processes should be checked. The outline of transverse processes in the lumbar spine should be smooth.

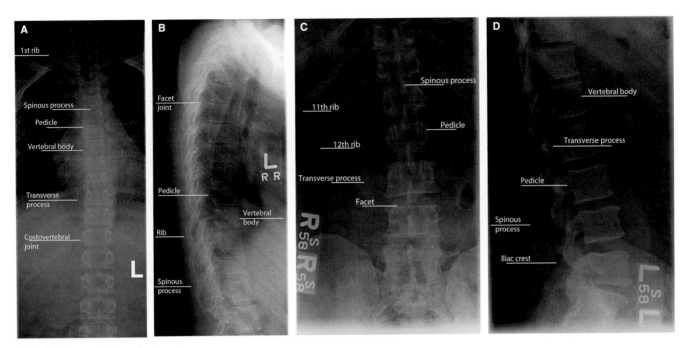

Figure 6.1. Normal thoracolumbar spine.
a. AP thoracic spine
b. Lateral thoracic spine
c. AP lumbar spine
d. Lateral lumbar spine

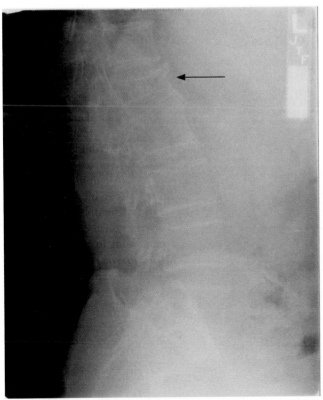

Figure 6.2. L1 compression fracture in patient with low back pain, lateral view. Note the decreased height of vertebral body.

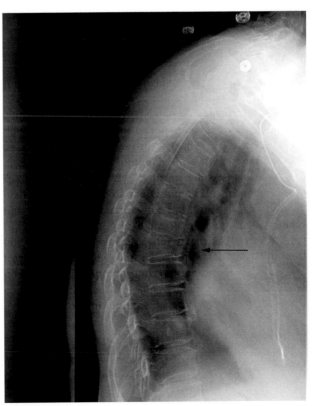

Figure 6.3. T8 compression/wedge fracture, lateral view.

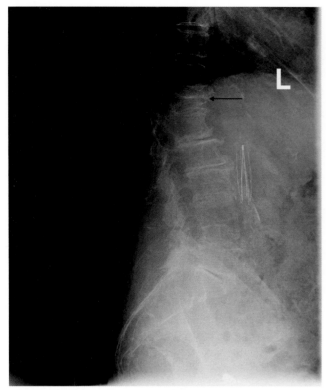

Figure 6.4. T12 compression/wedge fracture, lateral view. Note vertebral body has lost height anteriorly. Also note incidental finding of IVC filter.

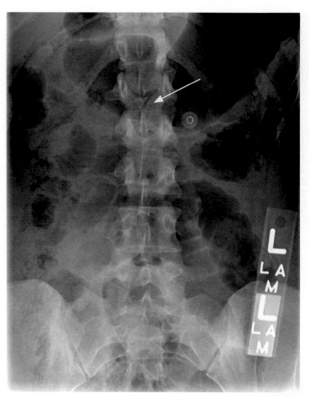

Figure 6.5. L1 superior end plate fracture after a fall from a second-story window, AP view.

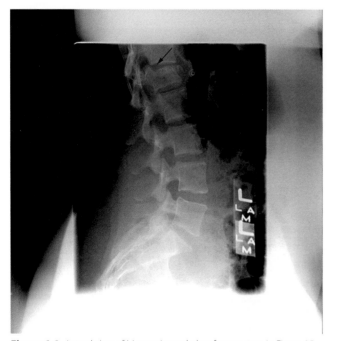

Figure 6.6. Lateral view of L1 superior end plate fracture seen in Figure 6.5.

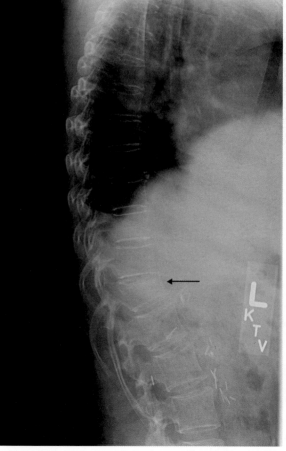

Figure 6.7. T12 superior end plate fracture after a fall, lateral view.

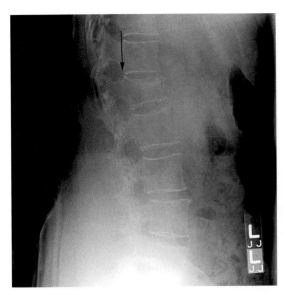

Figure 6.8. L1 fracture with retropulsion after a fall, lateral view.

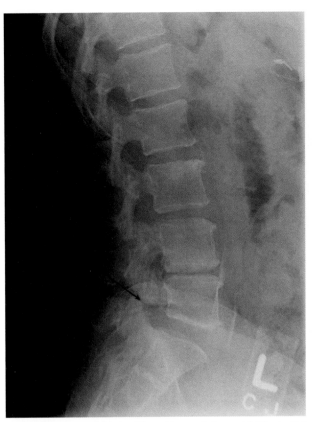

Figure 6.9. L5 spondylolysis with resulting grade 1 spondylolithesis of L5 on S1 after MVC, lateral view.

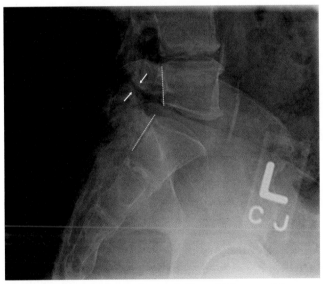

Figure 6.10. Magnified view of patient in Figure 6.9. Fracture of the posterior element of L5 has occurred (*arrows*). Discontinuity of posterior element of L5 allows it to slip forward on S1. The degree of slippage is ascertained by looking at the relation between the posterior portions of vertebral bodies (*dotted lines*).

Pelvis

Indications

Plain radiographs of the pelvis are ordered almost exclusively after a traumatic injury. Advanced Trauma Life Support (ATLS) protocols recommend all victims of trauma receive an AP pelvis radiograph. Subsequent studies (7, 8) question this indication and advocate more selective imaging based on clinical factors such as severity of injury and physical exam findings. All elderly patients who complain of hip or pelvic pain after even low energy

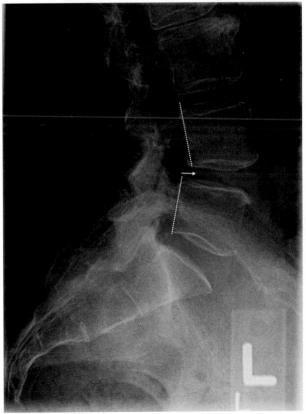

Figure 6.11. Grade 1 anterolisthesis L4 on L5 with degenerative changes, lateral view. The degree of slippage is ascertained by looking at the relation between the posterior portions of vertebral bodies (*dotted lines*).

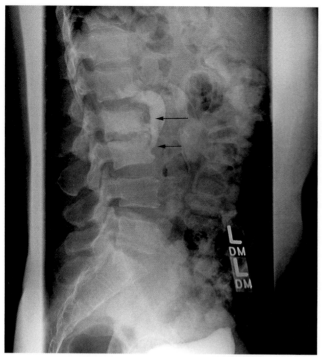

Figure 6.12. L2, L3 osteomyelitis in an intravenous drug abuser presenting with back pain, lateral view. Note loss of definition of vertebral end plate and narrowing of disk space.

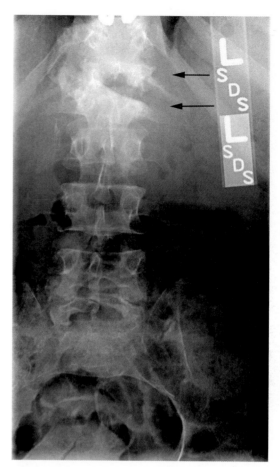

Figure 6.13. T12, L1 osteomyelitis, AP view.

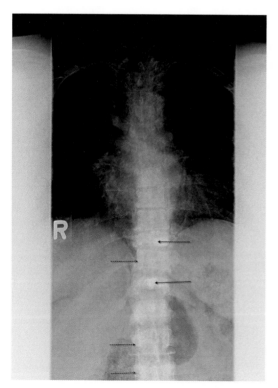

Figure 6.14. T11, L2, L3 diffuse sclerotic changes indicative of mestastic lesions in patient with breast cancer (*dotted arrows*), AP view. Also note vertebroplasty cement in compressed T10, T12 segments (*solid arrows*).

trauma, such as a fall from standing position, should be imaged. Fractures of the hip or pubic rami are not uncommon after minimal trauma in this cohort (9). In younger patients, other clear indications for radiographs include blood at the urethral meatus, a high riding prostate, perineal or inguinal ecchymosis, and instability or pain with compression of the pelvis (10). Another, less common indication is postpartum pelvic pain to evaluate for pubic symphysis diastesis from childbirth.

The pelvis is unusual in that a standard radiographic evaluation consists of only an AP view. Inlet and outlet views may be ordered to better visualize fractures of the main pelvic ring and sacrum (11). Asymmetry or discontinuity of sacral arcuate lines indicates uncomplicated sacral fractures while a more marked disruption is indicative of comminuted sacral fractures. Judet views can often visualize acetabular fractures better than an AP view. In both cases, however, CT is used much more commonly and provides more detailed images, especially when 3D reconstruction is used.

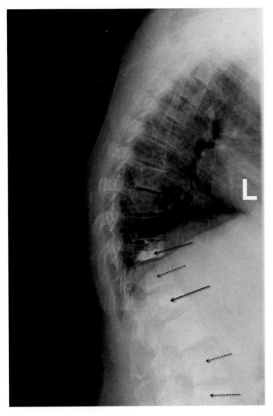

Figure 6.15. Lateral view on the same patient. T11, L2, L3 diffuse sclerotic changes indicative of mestastic lesions in patient with breast cancer (*dotted arrows*). Also note vertebroplasty cement in compressed T10, T12 segments (*solid arrows*).

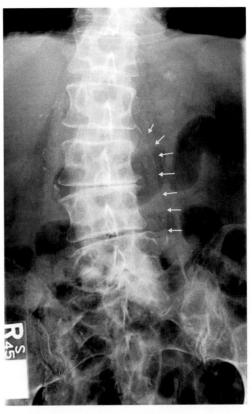

Figure 6.16. Degenerative changes in the spine in an elderly patient with back pain, incidental aortic aneurysm noted (*outlined by arrows*).

Diagnostic capabilities

Pelvic radiology is routinely used to diagnose fractures and ligamentous disruptions. Fractures may be noted in the inferior or superior pubic rami, sacrum, iliac wing, or acetabulum. Ligamentous disruption can be noted by widening or misalignment of the pubic symphysis or widening of the sacroiliac joint. Avulsion fractures from the iliac crest, iliac spines, and ischial tuberosity may be noted in athletic adolescents after vigorous activity. As with the spine, osteomyelitis, tumors, and Paget's disease may be noted if pelvic involvement is present.

Imaging pitfalls and limitations

Pediatric radiographs can be confusing due to the multiple ossification centers of the ilium, ischium, and pubis, as well as multiple apophyseal ossification centers that may mimic fractures. Consultation with an atlas of normal pediatric images may be necessary. The sacrum can be difficult to visualize due to overlying bowel gas on an AP radiograph. For better visualization, a lateral view, centered on the sacrum, can be added. Rotation of the patient may create asymmetries that may mimic subtle fractures. Acetabular fractures may produce only subtle findings on an AP pelvis radiograph and are easily overlooked. Coccygeal fractures are difficult to visualize on routine AP pelvis views, and the normal coccyx is often angulated or malformed. Coccygeal fractures, however, are of limited significance, can be diagnosed clinically, and require only pain control as treatment. Single pelvic fractures are unusual, unless they are of the pubic ramus, coccyx, or a transverse sacral fracture. Identification of one fracture should trigger careful reexamination for a second.

Clinical images

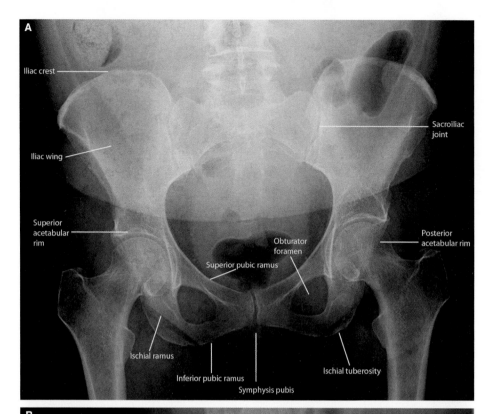

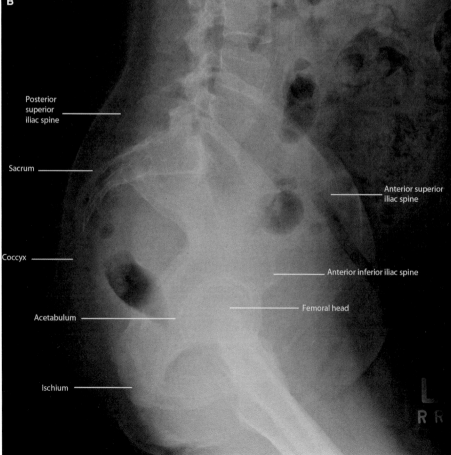

Figure 6.17. Normal pelvis. (a) AP view, (b) lateral view.

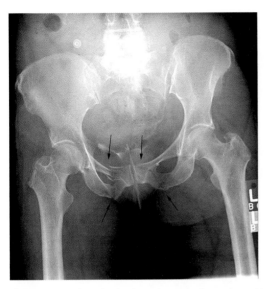

Figure 6.18. Bilateral pubic bone fractures after motor vehicle accident.

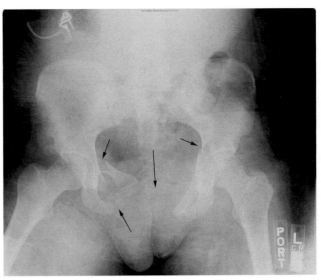

Figure 6.19. Inferior and superior right pubic rami fractures and diastasis of pubic symphisis after blunt trauma.

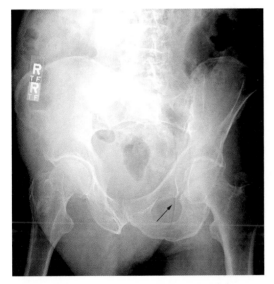

Figure 6.20. Left acetabulum fracture after fall, Judet view.

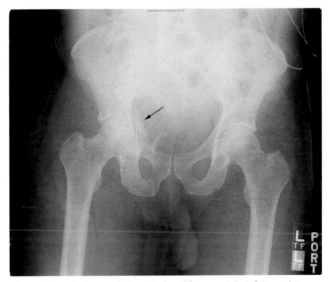

Figure 6.21. Right acetabulum displaced fracture, right inferior pubic ramus fracture after blunt trauma.

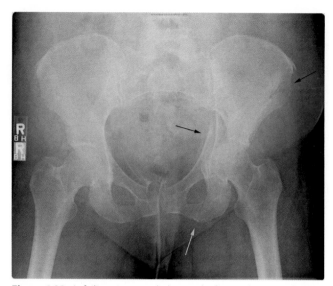

Figure 6.22. Left iliac wing, acetabulum, and inferior pubic ramus fracture.

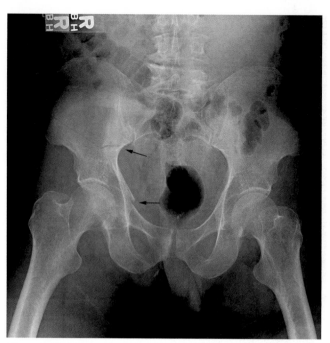

Figure 6.23. Right pubic ramus, acetabulum, and ilium fractures.

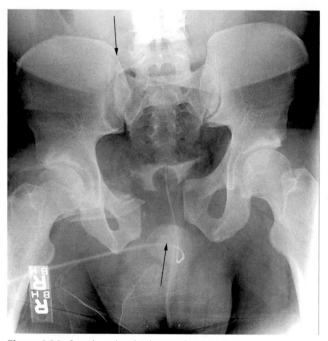

Figure 6.24. Symphyseal and right sacroiliac joint diastases.

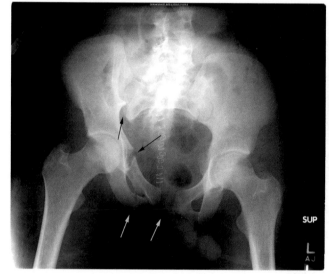

Figure 6.25. Symphyseal and right sacroiliac joint diastases with right pubic rami fractures, Judet view.

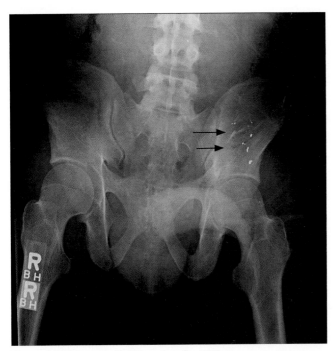

Figure 6.26. Fracture of left iliac wing after GSW.

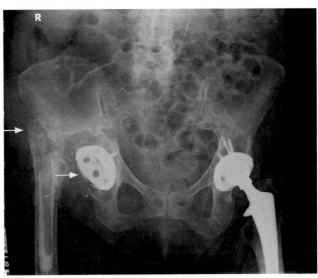

Figure 6.27. Superior displacement of femoral portion of right hip prosthesis with absent femoral component; fracture and superior displacement after a fall.

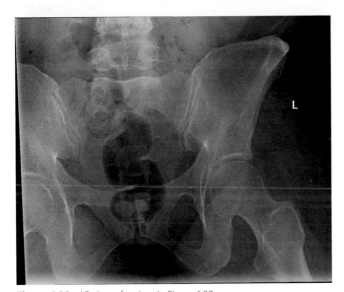

Figure 6.28. AP view of patient in Figure 6.27.

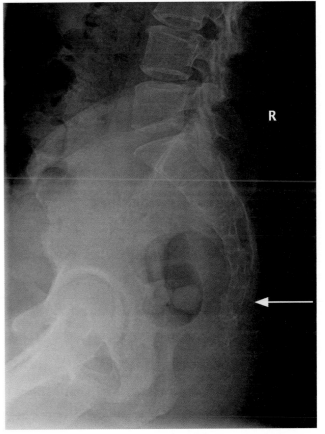

Figure 6.29. Lateral view of S5 transverse fracture with distal fragment displaced anteriorly and coccygel dislocation after a blunt trauma. Note the bowel/gas obstructing the view of the sacrum on the AP view, necessitating the lateral film for proper visualization.

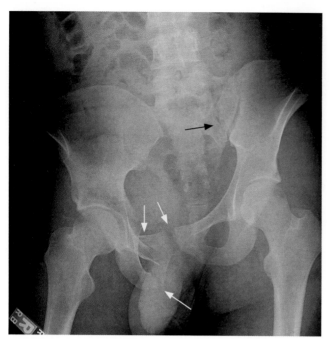

Figure 6.30. Fractures of the right superior and inferior pubic rami, fracture of the right pubic symphysis with borderline pubic symphysis diastasis, and fracture of the left sacral wing after blunt trauma.

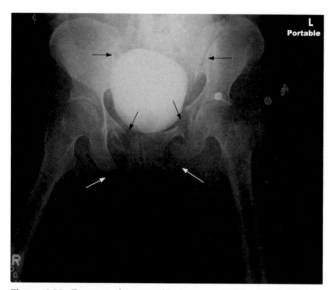

Figure 6.32. Transverse fractures of both superior pubic and inferior pubic rami with inferior displacement of the free segment, which contains the pubic symphysis status post MVA. Widening of both sacroiliac joints and contrast noted within the urinary bladder.

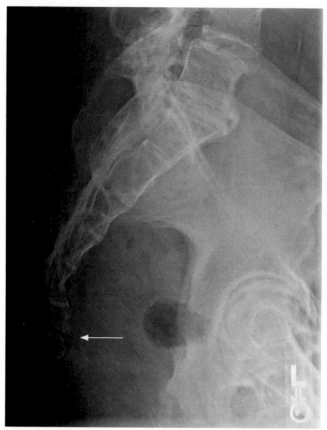

Figure 6.31. Coccygeal dislocation.

References

1. O'Connor E, Walsham J: Indications for thoracolumbar imaging in blunt trauma patients: a review of current literature. *Emerg Med Australas EMA* 2009;**21**(2):94–101.

2. Hsu JM, Joseph T, Ellis AM: Thoracolumbar fracture in blunt trauma patients: guidelines for diagnosis and imaging. *Injury* 2003;**34**(6):426–33.

3. Ballock RT, Mackersie R, Abitbol JJ, et al.: Can burst fractures be predicted from plain radiographs? *J Bone Joint Surg Br* 1992;**74**(1):147–50.

4. Dai L-Y, Wang X-Y, Jiang L-S, et al.: Plain radiography versus computed tomography scans in the diagnosis and management of thoracolumbar burst fractures. *Spine* 2008;**33**(16):E548–52.

5. Inaba K, Munera F, McKenney M, et al.: Visceral torso computed tomography for clearance of the thoracolumbar spine in trauma: a review of the literature. *J Trauma* 2006;**60**(4):915–20.

6. Sheridan R, Peralta R, Rhea J, et al.: Reformatted visceral protocol helical computed tomographic scanning allows conventional radiographs of the thoracic and lumbar spine to be eliminated in the evaluation of blunt trauma patients. *J Trauma* 2003;**55**(4):665–9.

7. Duane TM, Tan BB, Golay D, et al.: Blunt trauma and the role of routine pelvic radiographs: a prospective analysis. *J Trauma* 2002;**53**(3):463–8.

8. Kessel B, Sevi R, Jeroukhimov I, et al.: Is routine portable pelvic x-ray in stable multiple trauma patients always justified in a high technology era? *Injury* 2007;**38**(5):559–63.

9. Spaniolas K, Cheng JD, Gestring ML, et al.: Ground level falls are associated with significant mortality in elderly patients. *J Trauma* 2010;**69**(4):821–5.

10. Steele MT, Norvell, JG: Pelvis Injuries. In: Tintinalli, J (ed.), *Tintinalli's emergency medicine: a comprehensive study guide*, 7th ed. New York: McGraw-Hill, 2011, 1841–8.

11. Duke Orthopaedics: Radiology of Pelvic Fractures – Wheeless' Textbook of Orthopaedics. Dec. 14, 2013. Available at: http://www.wheelessonline.com/ortho/radiology_of_pelvic_fractures

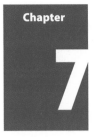

Chapter 7

Plain Radiography of the Pediatric Extremity

Kenneth T. Kwon and Lauren M. Pellman

Indications

Plain extremity radiographs are indicated in pediatric patients with significant mechanism of injury; pain; limitation of use or motion; or physical exam evidence of deformity, swelling, or tenderness. The joint above and below the site of injury should be carefully examined, and radiographs of adjacent joints should be obtained when indicated. Occasionally, parental pressure to exclude fractures is a contributing factor in determining the need for extremity radiographs.

Diagnostic capabilities

Pediatric extremities consist of growing bones and ossification centers, with wide variability in normal-appearing bones based on age. Despite these variations, a basic understanding of bone development physiology and time of onset of certain radiographic findings, particularly ossification centers of the elbow, is important to accurately interpret these films. Physeal injuries, which involve the growth plate, comprise up to one-third of all pediatric fractures. Because the physis itself is radiolucent, physeal fractures are not always evident on initial plain radiographs. Follow-up plain radiographs and, occasionally, imaging with magnetic resonance or nuclear bone scan may be necessary.

Minimum views of the extremity should include anteroposterior (AP) and lateral. Ensure that a true lateral of the elbow is obtained because fat pads may be obscured or distorted with any sort of rotated technique. Oblique views may be needed to define a fracture, particularly of the elbow or ankle. Comparison views with the contralateral extremity may be useful to determine normal variants, but they should not be ordered routinely on all patients.

Imaging pitfalls and limitations

Negative initial plain radiographs do not exclude a Salter–Harris type 1 physeal fracture. If a pediatric patient has negative films but significant swelling or point tenderness along the physis of a bone, assume a physeal fracture and splint accordingly. Also, resist the pitfall of diagnosing sprains in children with negative radiographs because ligaments tend to be stronger than the developing bones to which they are attached at the epiphyseal and perichondral areas. The incidence of sprains and dislocations are much less common in children than in adults.

Clinical images

Salter–Harris Classification

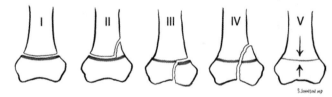

Figure 7.1. Physeal fractures: Salter–Harris classification. Physeal fractures occur at the physis, or growth plate. Approximately 18% to 30% of all pediatric fractures involve the physis. Physeal injuries are more common in adolescents than in younger children, with the peak incidence at 11 to 12 years of age. Most occur in the upper limb, particularly in the radius and ulna. Physeal fractures can be categorized from types 1 to 5 based on the Salter–Harris classification.

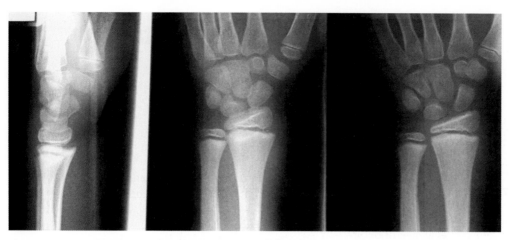

Figure 7.2. Salter–Harris type 1. This fracture involves separation of the metaphysis and epiphysis at the physis. It is suspected on clinical grounds if there is point tenderness or swelling at the physis. Radiographs are usually normal, but they may reveal some widening of the physis or mild displacement of the epiphysis. Note on the left image that the epiphysis appears slightly displaced dorsally and on the middle image that the epiphysis appears slightly displaced laterally. Follow-up radiographs at 1 to 2 weeks may reveal new bone formation at the physis.

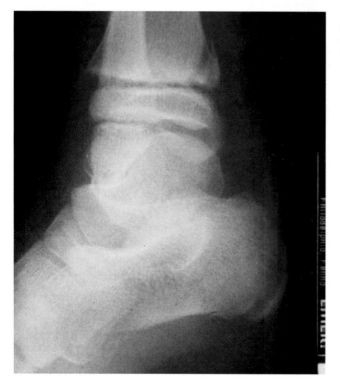

Figure 7.3A. Salter–Harris type 2. This fracture involves the physis and metaphysis. (It starts through the physis and then propagates across the physeal-metaphyseal junction into the metaphysis.) It is the most common physeal fracture (75%) and carries a good prognosis.

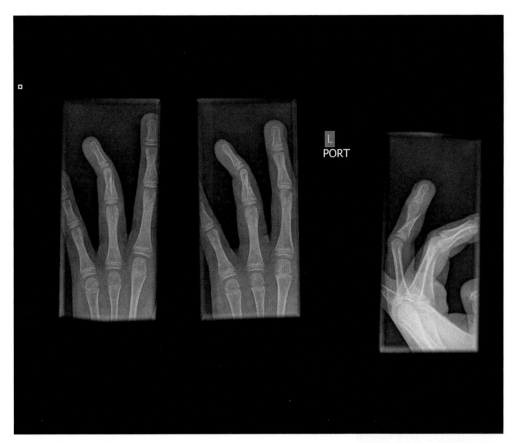

Figure 7.3B. Salter–Harris type 2. At first glance, this displaced spiral fracture of the middle phalanx may appear to be limited to the midshaft, but upon closer examination it is clear that it extends to the physis, definitive of a Salter–Harris type 2 fracture. Courtesy of Pablo Abbona, MD.

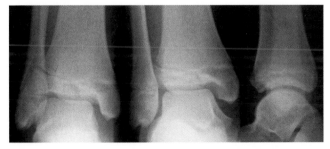

Figure 7.4. Salter–Harris type 3. AP, mortise, and lateral views of distal tibia shown here. Fracture through the physis and epiphysis, and intra-articular by definition. There is a vertical lucency through the distal tibial epiphysis extending to the mortise joint space. This can lead to growth arrest or chronic disability. ED orthopedic consultation is warranted. Courtesy of Loren Yamamoto, MD.

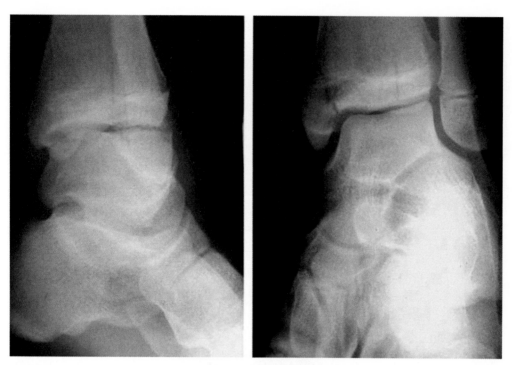

Figure 7.5. Salter–Harris type 4. Fracture through physis, metaphysis, and epiphysis, and intra-articular by definition. Same complications and management as type 3.

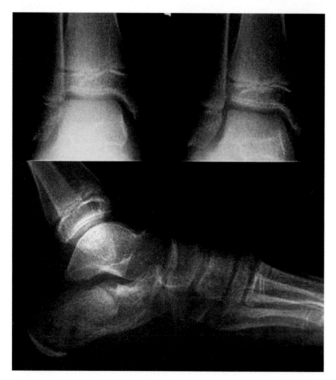

Figure 7.6. Salter–Harris type 5. Crush injury due to significant axial compression. This may appear obvious with distortion or marked narrowing of the physis, or it may be subtle and radiographically similar to a type 1 fracture. Note the narrowed tibial physis and concurrent calcaneal fracture in these images. If the mechanism is suggestive, consider a type 5 fracture. Comparison views may be needed. Courtesy of Loren Yamamoto, MD.

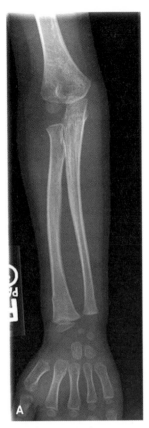
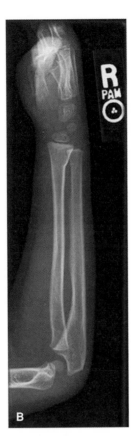

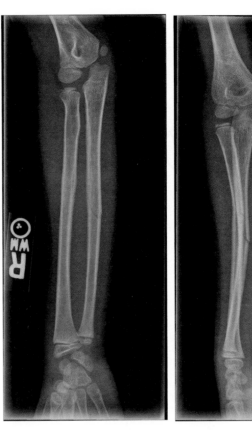

Figures 7.7A and B. Torus fracture. Also called a buckle fracture, this injury is common in younger children. It occurs in the metaphyseal region of bone from a compressive load injury. The cortex of bone "buckles" in a small area, resulting in a stable fracture pattern. The most common site of this fracture is the distal radius (frequently after falling onto an outstretched arm).
The fracture area may be seen on one side only or bilaterally. If a distal forearm torus fracture is unilateral and minor, a short arm splint is often adequate; if bilateral or more significant, use a sugar tong splint to immobilize the elbow joint as well.

Figure 7.8. Greenstick fracture of the mid–ulna shaft in a 9-year-old. A Greenstick fracture is an incomplete fracture that usually occurs at the diaphyseal-metaphyseal junction. Angulation of a bone causes a break on the convex side, while the periosteum and cortex on the concave side remain intact. To obtain an anatomical reduction, this fracture must often first be completed. Courtesy of Pablo Abbona, MD.

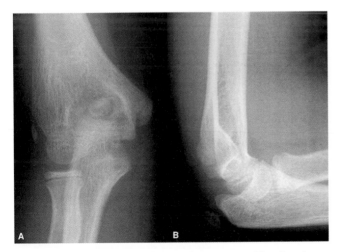

Figures 7.9A and B. Normal elbow ossification centers. The elbow is a common fracture site in a child, usually resulting from a fall onto an outstretched arm. Unfortunately, pediatric elbow radiographs appear intimidating due to the multiple ossification centers and various temporal–spatial relationships that need to be considered. In actuality, interpreting pediatric elbow x-rays is relatively straightforward if a simple, systematic approach is followed. Courtesy of Loren Yamamoto, MD.

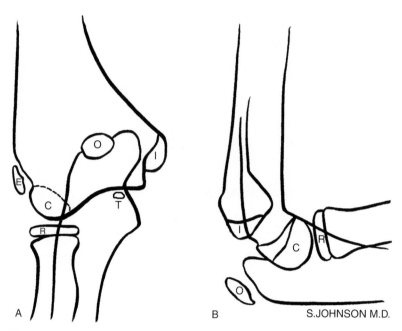

A   B   S.JOHNSON M.D.

Figures 7.10A and B. The normal ossification centers of the right elbow. They can be remembered using the mnemonic CRITOE, which stands for capitellum, radial head, internal (medial) epicondyle, trochlea, olecranon, and external (lateral) epicondyle. These ossification centers all appear at different ages and eventually fuse to adjacent bones. The ages at which they appear are highly variable, with the general guideline being 2, 4, 6, 8, 10, and 12 years of age for CRITOE, respectively. Although the ages at which they appear are variable in each child, it is critical to remember that these ossification centers always appear in a specific sequence, with only rare exceptions. Given this reasoning, if three bony fragments are seen, they should be the capitellum, radial head, and internal epicondyle. If the external epicondyle ossification center is seen but not the olecranon ossification center, what appears to be the external epicondyle ossification center is actually a fracture fragment. Also note that a true and reliable lateral of the elbow should give alignment and superimposition of the epicondyles, giving an "hourglass" or "figure 8" sign as highlighted in (B). If this hourglass sign is not seen, it may not be a true lateral and may be obscuring important fat pads or fracture lines. Looking at the lateral view, identify the anterior fat pad, which is a somewhat triangular-shaped dark lucency just anterior to the anterior border of the distal humerus. This is a normal anterior fat pad sign. If the elbow joint capsule becomes distended due to hemarthrosis from a fracture in the elbow joint space, that anterior fat pad will be displaced anterior and superiorly to form a more prominent lucency, or "sail sign." So a small anterior fat pad is considered normal, but a large one is considered abnormal and indicates an elbow fracture. A posterior fat pad located posterior to the distal humerus is normally not seen due to the deep olecranon fossa, but if a posterior fat pad of any size is seen, it is considered abnormal. Thus, a large anterior fat pad or a posterior fat pad of any size is considered abnormal, and an elbow fracture should be presumed, even if an obvious fracture is not seen.

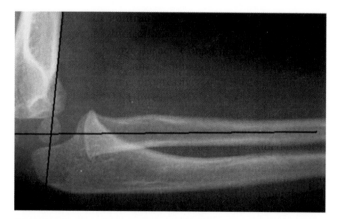

Figure 7.11. Anterior humeral and radiocapitellar lines. The anterior humeral line is an imaginary line along the long anterior axis of the humerus on the lateral view. This line should bisect the capitellum in the middle third. If the line intersects the anterior third of the capitellum or passes completely anterior, this most likely indicates a supracondylar fracture with posterior displacement. The radiocapitellar line is an imaginary line through the longitudinal central axis of the radius. This line should pass through the capitellum in both the AP and lateral views. If it does not, it most likely indicates a dislocation, usually of the radial head.

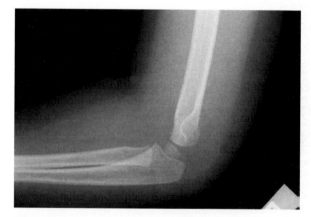

Figure 7.12. Supracondylar fracture. Note the cortical break in the posterior supracondylar area with the large associated posterior fat pad. Also note that the anterior humeral line is abnormal and crosses the anterior third of the capitellum, indicating mild posterior displacement of the fracture.

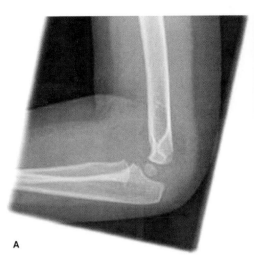
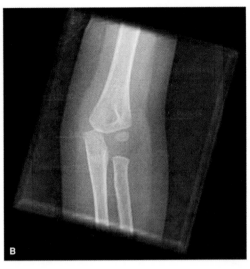

Figures 7.13A and B. Supracondylar fracture, occult. The only abnormality seen here is a posterior fat pad, indicating hemarthrosis and a presumed occult supracondylar fracture. In the pediatric population, supracondylar fractures are the most common type of elbow fracture, accounting for more than 50% of fractures of the elbow in this age group, whereas radial head fractures are more common in adults. Typical mechanism is a fall on the outstretched arm with hyperextension. Occasionally, distal pulses may be absent; most cases are due to vasospasm or arterial compression, which should resolve after reducing the fracture. It is extremely important to document neurovascular functioning of the distal arm with elbow fractures. Complications most commonly involve the brachial artery and median nerve, which may lead to Volkman's ischemic contracture if not properly managed. All supracondylar fractures warrant orthopedic consults in the ED for careful immobilization and close follow-up.

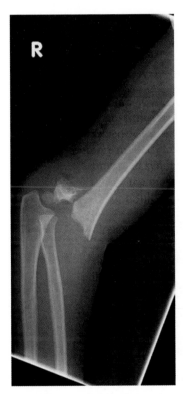

Figure 7.14. Supracondylar fracture, complete displacement. This is an example of a type 3 or completely displaced fracture.

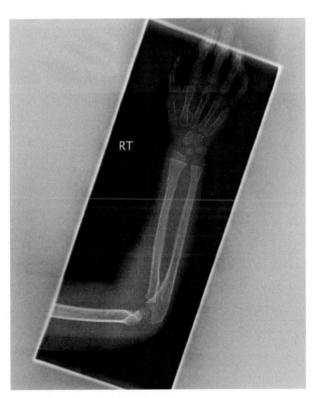

Figure 7.15. Supracondylar fracture with radius fracture. The obvious fracture is the transverse radius fracture. The subtle fracture is the associated occult supracondylar fracture, as indicated by the posterior fat pad sign.

113

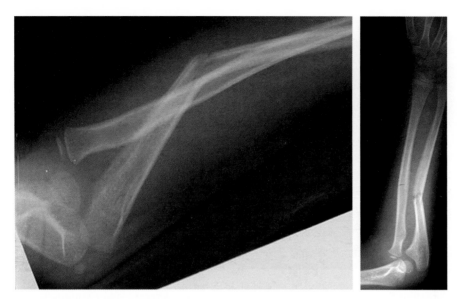

Figures 7.16 (left) and 7.17 (right). Monteggia's fractures. These two radiographs are examples of Monteggia's fracture, which is a combination of a proximal ulnar fracture and radial head dislocation. Notice the radiocapitellar line does not pass through the capitellum, thus revealing the dislocation. Monteggia's fractures comprise 2% of all elbow fractures in children. The usual mechanism is elbow hyperextension. If the radial head dislocation is not recognized early and properly reduced, it could lead to permanent radial nerve damage and limited elbow motion. Needless to say, emergent orthopedic consultation is required. Most of these fractures can be closed reduced, but some will require open reduction and fixation.

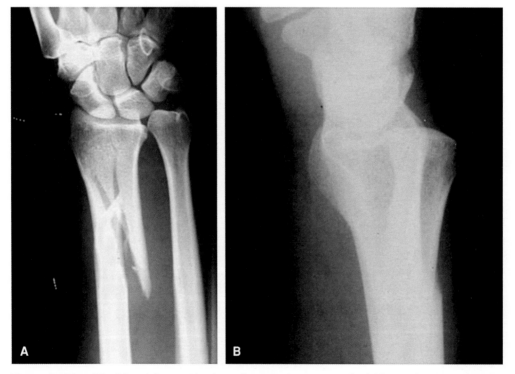

Figures 7.18A and B. Galeazzi's fracture. The obvious fracture is the comminuted radial fracture, but the more subtle injury is the dislocation of the distal ulna, seen clearly on the lateral view. This is an example of Galeazzi's fracture, which is classically described as fracture of the distal third of the radius with dislocation of the distal ulna. This fracture should be suspected with any angulated fracture of the radius. Like Monteggia's injuries, most of these fractures can be closed reduced.

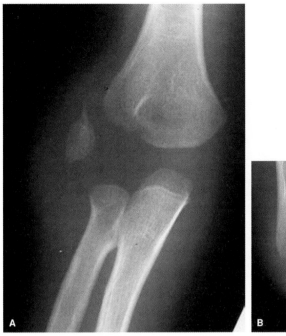
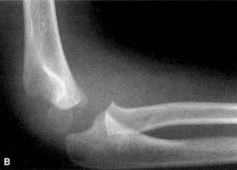

Figures 7.19A and B. Lateral epicondyle fracture. Note the fracture fragment off the lateral condyle, seen best on the AP view. This is not a normal ossification center because the lateral (external) epicondyle is the last ossification center to become visible. In this patient, no other ossification centers are visible, not even the capitellum, which should be the first ossification center to be seen.

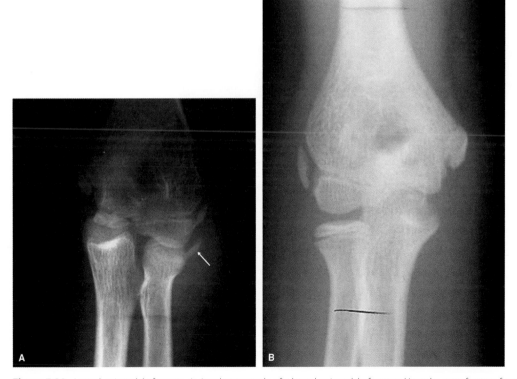

Figure 7.20. Lateral epicondyle fracture. A: Another example of a lateral epicondyle fracture. Note the extra fracture fragment (*arrow*) inferior to the normal lateral epicondyle ossification center. In this patient, all ossification centers are visible. B: Comparison view of the other normal elbow of the same patient.

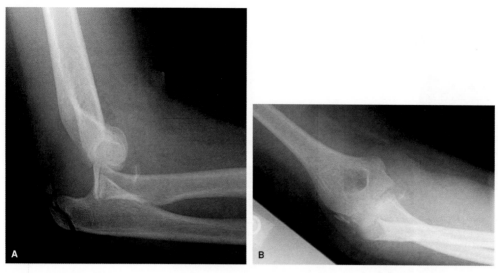

Figures 7.21A and B. Elbow dislocation with epicondylar fracture. This typical posterior elbow dislocation occurred in a child who fell onto his outstretched arm. Also note the small fracture fragments off both the lateral and medial epicondyles, confirming a distal humeral epicondylar fracture.

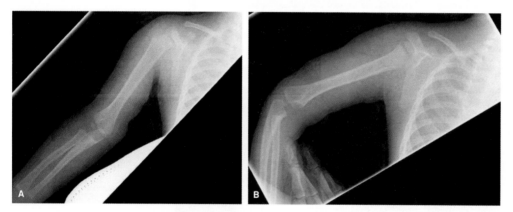

Figures 7.22A and B. Radial head subluxation (nursemaid's elbow). Note that the radiocapitellar line does not go through the capitellum in all views. This patient was being swung around playfully by dad with the arms extended. The annular ligament becomes partially detached from the head of the radius and slips into the radiohumeral joint, where it is entrapped. This injury usually occurs in children a few months to 5 years of age, after which the strength of the annular ligament is such that the injury is uncommon. The usual mechanism is axial traction on an extended and pronated arm, such as when a child is lifted up or twirled around by the arms. The child usually holds the affected arm in pronation with the elbow slightly flexed. Mild tenderness may be noted with palpation of the radial head. Significant point tenderness or swelling should suggest an alternative diagnosis, such as a fracture. Radiographs are not needed unless a fracture is suspected, and, certainly, closed reduction should not be attempted without films unless a fracture can comfortably be excluded on historical and clinical grounds alone. Closed reduction is attempted with your thumb on the radial head area and a combination of supination and flexion of the elbow. Frequently, you will feel a palpable "click." If supination/flexion does not appear to work, you can try rapid hyperpronation and extension. When reduction is successful, the child typically uses the arm normally within 5 to 10 minutes. Postreduction radiographs are not needed unless arm use continues to be limited.

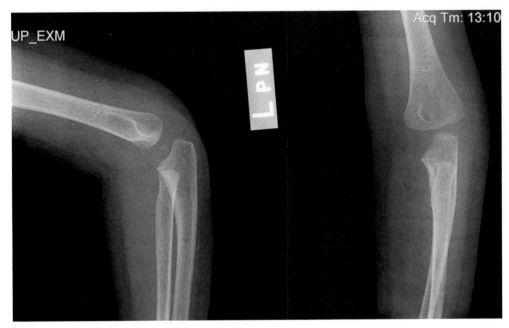

Figure 7.23. Lateral epicondylar fracture with radial head subluxation. The radiocapitellar line appears abnormal in both views. In addition, there is an avulsion fracture of lateral epicondyle. This radiograph was first interpreted as a normal lateral epicondylar ossification center, but on closer review, it is clear that the ossification centers of the radial head, medial (internal) epicondyle, trochlea, and olecranon are not yet visible radiographically (remember CRITOE); thus, the lateral epicondyle should also not be present. The only normal ossification center visible on this radiograph is the capitellum.

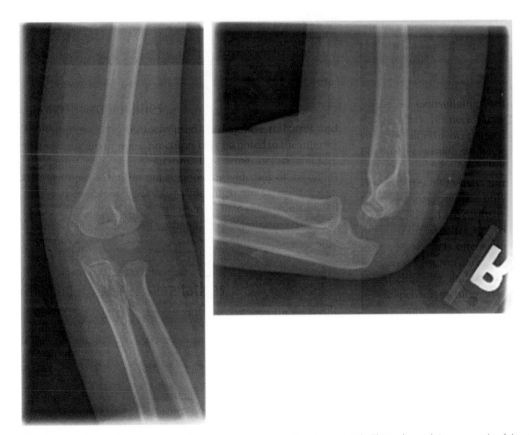

Figure 7.24. Ossification sequence variant. There are rare exceptions to every rule. This radiograph is an example of the medial epicondyle ossification center becoming visible prior to the radial head ossification center. This was confirmed by a comparison view of the other elbow. There is no fracture on this film.

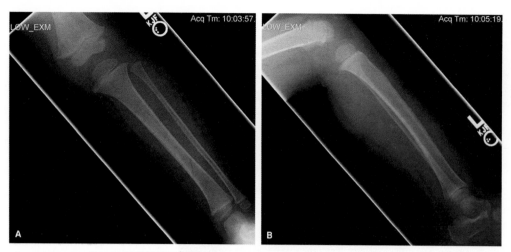

Figures 7.25A and B. Toddler's fracture. First described by Dunbar in 1964, this fracture is classically described as an oblique or spiral nondisplaced fracture of the distal tibia. It is most commonly seen in children 9 months to 3 years of age and occurs as a result of an axial loading and twisting injury on a fixed foot, which would maximize forces in the distal leg. Although any oblique or spiral fracture of a long bone in a child should raise the possibility of nonaccidental trauma, an oblique fracture of the distal tibia in a weight-bearing infant can be explained from normal accidental forces, such as a fall, which is frequently unwitnessed. More concerning would be a spiral fracture of the mid or proximal tibia, which may more likely suggest nonaccidental trauma, as a perpetrator holding and twisting the distal portion of a leg would maximize forces in the midshaft and proximal areas of the tibia. Isolated spiral fractures of the tibia neither confirm nor dismiss the possibility of abuse.

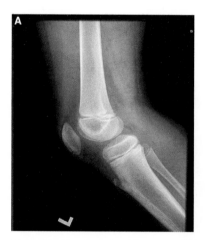

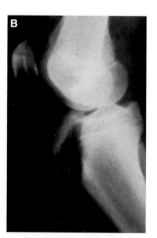

Figure 7.26A. Osgood–Schlatter disease. This adolescent developed acute knee pain while playing basketball and demonstrates an avulsion fracture and Osgood–Schlatter disease. Note the avulsion fracture of the tibial tuberosity. Osgood–Schlatter disease is inflammation or apophysitis of ossification centers (apophyses), mainly in the proximal tibia at the insertion of the patellar tendon. Repetitive stress due to strong muscular attachments to these apophyses can lead to microfractures, avulsions, or complete patellar tendon ruptures. Most are minor injuries and can be treated conservatively with symptomatic care and activity restriction.

Figure 7.26B. Osgood–Schlatter disease. This image depicts a mild case of Osgood–Schlatter disease with mild avulsion as seen in a 12-year-old boy with knee injury one week prior to presentation. Courtesy of Pablo Abbona, MD.

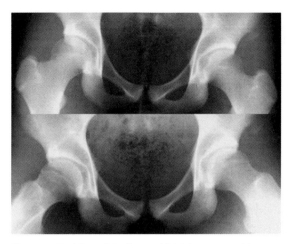

Figure 7.27. Hip avulsion fracture. This injury occurred in a teenage track sprinter while running and without direct trauma. Note the fracture off the superior iliac crest where the sartorius muscle inserts. These hip avulsion fractures occur in active adolescents due to jumping, running, or kicking. The most common sites of these avulsions are the superior iliac crest (insertion of the sartorius), inferior iliac crest (insertion of the rectus femoris), and ischial tuberosity (insertion of hamstring muscles). Many of these injuries are preceded by microfractures at these insertion sites, similar to Osgood–Schlatter disease. Most of these injuries can be treated conservatively and rarely require surgery. Courtesy of Loren Yamamoto, MD.

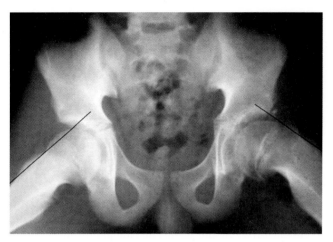

Figure 7.28. Slipped capital femoral epiphysis (SCFE). The lines demonstrate a Klein's line, which is a linear line drawn along the superior border of the proximal femoral metaphysis. This line should intersect the top part of the femoral epiphysis, which it does on the right hip. However, it does not pass through the epiphysis on the left hip, which is indicative of SCFE. This injury can present with chronic or acute pain in the hip, thigh, or knee, and up to 25% are bilateral. Most occur in older children and younger adolescents, which helps differentiate this disease from Legg-Calve-Perthes disease, which has a similar presentation but tends to occur in younger children. A frog leg view should always be included in any patient with suspected SCFE.

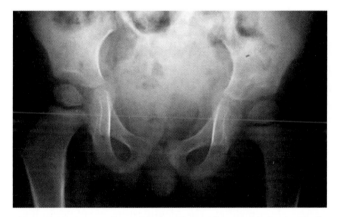

Figure 7.29. Septic arthritis of the hip. This toddler presented with refusal to walk and left hip pain. Note the widened joint space of the left hip compared with the right, indicating joint effusion and, in this case, pus. Hip aspiration grew out of *Staphylococcus aureus* in this patient. If hip radiographs are equivocal, other imaging modalities such as ultrasound, MRI, or bone scan are indicated.

Chapter 8

Plain Radiographs of the Pediatric Chest

Loren G. Yamamoto

Indications

Plain film radiographs of the chest ordered from the ED are indicated in stable patients to help diagnose health complaints potentially involving the chest. The radiographic findings on plain film chest radiographs are often nonspecific or subtle, but they serve as a useful screening measure to confirm or rule out various chest conditions.

Diagnostic capabilities

Plain film radiographs contrast differences in the standard five radiographic densities (metallic, calcific/bone, soft tissue/water, fat, and air) to assist in the diagnostic process. The dominant structures in the chest are the lungs (mostly air and soft tissue densities) and the heart (soft tissue density). In a standard chest x-ray (CXR), two basic views are generally obtained: the posteroanterior (PA) view and the lateral view. In most instances, these are both done with the patient upright. However, when the child is very ill, upright positioning is often not feasible. Although upright positioning in older children, teens, and adults is easy to achieve in most instances, upright positioning in infants and young children is difficult. Most imaging departments use some type of positioning device to keep the infant in the upright position with the infant's arms up in the air for proper positioning. These devices are universally unpopular with parents but necessary to achieve proper positioning. Portable CXRs or CXRs done in a supine position are generally anteroposterior (AP): the x-ray beam approaches the patient from the anterior to expose a film or sensing cartridge on the posterior side of the patient. This is the opposite of the PA view. It is important because the x-ray beam is not parallel. As the beam flares out slightly, the heart size on an AP CXR will appear bigger than the heart size on a PA CXR. Also the measurement of structures will be distorted, depending on how close the structure is to the x-ray beam. For example, an esophageal penny will always measure bigger than it actually is. This might lead the endoscopist to believe she will recover a nickel, when at endoscopy she recovers only a penny.

A single AP view is often obtained in a critical care setting to examine the lungs and to confirm placement of the endotracheal tube, central lines, and any other indwelling devices.

The CXR is generally taken during inhalation (inspiratory) to maximize the air content of the lung. This increases the sensitivity of identifying soft tissue or fluid density abnormalities (e.g., infiltrates, atelectasis). Preferably, 10 posterior ribs should be visible on a good inspiration. A suboptimal inspiration will result in a larger cardiac silhouette and greater accentuation of normal lung markings.

An expiratory view (preferably worded as taken during "exhalation" rather than "expiration" because the latter might imply that we will wait until the patient expires) can be specially requested if the possibility of air trapping (e.g., a bronchial foreign body) is suspected. Unfortunately, expiratory views require timing, and as with the inspiratory view, timing is not always perfect. The author's preference is to obtain bilateral decubitus views instead. Decubitus views (with the patient lying on his side) are useful to look for air trapping and to see if a pleural effusion will layer out.

Imaging pitfalls and limitations

Interpreting plain film radiographs is similar to identifying an object by examining only the shadow of the object. Unlike advanced imaging methods (CT, ultrasound, MRI), plain film radiographic abnormalities are often subtle. Serious pediatric conditions are uncommon, which limits the cumulative exposure of these findings, even for experienced clinicians. The subtlety of these findings makes identifying these important findings more difficult. On a radiology service, most of the plain film radiographs are normal or contain minor or obvious abnormalities. The identification of subtle findings identifying important and uncommon findings is best studied by viewing a collection of these abnormalities, which would ordinarily take the average clinician more than several career lifetimes to do.

Chest contents and diagnostic possibilities

Lungs

Pneumonia, atelectasis, pulmonary edema, lung abscess, tuberculosis, pleural effusion/empyema, bronchial foreign bodies, lobar emphysema, pneumothorax, respiratory distress syndrome (of prematurity), pulmonary interstitial emphysema, chronic lung disease, endotracheal tube placement, diaphragmatic hernia, pulmonary perfusion and congenital pulmonary vascular malformations

Heart

Cardiomegaly, congestive heart failure, congenital heart disease, myocarditis, pericarditis, pneumopericardium

Aorta

Aortic dissection, aortoesophageal syndrome, vascular ring/sling

Mediastinum

Pneumomediastinum, thymus enlargement, bronchogenic cyst, mediastinal mass

Bones

Clavicle fractures, rib fractures, thoracic spine fractures, discitis, osteopenia, osteomalacia, osteogenesis imperfecta

Clinical images

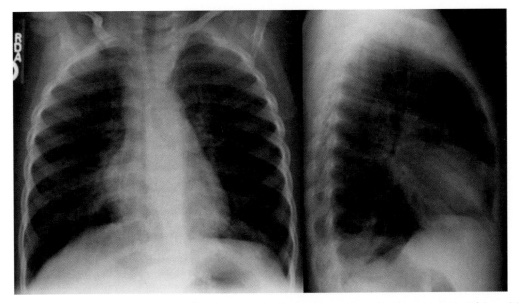

Figure 8.1. Bilateral central pulmonary infiltrates, most marked in the right middle and left lower lobes. The left lower lobe infiltrate is best seen on the lateral view inferiorly over the spine. The lungs are hyperaerated. Impression: right middle and left lower lobe infiltrates.

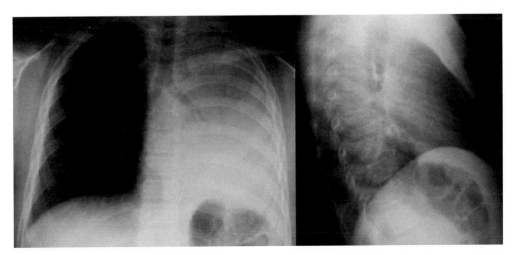

Figure 8.2. Consolidated left lung. This atelectasis results in a mediastinal shift to the left. Air bronchograms are evident over the left lung. On the original film, there is a suggestion of a 1.5-cm cylindrical foreign body in the left mainstem bronchus (not seen in this image).

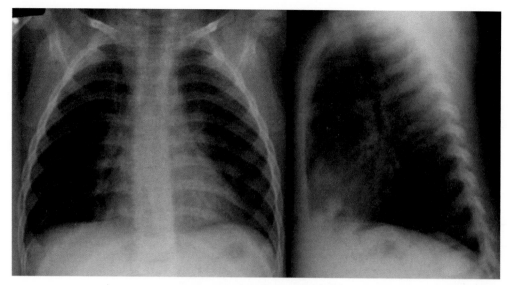

Figure 8.3. Small interstitial central pulmonary infiltrates most consistent with a viral pneumonia.

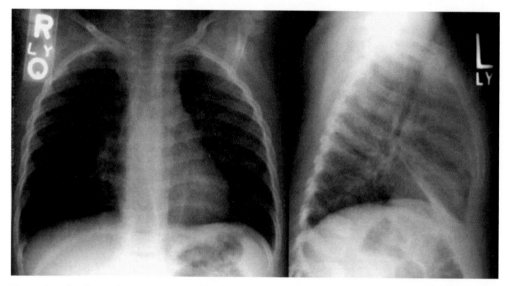

Figure 8.4. Small area of atelectasis in the right middle lobe. This is best seen on the lateral view as an oblique, flattened, wedge-shaped density over the heart. Instead of appearing in its normal triangular shape, the right middle lobe is flat and compressed, indicating atelectasis.

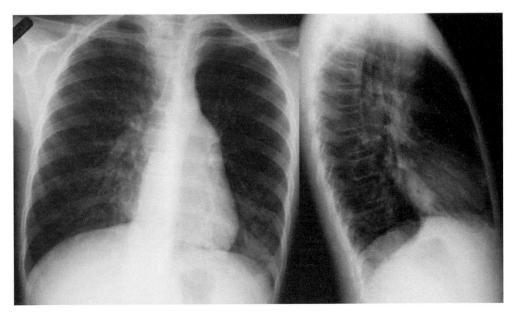

Figure 8.5. Patchy infiltrate at the left lung base. This is seen on the lateral view obliquely over the heart and on the PA view as haziness in the left lower lung. The prominence of the right perihilar region is probably due to rotation. Note the asymmetry of the spinal column and the ribs. This rotation exposes more of the right hilum in the radiograph, making it appear more prominent.

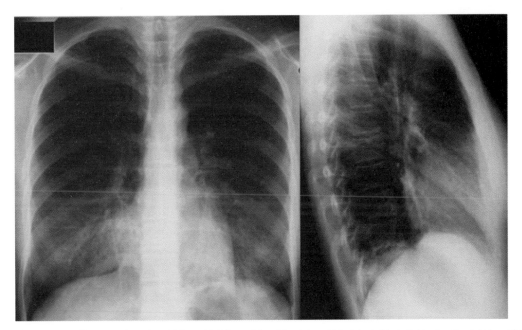

Figure 8.6. Infiltrates in the right middle and left lower lobes. The right middle lobe infiltrate is blurring the right heart border. It can also be seen on the lateral view as streakiness over the heart. The left lower lobe infiltrate is best seen on the lateral view posteriorly on the diaphragm. It can also be seen on the PA view as haziness in the lower lung on the left. The infiltrate in the right middle lobe was noted 2 years ago on a previous radiograph, and the possibility of a chronic infiltrate was raised.

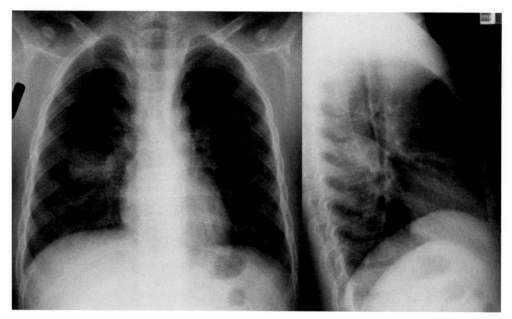

Figure 8.7. Circular density in the right lung. This is the superior segment of the right lower lobe. Although this has the appearance of a mass, it is most likely an infectious process. This is a spherical consolidation in the right lower lobe (round pneumonia).

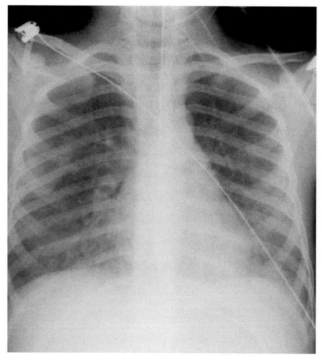

Figure 8.8. Near-drowning victim. The lungs show haziness consistent with pulmonary edema. Note the normal size of the heart, which suggests that the pulmonary edema is noncardiogenic. If the pulmonary edema was due to congestive heart failure, the heart would be enlarged.

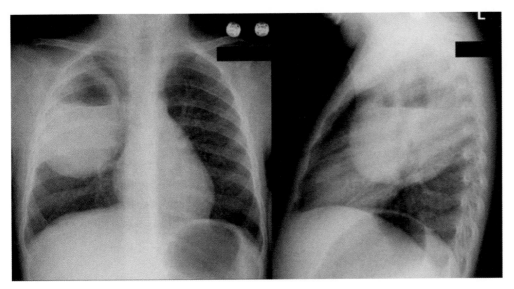

Figure 8.9. Mass with a large air-fluid level within the right lung. This is a large pulmonary abscess.

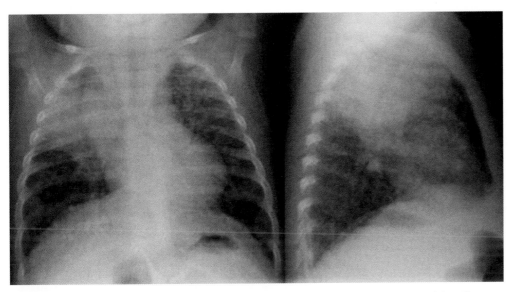

Figure 8.10. Infant with miliary tuberculosis. There are multiple small nodules throughout the lungs bilaterally.

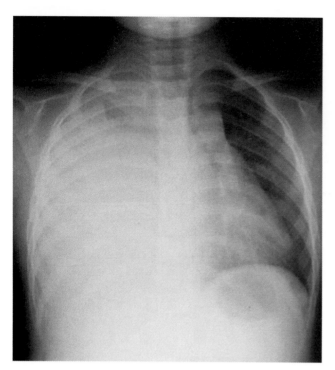

Figure 8.11. Three-year-old who presented with acute symptoms. This CXR demonstrates a complete opacification of the right hemithorax, with a shift of the mediastinal structures to the left. This patient's pulmonary etiology is also tuberculosis.

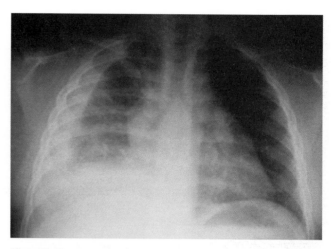

Figure 8.12. Large right pleural effusion in a 6-year-old. This patient had a previous CXR approximately 12 hours earlier that did not show a pleural effusion. The patient is very ill appearing, in respiratory distress. This rapid progression is highly suggestive of pneumonia due to *Staphylococcus aureus*. The pleural effusion is likely to be an empyema, requiring tube thoracostomy drainage.

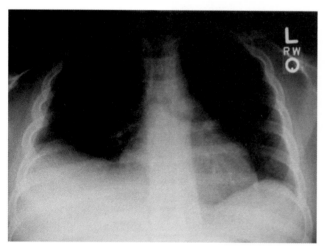

Figure 8.13. CXR from a 9-year-old demonstrates an unusual contour of both hemidiaphragms. Normally, the center of the hemidiaphragm is the highest portion of the diaphragm. However, in this case, the highest portion of the hemidiaphragm is the lateral portion of the diaphragm. This appearance is indicative of a pleural effusion. Blunting of the costophrenic angles is the classic radiographic sign of a pleural effusion.

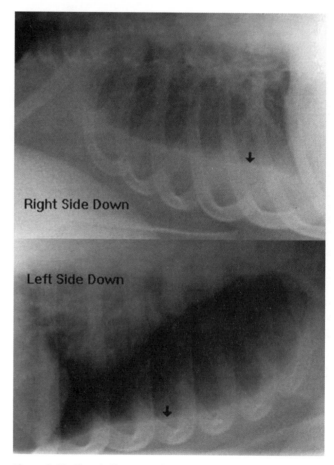

Figure 8.14. Pleural effusions are better demonstrated by obtaining lateral decubitus views, permitting the effusion to layer out. The effusion on the right is much larger than the effusion on the left.

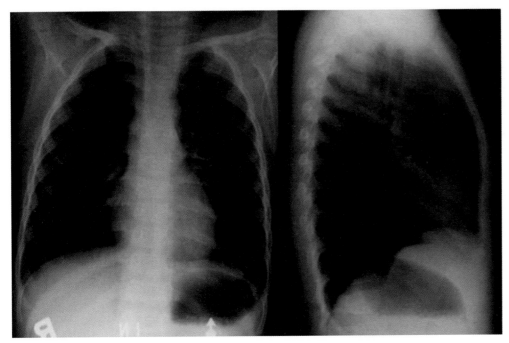

Figure 8.15. No infiltrates are noted. The right side is more lucent (darker) compared to the left. This is subtle and may be difficult to appreciate unless you step back and view the CXR from a distance. The right hemidiaphragm is slightly higher than the left hemidiaphragm; however, it should be higher than this. Both findings suggest right-sided hyperexpansion. More clinical history through a translator indicated that the patient was jumping on a bed while eating some food (believed to be meat), when she began choking. Since then, she has experienced respiratory difficulty. Further radiographs revealed bilateral air trapping. Bronchoscopy revealed bilateral bronchial peanut fragment foreign bodies.

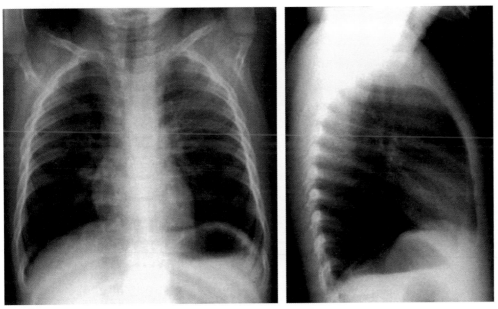

Figure 8.16. CXR from a 17-month-old with a history of choking while eating a chocolate nut bar. This CXR is highly suspicious for a bronchial foreign body. However, because it is nondiagnostic, expiratory and lateral decubitus views are ordered.

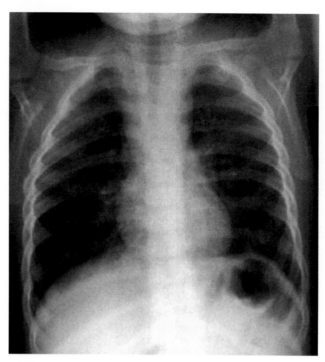

Figure 8.17. Expiratory view from the same patient as in Figure 8.16. Note that the PA views during inspiration (see Fig. 8.16) and exhalation look roughly the same. Counting posterior ribs is a more objective way of determining the degree of inflation. This figure suggests that bilateral air trapping is present. However, an expiratory view is highly dependent on the timing of the x-ray. If the x-ray is taken during inspiration but labeled as "expiratory," it will be substantially misleading.

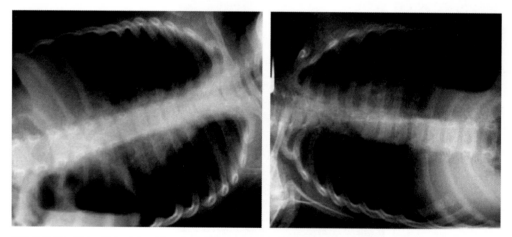

Figure 8.18. Bilateral lateral decubitus views. The appearance of the decubitus views does not rely on timing. Gravity should permit the mediastinum to fall toward the dependent side. In both lateral decubitus views, the mediastinum is exactly where it should be if the patient is upright. However, these views are abnormal because the patient is sideways. Both lateral decubitus views confirm bilateral air trapping. Bilateral bronchial foreign bodies were confirmed at bronchoscopy.

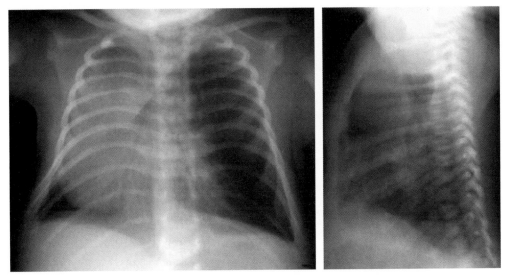

Figure 8.19. CXR of a 2-week-old male infant who presents with severe respiratory distress. This infant has had some respiratory symptoms since coming home from the newborn nursery, but he became much worse today. At first, this CXR was believed to demonstrate a tension pneumothorax. The left hemithorax appears to be pushing the mediastinum toward the right. However, on further consideration, a severe tension pneumothorax of this magnitude should result in the patient being severely hypoxic and hypotensive. Although the patient was mildly hypoxic in room air, his oxygen saturation is 100% while breathing supplemental oxygen. His blood pressure is normal, and his visible perfusion is good. He does not appear to be deteriorating. In addition, the factors that usually lead to a tension pneumothorax (positive-pressure ventilation or a penetrating chest wound) are not present. The CXR is examined more closely for lung markings in the left hemithorax. There is some suggestion of lung markings, but it is difficult to confirm. Because the patient is stable, a thoracentesis or a tube thoracostomy is *not* attempted. This patient has congenital lobar emphysema of the left upper lobe. The left upper lobe is filling the entire left hemithorax. The remainder of the left lung is compressed and is not easily visualized on the CXR. After the emphysematous left upper lobe is removed surgically, the patient recovers well.

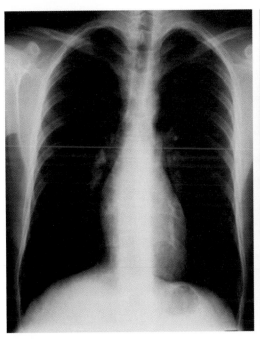
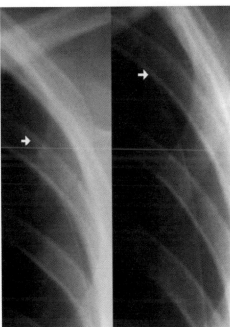

Figure 8.20. A tall, slender teen presents with a 1-hour history of pain in his chest and back occurring after lifting his mother. He describes the pain as knife-like and non-radiating. His pain worsens with deep inspiration. This CXR demonstrates how tall and slender he is. The lung fields appear to be hyperexpanded. However, lung markings are visible all the way to the periphery. A repeat CXR done as an expiratory view to help accentuate the pneumothorax reveals a small left apical pneumothorax (*white arrow*).

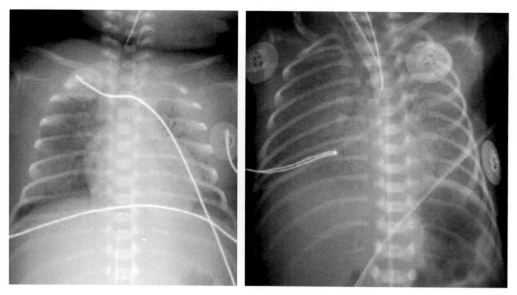

Figures 8.21 and 8.22. Hazy classic "ground-glass" (or "frosted glass") appearance of neonatal respiratory distress syndrome (RDS). Both CXRs show classic "air bronchograms." Air bronchograms occur because the air-filled bronchi normally overlie the air-filled lungs, rendering them invisible. However, because the RDS lungs have more fluid, the air-filled bronchi can be visualized. The denser the lungs are, the greater the visibility of the air bronchograms. Chest x-rays are frequently obtained to confirm endotracheal tube (ETT) position. In Figure 8.21, the ETT is high, and of the two vertical linear densities, the one on the patient's right is an umbilical venous catheter in the liver, whereas the other is a temperature probe wire on the patient's chest. In Figure 8.22, the ETT is in good position, but note that there is a nasogastric tube in the esophagus that is too high.

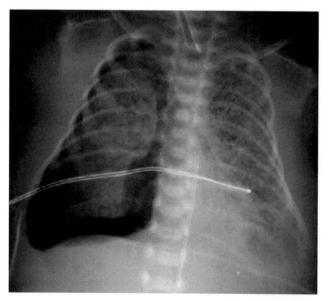

Figure 8.23. Neonate with a right pneumothorax. Also note that both lungs are very hazy with a speckled pattern of air. This appearance is due to pulmonary interstitial emphysema (PIE), in which tiny amounts of air have dissected into the lung parenchyma. PIE places the patient at high risk of pneumothorax. The ETT is high, and the umbilical artery catheter is at T7.

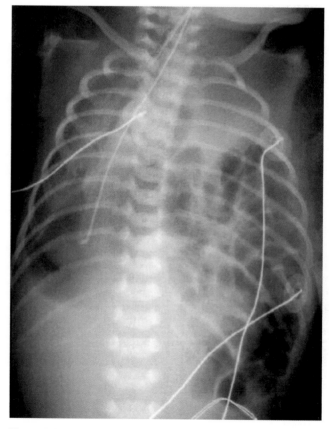

Figure 8.24. Diaphragmatic hernia. This figure shows the more common location on the patient's left.

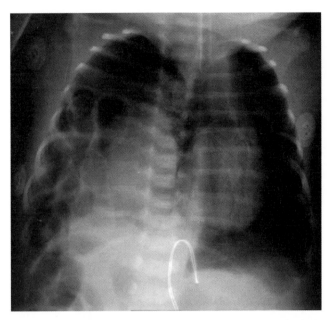

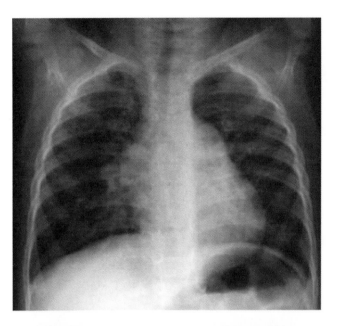

Figure 8.25. This diaphragmatic hernia is on the patient's right side (the less common side). This figure also shows a left pneumothorax, although this might be difficult to see on this image.

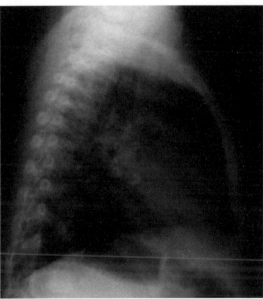

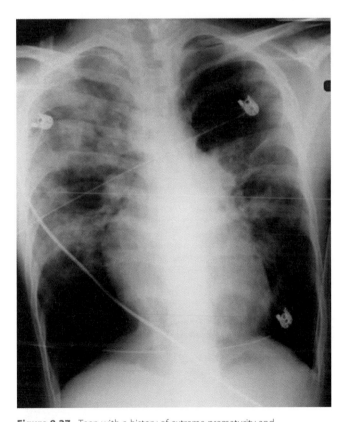

Figure 8.26. A 14-month-old with a history of extreme prematurity. This CXR shows chronic infiltrates from bronchopulmonary dysplasia.

Figure 8.27. Teen with a history of extreme prematurity and bronchopulmonary dysplasia. He has been hospitalized numerous times. This CXR demonstrates severe bronchopulmonary dysplasia and chronic lung disease with chronic infiltrates and focal areas of hyperexpansion.

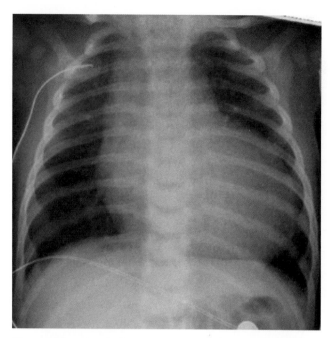

Figure 8.28. A 7-week-old with wheezing and coughing. This CXR shows cardiomegaly. The lung fields look relatively clear, but some early pulmonary vascular congestion might be present. Blood pressures were significantly higher in the upper extremities compared with the lower extremities. Echocardiography demonstrated aortic coarctation.

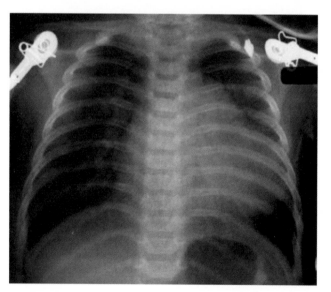

Figure 8.29. A 2-month-old with a ventricular septal defect (VSD). The cardiac silhouette is enlarged, and there is pulmonary vascular congestion. This CXR also shows thymic aplasia (DiGeorge syndrome).

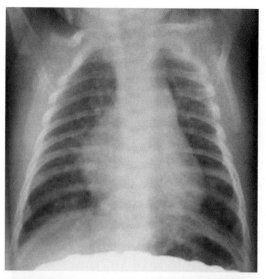

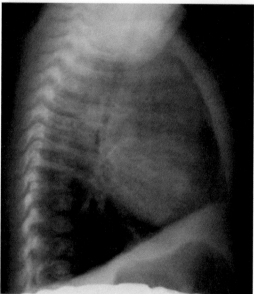

Figure 8.30. Borderline cardiomegaly with prominence of the right atrium and increased pulmonary vascularity. There are diffuse reticular markings fanning out from the hilum that suggest pulmonary venous congestion but are difficult to distinguish from perihilar infiltrates. These findings are suggestive of congenital heart disease. An echocardiogram confirmed cor triatriatum.

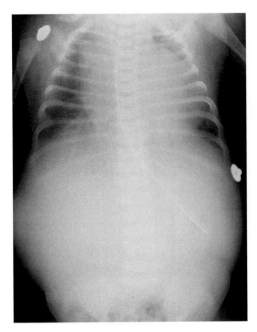

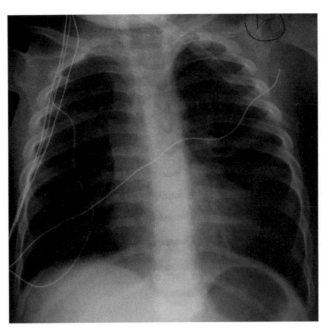

Figure 8.31. Cardiomegaly and a distended abdomen. This patient has multiple intrahepatic hemangiomas, resulting in arteriovenous shunting and high-output congestive heart failure.

Figure 8.32. A 6-month-old male infant presenting with wheezing and cyanosis. A heart murmur was previously noted and believed to be an isolated VSD. Administration of oxygen results in minimal improvement in his oxygen saturation. This CXR show a normal heart size. The lung fields look blacker than usual. Although this can sometimes be due to variations in CXR acquisition techniques, coupled with this clinical history suggestive of cyanotic congenital heart disease, it is likely that these lung fields are consistent with pulmonary hypoperfusion. This finding is seen in many of the cyanotic congenital heart disease conditions because bypassing the pulmonary circulation is common to most of these conditions. Plain film CXRs are not highly diagnostic in most congenital heart disease cases. However, an assessment of pulmonary perfusion is useful in establishing the diagnosis. The sudden change in appearance from pink to cyanotic is suggestive of tetralogy of Fallot, which was confirmed by echocardiography.

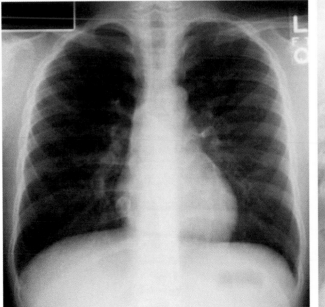

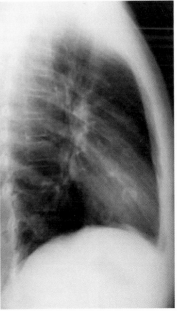

Figure 8.33. Circular calcification seen over the heart and in both PA and lateral views. This patient had a history of Kawasaki disease complicated by coronary aneurysms. The circular calcifications are calcified coronary aneurysms.

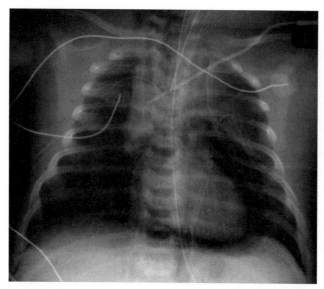

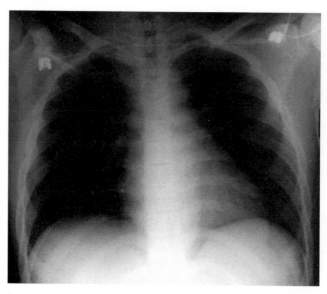

Figure 8.34. The patient is on a ventilator and has suddenly deteriorated, suggesting a tension pneumothorax. There is a lucency visible surrounding the heart, representing air dissecting into the pericardium, known as a pneumopericardium. Pneumopericardium is usually a serious emergency because it results in sudden cardiac tamponade. Immediate pericardiocentesis is required. This is a highly complication-prone procedure because it may lacerate the heart, and even if it temporarily relieves the tamponade, more air will continue to accumulate in the pericardial space, resulting in recurrent tamponade. Because of reaccumulation of air, inserting a plastic catheter into the pericardium using a catheter-over-needle or the Seldinger technique may be more effective in preventing reaccumulation of air and tamponade.

If a surgeon is immediately available, a pericardial window procedure may be more efficacious immediately following pericardiocentesis.

Figure 8.35. CXR from a 14-year-old presenting with severe back, chest, and abdominal pain. A family history of aortic dissection raises suspicion that the aortic shadow might be widened. A CT scan confirms aortic dissection.

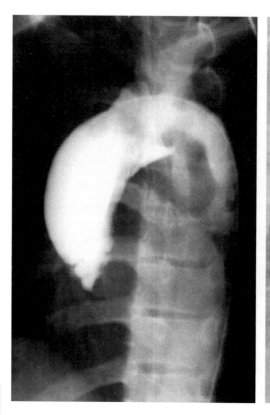

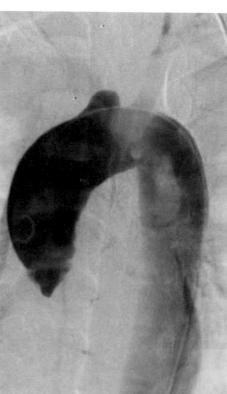

Figure 8.36. Aortogram that shows the catheter tip at the aortic root. The aortic root is irregular. Because contrast does not enter the carotid vessels, the catheter is presumed to be in the false lumen of the aortic dissection, which is dilated at the aortic root. An imprint of the brachiocephalic artery (a noncontrast-filled vessel impinging on the contrast-filled false aortic lumen) is seen overlying the aorta.

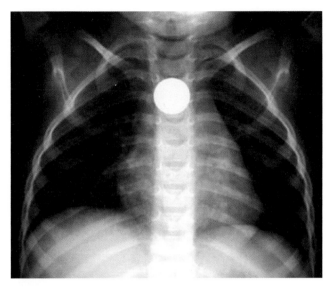

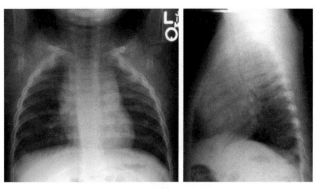

Figure 8.37. Esophageal coin. Although this is a very common problem, if the history suggests that the coin has been lodged in the esophagus for a long time, there is a significant risk that the coin has eroded through the esophagus. If the patient presents with hemoptysis, hematemesis, or melena, this suggests that the coin might have eroded through the esophagus into one of the great vessels, such as the vena cava or the aorta, known as aortoesophageal syndrome. If the coin is removed, vena cava or aortic hemorrhage could result in exsanguination and death. If aortoesophageal syndrome is suspected (i.e., the integrity of the aorta or vena cava is in question), a cardiovascular surgery team should be standing by for immediate surgical intervention should a perforation of a major vessel be present.

Figure 8.38. A 6-month-old with a history of frequent wheezing episodes. The PA view shows clear lung fields. The lateral view shows no infiltrates, but the tracheal air column is very narrow. From the hilum to the top of the image, the tracheal diameter is narrow. With a history of frequent wheezing episodes in an infant, a narrow tracheal diameter suggests the possibility of a congenital malformation involving the trachea. Possibilities include intrinsic tracheomalacia or a tracheal malformation, or extrinsic compression on the trachea. An esophagram (see Fig. 8.39) demonstrates a mass impinging on the esophagus. This is highly suggestive of a vascular ring with a large vessel impinging on the esophagus and the trachea.

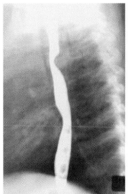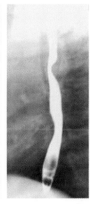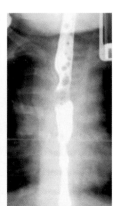

Figure 8.39. A vascular ring is a malformation in which a major vascular structure surrounds the esophagus and the trachea, compressing both structures. This is a diagram of a double aortic arch, which is one of the common vascular rings. In the double aortic arch, the aorta passes over both the left and the right mainstem bronchi. The vascular ring structure compresses the esophagus and the trachea.

Double Aortic Arch

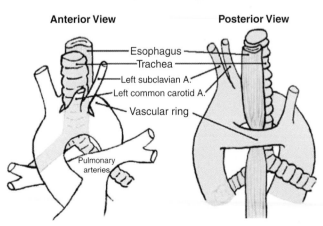

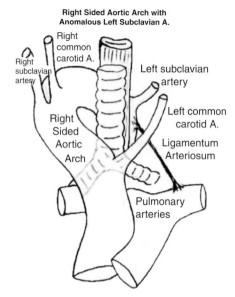

Right Sided Aortic Arch with Anomalous Left Subclavian A.

Figure 8.40. Diagram of a right-sided aortic arch with an anomalous left subclavian vein. The "ring" is formed by the right-sided aorta, the ligamentum arteriosum (formerly the ductus arteriosus), and the pulmonary arteries.

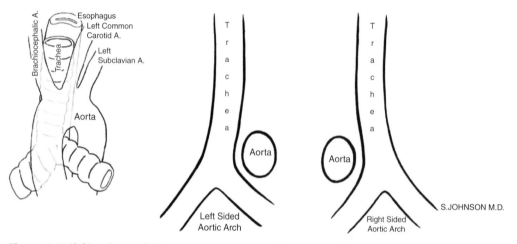

Figures 8.41 (*left*) and 8.42 (*right*). Figure 8.41 diagrams the normal left-sided aortic arch (i.e., the aorta arches over the left mainstem bronchus). Figure 8.42 diagrams the phenomenon of tracheal deviation. In the normal left-sided aortic arch, the distal trachea is deviated slightly to the right. This is sometimes evident on the PA view of a CXR. However, in a right-sided aortic arch, the distal trachea will often deviate to the left. This is an abnormal sign and should suggest a right-sided aortic arch. However, if the malformation is a double-sided aortic arch, then the trachea will be midline, which is not necessarily abnormal. In summary, the abnormal plain chest radiographic findings that suggest a vascular ring are a narrow tracheal shadow (suggesting tracheal compression) and deviation of the distal trachea to the left (if a right-sided aortic arch is present).

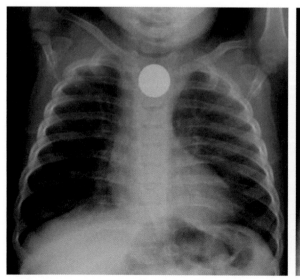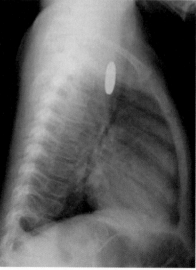

Figure 8.43. A 15-month-old who swallowed a coin. This CXR identifies the coin in the upper esophagus. However, note that on the lateral view, the tracheal air column is compressed. Although this could be due to the coin, the patient's history of chronic recurrent respiratory symptoms suggests a chronic condition. This patient also turned out to have a vascular ring.

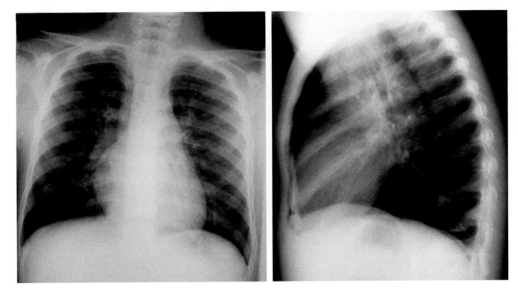

Figure 8.44. Pneumomediastinum. There are vertical air densities in the neck (subcutaneous emphysema). The lateral view reveals double outlining of the trachea. Normally, the tracheal air column is visible as a single air column. However, in the lateral view, the wall of the trachea has separate air outlines. This indicates air dissecting around the trachea. Additional air densities are noted in lower anterior chest (anterior to the heart).

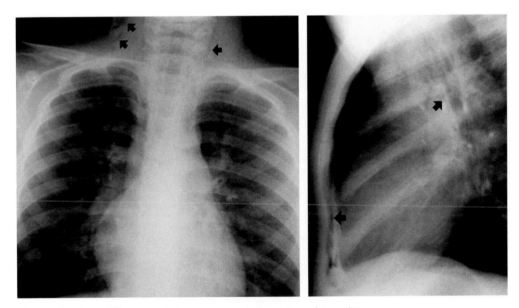

Figure 8.45. Same CXR as Figure 8.44, with arrows pointing at these abnormalities.

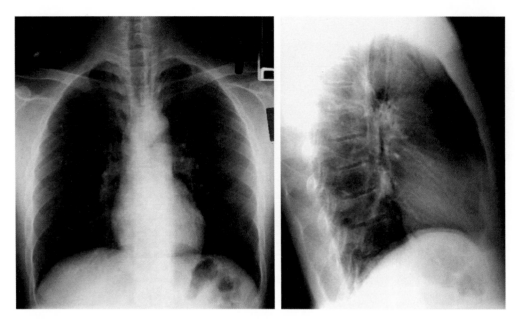

Figure 8.46. Teen presenting with chest pain who admits to substance abuse. The PA view shows vertical air densities in the upper mediastinum and neck. There is a triangular air density on the left aspect of the patient's aortic arch. This is due to air in the mediastinum that accentuates the aorta and the pulmonary arteries. The lateral view reveals a double outline of the tracheal air shadow similar to what is shown in Figures 8.44 and 8.45. Also visible are air densities in the anterior mediastinum (in the region of the thymus). Patients at risk of pulmonary air leaks (e.g., pneumomediastinum) often have a history of increasing intrathoracic pressure. Carrying something heavy, playing a musical instrument (e.g., the trombone), or inhaling illicit drugs (accompanied by a Valsalva) all result in increasing intrathoracic pressure.

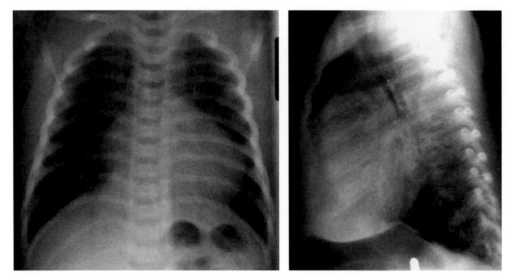

Figure 8.47. CXR from a newborn who is diagnosed with a VSD in the nursery. He presents a few days later with a seizure. The cardiac silhouette is enlarged (consistent with a VSD with mild congestive heart failure). The other significant radiographic abnormality is the absence of a thymic shadow, suggesting thymic aplasia. The "seizure" is found to be due to hypocalcemia (tetany). This patient has DiGeorge syndrome (thymic aplasia with hypoparathyroidism).

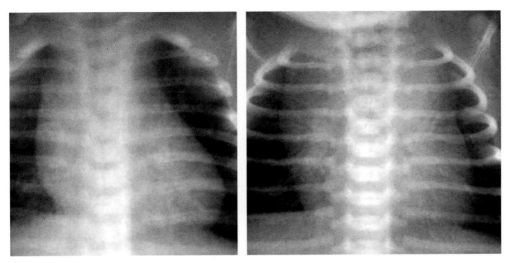

Figure 8.48. Two newborn CXRs with prominent thymic shadows, which is what is normally seen. Note that the upper mediastinum in Figure 8.47 shows a thin upper mediastinum.

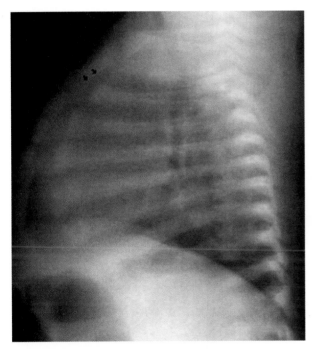

Figure 8.49. Normal lateral CXR in neonates. The mediastinum (*black arrows*) is normally filled with solid tissue (the normal prominent thymus) in the newborn. Note that in Figure 8.47 the lateral view shows lung tissue density (absent thymus). This is the normal pattern in older children, teens, and adults, but newborns should have a thymus in this area, as seen in this figure.

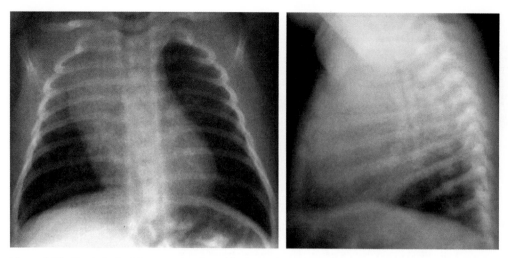

Figure 8.50. Density in the right upper chest is partially the usual prominent thymus for this age. The thymic shadow is larger on the infant's right than on his left. There is a density in the right upper lobe, but it is obscured by the thymus. Part of this density appears to be from the scapula, but on close inspection, there are densities suggesting infiltrates aside from the thymus and the scapula in the right upper lobe. This pneumonia is partially obscured by the thymus and the scapula.

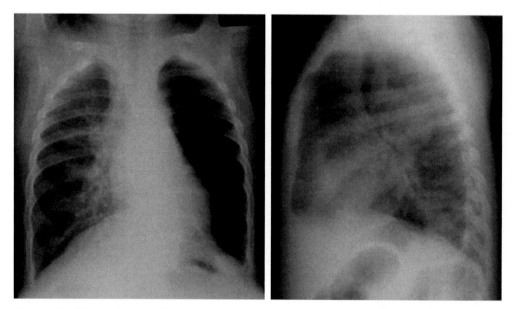

Figure 8.51. A 10-month-old male infant presenting with wheezing and coughing. He has a history of wheezing episodes. The PA view demonstrates decreased pulmonary vascularity and hyperlucency of the left lung. The right lung demonstrates increased pulmonary vascularity. The lateral view demonstrates a mass effect posterior to the lower portion of the trachea, which compresses and bows the trachea anteriorly, with considerable narrowing of the inferior portion. These findings are suspicious for a large mediastinal mass that is compressing the lower trachea and mainstem bronchus, causing obstructive emphysema of the left lung and decreased perfusion of this lung. A barium esophagram is ordered.

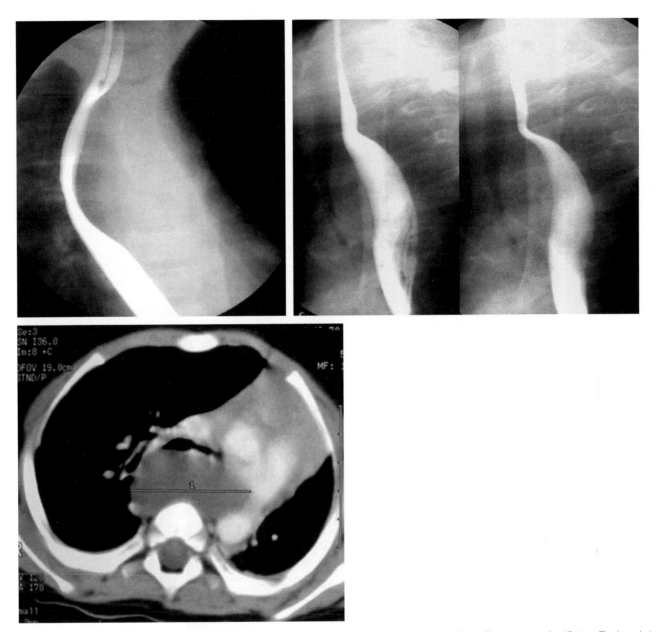

Figures 8.52 (*above*) and 8.53 (*below left*). Figure 8.52 is a barium study. The esophagus is displaced laterally, as seen on the AP view. The lateral views demonstrate the mass located between the trachea (the tracheal air column is compressed and displaced anteriorly) and the barium-filled esophagus (which is displaced posteriorly). A CT scan of the chest confirms the presence of a mediastinal mass identified as a bronchogenic cyst (Fig. 8.53).

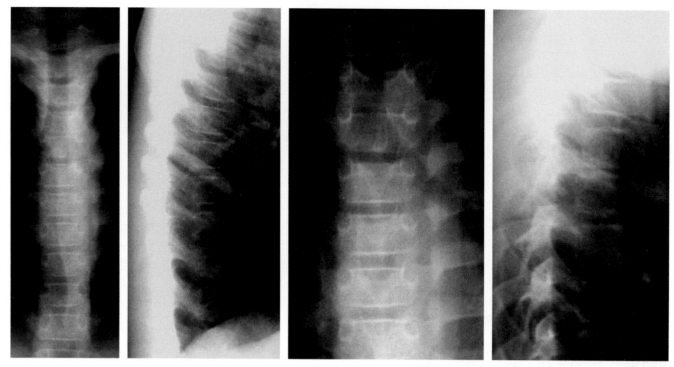

Figure 8.54. An 8-year-old boy presenting with fever. He is noted to have focal tenderness in his upper thoracic spine on exam. The two images on the left show AP and lateral thoracic spine views. Note the narrowed intervertebral space at the tracheal bifurcation. This is not easily appreciated on the lateral view. The pair of images on the right are enlargements of this area, and in both the PA and lateral views, intervertebral space narrowing is evident. These findings are consistent with discitis.

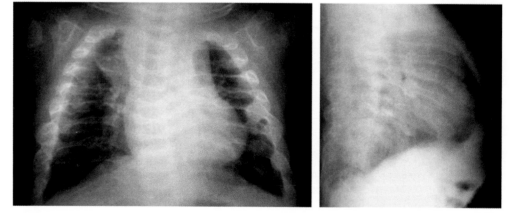

Figure 8.55. A 3-month-old male infant presenting with respiratory distress. He has a history of osteogenesis imperfecta diagnosed in the newborn period. This CXR shows severe osteopenia, multiple healing rib fractures (the bulbous deformities of the ribs), and severe irregularities of the vertebral column. There are multiple types of osteogenesis imperfecta. Most of the types diagnosed in the newborn period demonstrate multiple fractures and obvious severe osteopenia. The severe type is usually autosomal recessive and not compatible with long-term survival. The more occult types of osteogenesis imperfecta are autosomal dominant (so a positive family history of frequent fractures is usually present unless the patient is a new mutation) and not obviously osteopenic, yet the history suggests a greater-than-expected frequency of fractures.

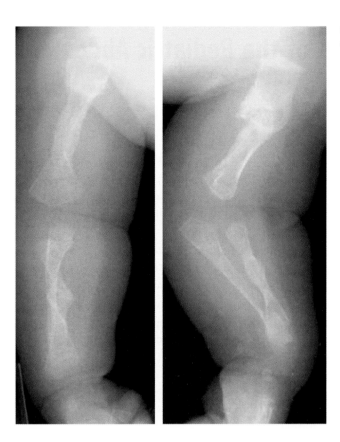

Figure 8.56. Patient's upper extremities, which demonstrate severe osteopenia and multiple fractures with the classic "crumpled" appearance of the long bones.

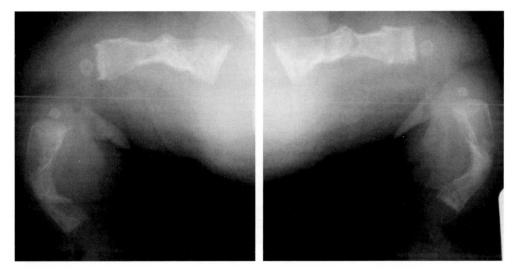

Figure 8.57. Patient's lower extremities, which demonstrate severe osteopenia and multiple fractures with the classic "crumpled" appearance of the long bones.

Plain Film Radiographs of the Pediatric Abdomen

Loren G. Yamamoto

Indications

Plain film radiographs of the pediatric abdomen ordered from the ED are indicated in stable patients to help diagnose abdominal medical complaints. The radiographic findings on plain film abdominal radiographs are often nonspecific or subtle.

Diagnostic capabilities

Plain film radiographs contrast differences in the standard five radiographic densities (metallic, calcific/bone, soft tissue/water, fat, and air) to assist in the diagnostic process. In an abdominal series, two basic views are generally obtained: flat (supine) and upright (erect). Other views include a prone view and an anteroposterior (AP) view of the chest. Occasionally, a single view is obtained to look for metallic foreign bodies, calcific urolithiasis, or other specific indications. The term KUB (kidney-ureter-bladder) is often used to order abdominal radiographs, but this term should be avoided because it is ambiguous as to whether one view or multiple views are desired. The standard upright view is useful to see the abdomen generally. It should be noted that gravity will make the liver and the spleen appear larger on this view than on the flat (supine) view. Air-fluid levels can only be viewed on the upright view because the air-fluid interface will be parallel with the x-ray beam. Free air is best viewed on the upright view because it has a tendency to collect under the diaphragm when the patient is upright. The flat view is useful to confirm the location of any suspicious findings. Soft tissue structures that were obliterated by overlying gas on the upright will be easier to see on the flat view because the gas will be layered perpendicular to the x-ray beam.

Imaging pitfalls and limitations

As noted in Chapter 8, plain film image abnormalities are subtle, and, especially with the abdomen, identifying these diagnostic abnormalities are greatly benefited by viewing examples of these subtle abnormalities in a chapter such as this.

Abdominal contents and diagnostic possibilities

Bowel: Ileus, bowel obstruction, midgut volvulus, bowel perforation, appendicitis, intussusception, pneumatosis intestinalis, foreign bodies

Liver: Abscess, intrahepatic air, hepatomegaly

Pancreas: Difficult to image with plain film radiographs; calcification might be evident

Spleen: Splenomegaly

Kidneys: Renolithiasis, staghorn calculus, ureterolithiasis

Bladder: Distended/dilated bladder, ruptured bladder

Peritoneum: Free air, neoplastic mass, abscess

Bones: Hip dysplasia, hip effusion, other hip pathology, leukemia, lymphoma, extramedullary hematopoiesis, fractures, dysplasia, osteopenia, osteomalacia, osteogenesis imperfecta, bony neoplasms

Muscles: Intramuscular abscesses, muscular calcification

Lungs (often overlooked): Lower lobe pneumonia, pleural effusion

Female reproductive tract: Most commonly nondiagnostic using plain film radiographs

Clinical images

Ileus versus bowel obstruction

There are several criteria that have been proposed to distinguish an ileus from a bowel obstruction. The term "ileus" means various things to different people (e.g., radiologist vs. gastroenterologist). However, the common feature is that suboptimal peristalsis results in radiographic abnormalities. An abdominal series is often obtained in patients with abdominal pain or patients who are vomiting. This is the most likely scenario in which an ileus is encountered.

The criteria for distinguishing a bowel obstruction from an ileus include roughly four findings. Because two of the findings are similar, some have suggested simplifying these to only three findings. However, for this discussion, all four are discussed:

1. *Gas distribution.* Does the gas pattern show distribution in all four quadrants of the abdomen? Is the overall quantity of gas best characterized as too much, just right, or too little (paucity). An example of "just right" is seen in Figure 9.1. A paucity of gas suggests a bowel obstruction, as seen in Figure 9.2. Too much gas can be normal in crying infants as long as the bowel is not distended, as seen in Figure 9.3. Thus, only a paucity of gas should be regarded as a positive finding toward a bowel obstruction.

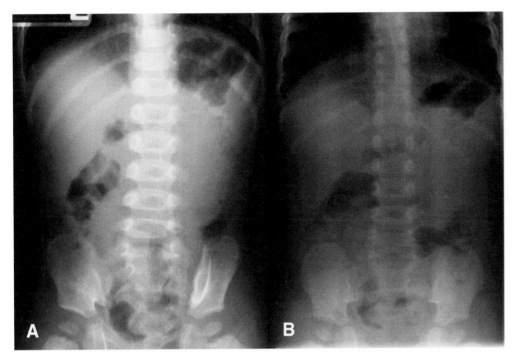

Figure 9.1. Gas distribution: unremarkable. The flat view does not have much gas in the central portion of the abdomen, but the upright view looks better.
Bowel distention: none. No smooth bowel walls.
Air-fluid levels: none.
Orderliness: disorderly like popcorn rather than orderly sausages.
Bowel obstruction: no.

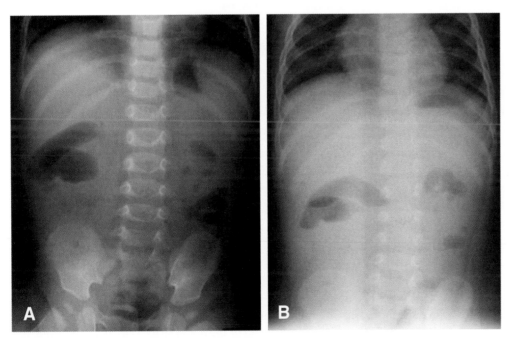

Figure 9.2. Gas distribution: best described as a paucity of gas.
Bowel distention: the few bowel segments that are seen are very smooth. The bowel walls resemble short hoses. Abnormal bowel distention is present.
Air-fluid levels: at first glance, this might not be obvious, but see Figure 9.6, which is the same x-ray, with white and black lines drawn. Note that these air-fluid levels are suggestive of an obstruction because two air-fluid levels are seen in the same segment of bowel (the J-turn, hairpin, or candy cane loop).
Orderliness: orderly. Looks more like sausages than popcorn.
Bowel obstruction: yes.

145

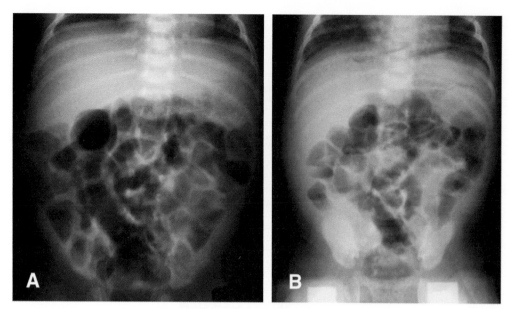

Figure 9.3. Gas distribution: a lot of gas in all parts of the bowel.
Bowel distention: although a lot of gas is present, there are no smooth segments that would suggest abnormal bowel distention.
Air-fluid levels: none.
Orderliness: disorderly. Looks more like popcorn than sausages.
Bowel obstruction: no.

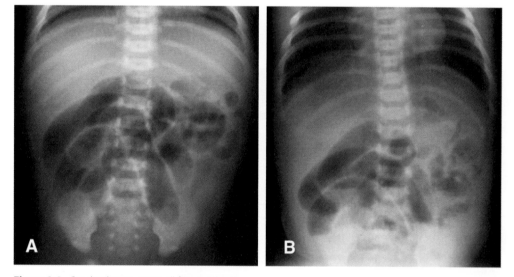

Figure 9.4. Gas distribution: gas in all four quadrants.
Bowel distention: yes. The bowel walls are smooth (resembling hoses or sausages).
Air-fluid levels: yes. If you carefully follow the bowel loops, at least one and probably two loops of bowel contain two air-fluid levels within the same bowel loop.
Orderliness: orderly. Looks more like sausages than popcorn.
Bowel obstruction: yes.

2. *Bowel distention.* Because children come in different sizes, measuring the diameter of the bowel does not result in reliable criteria. In normal bowel, the plicae in the small bowel and the haustra in the large bowel result in the normal bowel shape that is best characterized as irregular. This has also been described as resembling popcorn, especially the small bowel, as seen in Figure 9.3. However, when the bowel is distended, its walls become smooth, such that the bowel resembles smooth sausages or hoses, as seen in Figure 9.4. Distended bowel loses the irregularities of the bowel shape caused by plications and haustrations so that the bowel looks smooth. In children, the bowel distention feature is based on appearance and not diameter.

3. *Air-fluid levels.* Air-fluid levels are seen only on the upright view. An ileus tends to have multiple small air-fluid levels, whereas a bowel obstruction tends to have larger loops with J-turns (also known as hairpin

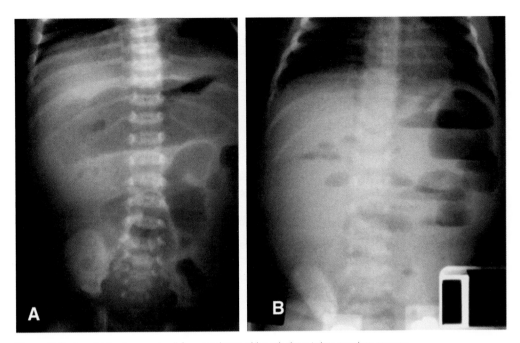

Figure 9.5. Gas distribution: gas in all four quadrants, although there is less gas than average.

Bowel distention: although there is one segment in which the diameter of the bowel is large, there is no segment that has smooth bowel walls resembling hoses or sausages.

Air-fluid levels: many air fluid levels, but note that they are all small and none can be clearly identified to be in the same bowel loop (no J-turn or candy cane phenomenon).

Orderliness: questionable. The flat view looks somewhat orderly, but the upright view looks disorderly. The flat view is best for determining this, which leans toward orderliness.

Bowel obstruction: no. This is more likely to be an ileus associated with gastroenteritis. The multiple small air-fluid levels are typical, and the other bowel obstruction findings are not present. The orderliness criterion is indeterminate.

turns and candy cane loops). The J-turn phenomenon is most indicative of a bowel obstruction when you can identify two separate air-fluid levels in the same loop of bowel. Note the difference in Figure 9.5, where there are multiple small air-fluid levels, as compared to Figure 9.6 (same x-ray as Fig. 9.2), which has large distended loops and visible air-fluid levels (two of which can be seen in the same contiguous loop of bowel). The white lines in Figure 9.6 show the two air-fluid levels in the same loop of bowel. The black lines in Figure 9.6 show the two air-fluid levels in another loop of bowel. Review Figure 9.2 to see this x-ray without the lines.

4. *Orderliness.* This is really a combination of the features described in the second and third criteria, which is why this might not be a characteristic by itself. This term is vague, but it is meant to describe whether there is a random or disorderly appearance of the bowel gas on a flat (supine) view versus an orderly view. The random or disorderly appearance is best described as a bag of popcorn (Fig. 9.3). The orderly appearance has been described as a step ladder, but a better description is a bag of sausages, as seen in Figure 9.4. Look at Figure 9.3. Does it look like popcorn (Fig. 9.7) or sausages (Fig. 9.8)? Look at Figure 9.4. Does it look like popcorn (Fig. 9.7) or sausages (Fig. 9.8)?

A bowel obstruction can present radiographically as a paucity of gas or a lot of gas. The differential diagnosis of a bowel obstruction can be remembered with the mnemonic AIM, actually double AIM, or A-A-I-I-M-M (adhesions, appendicitis, incarcerated hernia, intussusception, malrotation [with midgut volvulus], and Meckel's diverticulum [with a volvulus or intussusception]). It should be noted that non-bowel obstruction x-rays do not necessarily represent a benign diagnosis. Although an ileus picture is most often seen with gastroenteritis, more serious diagnoses can still be present, the most common of which is appendicitis.

Applying these four criteria to the x-rays that have been presented so far yields the diagnoses present in Figures 9.1 through 9.14.

Midgut volvulus and malrotation

The term "volvulus" by itself is used imprecisely in this condition. A sigmoid volvulus (due to redundant sigmoid bowel) occurs more often in elderly patients (Fig. 9.15), whereas a midgut volvulus is a true surgical emergency. The small bowel is lengthy, and it is amazing that it does not twist on itself more often. A normal bowel configuration suspends the small bowel to the posterior abdominal wall via broad mesenteric attachments. Figure 9.16 depicts this schematically. With this configuration, it is very difficult for the bowel to twist and infarct itself. However, in the

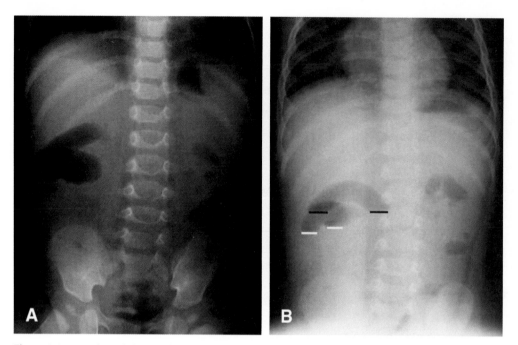

Figure 9.6. Large distended loops of bowel with visible air-fluid levels (two of which can be seen in the same contiguous loop of bowel). The white lines in this figure show the two air-fluid levels in the same loop of bowel. The black lines in this figure show the two air-fluid levels in the another loop of bowel. Figure 9.2 shows this same x-ray without the lines drawn.

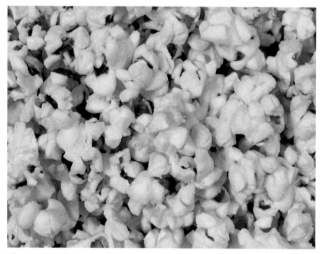

Figure 9.7. Example of popcorn. It may be helpful to think of this image when assessing an abdominal film for a normal bowel gas appearance.

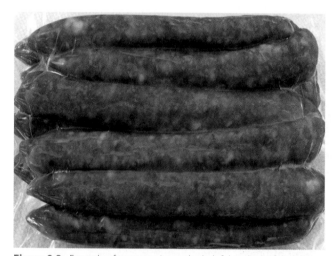

Figure 9.8. Example of sausages. It may be helpful to think of this image when considering a small bowel obstruction.

malrotation configuration, as shown in Figure 9.17, the small bowel is not suspended by a broad mesenteric attachment but rather a stalk of mesentery. The term "malrotation" places emphasis on the embryology of this malformation, seemingly reducing the importance of its clinical consequences. The malrotation malformation shown in Figure 9.17 should be renamed as "guts on a stalk" syndrome to refocus attention on the clinical consequence of this malformation. Guts on a stalk are prone to twisting as a midgut volvulus (illustrated in Fig. 9.18). A midgut volvulus is potentially catastrophic and is a true surgical emergency. The midgut volvulus involves the entire

small bowel, and if surgical reduction is delayed, the entire small bowel will undergo necrosis. It is imperative to make this diagnosis as soon as possible and to arrange for immediate surgical reduction to restore bowel perfusion.

Ladd's bands can also cause a bowel obstruction in malrotation. In Figure 9.17, the mesenteric attachment (the stalk in the LUQ) can compress the duodenum as it descends. This compression can also result in a high bowel obstruction. However, this does not compromise blood flow, and it is not nearly as emergent and serious as a midgut volvulus.

Patients born with a malrotation (guts on a stalk) are likely to sustain a midgut volvulus at some point in their lives.

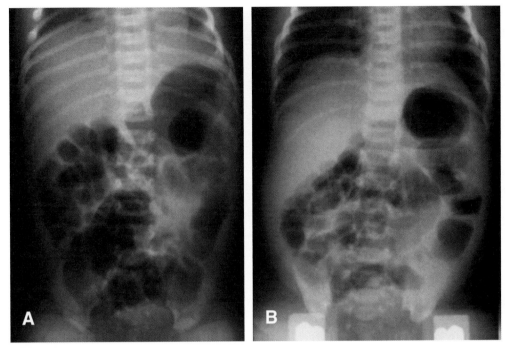

Figure 9.9. Gas distribution: a lot of gas in all four quadrants.
Bowel distention: possible, but not probable. The popcorn-like appearance is preserved so that, in most instances, the bowel is not distended. Bowel in the left lower quadrant (LLQ) might be smooth for a short segment, but the haustra appear to be preserved.
Air-fluid levels: no.
Orderliness: disorderly. Looks more like popcorn than sausages.
Bowel obstruction: no.

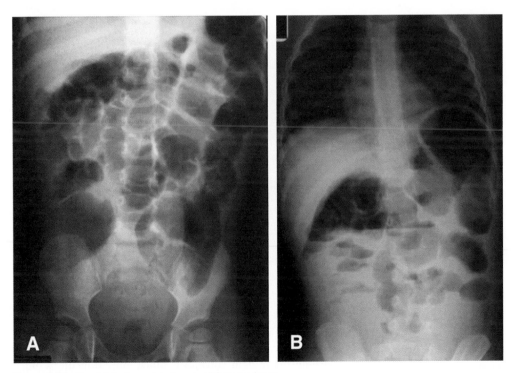

Figure 9.10. Gas distribution: a lot of gas in all four quadrants.
Bowel distention: possible, but not probable. In some areas, the bowel diameter is large, but this is not the criterion to determine bowel distention in children. Bowel distention is confirmed when the bowel walls are smooth (like hoses and sausages).
Air-fluid levels: many air-fluid levels, but note that they are all small and none can be clearly identified to be in the same bowel loop (no J-turn or candy cane phenomenon).
Orderliness: disorderly. Looks more like popcorn than sausages.
Bowel obstruction: no.

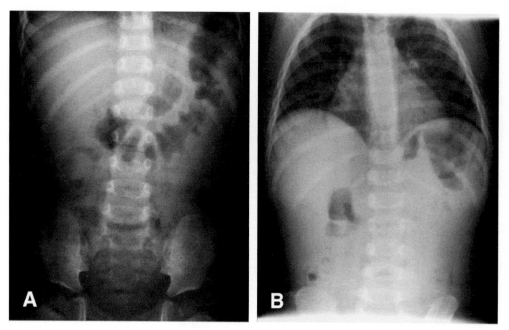

Figure 9.11. Gas distribution: a moderate amount of gas in most of the abdomen, except for the LLQ.
Bowel distention: no.
Air-fluid levels: no.
Orderliness: disorderly. Does not look like popcorn probably because the amount of gas is diminished.
Bowel obstruction: no.
The diagnosis is colitis. Note the transverse colon (mostly in the left upper quadrant [LUQ] of the flat view) has a finding described as thumbprinting. These indentations in the colon are found in colitis.

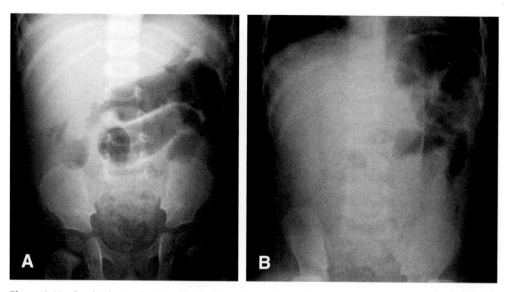

Figure 9.12. Gas distribution: limited to the upper quadrants. Not much gas in the lower quadrants. The upright view has gas limited to the LUQ.
Bowel distention: yes. The bowel walls are smooth. This looks like a twin pack of sausages.
Air-fluid levels: no.
Orderliness: orderly. Looks more like sausages than popcorn.
Bowel obstruction: yes.

Roughly 50% of malrotation patients will present with a midgut volvulus in the neonatal period. Most of the others will present in the pediatric age range. However, it is possible that a malrotation will not undergo a midgut volvulus until later in life. A midgut volvulus emergency should be immediately suspected in any neonate with bilious vomiting.

Diagnosing midgut volvulus is much more difficult in older children because the level of suspicion is lower.

Figures 9.19 and 9.20 show plain film x-rays of neonates with a midgut volvulus. In Figure 9.19, the x-ray is totally gasless. Coupled with a history of bilious vomiting, a gasless abdominal x-ray should prompt an immediate surgical

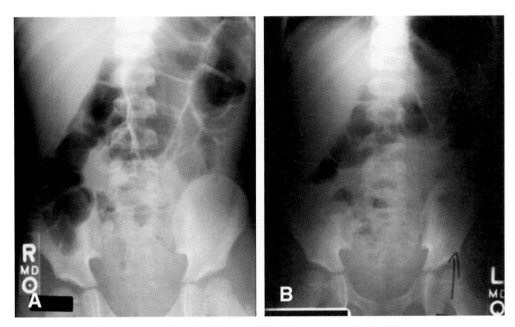

Figure 9.13. Gas distribution: gas is distributed in most of the abdomen except for the LLQ.
  Bowel distention: no.
  Air-fluid levels: no.
  Orderliness: disorderly. Looks more like popcorn than sausages.
  Bowel obstruction: no.
  Did you notice the circular appendicolith in the right lower quadrant (RLQ)? This patient has appendicitis.

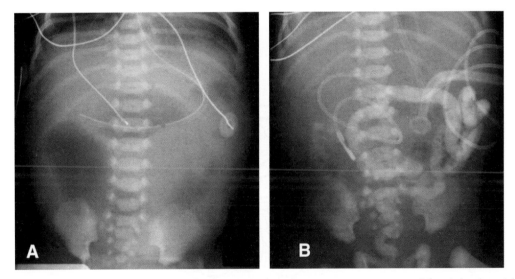

Figure 9.14. X-ray from a newborn. One of the concerns with newborns, neonates, or very young infants is that they might have a congenital malformation that has yet to reveal itself. The left image is a flat view, whereas the right image has contrast in the lower bowel.
  Gas distribution: poor. There are four large bubbles of gas, and the rest of the abdomen is fairly gasless. This should be regarded as a poor gas distribution, suggesting a bowel obstruction.
  Bowel distention: probably, but not definite. Considering the large gas collection on the right is unlikely to be the stomach, it is too large to be normal nondistended bowel.
  Air-fluid levels: no.
  Orderliness: orderly. This clearly does not resemble popcorn or sausages, but it is orderly and not random or disorderly.
  Bowel obstruction: yes.
  The contrast enema on the right shows a microcolon indicating the absence of bowel contents passing to the colon during gestation. In a proximal small bowel obstruction, a microcolon is usually not present. The presence of a microcolon suggests that the distal small bowel is also atretic.

consultation for a suspected midgut volvulus. In Figure 9.20, the x-ray gas pattern is fairly normal. Despite this, bilious vomiting in a neonate should still raise the suspicion of a midgut volvulus. An advanced imaging study is indicated to check for this possibility because of the emergent time-dependent nature of a midgut volvulus.

Figure 9.21 is an abdominal series of a 3-month-old infant presenting with bilious vomiting. Although not a neonate, the

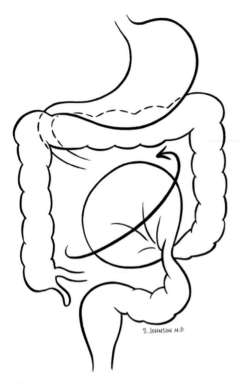

Figure 9.15.

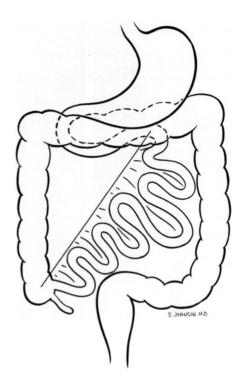

Figure 9.16.

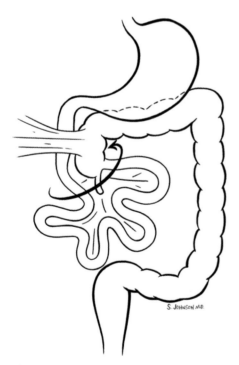

Figure 9.17.

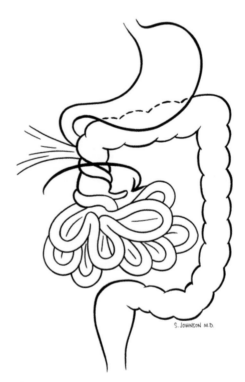

Figure 9.18.

infant is still very young, and bilious emesis should immediately raise the suspicion of a midgut volvulus. Figure 9.21 shows poor gas distribution. Most of the gas is trapped in the stomach, suggesting a high bowel obstruction. The small amount of residual gas in the LLQ should not be reassuring because this infant had been doing well for 3 months (plenty of time to feed, excrete stool, and form normal amounts of gas in the colon) prior to a midgut volvulus. This x-ray should be highly suspicious for a bowel obstruction. Although intussusception might also be possible, it generally obstructs in the

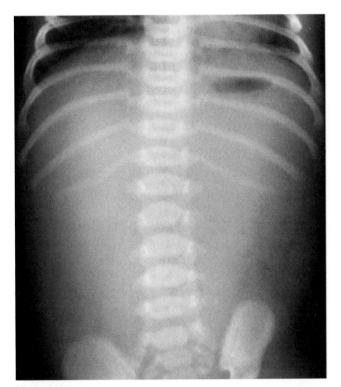

Figure 9.19.

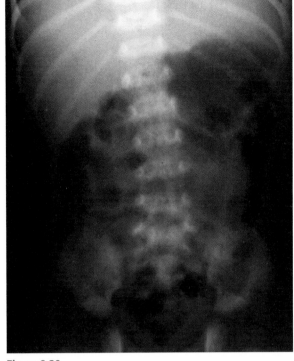

Figure 9.20.

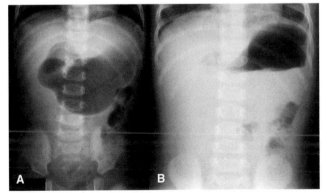

Figure 9.21.

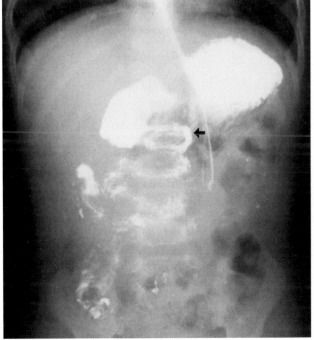

Figure 9.22.

ileocecal region (i.e., much lower). The dilated stomach seen here suggests a high obstruction, such as a midgut volvulus.

In Figure 9.22, a nasogastric tube has been placed, and thin barium has been administered into the stomach. Note the corkscrew appearance of the small bowel as the barium exits the stomach (*black arrow*). The corkscrew of the barium is the twist of the midgut volvulus, as illustrated in Figure 9.23. If the gastric contrast is unable to exit the stomach, the image will result in an abrupt halt of the advancing contrast. This "beak" appearance is indicative of a midgut volvulus.

Thin contrast such as thin barium or water-soluble contrast is more likely to demonstrate the corkscrew appearance in Figures 9.22 and 9.23.

153

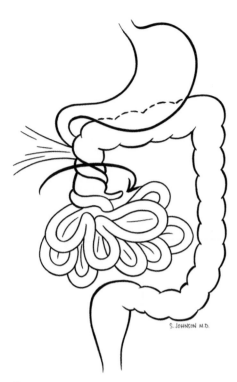

Figure 9.23.

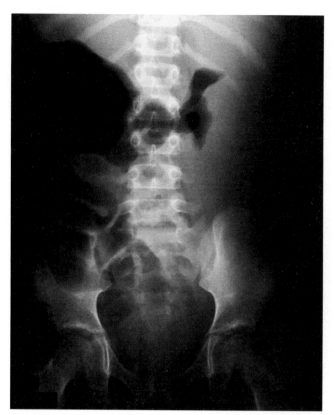

Figure 9.24.

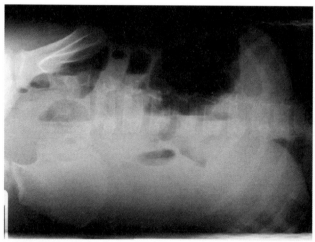

Figure 9.25.

Figures 9.24 and 9.25 are an abdominal series from a 7-year-old girl presenting with vomiting and abdominal pain of sudden onset. Figure 9.24 is the flat view. Figure 9.25 is a later decubitus view because the patient was too ill to stand.

In both figures, the distribution of gas is very asymmetric, with dilated bowel in the left and almost no bowel on the right. The lateral decubitus view demonstrates some air-fluid level in the same bowel loop (J-turn), which is highly suggestive of a bowel obstruction. This patient was diagnosed with a midgut volvulus due to malrotation. This patient's past history is interesting in that she had periodically complained of inter-mittent abdominal pain, as well as vomiting and dehydration that resolved. In a patient with a malrotation, the midgut could

undergo a volvulus at any time (guts on a stalk). As the volvulus initiates its first twist, there is roughly an even chance of twisting further (getting tighter) or untwisting itself. This twisting and untwisting result in "intermittent volvulus," which presents with pain and vomiting that resolves on its own. Patients with such a history should be imaged to determine if they have a malrotation that is intermittently twisting.

When a patient presents with severe acute symptoms, an imaging strategy should focus on confirming the presence of a midgut volvulus. However, if the patient is well on presenta-tion but gives a history of intermittent symptoms that suggest the possibility of an intermittent volvulus, then the imaging strategy should focus on confirming the presence of a malrotation. The best imaging study to confirm the presence of a malrotation is an upper GI series. As noted in Figure 9.16, the upper GI series will demonstrate contrast passing from the stomach into the duodenum. The duodenum crosses the mid-line from right to left. It is suspended on the left by the ligament of Treitz. In a malrotation, as diagrammed in Figure 9.17, the duodenum fails to cross the midline from right to left. This confirms the presence of a malrotation. A contrast enema can potentially identify a malrotation if the cecum is misplaced. However, in viewing Figure 9.17, it is possible for the cecum to be in the mid right abdomen, or even the RLQ. If the cecum is floating and just happens to be in the correct location when the contrast enema is performed, it will fail to identify the malrotation. An abdominal ultrasound can also demonstrate a malrotation by examining the vascular supply of the bowel.

However, the best imaging study to identify a malrotation is the upper GI series.

Appendicitis

Appendicitis is common. Roughly half of the patients with appendicitis will have an atypical presentation in which the diagnosis will be extremely difficult to establish clinically. Plain film radiographs have a limited role in diagnosing appendicitis. Ultrasound, CT scanning, and MRI are more advanced imaging modalities that are better suited to confirming the diagnosis of appendicitis.

The best known plain film sign of appendicitis is the presence of an appendicolith (sometimes called a fecalith). This radiographic sign is uncommon in acute appendicitis, but when it is present, it is highly suggestive of acute appendicitis. Because it is uncommon, most clinicians will encounter only a few appendicoliths in their career. Appendicoliths are generally in the RLQ of the abdomen, but their shape and appearance are highly variable. Figures 9.26 through 9.41 show a series of different appendicoliths.

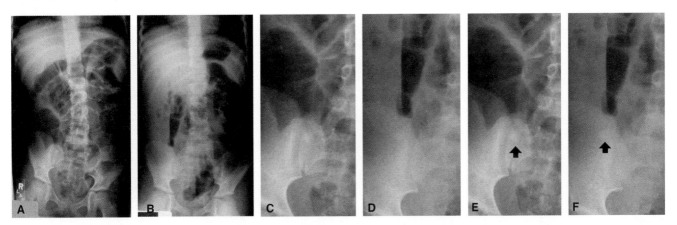

Figure 9.26. RLQ close-up RLQ appendicolith.

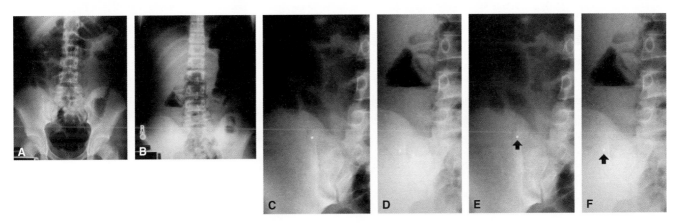

Figure 9.27. RLQ close-up RLQ appendicolith.

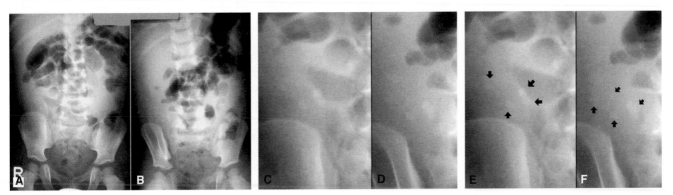

Figure 9.28. RLQ close-up RLQ appendicoliths.

155

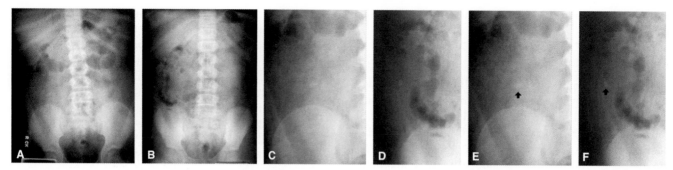

Figure 9.29. RLQ close-up RLQ appendicolith.

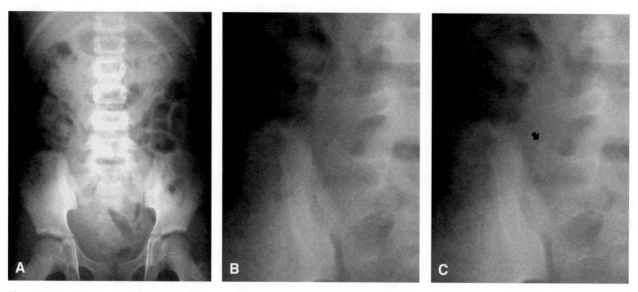

Figure 9.30. RLQ close-up RLQ appendicolith.

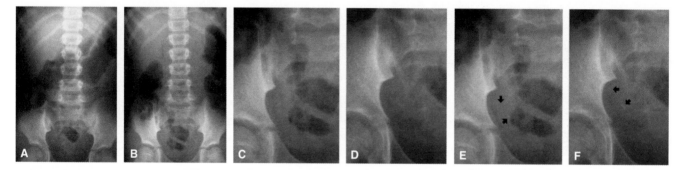

Figure 9.31. RLQ close-up RLQ appendicolith.

This case shows an x-ray of the appendix specimen that was removed at appendectomy.

This abdominal series shows diffuse gaseous distention of the colon and small bowel compatible with an ileus or an early obstruction. The distribution of gas is good. No free air is visible under the diaphragm. No appendicolith is visible. Compare the radiographic appearance of the LLQ with the RLQ. Can you appreciate any differences? Look at the peritoneal fat stripe on the left and on the right. The bowel should generally lie very close to this fat stripe (*white arrows*), which is what is seen on the

patient's left (right on image), but note that this is not the case on the patient's right (left on image). In the RLQ, the bowel is about 1 cm from the peritoneal fat stripe. In the LLQ, the bowel is about 1 to 2 mm from the fat stripe. This can be best visualized in the magnified focused view of the lower abdomen. Look at the peritoneal fat stripes on both sides just above the iliac crests (*white arrows*). Note that on the patient's left, there is a very narrow space between the fat stripe and the bowel. However, on the patient's right, the bowel is farther away from the fat stripe, suggesting that there is fluid, a mass, or thickened tissue pushing

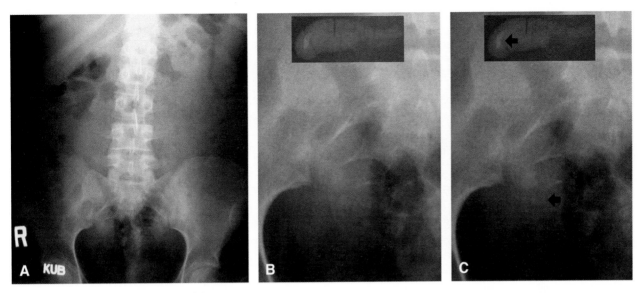

Figure 9.32. RLQ close-up RLQ appendicolith.

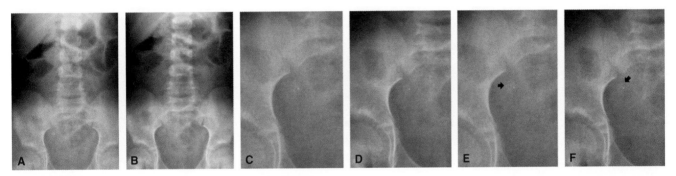

Figure 9.33. RLQ close-up RLQ appendicolith.

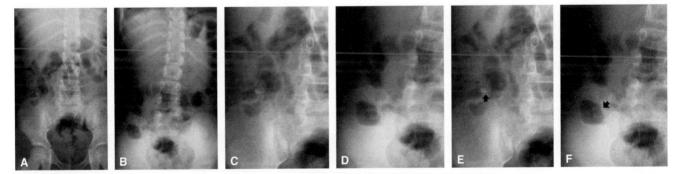

Figure 9.34. RLQ close-up RLQ appendicolith.

the bowel aside. There is a small gas pocket that does not appear to be within the bowel (*black arrow*). These findings together are highly suggestive of a ruptured appendix.

Intussusception

Most cases of intussusception occur in infants, but toddlers can be affected as well. Intussusception most often occurs in the ileocecal region. Plain film radiographs can be highly diagnostic of intussusception. Unfortunately, some patients with intussusception will have normal abdominal radiographs. It is generally not possible to rule out intussusception on plain film radiographs in most instances, although it is occasionally possible to conclude that ileocecal intussusception is not present if the ascending colon is conclusively filled with air or stool.

As a brief summary, the radiograph signs of intussusception are the target sign, the crescent sign, absence of the subhepatic angle, a bowel obstruction, and an RLQ mass effect.

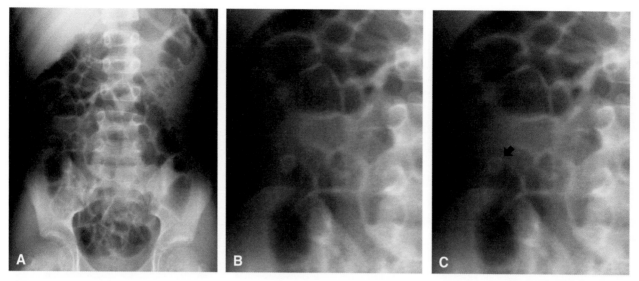

Figure 9.35. RLQ close-up RLQ appendicolith.

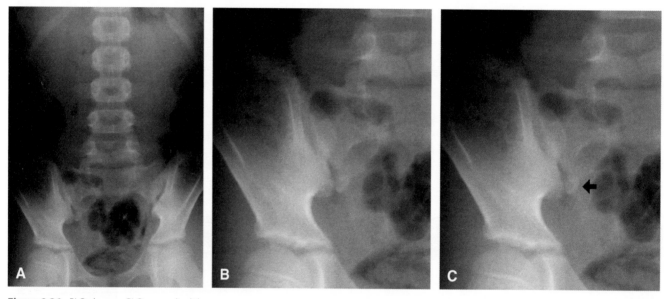

Figure 9.36. RLQ close-up RLQ appendicolith.

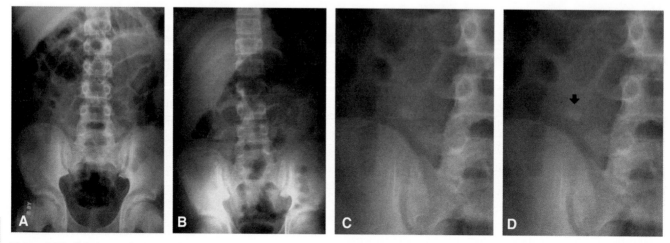

Figure 9.37. RLQ close-up RLQ appendicolith.

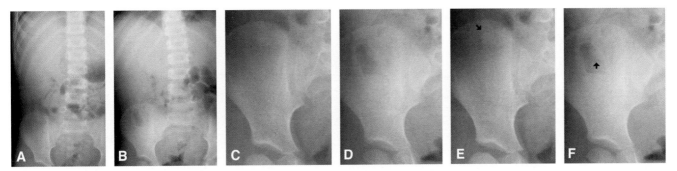

Figure 9.38. RLQ close-up RLQ appendicolith.

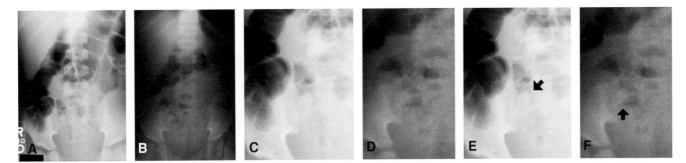

Figure 9.39. RLQ close-up RLQ appendicolith.

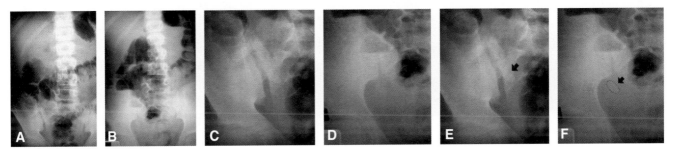

Figure 9.40. RLQ close-up RLQ appendicolith.

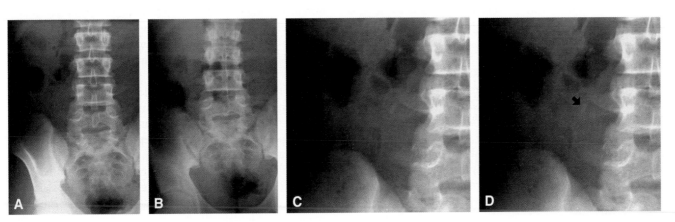

Figure 9.41. RLQ close-up RLQ appendicolith.

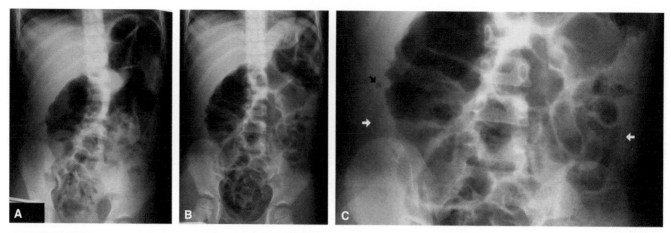

Figure 9.42. A 4-year-old child presents with signs and symptoms suggestive of appendicitis.

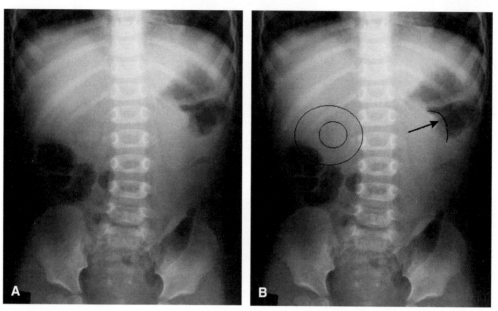

Figure 9.43.

Figure 9.43 illustrates the target sign and the crescent sign. The target sign is always found in the right upper quadrant (RUQ). It is due to alternating layers of fat and bowel. It resembles a donut with the center hole still filled in. It is very faint at best. To identify the target sign, one must search for it. If the target sign is identified, the likelihood of intussusception is extremely high.

The crescent sign occurs if the intussusceptum (the leading point of the intussusception) is protruding into a gas-filled pocket. If the gas pocket is large, the shape might not look like a crescent sign. This should more accurately be called the "intussusceptum protruding into a gas-filled pocket sign," but this is too difficult to say. The direction of the crescent sign (i.e., the point of the intussusceptum) must point in the proper direction, depending on where in the colon it is found. In other words, it must point superiorly in the ascending colon, to the left in the transverse colon, and inferiorly in

the descending colon. If the direction of the crescent is reversed, it is more likely that this is not a true crescent sign. If the crescent sign is identified, the likelihood of intussusception is very high.

Other signs of intussusception are the absence of the subhepatic angle, a bowel obstruction, and an RLQ mass effect. This simply means that the liver edge is not seen. Because intussusception usually occurs in the ileocecal region, the bowel in the RLQ, and potentially the RUQ, will become more edematous, thus obliterating the normal interface of the liver edge with non-gas-filled bowel. This is a less specific sign of intussusception. A target sign will almost always obscure the liver edge because the target sign is always in the RUQ, as seen in Figure 9.43. An RLQ mass effect is seen because of the edema of the intussusception. In Figure 9.43, there is no gas present in the RUQ suggestive of a mass effect.

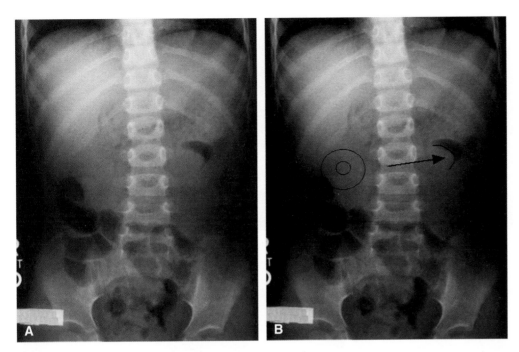

Figure 9.44.

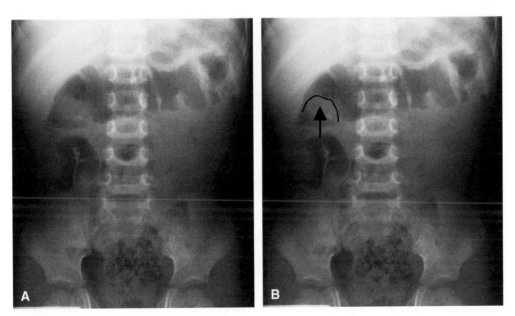

Figure 9.45.

In Figure 9.44, the target and crescent signs are again visible. This figure might actually have two target signs: one is circled, and the other is above this to the right of the spine. A crescent sign is also present in the LUQ. This x-ray is diagnostic of intussusception.

In Figure 9.45, a crescent sign is present. However, in this case, the crescent sign is not crescent shaped. Note the intussusceptum protruding superiorly into a gas-filled transverse colon at the hepatic flexure. This is why this phenomenon should more accurately be called the "intussusceptum protruding into a gas-filled pocket" sign.

In Figure 9.46, a bowel obstruction is present based on the criteria reviewed in the first part of the chapter. Note that the few air-fluid levels seen are in the same loop of bowel, which is highly suspicious of a bowel obstruction. The circled area shows a target sign, but it is not as obvious because some bowel loops overlie the target sign. In infants and very young children, bowel obstructions in intussusception tend to be shown on x-ray by a paucity of gas rather than a lot of gas obstructing the bowel.

In Figure 9.47, a target sign is present in the RUQ. The gas distribution is poor. The air-fluid levels are

161

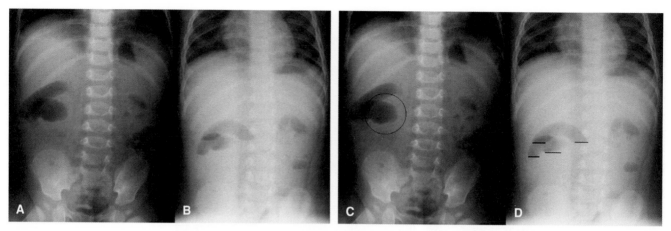

Figure 9.46.

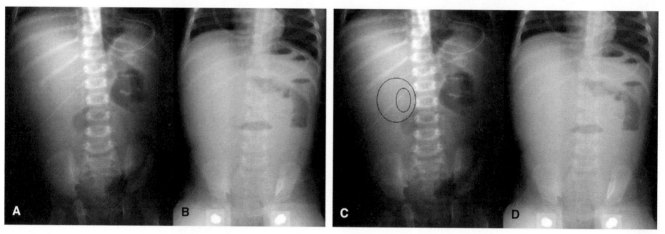

Figure 9.47.

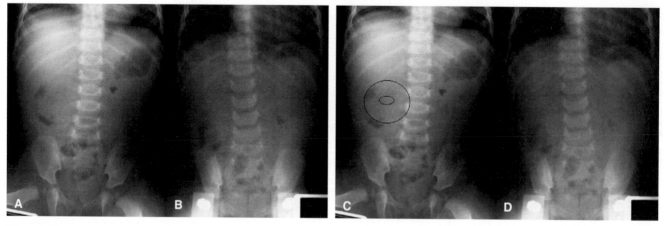

Figure 9.48.

not obviously indicative of an obstruction as in the previous case, but following the bowel loops indicates that there are air-fluid levels in the same loop of bowel in the LUQ. With the target sign and the paucity of gas bowel obstruction, this is highly indicative of intussusception.

Figure 9.48 demonstrates a very questionable target sign, but the more you stare at the RUQ, the more obvious the target becomes. Even if you cannot imagine a target there, you should be able to appreciate a circular mass effect in the RUQ. This target sign, along with the poor gas distribution, is highly suggestive of intussusception.

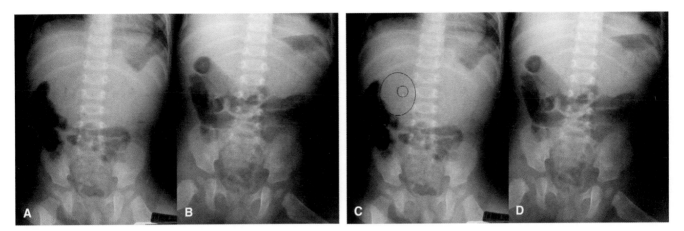

Figure 9.49.

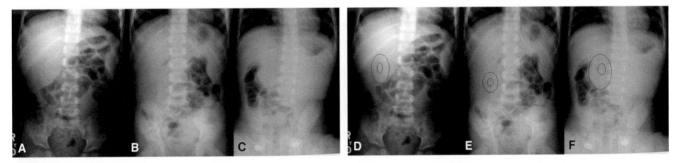

Figure 9.50.

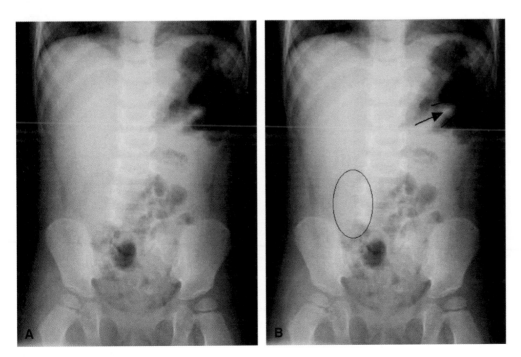

Figure 9.51.

In Figure 9.49, a RUQ target sign is present. The bowel walls are smooth and hoselike, indicating bowel distention. These two findings are highly suggestive of intussusception.

Figure 9.50 shows a subtle target sign in the RUQ on three different views of the same patient.

Figure 9.51 shows a target sign in the right middle portion of the abdomen, and a crescent sign in the LUQ. Again, the

163

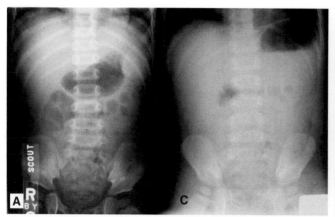
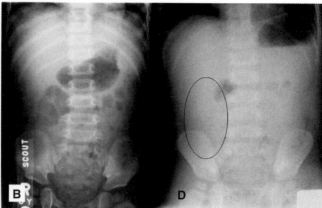

Figure 9.52.

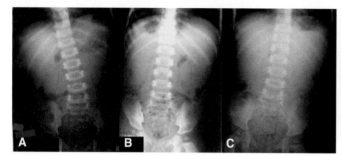
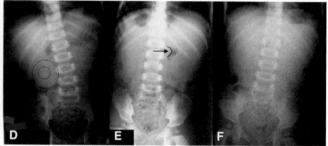

Figure 9.53.

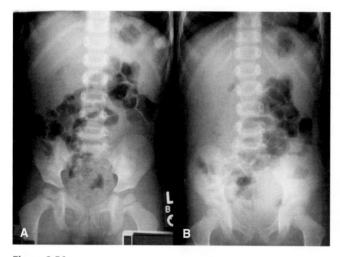
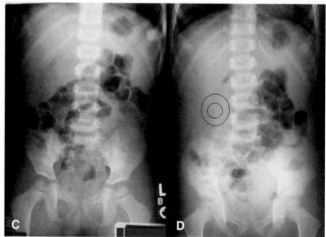

Figure 9.54.

crescent sign is not crescent shaped because the gas-filled pocket is large.

Figure 9.52 shows a suspicious bowel gas pattern in the RUQ. The upright view further demonstrates a suspicious target sign.

Figure 9.53 demonstrates a target sign in the RUQ and a crescent sign in the LUQ.

Figure 9.54 demonstrates a target sign in the RUQ. Although this might not clearly look like a target, it represents the same phenomenon in that intussuscepting bowel is forming a mass of soft tissue alternating with fat tissue densities.

Figure 9.55 demonstrates a target sign (or at least a mass effect) in the RUQ.

Figure 9.56 demonstrates a poor gas distribution, distended bowel, and air-fluid levels suggestive of a bowel obstruction. There is a RUQ mass effect and a target sign.

Figure 9.57 demonstrates a target sign on the right.

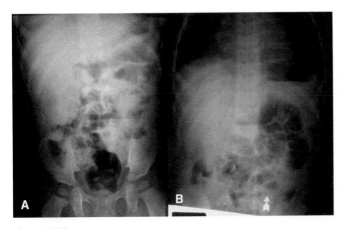

Figure 9.55.

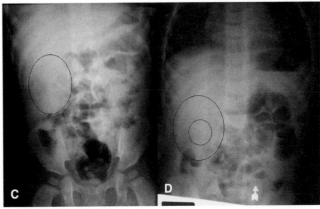

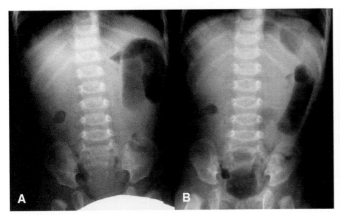

Figure 9.56.

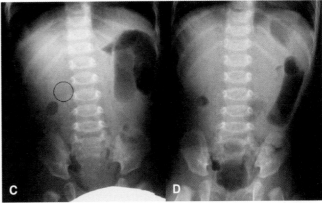

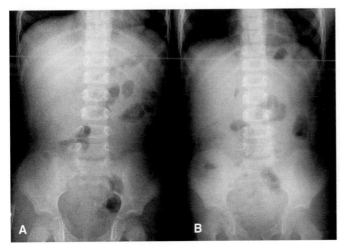

Figure 9.57.

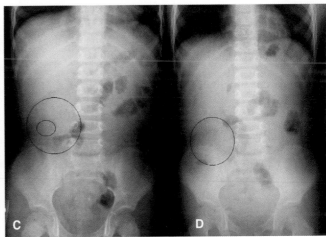

Pneumatosis intestinalis

Pneumatosis intestinalis is a radiographic finding resulting from air dissecting into the bowel wall. The bowel wall is normally a single soft tissue density, but when air dissects into the bowel wall, air bubbles are visible within the bowel wall, or the bowel wall looks like parallel soft tissue lines separated by a line of air ("train tracks"). More specifically, these are train tracks without the ties. Pneumatosis intestinalis is a radiographic sign of necrotizing enterocolitis (NEC) in the newborn. Patients with NEC are almost always premature infants. However, pneumatosis intestinalis is sometimes encountered in term

165

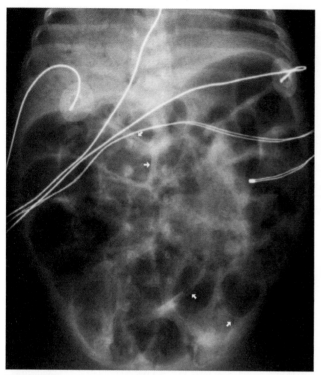

Figure 9.58.

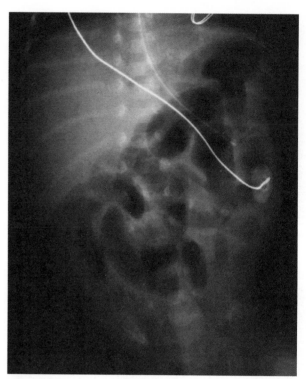

Figure 9.59.

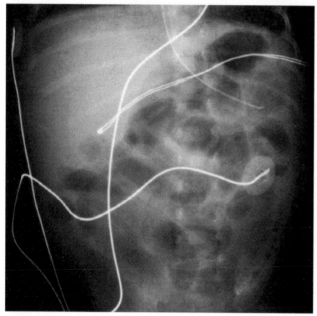

Figure 9.60.

In Figure 9.58, the white arrows point to the multiple areas of pneumatosis intestinalis. Air is dissecting into the bowel walls. Parallel lines are seen that represent the mucosal side of the bowel wall and the outer bowel wall sandwiching a layer of air between these two layers. Note that the liver is speckled with air densities as well. In NEC, air is often seen in the liver, and in severe cases, the biliary tree can be visualized. Ultrasound of the liver is the most sensitive means of identifying air bubbles circulating through the liver in NEC.

Figure 9.59 is a very dark x-ray of poor quality. What can be seen here is that the bowel walls are smooth and hose-like, indicating a bowel obstruction. It is not possible to see pneumatosis intestinalis on this x-ray, but air within the liver is visible, again indicating NEC.

Figure 9.60 demonstrates distended bowel and pneumatosis intestinalis. Double outlining of the bowel wall (train tracks) is identified in multiple bowel segments. In the LLQ, the cigar-shaped bowel segment demonstrates irregular bubble formation within the bowel wall.

Figure 9.61 is from a 5-month-old term infant who presented with bloody diarrhea. The first two images demonstrate pneumatosis intestinalis. The third image demonstrates large amounts of bowel wall gas with a double track of air.

Foreign bodies

Abdominal foreign bodies are usually not visible on plain film radiographs, with the exception of metallic and calcific

infants, older infants, and even adults. Chronic obstructive pulmonary disease or other conditions predisposing adults to soft tissue air dissection (pneumomediastinum, subcutaneous emphysema, etc.) are sometimes associated with pneumatosis intestinalis. However, in premature infants, pneumatosis intestinals should indicate the presence of NEC.

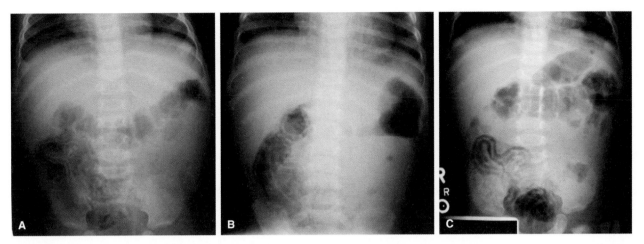

Figure 9.61.

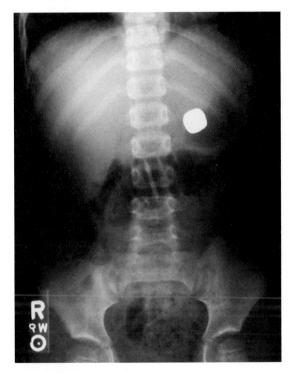

Figure 9.62.

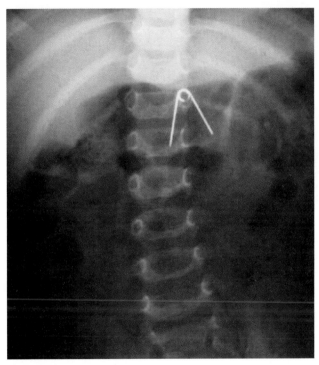

Figure 9.63.

foreign bodies. Ingestion of a coin is a common indication to confirm that the coin is in the stomach and not in the esophagus.

Figures 9.62 to 9.64 show obvious metallic foreign bodies. In Figure 9.62, it is a lead die (a single dice). In Figure 9.63, it is a safety pin. In Figure 9.64, what appears to be a coin is actually a disc battery, as the close-up view of this "coin" in Figure 9.65 demonstrates. Note the inner rim lucency of the battery, which is from the plastic insulator. Figure 9.66 demonstrates some of the radiographic characteristics of disc batteries compared with coins. The side view of a disc battery has a "frosting on the cake" appearance such that a top

layer is seen. The front view of the battery will often reveal an inner circle from the plastic insulator. However, if the metal in the battery casing is very thick, this inner circle is not always visible. If the battery is viewed obliquely, one may appreciate a cylindrical silhouette (as opposed to a flat disc).

A more recent foreign body concern is the high-strength rare earth magnets also known as neodymium magnets, which come in different shapes such as cylinder segments, spheres, disks, and rods. These magnets are often small and so strong that they can compress tissue between magnet pairs, which can perforate the bowel wall trapped between the two magnets. Figure 9.67 show a string of neodymium magnetic

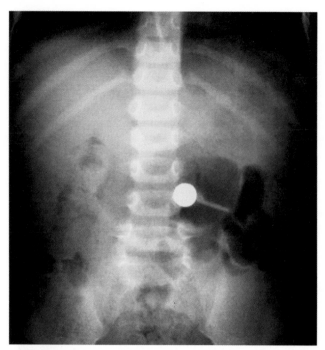

Figure 9.64.

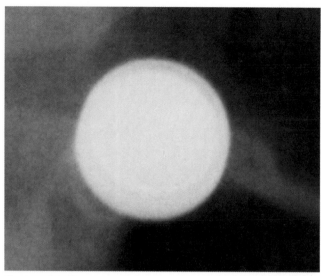

Figure 9.65. Close-up view of a battery initially thought to be a coin. Note the inner rim lucency characteristic of batteries.

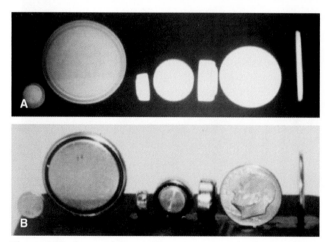

Figure 9.66. Commonly ingested batteries compared with coins.

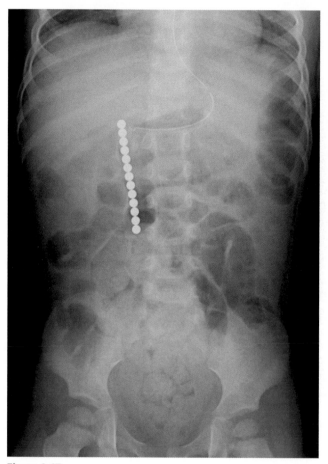

Figure 9.67.

beads. If these are all in a single line, such as in Figure 9.68, then it is fairly likely to pass through the GI tract. However, if the magnets are in separate bowel segments such that the bowel is being squeezed between the string of neodymium magnets, as in Figure 9.69, it will perforate the bowel and, thus, surgical removal is necessary to prevent this from occurring. In examining this long chain of magnets, it is not likely that the child swallowed all of these magnets at once. If enough time lapses between the ingestion of each sphere, the spheres will potentially be in different bowel segments as shown in Figure 9.69.

Figure 9.70 demonstrates faint calcifications in the RUQ. This is difficult to appreciate on the full abdominal images, but it is easier to see in this enlarged, focused view of the faint calcifications. Although not a foreign body, this calcification pattern is seen with the ingestion of bismuth subsalicylate (e.g., Pepto-Bismol). Other substances that may be radiopaque include ingested dirt, sand, and dental debris. Other agents that may be radiopaque include CHIPES (chloral

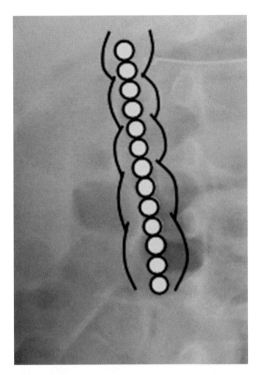

Figure 9.68.

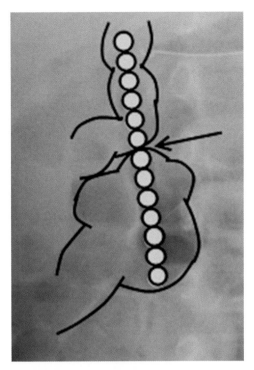

Figure 9.69.

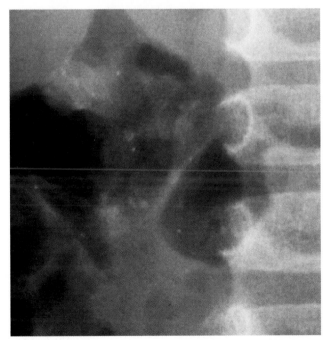

Figure 9.70.

hydrate/calcium, heavy metals [lead, arsenic, etc.], iodides/ iron [vitamin pills], phenothiazines and psychotropics, enteric-coated tablets, and slow-release capsules).

Urolithiasis

Kidney stones are relatively uncommon in children; however, they do occur. Kidney stones are composed of precipitated uric acid, calcium oxalate, or other calcium-containing compounds. Calcium-excreting diuretics such as furosemide can increase the concentration of urinary calcium. Uric acid and most calcium oxalate stones are not radiopaque on plain film radiographs. Struvite (magnesium ammonium phosphate) stone tends to form in the renal pelvis as "staghorn calculi," and these are usually radiopaque and visible on plain film radiographs.

CT scan can often identify the stone, but if contrast is administered, visualizing the stone will be obliterated by the excreted contrast in the ureter.

An intravenous pyelogram (IVP), also known as urogram, can identify the stone by locating the point of ureteral contrast obstruction, rather than visualizing the stone directly. This type of imaging study has largely been replaced by ultrasound and CT.

A suspicion of urolithiasis is often raised when a patient presents with a sudden onset of severe flank pain and severe costovertebral angle (CVA) tenderness. Occasionally, plain film radiographs ordered for other reasons will identify asymptomatic stones (usually in the renal pelvis).

Figure 9.71 is from a teen presenting with classic renal colic. A plain film abdominal x-ray demonstrates a questionable kidney stone (*black arrow*). Figure 9.72 is the patient's IVP. The first image is an early view. Prompt excretion is noted in the left kidney. The right kidney shows blunted calyces and delayed excretion. The next two images are delayed views, which show the blunted calyces and hydronephrosis in the right kidney. The last image is a close-up showing the location of the kidney stone demonstrated by a narrowing in the ureteral column of contrast excretion (*black arrow*).

Figure 9.73 is from a teen presenting with fever and CVA tenderness. An abdominal series demonstrates calcifications

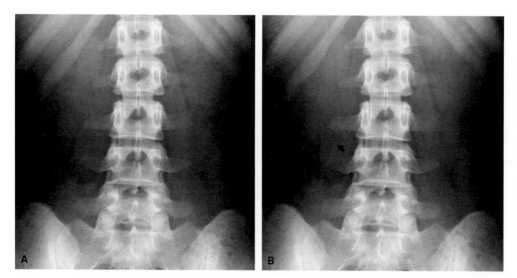

Figure 9.71.

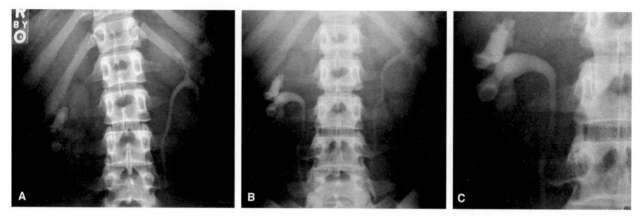

Figure 9.72.

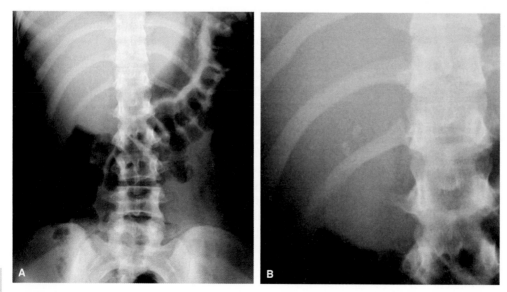

Figure 9.73.

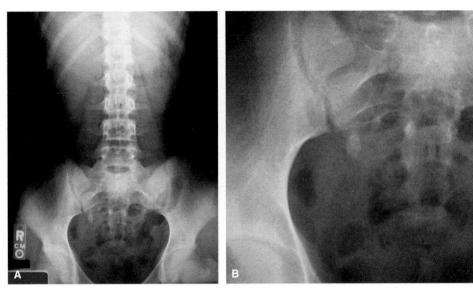

Figure 9.74.

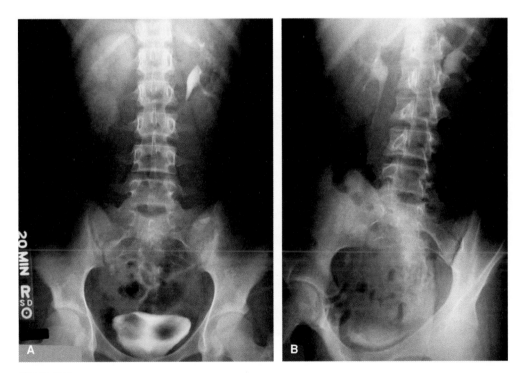

Figure 9.75.

overlying the renal shadow. A CT scan confirms that these are within the renal pelvis. A urine culture grew *Proteus* species. These findings are indicative of an early staghorn calculus composed of struvite (magnesium ammonium phosphate), which is usually caused by pyelonephritis due to a urea-splitting organism such as *Proteus*.

Figure 9.74 is from a teen presenting with classic renal colic. After analgesia, this abdominal x-ray shows a calcific density in the RLQ just inferior to the right sacroiliac joint. This ureteral stone appears to be very large, so a urologist was

consulted. Figure 9.75 is the patient's IVP. The initial image shows prompt excretion on the left but delayed excretion on the right, consistent with a ureteral obstruction. The delayed image shows delayed excretion on the right; however, the location of the ureteral obstruction does not appear to be where the RLQ calcification is located. Other views demonstrate that the calcification is not in the path of the ureter. The patient has a small ureteral stone that she subsequently passes. The RLQ calcification is an appendicolith, and the patient underwent an appendectomy for acute appendicitis.

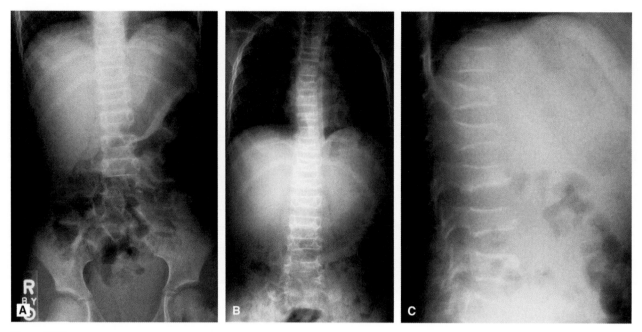

Figure 9.76.

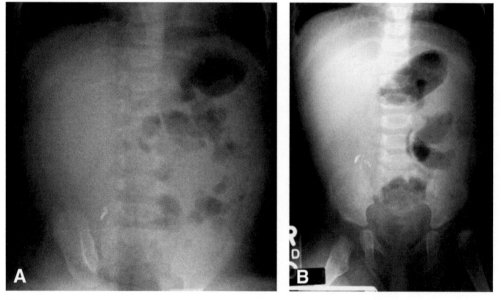

Figure 9.77.

Bony abnormalities

The abdomen contains bony structures, as well. The dominant structures here are the spine, the pelvis, and the hips. There is a tendency for clinicians to ignore the bones on abdominal radiographs; however, when bony abnormalities are present, these tend to be serious findings that should not be missed.

Figure 9.76 shows the first image obtained when the patient presented with abdominal pain. This was believed to be nonspecific. The patient returned, complaining of both abdominal and back pain. The second two images were obtained on the subsequent visit, at which point a close

examination of the vertebral bodies reveal that they are compressed. This is especially evident on the lateral view, which shows multiple compression fractures of the patient's lumbar spine. In retrospect, the vertebral compression fractures are evident on the initial abdominal x-ray, but it is not nearly as obvious. This patient was ultimately diagnosed with leukemia. Leukemia will often present with bony abnormalities on x-ray. Lucencies or indistinct bony margins could also be seen with malignancies.

Figure 9.77 is an abdominal series taken on day 2 of hospitalization. This is a 5-month-old infant who was diagnosed with intussusception at a general hospital. A barium enema at the hospital confirmed the intussusception, and a successful reduction was achieved. At that point, the patient was transferred to a children's hospital for overnight observation, despite the resolution of the patient's symptoms. After doing well overnight, orders for discharge were written; however, the patient vomited, and the discharge was cancelled. An abdominal series was obtained, which is shown in Figure 9.77. The gas distribution is poor. There is some residual barium present. The patient improves and does not have an intussusception recurrence. However, a different abnormality is incidentally noted on this x-ray.

Figure 9.78 is an enlargement of the lower portion of the patient's abdominal x-ray. A congenital dislocated left hip is noted. Because the femur heads are not ossified at an early age, it is not obvious that the hip is dislocated. There are many rules to help identify the dislocated hip, but the easiest rule is to use Shenton's arc. This is an arc (oval) drawn through the obturator foramen and the medial portion of the proximal femur. Note the normal Shenton's arc in the patient's right hip, whereas Shenton's arc is obviously disrupted in the patient's left hip. The radiologist at the previous hospital was so focused on diagnosing and then reducing the intussusception that the dislocated hip was missed. Only a methodical and compulsive approach to reviewing the bony structures of all x-rays will enable one to make such a diagnosis. Because the ED orders many abdominal x-rays, it is likely that a dislocated hip will be encountered in one or more of these x-rays.

Lungs (often overlooked)

The lower portion of the lungs should be visible on at least one view of an abdominal series. Because abdominal radiographs are usually ordered for abdominal complaints, there is a tendency to ignore the lung portion of the x-ray. However, it is well known that lower lung conditions can result in abdominal complaints. For example, lower lobe pneumonia commonly causes abdominal pain. Pleural effusions blunting the costophrenic angles should also be visible on the upright view of the abdomen if the diaphragm is properly included in the image. Always examine the periphery of the image because this is where things are often missed.

Figure 9.79 is an abdominal series of a teen presenting with abdominal pain. This patient has an infiltrate in the left lower lung. It is best seen on the left image, superimposed over the heart and spine as a triangular density.

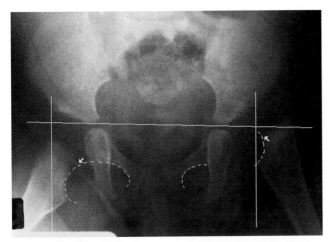

Figure 9.78.

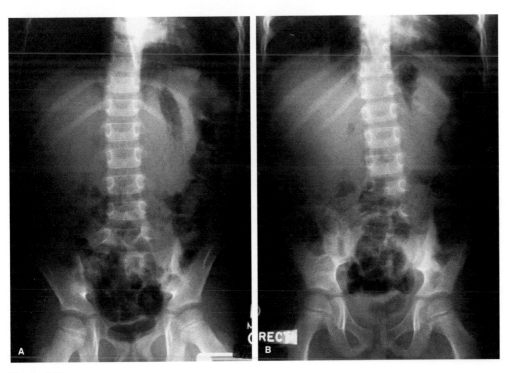

Figure 9.79.

Plain Radiography in Child Abuse

Chapter

10

Kenneth T. Kwon

Indications

Complete skeletal survey plain radiographs are essential in the evaluation of suspected child abuse, particularly in infants and toddlers. Extracranial abnormalities are detected in 30% to 70% of abused children with head injuries. Shaken baby syndrome is classically described as subdural hematoma, retinal hemorrhages, and long bone fractures with minimal external signs of trauma. Because of the close association of intracranial injuries with fractures in nonaccidental trauma, both CT of the head and complete bone survey radiographs should be minimal standard imaging in any suspected child abuse case.

Diagnostic capabilities

Fractures suggestive for nonaccidental trauma can be categorized based on specificity for abuse:

1. High specificity: metaphyseal corner or bucket handle fracture, posterior rib fracture, sternal fracture, spinous process fracture, scapular fracture, bilateral acute long-bone fractures
2. Medium specificity: complex skull fracture, vertebral body fracture, multiple fractures of different ages
3. Low specificity: linear skull fracture, long bone shaft fracture in weight-bearing age

These injuries need to be taken within the context of clinical history and mechanism reported (if any), physical exam findings, developmental age, and assessment of family and social dynamics. Any injuries considered medium or high specificity should warrant notification to the appropriate reporting agency, as should any low-specificity injuries with unclear mechanisms.

Imaging pitfalls and limitations

Subtle injuries may be missed on initial acute skeletal survey. Delayed repeated skeletal radiographs 1 to 2 weeks after initial survey or radionuclide bone scans may be needed in these children where there is high suspicion of child abuse but initial screen is negative. Negative skull radiographs as part of the skeletal survey do not obviate the need for obtaining CT

of the brain to investigate for intracranial bleeding or injury in suspected abuse cases.

Clinical images

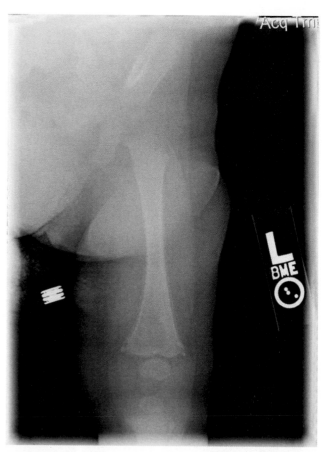

Figure 10.1. Metaphyseal corner and "bucket handle" fractures. This 3-month-old presented with unexplained bruises and irritability. Abuse was suspected, and a skeletal survey was performed. Figure 10.1 shows the classic metaphyseal corner fractures, which are evident on both medial and lateral aspects of the left distal femur. These avulsion like fractures are due to the strong ligamentous and periosteal attachments to the ends of young growing bones. Sudden traction or torsional forces, as can occur by a perpetrator violently twisting or pulling an extremity, are typically not seen in accidental traumatic circumstances and can generate the necessary forces to create such injuries.

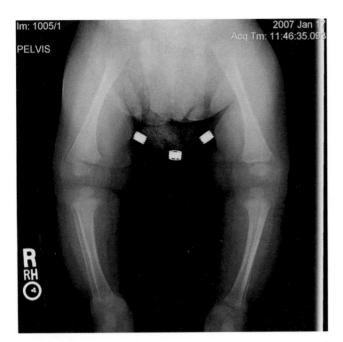

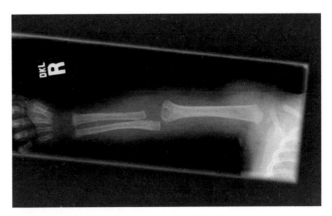

Figure 10.3. Bucket handle fracture of the distal humerus.

Figure 10.2. A different angle of the same patient in Figure 10.1, showing the medial distal femur metaphyseal fragment to resemble more of a bucket handle than a corner. As periosteum is torn from the underlying cortex, subperiosteal bleeding can occur. The resultant periosteal reaction can create a new external layer of bone away from the cortex, resembling a thin handle of a bucket. Because the periosteum is more loosely attached at the diaphysis than at the physis of growing bones, this layering of periosteal new bone may be seen extending into the diaphysis. In this case, note the thin layer of new bone extending proximally on both medial and lateral aspects of the femoral diaphysis.

Metaphyseal corner and bucket handle fractures are perhaps the most highly specific for abuse. They are virtually pathognomonic but can also be seen in rare congenital or acquired orthopedic conditions.

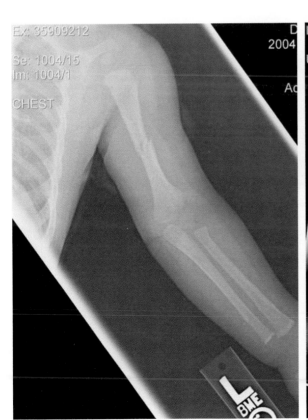

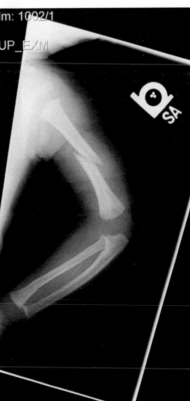

Figures 10.4 and 10.5. Multiple fractures of varying age. This is part of the same skeletal survey of the 3-month-old patient in Figures 10.1 and 10.2. The obvious finding is the acute transverse fracture of the midhumerus, which is highly suggestive of abuse in an infant who is not bearing weight or even crawling. The more subtle fracture is the bucket handle fracture of the proximal humerus. Also, in the distal radius and ulna, there is thickening of the cortexes with slightly sclerotic edges, which represents healing fractures.

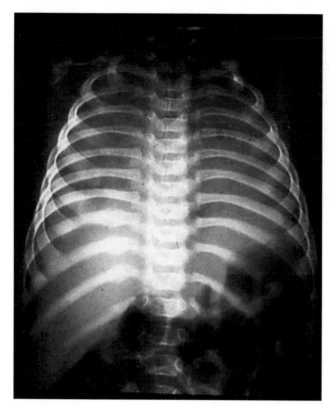

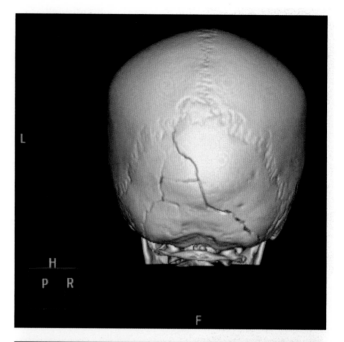

Figure 10.6. Posterior rib fractures. Note the healing posterior rib fractures of the right thoracic ninth to twelfth ribs with callus formation. This infant had been physically abused a few weeks prior to presentation. Posterior rib fractures are highly suggestive of abuse and usually occur as a result of arms or hands wrapped around the thorax while shaking or squeezing. Rib fractures due to accidental trauma tend to occur in the anterior aspect of the ribs.

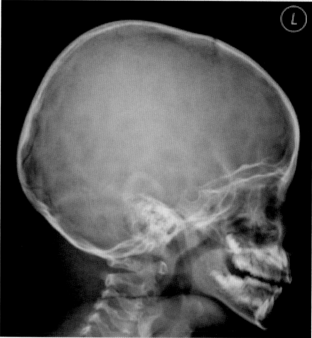

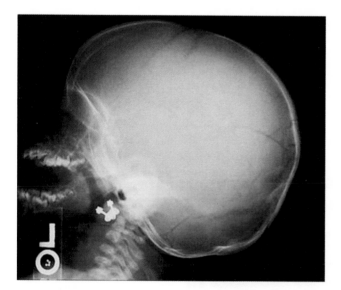

Figures 10.7A and B. Linear skull fracture. The occipital bone demonstrates a simple, linear, nondisplaced fracture. Fractures resulting from accidental falls or trauma are usually linear and uncomplicated. Linear skull fractures have a low specificity for child abuse.

Courtesy of Pablo Abbona, MD.

Figure 10.8. Complex skull fracture. Note the multiple fracture lines emanating from the midoccipital region and coursing anteriorly to the parietal-temporal area. The symmetric lucencies on the superior parietal areas represent normal coronal sutures, and the lucencies in the inferior occipital area represent normal lambdoid sutures. Skull fractures are considered complex if multiple, stellate, depressed, or cross suture lines. Complex skull fractures are more specific for abuse than linear skull fractures, but they are less specific than metaphyseal corner/bucket handle fractures or posterior rib fractures. Up to 50% of infants suffering from nonaccidental head injury will have skull fractures.

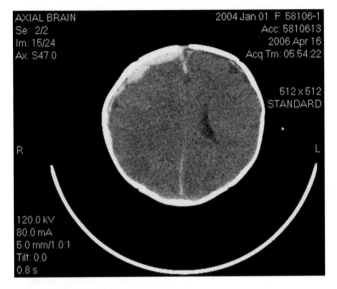

Figure 10.9. Subdural hematoma. This CT image is from the same patient seen in Figure 10.1 and confirms shaken baby syndrome. Note the bilateral subdural hematomas, right greater than left, with no definite skull fracture identified. Although subdural hematomas like these are commonly seen in abuse cases, the most characteristic subdural hematoma for shaken baby syndrome is in the posterior interhemispheric area, with blood layering in the interhemispheric fissure, causing the posterior falx to appear more dense than normal. Subdural hematomas can be caused by direct trauma or severe acceleration-deceleration forces, such as from shaking. These injuries are associated with significant morbidity and mortality due to the high rate of associated irreversible brain damage. It is the most common intracranial hemorrhage seen on autopsy in shaken baby deaths.

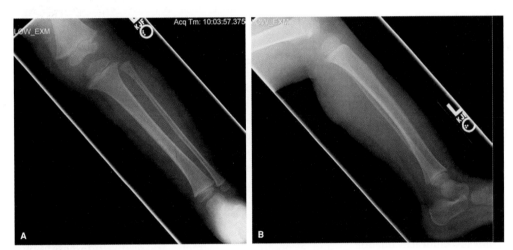

Figure 10.10. (same as Figs. 7.25A and B in Chapter 7): Toddler's fracture. First described by Dunbar in 1964, this fracture is classically described as an oblique or spiral nondisplaced fracture of the distal tibia. It is most commonly seen in children 9 months to 3 years of age and occurs as a result of an axial loading and twisting injury on a fixed foot, which would maximize forces in the distal leg. Although any oblique or spiral fracture of a long bone in a child should raise the possibility of nonaccidental trauma, an oblique fracture of the distal tibia in a weight-bearing infant can be explained from normal accidental forces, such as a fall, which is frequently unwitnessed. More concerning would be a spiral fracture of the mid or proximal tibia, which may more likely suggest nonaccidental trauma, as a perpetrator holding and twisting the distal portion of a leg would maximize forces in the midshaft and proximal areas of the tibia. Isolated spiral fractures of the tibia neither confirm nor dismiss the possibility of abuse.

Plain Radiography in the Elderly

Ross Kessler and Anthony J. Dean

Indications

The indications for plain film radiography in the elderly are modulated by the pathological effects of age. Radiographic indications that are particular to older patients could be summarized by stating the indications for ordering imaging studies are broader, and the threshold for ordering them is lower. Imaging considerations unique to older patients generally fall into one of the following categories:

1. Some common disease processes and mechanisms of trauma afflict the elderly more severely. A fall that might cause a wrist sprain in a 35-year-old might result in a significant fracture in a 75-year-old with osteoporosis. This clinical consequence of senescence is reflected in the American Thoracic Society pneumonia score and the age-based exclusion criteria of the Ottawa knee and ankle rules.

2. Attenuated responses to systemic insults are common in the elderly. Therefore, "typical" signs and symptoms may not be as apparent in this population. The clinical exam may also be compromised by altered sensorium or mobility in the elderly.

3. Many diseases of adulthood become increasingly prevalent with age (e.g., cancer, atherosclerosis, heart disease, lung disease). In this context, a clinical evaluation that is the basis for an extremely low pretest probability in a younger patient might in the elderly be associated with a much higher pretest probability, mandating further diagnostic or imaging tests. Thus, signs or symptoms relating to the chest – including pain, pressure, cough, dyspnea, and hypoxia – may all warrant plain chest radiography in this population.

4. The constitutional effects of aging make the consequences of misdiagnosis direr in the elderly.

Diagnostic capabilities

In general, the capabilities of diagnostic radiology in the elderly are similar to those noted in the previous chapters. Not infrequently, radiographs of the elderly reveal incidental findings such as vascular and soft tissue calcifications, arthritic conditions, pulmonary nodules, or vertebral fractures. These may warrant follow-up or further imaging on either an emergent or non-emergent basis. A close examination of bony structures may reveal chronic but clinically important bony irregularities (e.g., lytic or blastic lesions).

Further imaging options include CT, MRI, or nuclear scans. The latter are of use in identifying metabolically active lesions. However, the widespread availability of plain film radiography in emergency departments make it an ideal initial study in many instances, particularly those with time-sensitive treatments in which a screening test to rule out contraindicated therapies is quickly needed.

What follows is a brief outline of some of the ways that plain film radiography is modulated by the special diagnostic considerations and clinical concerns relating to elderly patients.

Spine plain film imaging

Many findings on plain spinal films in the elderly are degenerative changes from either normal aging or accelerated bony change from disease or injury. The most common include osteoporosis and osteophytes. Osteoporosis is a systemic skeletal disorder characterized by low bone mineral density and is generally seen radiographically as an overall increase in bone lucency and thinning of the cortex. Factors that lead to osteoporosis include age-related loss of total bone mass, post-menopausal increase in bone resorption, exogenous steroid administration, Cushing's disease, decreased physical activity, and alcoholism. Radiographs are relatively insensitive for detecting osteoporosis, requiring almost 50% of bone mass to be lost before radiographic changes can be detected on plain x-rays. Currently, the DEXA scan using densitometric-imaging techniques is the most accurate and sensitive method for measuring bone mineral density. Osteophytes are bony growths at the joint margins that result in joint space narrowing and are usually the result of degenerative arthritis.

Whereas spinal fractures are almost always the consequence of a traumatic event in younger patients, in the elderly fractures can occur even in the absence of trauma, so clinicians should have a low threshold for performing spine imaging. Fractures or suspected fractures may warrant additional advanced imaging, such as CT or MRI, either in the ED or on an outpatient basis.

Degenerative spinal disease includes joint narrowing, calcifications of ligaments, sclerotic changes, osteophyte formation, and fusion. Many of these are broadly termed as degenerative joint disease (DJD). Involvement of the endplates, as with osteophytes, can result in degenerative changes with sclerosis or narrowing. Osteoarthritic changes occur through the loss of hyaline cartilage and chronic inflammation. Some disease processes such as rheumatoid arthritis and ankylosing spondylitis are associated with specific abnormalities, the most important of which include destabilization and subluxation of the atlanto-occipital joint. Diffuse idiopathic skeletal hyperostosis (DISH) is a relatively uncommon condition in which there is prominent and diffuse calcification of the anterior cervical longitudinal ligaments, which bridge the vertebral bodies. Spondylolysis results from a defect in the pars interarticularis and allows spondylolisthesis, or the anterior slippage of one vertebral bony on another, to occur. Among the elderly, spondylolisthesis may occur due to degeneration of the interosseous elements in the absence of spondylolysis, in which case it is referred to as degenerative spondylolisthesis. In most patients complaining of severe pain or trauma, severe degenerative changes identified on plain films are sufficiently confounding to prevent exclusion of serious injury, so that additional diagnostic studies are needed.

The spine can be the site of any type of tumor, but among the most common are metastatic lung, breast, and prostate cancers. Osteolytic lesions cause destruction of the spine and are commonly seen with multiple myeloma and metastatic breast, lung, renal, and thyroid cancers. Prostate cancer is most frequently osteoblastic, which causes the radiographic appearance of dense radiopaque densities in the bone. In some cases, changes to the bony spine may cause spinal cord compromise. In the setting of neurological deficits with known or suspected metastatic spinal lesions, MRI to evaluate the spinal cord is indicated.

Pelvic imaging

Imaging of the pelvis is most commonly prompted by pain or trauma. In addition to identification of fractures, emergency physicians should look for neoplastic lesions and degenerative changes of the hip joints or sacroiliac joints. Calcifications may be seen in the bladder or uterus (leiomyomata), in the vasculature, and in the overlying soft tissues.

Most commonly involving the pelvis, Paget's disease (osteodystrophia deformans) is a chronic bone disease of the elderly that is caused by disregulated bone metabolism with increased bone resorption and abnormal bone formation. Usually referred to by its eponym, the findings on plain radiography include thickening of the cortex, coarsening of the trabeculae, and an increase in size of the involved bone. This denser bone is mechanically inferior to normal bone and therefore prone to pathologic fractures.

Chest imaging

Diagnostic considerations that will prompt chest radiography among the elderly are similar to those for other adults. However, the high prevalence of cardiopulmonary diseases identifiable by radiography among older patients is likely to prompt a lower threshold for testing in this group. An incomplete list of such diagnoses would include pneumonia, pulmonary embolus, chronic obstructive pulmonary disease, malignancy, pleural diseases, aortic disease, pericardial disease, and congestive heart failure. In many of these, the chest radiograph (CXR) may give only indirect evidence of the disease process (e.g., pulmonary embolus, aortic dissection, pericardial effusions) and is insufficiently sensitive to rule out disease. Therefore, with anything more than a low pretest probability of disease, more sophisticated (also more time-consuming and resource-intensive) imaging studies are likely to be needed. However, the ease with which a CXR can be obtained – along with its availability, noninvasiveness, and low cost – make it highly valuable in the initial evaluation of undifferentiated thoracic conditions.

Rheumatologic conditions and extremity imaging

Rheumatologic conditions are increasingly common with age. Because their radiological findings are protean and their diagnosis is not a primary responsibility of the emergency physician, the examples presented here are limited in scope and number. Emergency physicians should become familiar with some of the more common radiographic manifestations of rheumatologic disease so they can recognize them when the physicians encounter them in films obtained to evaluate an acute condition.

Abdominal imaging

The limitations of plain radiographs in the evaluation of abdominal pathology are the same in the elderly as in other adults, with the because that CT is often the imaging modality of choice, particularly because the prevalence of serious pathology is much higher in the elderly and the long-term effects of radiation exposure are of diminishing concern. In addition to the issues regarding general plain abdominal imaging discussed in Chapter 4, clinicians are often called on to replace dislodged feeding tubes (g-tubes, j-tubes, etc.) or verify placement of feeding tubes placed via the naso- or orogastric route. Abdominal images may also reveal abnormal calcifications or air in the vascular system, peritoneum, biliary tract, pancreas, kidney, ureters, bladder, or uterus.

Imaging pitfalls and limitations

Most of the limitations of plain radiography in the elderly are the same as those for other adults. Osteoporosis or chronic degenerative changes may make the identification of fractures more difficult. Radiographs may be limited by the patient's inability to cooperate with the exam. Elderly patients may have difficulty with positioning due to physical (e.g., contractures from prior stroke) or neurological (e.g., paralysis, altered mental status) constraints.

Clinical images

The following images depict radiographic findings and pathology that clinicians should be familiar with in the elderly patient.

Plain film images in the elderly

Spine imaging

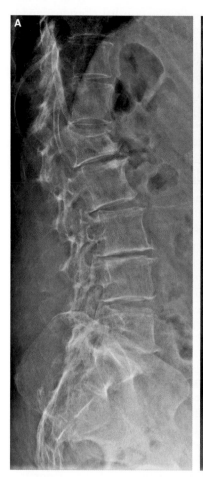
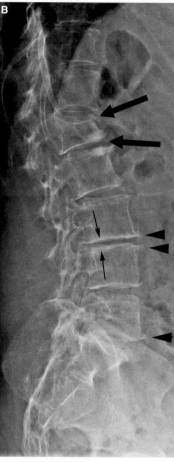

Figures 11.1A and B. An osteoporotic lumbar compression fracture of L1 (*large arrows*) was found in a patient presenting with back pain. Note the diffuse osteopenia, which suggests osteoporosis. Osteoporotic compression fractures are common in the elderly. The radiographic appearance typically involves compression of the anterior and superior aspects of the vertebral body with sparing of the posterior aspect, producing a wedge-shaped deformity. There is usually no neurological deficit because the fracture does not extend posteriorly, and no specific treatment is usually required. Osteophytes (*arrowheads*) and sclerosis of the endplates (*small arrows*) due to degenerative joint disease are also seen.

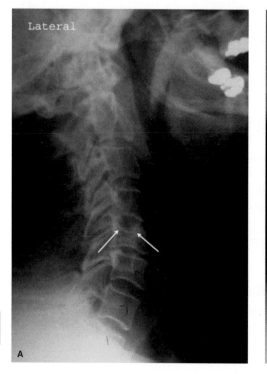
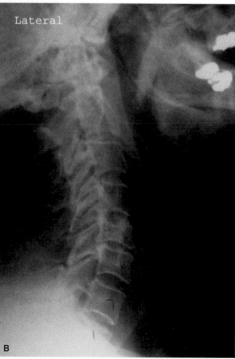

Figures 11.2A and B. Cervical compression fracture secondary to multiple myeloma. This is a good-quality lateral cervical x-ray showing C1 to the top of T1. There is a compression fracture (*arrows*) with loss of the vertebral body height of the fifth cervical vertebral body secondary to multiple myeloma. In contrast to compression fractures caused by osteoporosis, this pathologic fracture involves the entire length of the vertebral body. Note the sclerotic margins of the lesion indicating it is chronic. There are other lesions in the fourth and sixth cervical vertebrae as well (*arrowheads*).

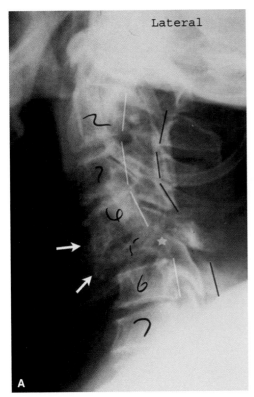
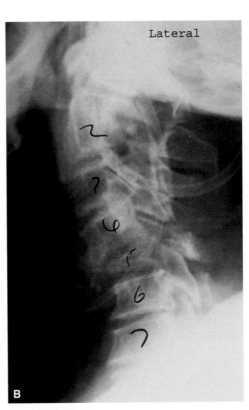

Figures 11.3A and B. Cervical vertebral body destruction. Lateral view of the cervical spine in a patient with severe neck pain. The arrows indicate bony destruction of the vertebral body. The posterior vertebral line (*white lines*), which should normally be traced as you inspect the posterior aspect of the vertebral bodies, is not well defined around the fifth cervical vertebra. The bony fragment (*white star*) is concerning for retropulsion into the spinal canal, which is marked anteriorly by the posterior vertebral line and posteriorly by the spinolaminar line (*black lines*). This is an unstable cervical spine and may lead to spinal cord impingement and paralysis if not stabilized.

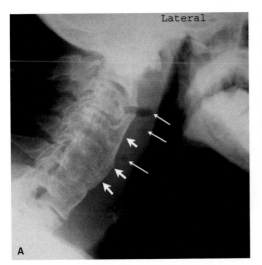
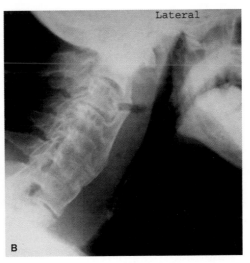

Figures 11.4A and B. Cervical hyperostosis. An elderly patient presents from the nursing home with a fever. The lateral view of cervical spine shows diffuse, thick bridging calcification of the anterior longitudinal ligament (*large arrows*). This condition, termed diffuse idiopathic skeletal hyperostosis (DISH), is more common in the thoracic and lumbar spine but can be found anywhere. Unlike degenerative disk disease, the disk spaces and facet joints are usually preserved. Despite the bridging of the vertebral bodies, it is typically not a major cause of pain. This image also depicts mild thickening of the prevertebral soft tissue and air in the prevertebral soft tissue (*small arrows*), raising concerns of infection, esophageal injury, mediastinitis, or less likely trauma.

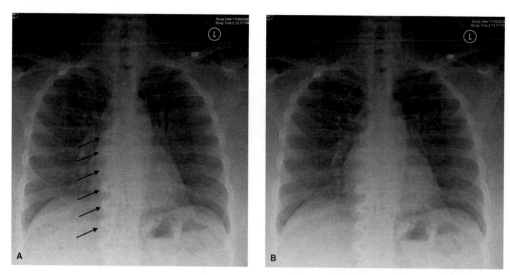

Figures 11.5A and B; Figures 11.6A and B. A PA and lateral chest radiograph revealing DISH of the thoracic spine in a 60-year-old being evaluated for shortness of breath. These images show the smooth contours of the bulky, bridging calcifications of DISH. In severe cases such as this, there may be some limitations of movement. Despite the striking radiographic deformities, it is not usually a cause of back pain.

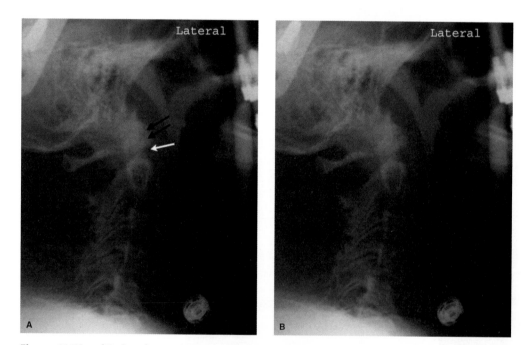

Figures 11.7A and B. Dens fracture. A 75-year-old female presents ambulatory for the second time with worsening neck pain after falling out of bed 3 days ago. On the first ED visit, the cervical spine was interpreted as normal. On the second visit, the lateral view of the cervical spine reveals loss of normal lordosis, degenerative changes in all cervical vertebrae, a cortical defect involving the low dens (*white arrow*), and a linear lucency located at the anterior arch of the first cervical vertebra (*black arrows*). The latter may be chronic, as suggested by the corticated margins and the absence of swelling in the prevertebral soft tissue. However, the dens fracture was certainly acute and unstable (based on films showing movement after placement of a halo cervical immobilizer). There is also apparent fracture of the facet of C2 (*arrowhead*), which may be chronic based on its sclerotic margins, in addition to a compression fracture of the facet of C3 (*asterisk*). This case demonstrates some of the difficulties both with clinical assessment and radiographic interpretation in the elderly. In the lower cervical spine, sclerosis and loss of vertebral height are also seen at several levels.

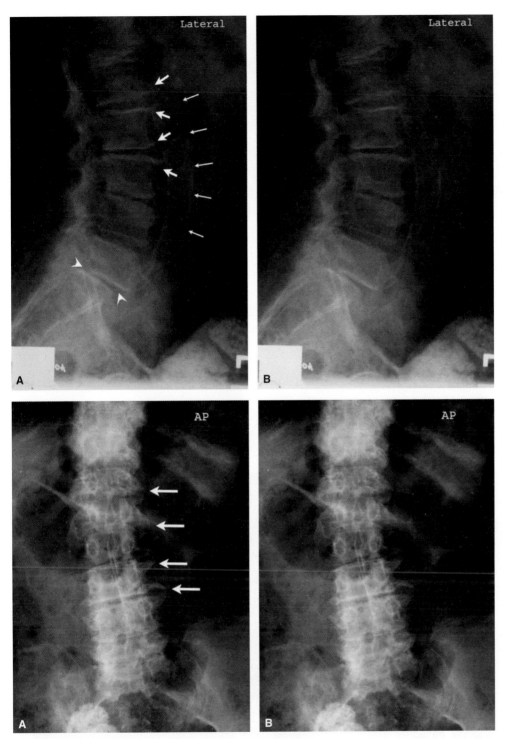

Figures 11.8A and B; Figures 11.9A and B. Lumbar spine DJD and aortic calcification. Lower back pain prompted this lumbar spine plain film series. The lateral image shows significant aortic calcifications (*small arrows*) without evidence of aneurysm. The anterior aspects of the lumbar vertebral bodies have characteristic osteophytes (*large arrows*) that appear to bridge with the adjacent osteophytes (lateral and AP views). The *arrowheads* denote spondylolisthesis of L5 on S1 with the slippage of less than 25%. A grading scale exists that also corresponds to treatment recommendations: grade I = 1%–25% slippage, grade II = 26%–50% slippage, grade III = 51%–75% slippage, and grade IV = 76%–100% slippage. Treatment for grades I and II is generally conservative, with surgical options usually reserved for grades III and IV. Ninety percent of spondylolisthesis occurs at the L4–5 and L5-S1 levels. The AP view also demonstrates mild scoliosis.

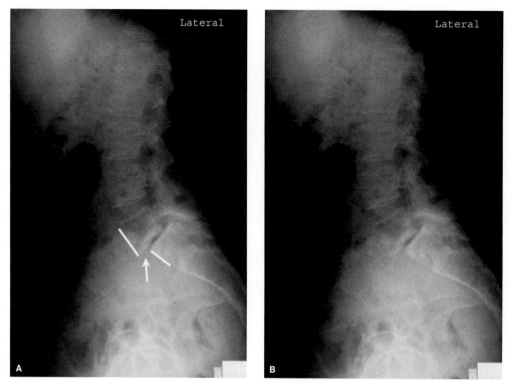

Figures 11.10A and B. Lumbar spondylolisthesis. A common cause of low back pain, this lateral lumbar spine demonstrates the anterior translation of L5 on S1 (*arrow*). When examining spine films, the anterior vertebral line should form a smooth contour.

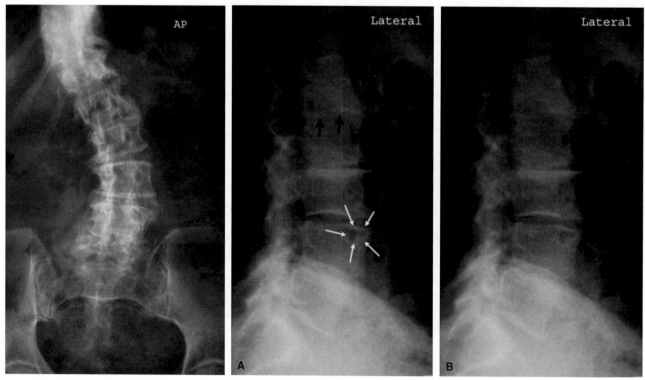

Figure 11.11; Figures 11.12A and B. Lumbar scoliosis with DJD. These AP and lateral lumbar spine films demonstrate severe scoliosis, DJD (*black arrows*), several osteophytes, and a cyst (*white arrows*) in the superior/anterior fourth lumbar vertebrae. Overlying bowel gas can be mistaken as a cyst. Note the sclerotic margins that differentiate the cyst from overlying bowel gas.

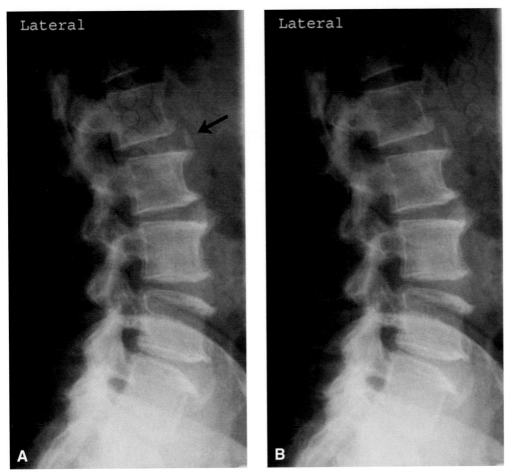

Figures 11.13A and B. Annular calcification. Calcification of the L1-L2 intervertebral disk (*arrow*) can be confused with vertebral fractures or osteophyte fractures. These structures are found anterior and between two adjacent vertebral bodies. The calcifications have well-defined smooth edges and do not make contact with either endplate of the adjacent vertebral bodies. Another can be seen in the L4-L5 interspace. There are numerous osteophytes throughout the lumbar spine.

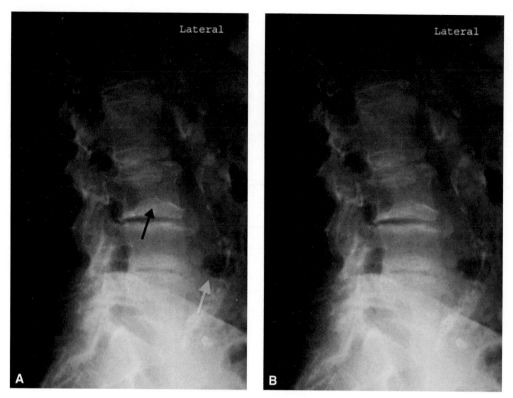

Figures 11.14A and B. Schmorl's node of L3. Defects in the endplates of the vertebral bodies, most frequently in the lumbar spine, are common nontraumatic findings. The defect, known as a "Schmorl's node" (*black arrow*) appears as a defect in the vertebral body with sclerotic margins in the anterior or midportion of either endplate. It is believed to arise from protrusion of the nucleus pulposus. This patient also has marked aortic calcification (*star*), bowel gas adjacent to the anterior portion of the midlumbar vertebrae (*white arrow*), and loss of L4 vertebral height and collapse of the L3-L4 and L4-L5 intervertebral disk spaces.

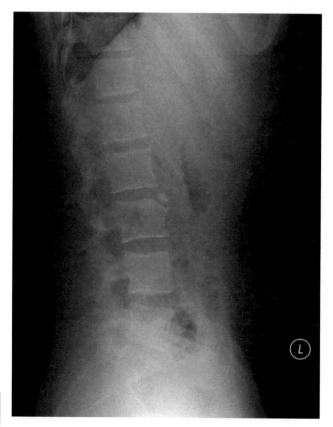

Figure 11.15. Limbus vertebra. In the lateral projection of the lumbar spine of a 43-year-old, a limbus vertebra can be seen involving the superior anterior aspect of L3. It is believed to result from herniation of the nucleus pulposus through the ring apophysis prior to fusion of the vertebral body. It is isolated to a small corner segment of the vertebral rim, most commonly affecting the anterosuperior corner. Note the well-corticated edges, indicating this is not an acute process. Also note that the intervertebral disc spaces are similar and that there is a lack of pathology of the contiguous vertebral bodies, distinguishing this from a fracture. As this radiograph indicates, this finding can be seen in patients of any age.

Pelvis imaging

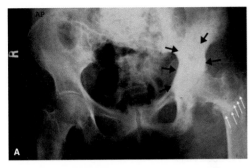
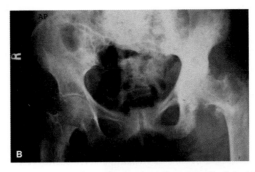

Figures 11.16A and B. Paget's disease of bone. Paget's disease is a chronic bone disease that affects 1%–2% of the U.S. population older than 55 years. It is a disorder of disregulated bone remodeling characterized by lytic-appearing lesions (early) or dense sclerotic lesions (late). It is most commonly found in the pelvis but also in the skull, proximal femurs, tibia, and humerus. In this image, the left os coxa and proximal femur are diffusely radiodense compared to the right. The bone is also enlarged, with loss of trabecular markings and cortico-medullary differentiation (*black arrows*), making it mechanically flawed and prone to fractures. A left intertrochanteric fracture is seen (*white arrows*) in addition to severe degenerative changes of the hip joint with joint space narrowing and probable collapse of the femoral head.

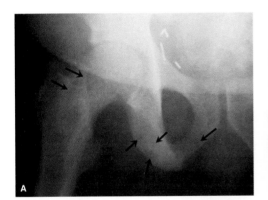
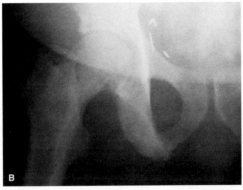

Figures 11.17A and B. Bony metastases. In a 65-year-old male with prostate cancer presenting with pelvic pain, this close-up shows numerous small lytic lesions in the pelvis and right hip (*arrows*). Surgical clips are noted status post prostatectomy.

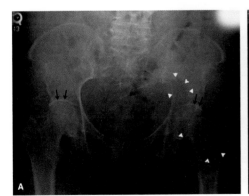
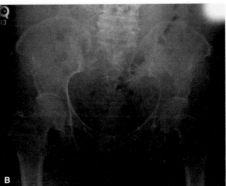
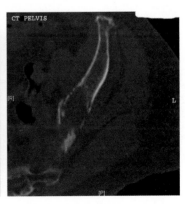

Figures 11.18A and B; Figure 11.19. Metastatic colon cancer. A 73-year-old female with history of colon cancer and resection presents several years later with pelvic pain. This AP pelvis shows diffuse left pelvic and humeral head and neck lytic lesions (*white arrowheads*). This patient also has degenerative sclerotic changes of both hip joints (*black arrows*), with erosions and collapse of the medial aspect of the femoral heads bilaterally. The pelvic CT (Fig. 11.19) demonstrates the lesions in the left pelvis.

Abdominal imaging

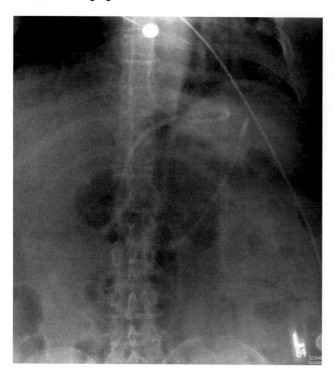

Figure 11.20. Feeding tube placement verification. Following blind nasal placement, ideally the plain radiographs should demonstrate the tip in the proximal small bowel. This portable AP view of the abdomen shows the bowel gas pattern to be normal. The Dobhoff tube crosses the midline, coursing through the duodenum, and probably ends in the proximal jejunum.

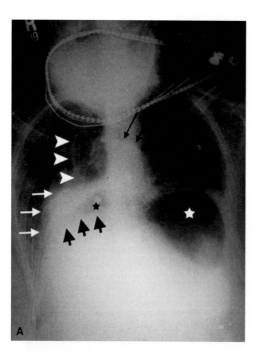
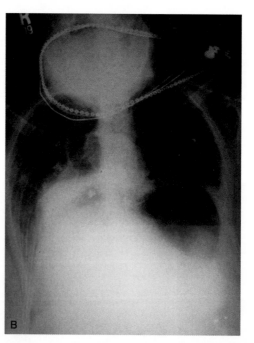

Figures 11.21A, B. Hiatal hernia. This elderly patient complained of burning chest pain. A PA chest radiograph demonstrates a gas-filled (*star*) soft tissue mass within the mediastinum just superior to the medial left diaphragm (*arrows*), suggesting a hiatal hernia. This may be difficult to distinguish from a thoracic aortic aneurysm, although in this case, the structure appears to contain gas, and the aortic knob is entirely normal. The lateral view demonstrates a normal aortic contour and a suggestion of a hiatal hernia at the medial portion of the diaphragm. A subsequent CT was performed, which demonstrated a large hiatal hernia.

Chest imaging

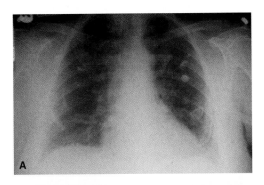
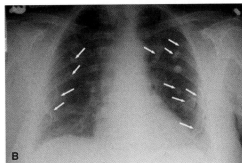

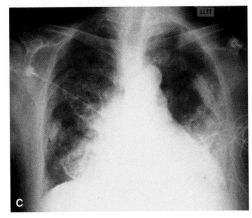

Figures 11.22A, B, and C. Asbestosis. An elderly patient presents with worsening shortness of breath and a history of "lung problems." He has a chronic cough productive of white sputum. This film shows scattered "veillike" densities of pleural plaques associated with asbestos exposure *(white arrow)*. Asbestos-related plaques can take many forms, from thin linear calcifications only seen when the x-ray beam is tangential to the pleura at that location, to large disorganized masses, easily seen *en face*, such as those seen in Figure 11.22C. The plaques can be associated with extensive pleural thickening. Figure 11.22C also shows loss of lung markings in the apices, which is suggestive of advanced emphysema.

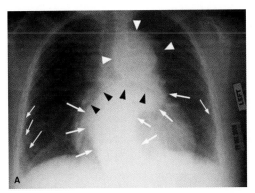
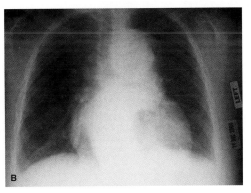

Figures 11.23A and B. Thoracic aortic aneurysm. An 83-year-old patient presents with a month-long persistent dry cough. He has also noticed some difficulty swallowing anything but liquids. The patient has a history of CHF, but he says "it doesn't feel like that." His lungs are clear, although systolic and diastolic murmurs are noted. CXR shows several abnormalities. First, his aortic knob is enlarged *(arrowheads,* measured at 6.3 cm), leading into an ectatic thoracic course *(large white arrows,* often referred to as "uncoiling" of the aorta). Second, cardiomegaly, splaying of the carina *(black arrows)* suggestive of left atrial enlargement, and Kerley B lines *(small white arrows)* all suggest the patient's chronic CHF. Aneurysms, in addition to the well-known syndromes of acute instability, can present more chronically. In this case, the aneurysm was having a mass effect in the chest and causing aortic insufficiency with secondary mitral regurgitation. Kerley B lines are caused by increased interstitial fluid in the lungs and can be seen in the absence of rales on exam.

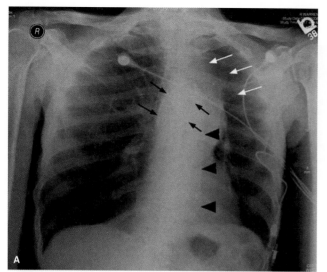

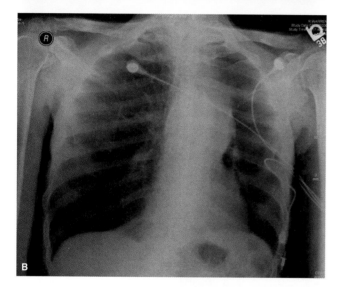

Figures 11.24A and B. Left upper lobe atelectasis secondary to obstructing tumor. An 80-year-old man, who quit one week ago after 60 years of smoking, presents with poorly defined chest pain and possible weight loss. His CXR is shown. Initially, the large mass in the upper left hilum might be mistaken for an aortic aneurysm, but the calcifications in the ascending aorta (*black arrows*) and the left wall of the descending aorta (*arrowheads*) suggest that it is not enlarged. The entire mediastinum is shifted to the left, with attenuated lung markings seen in the left lung fields (*white arrows*). Although it might be expected to have a distinctly more radiodense lung field in this situation, the findings suggest atelectasis of the left upper lobe possibly due to bronchial obstruction. CT confirmed a left hilar mass, and carcinoma was identified by subsequent endobronchial biopsy.

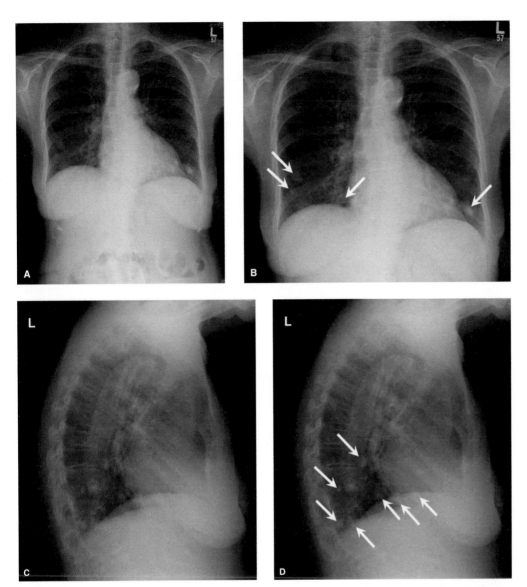

Figures 11.25A, B, C, and D. Pulmonary nodules. A 75-year-old female presents to the ED after being involved in a frontal motor vehicle crash while driving to a doctor's appointment. She is complaining of chest pain. Upright posteroanterior (PA) and lateral radiographs are obtained and shown here. There is no evidence of acute injury, but multiple pulmonary nodules are seen in both views (*arrows*). Differential for these nodules include scarring from prior granulomatous disease (e.g., tuberculosis, fungal infections, or sarcoidosis) or acute metastatic disease. Old films of the patient were found, and they demonstrated these nodules to be unchanged from previous films. If these had not been available, the patient would have been referred for further outpatient evaluation with possible CT, biopsy, or serial imaging studies to monitor for growth in the nodules.

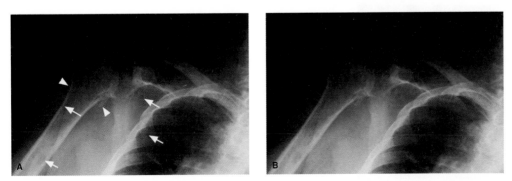

Figures 11.26A and B. Multiple myeloma. A 67-year-old patient presents to his primary care physician after a 3-day history of nonproductive cough. An upright chest x-ray does not demonstrate a lung consolidation. However, there is a large lytic lesion in the left distal clavicle (*white arrows*), consistent with the patient's known history of multiple myeloma.

Extremity imaging and rheumatologic conditions

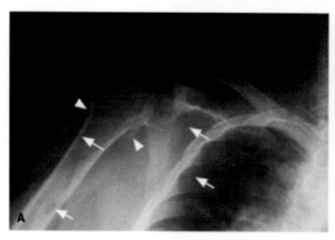

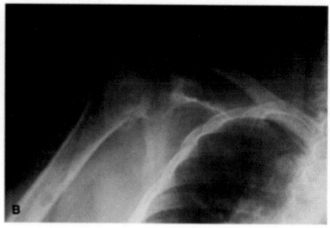

Figures 11.27A and B. Pathological fracture, right shoulder. A 65-year-old female presents after a minor bump to her shoulder 3 days ago. She complains that "the pain just won't go away, and I can't seem to use it properly." She had treatment for breast cancer 5 years ago with no known recurrence. Her x-ray demonstrates a nondisplaced surgical neck fracture (*arrowheads*). In addition, there are multiple lytic lesions of varying sizes in the humerus and scapula (*arrows*). These become confluent in the humeral head, making it appear osteopenic. The patient was subsequently managed for metastatic recurrence of her breast cancer.

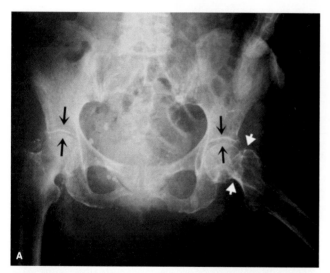

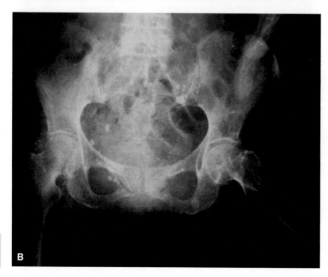

Figures 11.28A and B. Osteoarthritis and septic joint. Comparison of the two hips demonstrates asymmetry of the joint spaces (*black arrows*) with widening on the left side. Also note the position of the limbs: the left femur is flexed and externally rotated. The intertrochanteric line (*white arrows*) should not be mistaken for a fracture line. A septic joint must be considered with such prominent joint-space asymmetry. Other incidental findings include various calcifications in the pelvis: these regular, smooth, often corticated densities are termed phleboliths. There is also vascular calcification seen in the proximal right leg medial to the femur.

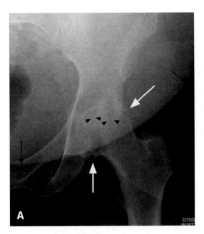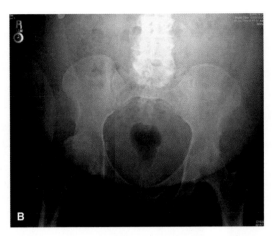

Figures 11.29A and B. Severe osteoarthritis of hips. An obese patient presents with complaints of severe pain down her posterior left thigh that awoke her from sleep 4 days ago. The pain has been continuous since then. In addition to evaluation for deep vein thrombosis (DVT), the patient had a plain film of the pelvis. A close-up view of the left hip is shown. The entire joint is narrowed. Osteophytes have formed around the rim of the acetabulum (*white arrows*). The bone on both sides of the joint shows areas of sclerosis (radiodense areas of increased calcium deposition). There are also subchondral "cystic" (radiolucent) areas (*arrowheads*) that suggest osteonecrosis, with resultant collapse of bone and flattening of the femoral head. Osteonecrosis can be both a cause and effect of severe DJD. The soft tissue density overlying the film is the patient's pannus (*black arrows*). The patient's ED workup was negative for DVT and other soft tissue processes. Of note, hip injury can present with pain in the back, buttocks, thighs, or knees. The patient subsequently underwent a hip replacement.

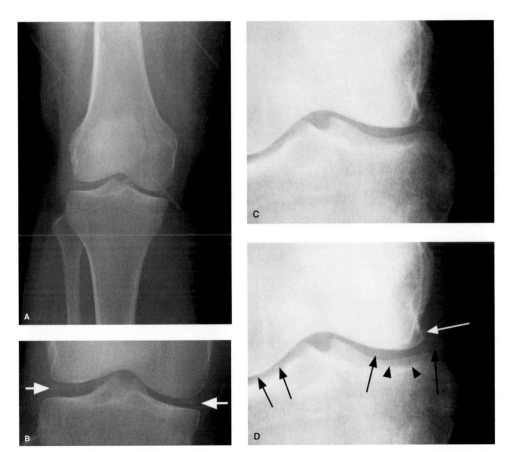

Figures 11.30A, B, C, and D. Chondrocalcinosis of the knee. A 55-year-old woman presents with pain and swelling in her right knee after "twisting" it while walking up stairs 4 days ago. She states that the swelling is not as bad as it was 2 days ago. A radiograph of her knee is shown in Figure 11.30A, with a detailed image of the joint in Figure 11.30B. Fine radiodense deposits can be seen in the meniscus on either side of the joint (*white arrows*). These are characteristic of the calcium pyrophosphate deposits of chondrocalcinosis, which have a predilection for hyaline cartilage and fibrocartilage (as in this case). The majority of these deposits are asymptomatic, although they can cause symptoms such as acute pain, redness, and swelling (sometimes precipitated by trauma, as in this case), referred to as pseudogout. They occur most commonly in the hands, knees, and wrists. With the absence of signs of an infectious process and relatively mild symptoms, she was treated empirically with nonsteroidal anti-inflammatory agents and referred to follow-up with her primary care physician. Another case of more advanced chondrocalcinosis is shown in the right knee film seen in Figures 11.29C and D. Again, the outline of the meniscus can be seen, but there are also calcium pyrophosphate deposits in the joint space (*black arrows*). The joint space is narrowed with osteophyte formation (*white arrow*), and there are areas of subchondral cysts (*black arrowheads*), characteristic of this arthropathy.

193

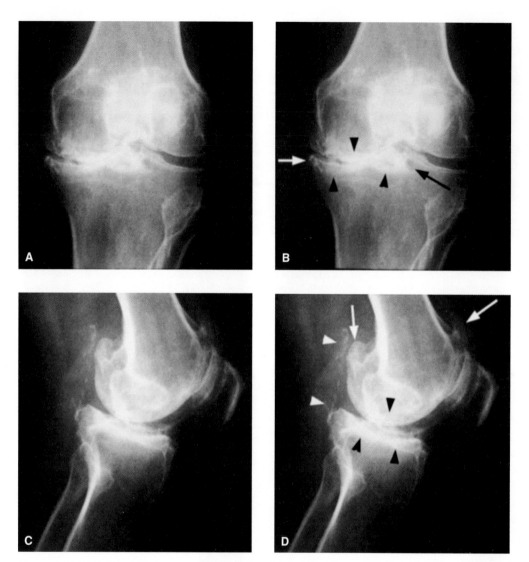

Figures 11.31A, B, C, and D. Degenerative joint disease of the knee. A 74-year-old male presents complaining of left knee pain after slipping and falling on a patch of ice. He says his knees are "always a bit creaky, but now this one's really paining." Physical exam reveals a mild effusion, diffuse joint line tenderness, and characteristic osteoarthritic deformities. Figures 11.31A and B show his AP knee films, and Figures 11.31C and D show the lateral films. The medial side of the knee joint is often more severely affected by DJD, as is the case here. There is severe joint space narrowing, subchondral sclerosis (*black arrowheads*), osteophytes and periarticular calcifications (*white arrows*), and subchondral bone cysts (*black arrow*). The soft tissue density seen posterior to the joint on the lateral view is a calcified popliteal artery (*white arrowheads*). Significant fractures can be occult on plain films of the knee, and severe osteoarthritis such as this further impedes interpretation. Depending on one's clinical suspicion, consider CT or arthrocentesis, looking for fat globules, which will identify an occult fracture. The latter approach has the additional advantage of also relieving the pain of an effusion.

Introduction to Bedside Ultrasound

Michael Peterson and Zahir Basrai

Nothing has generated as much change in emergency medicine in the past 20 years as the introduction of bedside ultrasound. Why? Because physicians who have embraced this new tool realize how important it is to their everyday practice and how lost they would be without it. "Bedside ultrasound" means ultrasound examinations performed and interpreted by the treating physician at the time of the patient encounter. Clinical questions can be answered immediately, accelerating both decision making and treatment. In acute situations where time to diagnosis directly affects treatment and outcome – such as with penetrating cardiac trauma, pericardial tamponade, intraperitoneal hemorrhage due to trauma or ectopic pregnancy, or leaking abdominal aortic aneurysm – ultrasound can be a critical adjunct. As newer applications of ultrasound have found their way into emergency medicine practice, the core applications of the ultrasound have expanded to include thoracic, soft tissue, musculoskeletal, and ocular systems (1).

Ultrasound also benefits many procedures commonly performed in the ED. The use of ultrasound for procedures was underemphasized until recently, but it appears that it may now be a major driving force behind the desire of practicing emergency physicians (EPs) to learn ultrasound. No longer does one have to rely on inaccurate clinical judgment to guide the decision to perform time-consuming, expensive, and potentially hazardous procedures. Central lines go in on the first attempt with a reduced risk of puncturing an artery or having an unsuccessful procedure; suspected abscesses are not needled or drained without knowing whether there is a fluid collection present; paracentesis is nearly 100% successful with little risk of puncturing tethered bowel; and pericardiocentesis is done only when there is pericardial fluid to drain, with the needle placed exactly where it is wanted (2, 3). Before bedside ultrasound, EPs were forced to make initial critical clinical decisions entirely on information from the often imprecise history and physical examination. Now EPs can directly visualize important internal signs of illness and injury rapidly, conveniently, inexpensively, and noninvasively. Likewise, procedures previously done in a blind percutaneous fashion can be guided by direct visualization with ultrasound. Just as important, ultrasound can prevent costly and hazardous attempts at procedures that are unnecessary or have a low likelihood of success.

The reach of ultrasound application in the emergency department has spread to developing countries and new economic powers. It is in these settings that the benefit of ultrasound is seen the most as its use has replaced more expensive diagnostic modalities. On the battlefield, emergency ultrasound has become a mainstay for the evaluation of those injured during military conflict (1).

The most important question we now face is how to best disseminate these skills to the practicing physician. Ultrasound training is currently a requirement in emergency medicine residency. Many (unfortunately, not all) residents will finish residency as skilled sonographers, but training requires a significant investment of time. Ultrasound cannot be learned from reading a textbook or even going to a course; learning it requires practical experience under guidance. Physicians already in practice are struggling with the fact that more of their newly trained colleagues have ultrasound skills and that the standard of care in emergency medicine is evolving toward requiring ultrasound skills in many clinical situations. According to the American Board of Emergency Medicine's longitudinal study, half of EPs now perform bedside ultrasound, and this number has grown steadily (4). As of yet, the ability to perform bedside ultrasound is not the standard of care in the ED, but it is likely to become so in the near future. The American College of Emergency Physician's (ACEP's) Section on Ultrasound currently has more than 500 members. In 2000, there were approximately three fellowships in emergency ultrasound, whereas the Society for Academic Emergency Medicine now lists 61 fellowships. It is clear that interest in bedside ultrasound in emergency medicine is rapidly expanding.

This chapter presents a general overview of the pathway for physicians to become skilled in the use of bedside sonography and the elements required to implement a bedside ultrasound program. Although bedside ultrasound requires a definite commitment to training, it is not overwhelming. In the end, physicians will likely be very pleased with the effort made and time spent to advance their ultrasound skills to the benefit of their practice and patients.

Selecting an ultrasound machine

A comprehensive discussion of the differences in ultrasound machines is beyond the scope of this chapter. For this, the reader is directed to other, more comprehensive emergency ultrasound textbooks and the ACEP Clinical and Practice Management Resource website (5). There are, however, some general points and a few tips worth considering when thinking about purchasing an ultrasound machine. The first is cost: a typical ultrasound machine used for emergency bedside ultrasound costs between $5,000 and $50,000. This is significantly less than the more comprehensively equipped machines that the radiology department typically uses. Less complex machines are now marketed specifically for bedside ultrasound. List prices are often deeply discounted, and package purchases that include extra probes, printing devices, and even maintenance contracts can save thousands of dollars. Furthermore, machines do not have to be purchased; they can also be leased. Some departments even borrow or inherit old machines from elsewhere in the hospital.

The hospital typically purchases the ultrasound machine for the ED. Hospitals can charge a "technical" fee, separate from the physician's fee, to recover machine and consumables costs. Physicians should be involved in ultrasound equipment purchase decisions, especially when it comes to probe selection and features (such as color flow Doppler). Equipment options will dictate what exams can be performed.

All ultrasound machines have the same basic controls, and once you learn where the controls are, you can operate just about any machine. Ultrasound machines also have many features that you are unlikely to use, including reporting functions and complicated calculations packages. Do not let the complexity of the keyboard put you off. If you are familiar with the following few adjustments, you will be able to operate even the most complex of equipment. The Preset or Exam Type button allows you to tell the machine what kind of exam you are doing so it can adjust to give you the best picture. The Gain adjustment changes the brightness of the whole screen at once. The Time Gain Compensation (TGC) sliding switches adjust the screen brightness at various depths on the image. The Depth adjustment shrinks or enlarges the image, and the Freeze button freezes the image so you can examine or print it. The Trackball or Cine Loop adjustment allows you to scroll back through previous images in case you were not quite fast enough on the Freeze button, and the Calipers or Measurement function allows you to measure things on the screen. Knowing these functions will allow you to perform 95% of what you need to do with an ultrasound machine.

The point of ultrasound is to create interpretable pictures of internal anatomy, so the primary goal is to select a machine that makes the best pictures possible. The best way to decide which machine has the best picture is to compare two or more optimally adjusted machines side by side while scanning a standard patient. This is easier to achieve than you might think, especially if you visit a specialty conference or attend an ultrasound course where ultrasound training or marketing is occurring. These venues rely on ultrasound manufacturers to bring equipment and technicians to assist with training and marketing; in return, manufacturers hope to interest prospective buyers. Compare machines by allowing the ultrasound technician (also known as an "application specialist") to scan you. You are the standard patient, and the technician ensures the machine is adjusted for the best possible picture. Have the technician demonstrate different types of exams because the same machine may perform differently with different probes and in different anatomical areas. Comparing how the heart looks on various machines is especially important if you plan

on imaging the heart (an examination of the heart is part of the focused abdominal exam for trauma, or FAST, exam). If you do not know much about ultrasound, bring along someone who can help you judge the quality of the images. Once you have narrowed down machines based on picture quality, start asking about features. For general diagnostic use, avoid machines with very small or grainy displays; they make interpretation difficult, especially from a distance. Such machines may be useful as second machines for specific uses, such as vascular access, where a small machine that can fit easily next to a patient and a procedure tray is handy.

Some important considerations that are sometimes overlooked include how long it takes for the machine to be ready for scanning after it is turned on. Machines were originally designed to stay in one place and to be turned on in the morning and turned off after the scanning day was over, so startup time was not critical. Machines in the ED will be moved constantly and will be turned on and off many times a day. Under these circumstances, a startup time of 1 minute or longer can be quite annoying. Also, because the machine needs to be mobile, machine size should be considered. Will the machine fit easily in the exam areas in your ED? To comfortably scan, a machine needs to be placed next to a patient's bed with enough room left to get behind the machine and plug it in. The desire for a smaller machine should be balanced against screen size and machine durability. The more people who use your machine and the more exams it performs, the more likely it will be handled roughly and damaged.

Once ultrasound is integrated into the ED, you will find it rapidly becomes an essential piece of equipment. Manufacturer support is the key to minimizing machine downtime. Equipment failures are not uncommon, usually from dropped probes or probe cord damage from the ultrasound wheels. The quality of support varies by manufacturer and depends to a great extent on the specific repair person for any geographic area. Find out if other services in the hospital or other hospitals in your area use equipment from the same manufacturer. If so, has their experience with service and repairs been satisfactory? Does the manufacturer respond promptly to requests for repair? Remember that the ED operates around the clock, which encompasses four times as many hours as are in the typical business week. This translates to higher ultrasound utilization and repair needs. Unless you have ready access to funding for intermittent repair service, consider investing in a maintenance contract. Remember, however, that these contracts do not cover "abuse"; the best protection against loss due to abuse is to educate and continually remind physicians about machine care.

Options

The most important options you will consider are probes. Probes, based on their shape and frequency (frequency relates to depth of visualization and picture detail), will dictate what you can do with your machine. The four basic probe types are as follows:

- *Small curved linear array* – for abdominal examination and FAST in large children and adults, as well as cardiac examination
- *Endovaginal* – for evaluations of early pregnancy
- *High-frequency linear array* – for high-resolution imaging of superficial structures, used in vascular access, foreign body detection, abscess evaluation, and for abdominal exams on smaller children
- *Phased array* – for higher-quality cardiac examination

It is generally cheaper to get all the probes you need when buying the machine because individually purchased probes can be very expensive ($5,000–$10,000). However, probes can often be added later if you are not sure of your needs. Make sure the machine you purchase will support probes you might be interested in in the future. I recommend purchasing at least the first three probes mentioned above and the fourth (phased array) if your budget allows. The phased array probe will help reduce the number of false-positive pericardial fluid exams.

Next consider if you want options such as color flow Doppler, which is helpful when trying to differentiate a vessel from a static fluid collection, although this can also be done with the pulsed wave Doppler found on less expensive machines. Power Doppler is essential if you want to look for blood flow in low blood flow areas, such as the testes or ovaries, to rule out torsion. Even if you think you will not be doing these exams, I suggest you purchase these options if you can afford them. Ultrasound applications in emergency medicine are rapidly expanding, and, assuming an ultrasound machine's life expectancy is about 5 years, you may not get the chance to upgrade for some time.

Training

The goal of US training is to make EPs knowledgeable in the indications for ultrasound applications, competent in image acquisition and interpretation, and capable of integrating the findings appropriately into the clinical management of their patients (3). In 2008, ACEP published the most widely used training guidelines in emergency bedside ultrasound. The guidelines outline the type and amount of experience a physician needs to be considered competent in "limited" emergency ultrasound (1). The ACGME mandates procedural competency for all EM residents in emergency ultrasound (6).

"Limited" exams do not look for all pathology but only for certain specific findings that assist with immediate patient care decisions. The advantage of limited exams is that they require limited training. ACEP also published the *Emergency Ultrasound Imaging Criteria Compendium*, which describes the indications and methods of examination for many of the limited exams EPs do (7). Both documents are available free of charge from the ACEP.

Training generally starts with classroom work, including lectures and hands-on ultrasound practice on model patients. After the class work, physicians practice their exam skills in the ED by performing additional exams and confirming their results ("experiential training"), until they have performed 25 to 50 exams of any given type. Although some experts suggest specific testing of competency after the completion of the experiential training, the ACEP guidelines do not require it. Each individual ED group should develop a plan outlining the requirements for the amount of training needed for privileging in ultrasound.

Procedural ultrasound applications are simpler to master, so training requirements are generally less. According to the ACEP training guidelines for procedural ultrasound, as long as a physician is privileged in the procedure and in some other application in ultrasound, no additional experience is required (1). The ACEP gives no specific guidance for physicians who want to learn only procedural ultrasound and hold no other ultrasound privileges. At our institution, we require three proctored exams for each procedural ultrasound application, in addition to being trained in one diagnostic ultrasound application.

The experiential component of training is the most difficult to complete because practicing physicians are often left to their own devices to collect practice exams during busy ED shifts. Rarely are more experienced individuals available to assist if there are difficulties in performing the exam. Although some logistic difficulties with this part of the training remain, there are ways to get assistance with experiential training. You can hire an expert teacher; this can be an experienced physician from a training program who will travel to teach or a moonlighting ultrasound technician. There are also services that will review videotaped exams for accuracy. Physicians may want to gain experience by sitting and performing exams with sonographers in the ultrasound department at their hospital. Some ultrasound training programs offer on-site "mini fellowships" that give intensive ultrasound training over days or weeks. One-year fellowships are also available for those EPs looking for more in-depth knowledge of how to optimally use the ultrasound. ACEP established Guidelines for Emergency Ultrasound Fellowships in 2011 (8). Once you build up a pool of trained physicians within your organization, teaching duties can be transferred to them.

Policies

A well-structured ultrasound program should have training and usage policies, and it should be created with the cooperation and approval of the hospital governing body. Example policies from other facilities using ultrasound can be acquired and modified to your needs. The following policies should be in place before beginning any training:

- Training
- Privileging
- Results reporting and archiving
- Quality improvement
- Billing
- Equipment care

Training

The exact training requirements should be laid out for each type of exam. Requirements should include the amount of introductory and application-specific didactic education, as well as the number of practice exams required for training in each application. I recommend requiring that a minimum number of practice exams have the abnormal finding (gallstones, abdominal aortic aneurysm, etc.) of interest. Consider instituting a competency assessment after training to ensure competency. This could be a written exam, image interpretation test, practical assessment, or a combination of these. Program requirements should meet or exceed the ACEP training guidelines.

Privileging

A privileging policy should define eligibility for hospital privileges for bedside ultrasound and the process for obtaining both provisional and full privileges. It should address the training and experience requirements for both those who are training at the hospital and those who were previously trained, and it should define what having privileges allows the physician to do. Will each exam type be a separate privilege requiring multiple submissions to the hospital governing body? A better method is to have a general privilege in limited emergency ultrasound at the hospital level and to regulate which exams providers are allowed to do (based on their specific experience and training) at the department level.

Results reporting and archiving

This policy should outline the method for reporting results to the medical record and delineate who is allowed to report. It is a good idea to restrict unprivileged providers from using and reporting their ultrasound results. The policy should also define the method of image storage.

Quality improvement

Once physicians begin performing ultrasounds that influence patient care, there should be a method of evaluating the accuracy of the interpretations and the degree to which physicians are following documentation procedures. The QI program serves to identify problems with the program in general and individual physicians in particular. Specific feedback should be given to providers about their compliance with image labeling, image quality, image interpretation, and documentation policies. Bedside ultrasound results can be compared with other clinical information to assess the quality of interpretations. Providers will benefit from feedback about areas for improvement. Certain providers may be identified as needing additional training.

A QI program can consist of specific reviews of problem cases, a random selection of cases, or, better yet, a combination of both. A random review can be of a defined percentage of cases examined for overall quality. Exam reports, images, and the patient's chart are pulled and reviewed for

discrepancies. Records of QI activities and provider feedback should be kept.

Billing

This policy should define when exams are to be billed. Clearly, exams done by unprivileged providers should not be billed to patients, except in extreme circumstances (e.g., in a truly emergent situation where an unprivileged provider used ultrasound in a clearly lifesaving role). Ethically speaking, exams should be billed only when they add value to the patient's visit. There may be times when, because bedside ultrasound carries no significant risk, an exam is performed for a marginal indication. Providers should have the right to request such exams not be billed if, in their judgment, the exam did not add value to the patient's visit.

Equipment care

The very nature of ultrasound use in the ED – where multiple users move and use the equipment frequently in a time-pressured manner – tends to lead to innocent abuse of ED ultrasound machines. The equipment care policy should include tips for keeping the ultrasound safe from damage, including probe and cord usage and storage, and ultrasound machine placement when not in use. An exposed ultrasound machine is vulnerable to being hit by other mobile equipment, including portable x-ray machines and gurneys. Probes are easily damaged by being dropped, and cords are lacerated when run over by the ultrasound machine wheels.

The policy should also include specific instructions for cleaning probes to prevent disease transmission. Care must be taken to make sure the cleaning plan is consistent with hospital infection control policies and the American Institute for Ultrasound in Medicine's probe cleaning policies (9, 10). To ensure the ultrasound machine warranty is not voided, the cleaning protocol must use agents and techniques approved by the ultrasound manufacturer. Model the policy after those from other services in the hospital, such as obstetrics and gynecology or cardiology.

Privileging process

The hospital governing body controls the right to grant privileges to EPs in bedside ultrasound. Physicians may encounter resistance at the hospital level when trying to acquire privileges. When dealing with this resistance, it is helpful to know that the American Medical Association supports the right of individual specialties to use ultrasound and to set their own standards in doing so (11). The ACEP considers ultrasound a skill that falls under the scope of practice of emergency medicine, as does the Accreditation Council for Graduate Medical Education, which requires ultrasound training during residency in emergency medicine (1, 6). Occasionally, hospitals require or request that radiologists assist with the implementation of training or quality improvement (QI) programs for bedside ultrasound. This should be seen as a positive development and an opportunity to build a relationship with a valuable partner. That being said, training programs can function well without the assistance of radiology departments, and many do.

Some programs opt to do bedside ultrasound without a formal privileging process. This is a suboptimal approach; at a minimum, it leaves an ultrasound program vulnerable to termination without due process, and at its worst, it may put ultrasound in the hands of undertrained physicians and lead to medical misadventure.

Documentation and archiving of interpretations

Documentation of the results of a bedside ultrasound can be as simple as a note in the patient's medical record. Many programs have developed forms to assist with documentation. The advantage of a form is that, when designed to limit what can be reported, it can prevent physicians from interpreting ultrasound exams beyond their expertise and privileging. A form can also contain an explanation about the limited nature of the examination. At our facility, we use an electronic form that archives our interpretations on the hospital information system, making exam results available to all physicians in the hospital. Electronic documentation of exams makes possible queries for compliance (e.g., are unprivileged providers doing exams?) and QI purposes. Regardless of their format, results from exams used to make decisions about patient care need to be placed in the medical record.

Image archiving

Images of examinations need to be documented both for training and for medical record and billing purposes. There are a variety of methods to document images. The method used needs to be determined before purchasing an ultrasound machine because the machine must be configured correctly. Imaging documentation can be done on paper using a thermal imager (common) or a computer printer (less common). Choose a method that retains image quality for the length of time required by law for retention of medical records. Although it was originally believed that thermal images degraded relatively quickly, we have found that images taken more than 10 years ago have survived relatively unchanged.

How you archive images depends on who needs to access them. Paper images can be saved locally (in the ED) or placed in the patient's medical record. Digital images can be saved locally or uploaded to the hospital information system using a compatible interface. Make sure your machine has the correct options installed to provide you with the desired archiving capability.

Hospitals that are equipped with wireless Internet capabilities can have ultrasound images directly downloaded to a picture archiving and communication system for review and storage into the medical record. This leads to faster integration of bedside ultrasound images into the medical record and allows for faster review of the images by specialists and other consulting services. Appropriate firewalls and secure connections are required when storing images in this fashion to prevent HIPPA violations.

Continuing education

Although the ACEP training guidelines suggest that physicians receive continuing medical education (CME) in ultrasound, there are no specific recommendations. Individual physicians are free to decide the type and quantity of CME related to ultrasound they acquire. Ever-increasing demands on EPs for specific CME make it impractical to expect more than a small amount of a physician's time to be spent in ultrasound-related CME. One exception is when learning a new ultrasound exam type: physicians must take a minimal didactic component to become trained, generally consisting of at least 1 hour of didactic education followed by 1 hour of hands-on education. Experiential requirements for the exam must then be met.

Billing

EPs are entitled to bill for ultrasound exams that they do. The exams are generally billed as procedural or limited diagnostic exams. A limited exam done by an EP does not necessarily preclude a radiologist from performing and billing for a complete exam of the same organ system or anatomical area, even on the same day. EPs may also bill for multiple exams of the same type (e.g., serial FAST exams) done on the same visit, as long as they are clinically indicated. For a more detailed discussion of billing, see the report on ultrasound billing published by the ACEP (12). There are still some unresolved issues about billing, and the reader is advised to consult with billing professionals prior to billing for bedside ultrasound.

Troubleshooting and pitfalls

There are predictable areas of difficulty in establishing and running an ultrasound program. Some common issues and concerns are as follows:

1. *How can I get an ultrasound machine?* There are many options, including looking for an ultrasound machine in the hospital that is not being used by whomever it belongs to. Ask the obstetrics and gynecology and radiology departments if they have an old machine they are willing to loan. Radiologists may like the idea of reducing the amount of calls the often-overworked on-call ultrasound technician gets after hours.

   Eventually, you will want state-of-the art equipment. Hospitals may find the expense of buying or leasing equipment for the ED a reasonable investment when they evaluate their potential income from the technical charge generated by each exam. To help persuade hospital leadership, present them with the documents mentioned previously in this chapter that suggest bedside ultrasound is rapidly becoming the standard of care in the ED.

2. *How do we motivate physicians in our group to become trained?* This is a ubiquitous problem because clinicians are often too busy to concentrate on collecting practice ultrasounds. One suggestion is to get physicians trained quickly in at least one application; additional applications take less effort to learn after the first. Procedural uses are perfect as first applications because training requirements tend to be less demanding. Hopefully, once the utility of performing ultrasound is evident, physicians will see the benefit of expending the effort.

3. *The radiologists in our hospital do not support doing ultrasound exams in the ED.* Despite the arguments supporting bedside ultrasound, some still harbor a misunderstanding about the economics. Some radiologists believe that physicians performing bedside ultrasonography will cause radiologists to lose revenue, although this has never been shown. In some institutions, radiologists have contracts as "exclusive providers" of ultrasound. However, an argument can be made that radiologists are not providing some exams that are needed in the ED, either in terms of the exam type (e.g., ultrasound guidance for central lines in the ED is usually not done by the radiology department) or the timeframe in which the exam is needed. Is the radiology department able to provide FAST exams within the necessary timeframe, often 5 to 10 minutes, to make critical operative decisions on a 24-hour, 7-day-a-week basis? It follows that the radiology department should either provide these exams or allow exceptions to the contract.

4. *Unprivileged physicians are using ultrasound for patient care decisions.* One of the functions of the QI program is to identify this activity and correct it. Untrained physicians are at risk of making medical errors based on inexperienced interpretation of exams; this places patients at risk and jeopardizes the integrity of the ultrasound program.

5. *Consultants are confusing a "practice" exam done by a physician-in-training with an "official" exam done by a trained and privileged physician.* Consultants may assume that anyone who is performing an ultrasound exam in the ED is trained and qualified to interpret their exam. It is up to the physicians-in-training to make it known that they are not privileged in ultrasound. Better yet, physicians-in-training should not communicate interpretations of practice exams to anyone, including patients.

Conclusion

Ultrasound is an incredibly useful tool in the practice of emergency medicine. Although requiring more than a small amount of time to learn, the effort is well worth it. Half of all practicing EPs and almost all currently graduating emergency medicine residents possess ultrasound skills. Physicians

planning on staying in emergency medicine for longer than a few years are likely to be faced with a practice and medico-legal environment where the ability to perform and interpret bedside ultrasound examinations is no longer optional. This aside, there is still plenty of time to seek out and take advantage of educational opportunities in bedside ultrasound.

References

1. American College of Emergency Physicians (ACEP): ACEP policy statement: emergency ultrasound guidelines. Dallas, TX: ACEP, October 2008. Available at: www.acep.org/workarea/downloadasset.aspx?id = 32878

2. Squire BT, Fox JC, Anderson C: ABSCESS: applied bedside sonography for convenient evaluation of superficial soft tissue infections. *Acad Emerg Med* 2005;**12**:601–6.

3. Denys BG, Uretsky BF, Reddy PS: Ultrasound-assisted cannulation of the internal jugular vein: a prospective comparison to the external landmark-guided technique. *Circulation* 1993;**87**:1557–62.

4. American Board of Emergency Medicine: Longitudinal survey of emergency physicians. 2009. Available at: www.ABEM.org

5. American College of Emergency Physicians (ACEP): Clinical and practice management resources: ideal ultrasound machine features for the emergency medicine and critical care environment. Dallas, TX: ACEP, 2008. Available at: www.acep.org/Clinical--Practice-Management/Ideal-Ultrasound-Machine-Features-for-the-Emergency-Medicine-and-Critical-Care-Environment-2008/

6. Accreditation Council for Graduate Medical Education (ACGME): ACGME program requirements for graduate medical education in emergency medicine. September 2012. Available at: www.acgme.org/acgmeweb/Portals/0/PFAssets/2013-PR-FAQ-PIF/110_emergency_medicine_07012013.pdf

7. American College of Emergency Physicians (ACEP): ACEP policy statement: emergency ultrasound imaging criteria compendium. Dallas, TX: ACEP, April 2006. Available at: www.acep.org/workarea/downloadasset.aspx?id=32886

8. American College of Emergency Physicians (ACEP): Emergency ultrasound fellowship guidelines: an information paper. Dallas, TX: ACEP, July 2011. Available at: www.acep.org/WorkArea/linkit.aspx?LinkIdentifier=id&ItemID=80954&libID=80981

9. American Institute of Ultrasound in Medicine (AIUM): Guidelines for cleaning and preparing endocavitary ultrasound transducers between patients. Laurel, MD: AIUM, June 4, 2003. Available at: www.aium.org/officialStatements/27

10. American Institute of Ultrasound in Medicine (AIUM): Recommendations for cleaning transabdominal transducers. Laurel, MD: AIUM, June 22, 2005. Available at: www.aium.org/officialStatements/22

11. American Medical Association (AMA): H-230.960 Privileging for ultrasound imaging. Chicago: AMA, 2000. Available at: www.ama-assn.org/ssl3/ecomm/PolicyFinderForm.pl?site=www.ama-assn.org&uri=/resources/html/PolicyFinder/policyfiles/HnE/H-230.960.HTM

12. American College of Emergency Physicians (ACEP): Ultrasound section, emergency ultrasound coding and reimbursement. Dallas, TX: ACEP, 2009. Available at: www.acep.org/content.aspx?id=33280

Chapter 13

Physics of Ultrasound

Seric S. Cusick and Theodore J. Nielsen

Ultrasound provides unique advantages in the diagnostic imaging of patients in the ED. A comprehensive understanding of the physical principles supporting this modality is not mandatory for incorporation into an emergency medicine practice. However, an appreciation for several fundamental concepts and a solid grasp of the system controls will allow improved image acquisition at the bedside and facilitate precise image interpretation.

Principles of ultrasound

The fundamental principle of diagnostic ultrasound relies on the transmission of sound into the patient's body and reception of reflected sound – which is then displayed as data for interpretation. The sound energy used in diagnostic ultrasound generally ranges from 2 to 13 MHz, far outside the range detectable by the human ear (20–20,000 Hz). A simple analogy to assist in understanding ultrasound is the use of sonar, in which sound waves are emitted and the sonar device awaits the return of these impulses. Based on an assumed rate of travel, the sonar device may then determine the distance of objects by the time lapse from emission to return of a pulse of sound.

The modern use of diagnostic ultrasound can be traced back to the 1950s. Although the application of these early systems differs significantly from the units in use in today's EDs, several important physical principles have remained the same.

The creation of the ultrasonic energy is dependent on the piezoelectric effect in which electricity is transmitted into the probe, vibrating the crystals, and leading to the emission of sound. These sound waves then travel into the body at the assumed rate of 1,540 m/s, are reflected off structures, and return to the probe. This returning sound then vibrates the crystals, which transmit this energy to electrical impulses. In A-mode ultrasound – used in early diagnostic applications – stronger returning signals were depicted as larger deflections on the Y-axis of a graphical display. Modern B-mode imaging uses a gray scale of at least 256 points to depict the strength of the returning sound, with stronger signals being hyperechoic (brighter or whiter) and the absence of returning signals being depicted as anechoic (jet black), with intermediate strengths being assigned shades of gray. The use of a time–distance relationship to plot the location of a data point and a gray scale to depict the strength of a given returning impulse allows the creation of a 2D image. The relative intensity of the returning echoes is determined by the acoustic impedance of the encountered tissues. Objects of high acoustic impedance – such as gallstones – reflect most of the sound back to the transducer and permit very little sound to travel to deeper structures (described further in the "Image artifacts" section). Conversely, those of low impedance – such as the urinary bladder – permit much of the sound to travel through, reflecting little and resulting in a hypoechoic or anechoic signal on B-mode imaging. Real-time ultrasound images are thereby created through the repetition of this process multiple times per second, allowing our minds to view motion as 11 to 60 frames per second. The basic process outlined here can then be hindered by imaging artifacts and modified by the system controls available to the sonographer.

System controls

An understanding of basic system controls will allow the operator to obtain a quality diagnostic ultrasound image while reducing unnecessary echo information and patient risk. This section addresses the operation of fundamental controls for image acquisition; however, each manufacturer may have specific technology and adjustments to enhance transmit and return echo information. An ultrasound manufacturer's clinical representative or system manual may provide alternate means for understanding controls specific to a particular system.

Time gain compensation

Two fundamental controls allow the operator to adjust the brightness or image intensity of returning echo information. Although some systems may also permit an auto adjustment of image intensity, prudent use would dictate an understanding of the available manual adjustments.

Time gain compensation (TGC) adjusts returning echo information relative to depth within the ultrasound image. Effects of acoustic attenuation cause the ultrasound waves to continually weaken as they propagate through the anatomy. If no control was available, ultrasound images would generally appear hyperechoic near the origin at the top of the screen and display less echo information as the wave travels through the tissue to the far field of the image. The TGC control allows the operator to manually adjust or compensate the intensity of the returning echoes for depth because additional time is required for the echoes to return to the transducer from

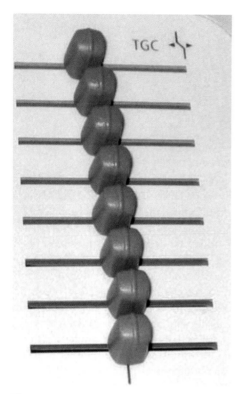

Figure 13.1. Example of standard controls for time gain compensation.

deeper structures. This control permits an equal display of the intensity of echo information from the top of the screen to the bottom. The goal of the TGC control is to provide uniform amplification of returning echo information, regardless of depth or distance from the transducer.

The actual operation of this control may vary among manufacturers. Traditionally, TGC incorporates multiple sliding controls that correspond to a particular depth within the imaging field (Fig. 13.1). Some manufacturers may elect to replace the sliding controls with two controls simply labeled "Near" and "Far." The sliding controls allow the sonographer to determine the image intensity at specific depths within an image, whereas near and far settings are, by design, targeting the relative near half (closer to the probe and top of the screen) and far half (away from the probe and closer to the bottom of the screen). Furthermore, several newer machines offer a feature that allows the user to depress a single button that attempts to create uniform gain throughout the image. Regardless of which design is incorporated into the system being used, the intent or correct operation of the control is to maintain a uniform balance of echo intensity information.

Gain

As with the TGC control, the gain control allows a manual adjustment of the intensity of the returning echoes. The difference, however, is the location at which the amplification occurs. As defined in the previous section, the TGC control allows amplification of the returning echoes at specific depth intervals or at the near and far components of the image

display. In contrast, the gain control amplifies all returning echoes equally, regardless of depth.

The unit of measure is the decibel and may be displayed on the screen as "db" or as a numeric value. This control may be compared with a volume control on a radio. When the volume or gain is increased, the "louder" or "brighter" returning echo information will be displayed on the screen. A common error for the novice sonographer is to employ excessive gain settings, which reduce contrast resolution and the ability to appropriately distinguish the presence of structures, their echogenicity, and related borders. To minimize the perceived need for increased gain, create a dimly lit environment for accurate sonographic examination.

Resolution

Resolution may be most simply described as the ability to differentiate among two distinct objects in the scanning plane. Axial resolution refers to the discriminatory limits for objects that lie within the beam axis and is directly related to the frequency. Lateral resolution is the resolution among points perpendicular to the imaging plane and is inversely related to the beam width.

Frequency

Transducers are designed for various applications and are manufactured in a variety of sizes and shapes. Physical shape and technology are dictated by each manufacturer and may incorporate a variety of arrays, including mechanical, phased, convex, and linear designs. Transmit frequency remains one of the fundamental features of all transducers. Many transducers allow multiple transmit frequencies to be incorporated into a single transducer and selected by the sonographer. The number of available frequencies in a specific transducer is determined by its manufacturer and is related to its intended application. It is important to remember that imaging frequency and Doppler frequency are independent of each another. Higher imaging frequencies will produce an image of increased resolution while sacrificing signal penetration.

Higher frequencies are used to image superficial structures, whereas lower frequencies are used for deeper structures. Although an increase in frequency generally improves image resolution, other factors must also be considered, including internal focusing of the beam and the pulse length of the wave. The pulse length is dependent on transducer characteristics designated by the manufacturer. This may partially explain the finding that simply increasing the transmit frequency of a transducer may not always result in perceived increased resolution. Selecting the transducer designed for the intended application *and* using the highest imaging frequency that will penetrate to the targeted area of interest will contribute to the best resolving capability.

Beam width

If we consider the 2D profile of the ultrasound beam, we may take creative license and compare it to the shape of an hourglass. The center point of the glass may be considered the point at which the greatest degree of beam convergence occurs. It is at this level that anatomical structures will be displayed with greatest lateral resolution. A user-modifiable focal zone may allow the operator to adjust the width of the ultrasound beam relative to depth, or more simply, where the greatest degree of convergence will occur relative to the anteroposterior depth within the image. Ideally, the focal zone should be positioned on the display adjacent to the targeted area of interest because the ultrasound beam profile will be the narrowest at this point. Multiple focal zones may be selected, thereby increasing the resolving capability throughout the image; however, multiple zones will decrease the displayed frame rate, as additional processing time is required. The resulting image will have less of a "real-time" appearance. Single focal zone selections are usually sufficient for most cardiac and abdominal examinations, although multiple focal zones may be of greater value with superficial imaging when speed of transducer movement is at a minimum. Systems that do not offer a user-selectable focal zone may possess technology that automatically adjusts beam width to improve resolving capability when the desired anatomy is positioned in the center of the display.

Depth, magnification, and zoom

The depth control allows the operator to manually adjust the field of view, determining the depth or range of the information that is displayed. This adjustment results in the perceived increase or decrease in overall size of the image. When an increase in depth is selected, the resulting anatomical structures must appear smaller on the screen, so a greater absolute depth may be displayed within a fixed monitor size. If less depth is displayed, targeted structures within the image will appear larger while sacrificing the interrogated depth of tissue. Beginning an examination with a maximum depth setting will ensure all anterior-to-posterior information will be displayed, thus allowing the operator a large field of view to ensure the desired anatomical structures are not missed. Once the anatomical region of interest is identified, the depth setting may be reduced to ensure the viewing area is focused on these structures.

The zoom function is an additional control that allows an increase in the size of the anatomical structures displayed on the screen. To zoom an image often refers to the operator selecting a targeted area of interest within the image. Once the area is identified, the zoom function allows a magnification of only the selected area. The amount of zoom may be a fixed or adjustable depending on the system. Using this function may be of particular interest when attempting to view small structures within an image. Some systems may allow for the zoom function to be used only during real-time scanning, whereas others may allow this function to be used on a still or frozen image on the screen.

Acoustic power

Acoustic power is defined as the amount of transmitted power or amplitude incorporated to provide the pulse to the transducer. Remember that TGC and gain are controls that affect the display of returning echo information via amplification or modification of the obtained information. The power emitted from the transducer affects all aspects of scanning from image acquisition to Doppler. The amount of power may be displayed on the ultrasound screen as a numerical value or simply identified as a percentage value. Some ultrasound systems do not allow an adjustment of acoustic power, with power output values internally assigned by the manufacturer for each mode of operation. Indices of transmitted power are often displayed on the ultrasound screen as mechanical index (MI) and thermal index (TI). Multiple system controls may affect the calculated values associated with MI and TI, including acoustic power, scanning mode, and pulse repetition frequency, among others. In the event that manual adjustment of the power is afforded, the sonographer should attempt to modify other parameters prior to increasing transmitted power in accordance with the "as low as reasonably achievable" (ALARA) principle described in the "Biological effects" section.

Measurement and analysis

Basic distance measurements are among the most commonly used calculations on an ultrasound system. Many systems allow for multiple calipers to be displayed simultaneously, with shape-specific (+ and ×) or alphabetically labeled (A and B) caliper end points allowing measurements to be easily differentiated. The calipers automatically calibrate as adjustments are made, with distances displayed on the system monitor. Additional analysis packages available in each exam type or preset allow calculations using standardized charts associated with previously researched data. Examples of these parameters include gestational age, cardiac output, urinary bladder volume, and fetal heart rate. This measurement data may also be associated with report pages designed to provide a summary of information on conclusion of the examination.

Doppler

A detailed discussion of Doppler physics and appropriate application is beyond the scope and intent of this chapter. That which follows is an introduction to the modes of Doppler available on common ED systems and possible indications. The use of Doppler in clinical imaging is largely dependent on pulsed wave technology. Pulses of sound are emitted into tissues and reflected back to the probe. In addition to the information of intensity and time used to establish B-mode images, Doppler modes assess the frequency of the returning sound. Due to the *frequency shift* that occurs when the ultrasound beam is reflected off moving particles, the unit is able to determine direction and velocity of the moving particles by incorporating the change in frequency

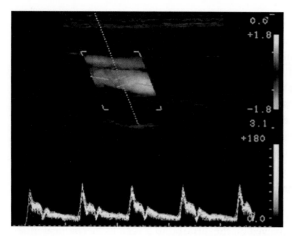

Figure 13.2. This image demonstrates the appearance of both color Doppler – visualized as directional signal within the lumen of the vessels – and pulse wave Doppler, which is the graphical display demonstrating rate of movement over time.

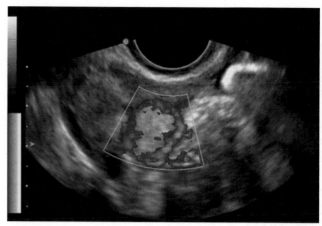

Figure 13.3. Color power Doppler – used here to demonstrate a "ring of fire" around an ectopic pregnancy – indicates movement using a color overlay but lacks directional information.

into the Doppler equation. The most clinically relevant feature of this calculation – which is not discussed in detail here – is the cos Θ present in the numerator. As the cos 90 = zero, the Doppler signal created by moving particles assessed at 90 degrees is nil. Absence of Doppler signal when imaging vascular structures at a perpendicular angle may be overcome by gentle angling of the probe.

Color Doppler places a bidirectional color signal over standard B-mode imaging, indicating the presence of movement and its direction in relation to the transducer (Fig. 13.2). Note that the color (red or blue) of the signal represents movement toward or away from the transducer, is modifiable via the units settings, and does not necessarily correspond to expected arterial or venous conventions (red = artery, blue = vein) established by anatomy texts.

Power Doppler uses a range of a single color – typically orange – to indicate movement with the absence of a directional component (Fig. 13.3). Due to characteristics of this technology that limit background noise and artifact, power Doppler may be employed with higher gain settings, enabling the sonographer to assess anatomical regions with lower flow velocities.

Spectral Doppler allows placement of a sampling gate within a region of interest and subsequent graphical representation of the flow velocities plotted over time (Fig. 13.2). Characterization of arterial and venous waveforms may then be performed, allowing analysis of physiological conditions.

M-mode

M-mode is a simple, alternative display to real-time B-mode imaging that has limited, focused application in the emergency setting. In this setting, motion of gray scale reflectors is plotted against time in a graphical display (Fig. 13.4). This allows for interpretation and quantitative assessment of anatomical and temporal patterns in applications such as cardiac

ultrasound, determination of fetal heart rate, and interpretation of lung sonography in the detection of pneumothorax.

Transducer selection

The sonographer must select a transducer for each exam with consideration of the patient's body habitus and the anatomy to be visualized. Transducers hold varied footprints – areas that participate in sound transmission and are intended to maintain contact with the surface imaged – that may lend to use in certain anatomical regions. In addition, each transducer determines the range of frequencies available to the sonographer, affecting both tissue penetration and resolution.

Mechanical transducers

Historically, the piezoelectric effect described previously was created via the mechanical oscillation of an individual crystal within the transducer head. This resulted in a palpable vibratory sense within the sonographer's hand and afforded good imaging characteristics obtained at a reasonable economic cost but limited by a fixed focal zone. An adjustable focal zone was obtained in these probes through the use of an annular array, but these transducers remain less common in the emergency setting today.

Array transducer

Array transducers electronically "fire" probe elements in sequence, creating the imaging field as displayed on the unit monitor. The orientation of the crystals and the contour of the probe footprint determine the shape and size of the image obtained. A *linear array* transducer (Fig. 13.5) emits and receives sound only in the field directly under the footprint of the probe. Often, these possess high frequencies and are used in superficial and vascular applications. A *curved, convex,* or *curvilinear* transducer maintains this rowlike orientation of elements but places it along a curved footprint. Therefore, the sound travels into

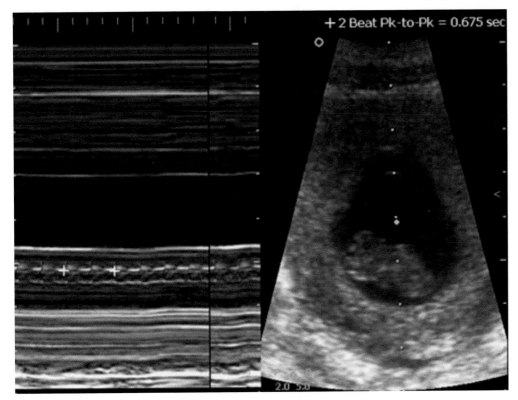

Figure 13.4. The sampling gate for M-mode is placed over the cardiac activity of a first-trimester fetus, yielding a graphical representation of movement. Using the system's software package allows quantification of the fetal heart rate by measuring the distance between two peaks.

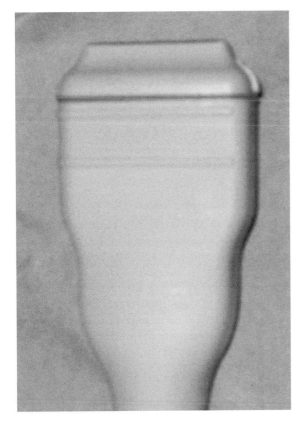

Figure 13.5. Linear array transducer.

a sector-shaped region and produces an image that is wider in the far field than the probe footprint. The relative width of this far field is dependent on the depth of the image and the degree of the footprint's curvature. A standard *curvilinear* abdominal probe (Fig. 13.6) places a gentle curvature across a broad footprint. Conversely, a tighter curvature is placed over a small footprint for an *intracavitary* probe (Fig. 13.7), maintaining a broad imaging field despite the required slim form factor.

Phased array transducer

Rather than align crystals in a linear fashion to determine the scanning field, phased array transducers rely on the electronic "steering" of sound impulses emitted under precise timing from multiple elements. Among other benefits, this allows a transducer with a small footprint to produce a sector-shaped image with a relatively wide far field. This has been most commonly employed in *cardiac* transducers (Fig. 13.8), permitting intercostal probe placement for echocardiography.

Image artifacts

Image artifacts may result from transducer design, anatomical interfaces and their reflections, body habitus, and ultrasound beam properties. Understanding and recognizing image artifacts increases the knowledge of the sonographer, while minimizing

205

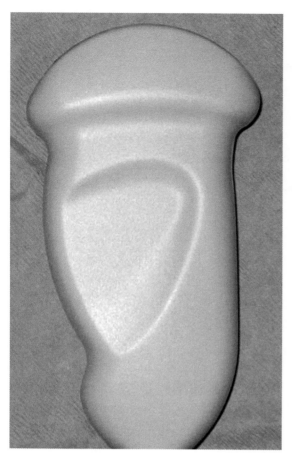

Figure 13.6. Convex (curvilinear) array transducer.

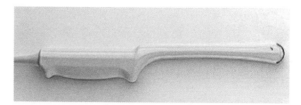

Figure 13.7. Intracavitary (curvilinear) transducer.

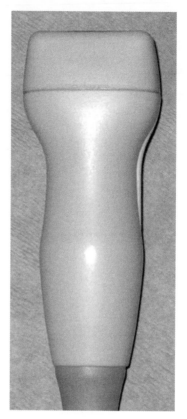

Figure 13.8. Phased array transducer.

the risk of interpreting misleading information. Some of the more common imaging artifacts are explored in this section.

Attenuation

The process of attenuation refers to the loss of sound energy as it passes through a medium. The rate at which this occurs is dependent on the medium through which the sound is traveling and the inherent frequency of the sound – with higher frequencies attenuating more rapidly. A small portion of this energy is lost to the tissues and converted to heat in the process of absorption, while the remainder of this attenuation is due to reflection and scattering of the initial sound energy.

Acoustic shadowing

One of the more common ultrasound imaging artifacts is acoustic shadowing. The reasons for shadowing include anatomical reflections, certain pathological conditions, and associated sonographic properties. When the ultrasound beam interacts with a highly attenuating structure, much of the energy is reflected back to the transducer with little or no acoustic energy continuing to travel to deep structures. Because no sound is able to travel to deeper structures, an anechoic region is displayed posteriorly. Bone, calcifications, and gallstones

are examples that demonstrate this phenomenon, as seen in Figures 13.9 and 13.10.

Refraction

Directional changes of the ultrasound beam may also be associated with perceived shadowing. As the sound passes through a boundary of two tissue types – particularly of varied impedance – an artifact termed *lateral cystic shadowing* or *edge artifact* may result. Significant differences in the propagation speed of sound through these tissues result in deflection of the path of sound. The absence of echoes returning from the region deep to the point of this refraction results in the appearance of an "acoustic shadow" (Figs. 13.9 and 13.11).

Acoustic enhancement

In contrast to acoustic shadowing, posterior acoustic enhancement occurs when sound crosses a tissue that

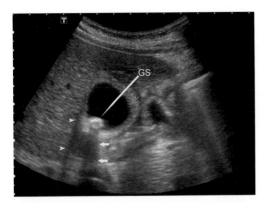

Figure 13.9. Image of the right upper quadrant demonstrating features of cholecystitis. Note the hyperechoic gallstone (GS) causing posterior acoustic shadowing (*arrows*). The interface between the hepatic parenchyma and the gallbladder wall frequently results in refraction, which is seen here as lateral cystic shadowing (*arrowheads*).

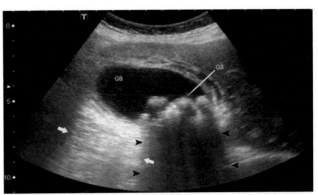

Figure 13.10. Ultrasound of the right upper quadrant in a patient with cholecystitis. Two artifacts may be appreciated here: posterior acoustic shadowing (*black arrowheads*) deep to the multiple gallstones and posterior acoustic enhancement (*white arrows*) seen relative to surrounding hepatic tissue as sound travels through the lumen of the gallbladder (GB).

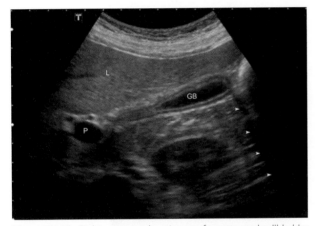

Figure 13.11. Right upper quadrant image of a contracted gallbladder (GB) in long axis seen adjacent to the portal triad (P), demonstrating lateral cystic shadowing (*arrowheads*).

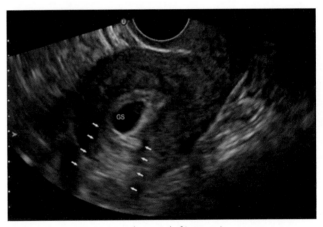

Figure 13.12. Intracavitary ultrasound of intrauterine pregnancy demonstrating gestational sac (GS) with yolk sac and posterior acoustic enhancement (*arrows*).

attenuates the signal less when compared to the surrounding anatomy. Anatomical structures of low impedances often result in acoustic enhancement – identified as a hyperechoic area displayed immediately posterior to the structure and following the same angle of interrogation (Figs. 13.10 and 13.12). This is commonly associated with fluid-filled objects and is often appreciated when imaging cysts, urinary bladders, and gallbladders. In addition, enhancement may occur when the ultrasound beam encounters any type of tissue that simply does not attenuate the signal with the same degree when compared to the surrounding structures.

Scatter

Bowel gas represents a frequent cause of scatter – an artifact that plagues many attempts at abdominal sonography. Partly due to the large differences in density that exist between gas molecules and soft tissue, the ultrasound beam that encounters bowel is often scattered and reflected at unpredictable

angles, resulting in little diagnostic information returning to the probe (Fig. 13.13). Changes in the transducer angle of interrogation, slight transducer pressure to displace bowel gas, or repositioning of the patient may improve visualization through an alternate acoustic window.

Reverberation

Reverberation artifacts may appear as recurrent bright arcs displayed at equidistant intervals from the transducer. When two highly reflective objects are positioned in close proximity to each other, the returning echo may reverberate, or "bounce," between the two structures, and the resulting reverberation artifact will lose energy with each propagation. Often, the reverberation artifact will appear at or near the anterior wall of a distended urinary bladder (Fig. 13.14), across the anterior portion of the gallbladder, or even deep to reflective foreign objects (Fig. 13.15). Changes in transducer frequency, patient positioning, or angle of

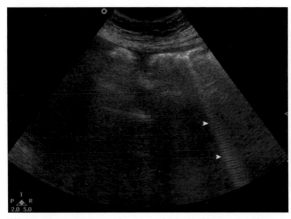

Figure 13.13. Abdominal sonography limited by commonly encountered artifact of scatter, obscuring visualization of anatomical structures. Also note excellent example of reverberation artifact (*arrowhead*).

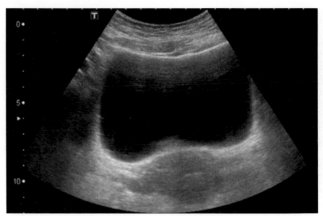

Figure 13.14. Urinary bladder sonography notable for reverberation artifacts in the near field; note the repetitive hyperechoic artifacts mirroring the probe curvature and crossing tissue boundaries.

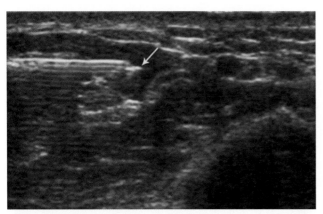

Figure 13.15. Dynamic ultrasound of median nerve block. The needle (tip indicated by *arrow*) is associated with reverberation artifact and seen as evenly spaced, repetitive echoes into the far field.

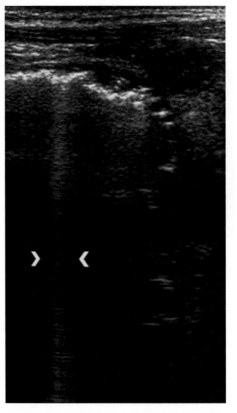

Figure 13.16. Ring-down artifact originating from normal bowel during an abdominal ultrasound.

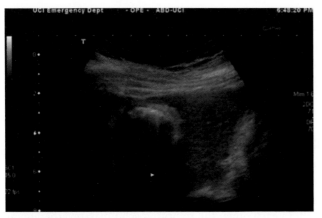

Figure 13.17. Right upper quadrant ultrasound in gangrenous cholecystitis. Air in the anterior wall of the gallbladder results in comet tail artifact (*arrowhead*).

interrogation may reduce or minimize their appearance; however, reverberation artifacts are generally not confused with a pathological condition.

Ring-down artifact is a type of reverberation artifact that is often seen when imaging the abdomen. The interface between air and visceral structures may result in projection of tightly spaced echoes deep to the origination of this artifact secondary to the reverberation of sound caused by air trapped within a fluid collection (1). This may originate at the normal interface that occurs within bowel (Figs. 13.13 and 13.16.), or in pathological intraabdominal conditions (Fig. 13.17). The term "ring-down" is also used to describe the artifact

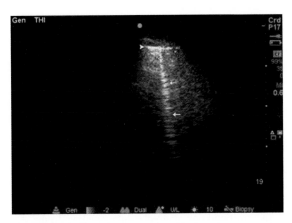

Figure 13.18. Thoracic sonography with phased array transducer demonstrating single comet tail artifact (*arrow*) emanating from the pleural line (*arrowhead*).

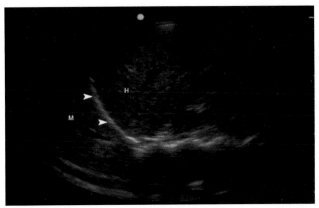

Figure 13.19. Right upper quadrant image obtained during a focused assessment with sonography in trauma (FAST). The diaphragm (*arrowheads*) creates a highly reflective surface when adjacent to normal lung. The true image of hepatic tissue (H) is also displayed on the left side of the image – superior to the diaphragm – as a mirror image artifact (M).

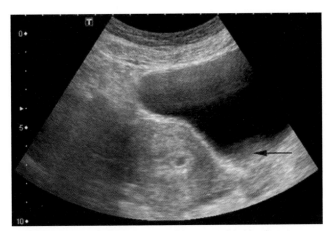

Figure 13.20. A longitudinal image of the urinary bladder demonstrates two common artifacts. In the near field, again seen is reverberation artifact, shown more clearly in Figure 13.14. In addition, side lobe artifact (*black arrow*) is seen near the apex of the bladder as a collection of hyperechoic signals.

that may occur deep to metallic objects, such as a foreign body or a needle during procedural ultrasound.

Comet tail artifact is another term used to describe a specific form of reverberation. The initial description of this phenomenon was in association with a metallic foreign body (2) but has more recently been applied to artifacts occurring in thoracic ultrasound (3–6). Repetitive reflections originating at the pleural interface extend deep into the imaging field, widening as they progress when performed with a phased or curved array transducer as seen in Figure 13.18.

Mirror image artifact

Mirror image artifact refers to the appearance of identical echoes – one being false – on either side of a strong reflector due to changes in the path of the ultrasound beam. Recall that the ultrasound system identifies the depth and position of reflected sound relative to speed of sound in tissue and the time necessary to return to the transducer – all assuming a direct line of travel. If the ultrasound beam performs multiple reflections during its course, the correct signal timing is interrupted and results in the placement of this echo deeper into the field than the actual source (the explanation of this phenomenon has also led to it being termed a "multipath artifact"). The duplicate echoes occurring deeper are the mirror, or "false," echoes. Mirror image artifacts are often visualized around the diaphragm, resulting in the appearance of hepatic tissue on either side of the diaphragm (Fig. 13.19).

Side lobes

Although we describe a solitary sound wave of uniform frequency that is transmitted from the transducer along a plane parallel to the central axis of the transducer, ultrasound beams of lower intensity (side lobes) may actually originate at various angles to the primary beam. These side lobes may result in inaccurate information being displayed that is associated with highly reflective interfaces and may appear as an oblique line of acoustic reflections or result in inaccurate placement of echoes (Fig. 13.20). Minor adjustments in the angle of interrogation will often abate these artifacts and confirm the returning echoes as side lobes.

Biological effects

Diagnostic ultrasound is generally regarded as a safe modality with no harmful bioeffects to humans reported in the literature. Considered a noninvasive imaging modality, potential risks associated with the various modes of ultrasound do exist, and prudent use dictates that the sonographer incorporate an understanding of those effects while minimizing patient risk. The American Institute of Ultrasound in Medicine (AIUM) has adopted the acronym ALARA, "as low as reasonably achievable," designed to guide the sonographer toward practicing ultrasound parameters that minimize the patient risk potentially associated with higher output levels and the effects of increased time for various modes of ultrasound (7). For example, controls such as frequency, TGC, and gain should be optimized prior to increasing acoustic power capabilities in an attempt to produce a high-quality diagnostic ultrasound image. Furthermore, due to the increase in transmitted power associated with Doppler technology, these modes should be avoided in general obstetrical imaging. MI and TI values provide information to the operator to determine if the current system settings may be adjusted to reduce the potential risk of biological effects to the patient. Current statements from the AIUM report the absence of data indicating risk of bioeffects at MI <0.3 and TI <2 (7).

Summary

This chapter introduces the physical fundamentals that form the foundation for the use of diagnostic imaging in the emergency setting. For providers interested in a more detailed discussion of Doppler physics, bioeffects, and imaging artifacts, the authors have provided a select list of references (8, 9). However, an understanding of the concepts presented in this chapter will allow improved image acquisition, effective management of system controls, and enhanced accuracy in image interpretation.

References

1. Avruch L, Cooperberg PL: The ring-down artifact. *J Ultrasound Med* 1985;**4**(1):21–8.

2. Ziskin MC, Thickman DI, Goldenberg NJ, et al.: The comet tail artifact. *J Ultrasound Med* 1982;**1**(1):1–7.

3. Lichtenstein D, Meziere G: A lung ultrasound sign allowing bedside distinction between pulmonary edema and COPD: the comet-tail artifact. *Intensive Care Med* 1998;**24**(12):1331–4.

4. Lichtenstein D, Meziere G, Biderman P, Gepner A: The comet-tail artifact: an ultrasound sign ruling out pneumothorax. *Intensive Care Med* 1999;**25**(4):383–8.

5. Lichtenstein D, Meziere G, Biderman P, et al.: The comet-tail artifact: an ultrasound sign of alveolar-interstitial syndrome. *Am J Respir Crit Care Med* 1997;**156**(5):1640–6.

6. Thickman DI, Ziskin MC, Goldenberg NJ, Linder BE: Clinical manifestations of the comet tail artifact. *J Ultrasound Med* 1983;**2**(5):225–30.

7. Holland CK: Mechanical Bioeffects from Diagnostic Ultrasound: AIUM Consensus Statements. *J Ultrasound Med* 2000;**19**(2):69–72.

8. Rumack CM, Wilson SR, Charboneau JW, Johnson JA: *Diagnostic ultrasound*, 3rd ed. St. Louis, MO: Mosby, 2005.

9. Middleton WD, Kurtz AB, Hertzberg BS: *Ultrasound—the requisites*, 2nd ed. St. Louis, MO: Mosby, 2004.

Chapter 14

Biliary Ultrasound

William Scruggs and Laleh Gharahbaghian

Indications

Gallbladder disease affects 8% to 17% of people (varying by gender) and is a common cause of emergency department visits, hospital admissions, and operative interventions (1, 2). The accepted initial imaging study for biliary evaluation is gallbladder ultrasound. While other imaging modalities offer comparable or even better overall accuracy, ultrasound offers significant advantages in cost, time, and radiation exposure (3, 4).

The most common indication for biliary ultrasound is right upper quadrant or epigastric pain concerning for cholelithiasis and acute cholecystitis. Ultrasound of the biliary system is also indicated for evaluation of the jaundiced patient, newly elevated liver function tests, and newly diagnosed pancreatitis, and it can be considered in the evaluation of liver lesions including suspected metastases and abscesses (5).

Diagnostic capabilities

Cholelithiasis and cholecystitis are both accurately diagnosed by ultrasound. Meta-analysis study of the diagnosis of cholelithiasis with ultrasound, adjusted for verification bias, suggests a sensitivity of 84% and specificity of 99% (6). Two such studies reviewing the test characteristics of ultrasound for acute cholecystitis find the sensitivity of ultrasound to be 81% and 88% (6, 7).

Other imaging modalities offer a more accurate diagnosis of acute cholecystitis. Cholescintigraphy appears to be the most accurate, demonstrating a sensitivity of 96%. MRI is also an acceptable alternative, with a sensitivity for acute cholecystitis of 85% (7). CT is poorly studied but is generally considered inferior in the evaluation of acute biliary disease (8, 9).

A growing body of literature supports emergency physician and surgeon-performed ultrasound for the diagnosis of cholelithiasis and acute cholecystitis. Pooled analysis of emergency physician ultrasound for cholelithiasis finds a sensitivity of 90% and specificity of 88%, though most of these studies are limited because they use radiology ultrasound as criterion standard (10). When compared with surgical pathology, emergency physician ultrasound has been found to be equal in accuracy to radiology ultrasound for acute cholecystitis (11).

Abscesses and neoplasms of the liver are accurately diagnosed by ultrasound, and ultrasound is used to guide abscess drainage and biopsies of the liver. However, CT is generally considered the first-line imaging study where available (12, 13).

Imaging pitfalls and limitations

Ultrasound of the biliary system is generally more difficult in obese patients, as increased abdominal girth moves the probe farther from the organs of interest. However, body habitus is not a reason to abandon ultrasound evaluation, and many obese patients produce excellent images.

Increased abdominal gas is much more detrimental to biliary ultrasound. Air in the hepatic flexure (sitting just inferior to the liver) and the duodenum (directly inferior and posterior to the gallbladder and anterior to the pancreas) scatters sound waves, making visualization of surrounding structures difficult or impossible. Air can be particularly problematic in acute cases when adynamic ileus in bowel develops due to local inflammation. Adequate analgesia is imperative for abdominal ultrasound. Sonologists may be able to push bowel gas out of the way with slow, constant pressure that an unmedicated patient may not tolerate. Changing the position of the patient (left lateral decubitus) or giving the patient a small amount of water to drink may help to displace duodenal air and improve visualization.

There are significant potential limitations to ultrasound of the biliary tract. The quality of any ultrasound examination is dependent on the experience and ability of the provider. In difficult-to-image patients, CT and MRI may better evaluate the overall structure of the liver, biliary tract, and pancreas. Given the difficulties of imaging around the duodenum, these two modalities are generally more effective in evaluating pathology related to the common bile duct.

Ultrasound does not evaluate organ function, and cholescintigraphy is more accurate for cystic duct obstruction and cholecystitis. When ultrasound is negative for pathology but clinical suspicion is high for outlet obstruction, clinicians should consider using cholescintigraphy.

Clinical images

Gallbladder

The gallbladder is a pear-shaped organ that accumulates and excretes bile to assist in digestion of fat within the small bowel. It most commonly lies on the caudal surface of the liver but may be found within the liver parenchyma. The upper limit of normal length is 10 cm and width 4 cm. The wall of the gallbladder should be homogenous in appearance and less than 3 mm in width. The bile that normally fills the gallbladder is anechoic.

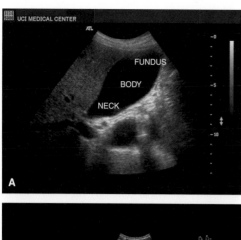

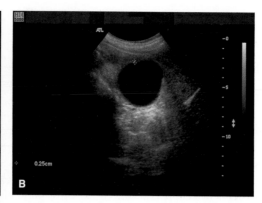

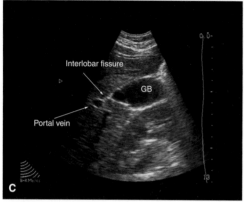

Figure 14.1. Gallbladder anatomy: The fundus of the gallbladder is a blind pouch that tapers toward the neck of the gallbladder, which further narrows to the cystic duct (A, B). In the short axis, the gallbladder appears circular (B). Both long- and short-axis views are needed for complete visualization. The main lobar fissure (MLF) is an important landmark. With the gallbladder in the long axis, the MLF will appear to connect the gallbladder to the portal vein. The tapered gallbladder in the long axis and portal vein in the short axis create the classic "exclamation point" (C).

The biliary tract

The biliary system is made up of the gallbladder along with the intra- and extrahepatic biliary ducts. The ducts are found within the portal triad, along with the portal veins and hepatic arteries. The intrahepatic ducts form in the subsegments of the liver and run toward the porta hepatis, where they form the common hepatic duct (CHD). The CHD then meets the cystic duct from the gallbladder to form the common bile duct (CBD). The CBD makes its way behind the duodenum and into the pancreas, usually joining the pancreatic duct at the ampula of Vater, where bile is expressed into the duodenum.

It is very difficult to identify the confluence of the hepatic duct and cystic duct. Therefore, we generally refer to the entire CHD and CBD as the common bile duct and divide it into the proximal duct, mid duct, and distal duct. The proximal CBD is found anterior to the right portal vein. The mid-CBD is posterior to the duodenum. The distal CBD lies in the head of the pancreas and meets the pancreatic duct. The CHD may be measured as a surrogate for the CBD.

The CBD is measured from inner wall to inner wall. A normal CBD will be less than 6 mm in diameter, while 6–8 mm is considered equivocal. A CBD greater than 8 mm in diameter is abnormally dilated. The CBD does gradually dilate with age. A rule of thumb is to add 1 mm for every decade above the age of 60. However, given the frequency of gallbladder disease in this age group, it is wise to be cautious in attributing a dilated CBD to age alone. After a cholecystectomy, the CBD will often dilate to as much as 1 cm in diameter.

The intrahepatic ducts are more difficult to evaluate because they are normally very narrow (<2 mm). They should never be more than 40% of the diameter of the adjacent portal vein. Vessels and ducts also differ in that the diameter of bile ducts varies through its course while arterial diameter remains consistent. Bile ducts tend to create stellate patterns at their confluences when they join into larger ducts (generally only visualized when dilated).

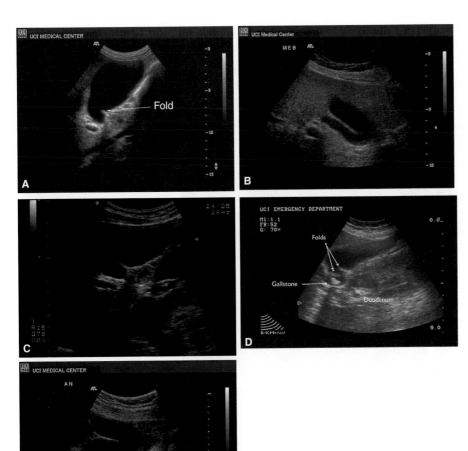

Figure 14.2. Gallblbladder variations:
The gallbladder has many normal variations. Folds are common and are most often found near the neck but may occur anywhere within the gallbladder (A–C). Multiple folds can develop (D). The term "phyrigian cap" refers to a fold in the fundus of the gallbladder (E). The gallbladder may be compartmentalized by septations or duplicated.

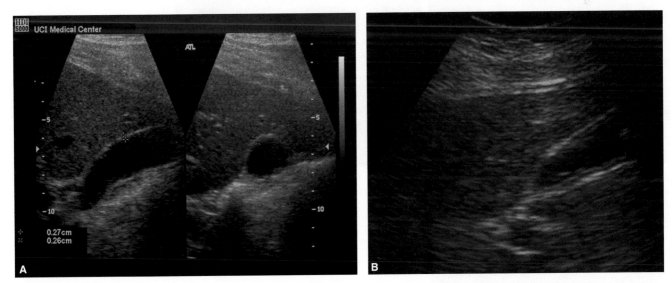

Figure 14.3. Gallbladder wall: The normal gallbladder wall is homogenous and echogenic (A). When contracted, the gallbladder wall demonstrates three layers – mucosa, muscularis, and serosa. The normal wall is <3 mm in width. A measurement of 3–4 mm is equivocal, and a measurement of >4 mm is considered abnormal. There are many possible causes of gallbladder wall thickening, acute cholecystitis being the most common cause (Table 14.1).

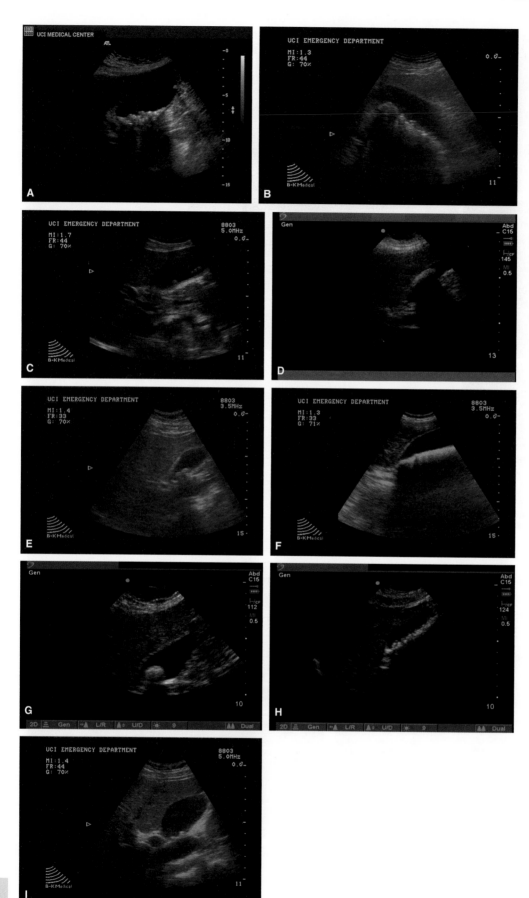

Figure 14.4. Gallstones: Gallstones are readily identified on ultrasound (A–H). Most are echogenic, meaning almost all ultrasound waves directed toward a gallstone will reflect from the stone creating an echogenic rim with dense shadowing beyond it. Stones as small as 1–2 mm can be identified with ultrasound. Imaging with higher frequency improves shadowing and the ability to visualize gallstones. The type of stone cannot be determined based on ultrasound. However, pigmented stones are typically softer and more likely not to shadow (I).

Gallstones vary in size, will occur in isolation or as multiples, and may be found in any location within the gallbladder. Most stones are mobile and gravitationally dependent, meaning that as patients are moved their gallstones will drop to the "lowest" point in the gallbladder. However, gallstones may adhere to the gallbladder wall making it difficult to distinguish between stone and polyp. Polyps generally do not cause shadowing.

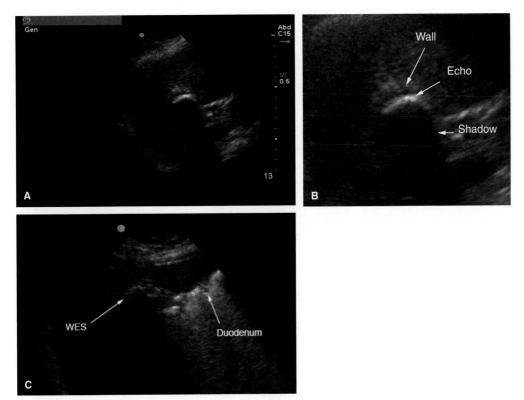

Figure 14.5. WES sign: Gallstones can be difficult to identify when the gallbladder wall is contracted around a gallstone. The wall-echo-shadow (WES) sign is uncommonly found and can be difficult to identify. It is created when the gallbladder completely contracts around a gallstone. The **w**all is identified, followed immediately by the **e**chogenic rim of the stone, and then the dense **s**hadowing of the stone.

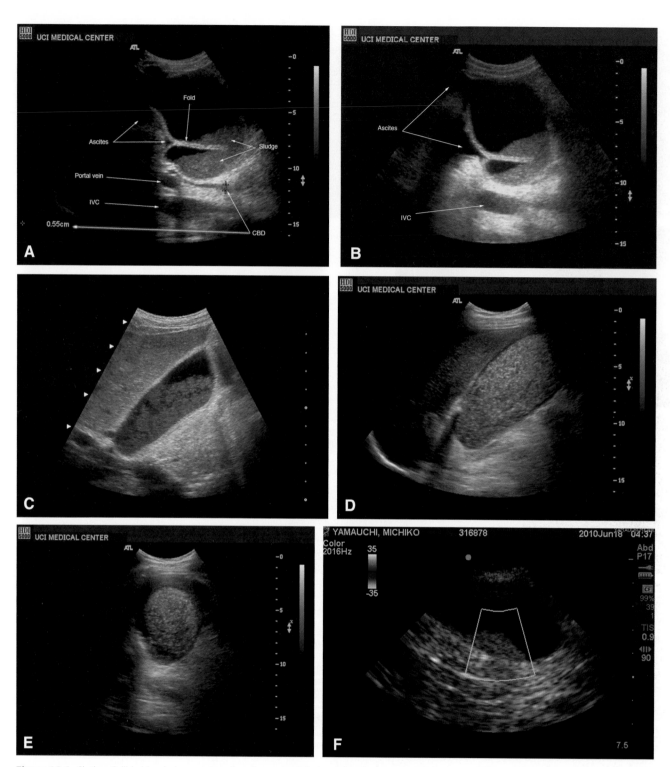

Figure 14.6. Sludge: Gallbladder sludge consists of small crystals of cholesterol and calcium. It appears as non-shadowing, moderately echogenic particles within the gallbladder. Often sludge will form a meniscus as it layers in the gallbladder (A–E). Tumefactive sludge is more dense and coalesces into structures that take shape rather than layering (F). Sludge and soft tissue masses can be difficult to tell apart. Color Doppler can assist in differentiating between the two, as soft tissue masses will exhibit blood flow. The clinical significance of sludge is poorly studied, though it is considered to be as great a risk factor for complications as gallstones.

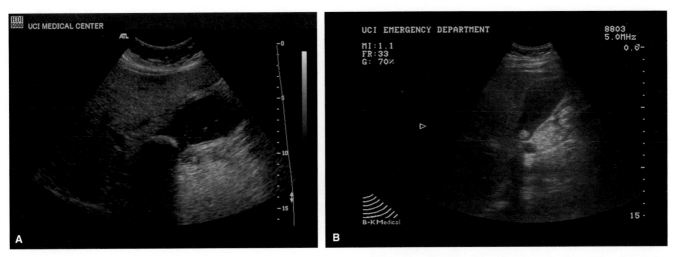

Figure 14.7. Stone in the neck (SIN) sign: Although it has not been well studied, the SIN sign is considered a marker for acute cholecystitis in the symptomatic patient. SIN indicates a gallstone impacted in the neck of the gallbladder (A, B) (14).

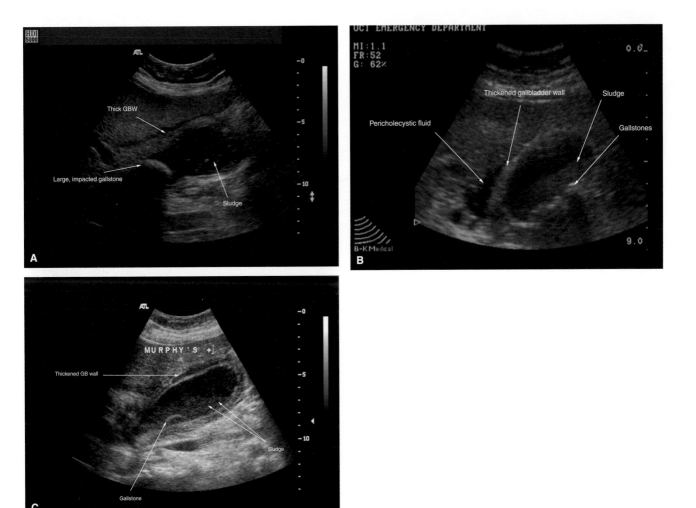

Figure 14.8. Acute cholecystitis: Acute cholecystitis is caused by outlet obstruction of the gallbladder. Most often, a gallstone or sludge obstructs the outflow of bile leading to increased pressure, inflammation, and ischemia of the gallbladder wall. Polyps, tumors, and certain systemic diseases can also lead to obstruction and inflammation. This group is lumped into the term acalculous acute cholecystitis and comprises 5% to 10% of acute cholecystitis cases.

There are five sonographic signs of acute cholecystitis, as shown in Table 14.2. There is no specific number of these findings that determines when acute cholecystitis is present. Rather, each additional finding makes the diagnosis more likely.

Sonographic Murphy's sign: A sonographic Murphy's sign occurs when maximal tenderness is elicited by pressing on the gallbladder with the probe. The combination of gallstones and a sonographic Murphy's sign has a positive predictive value of 92% (15).

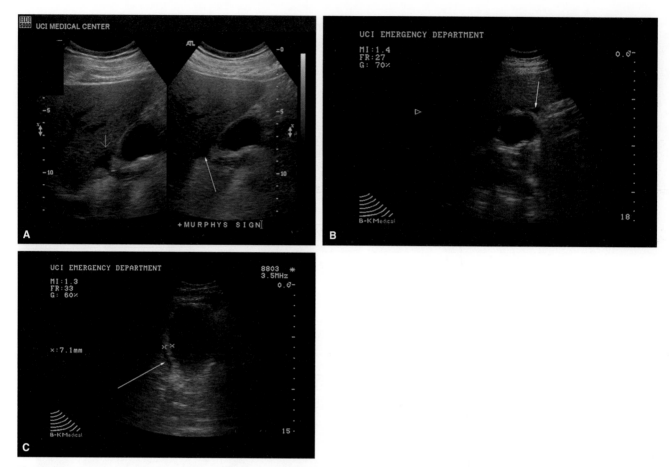

Figure 14.9. Pericholecystic fluid: Fluid surrounding the gallbladder is identified in only 20% of acute cholecystitis cases but is an important finding and may indicate more advanced disease. Findings of fluid can be very subtle (A–C). The initial site of accumulation is usually around the neck of the gallbladder, but larger amounts of fluid can track to the fundus.

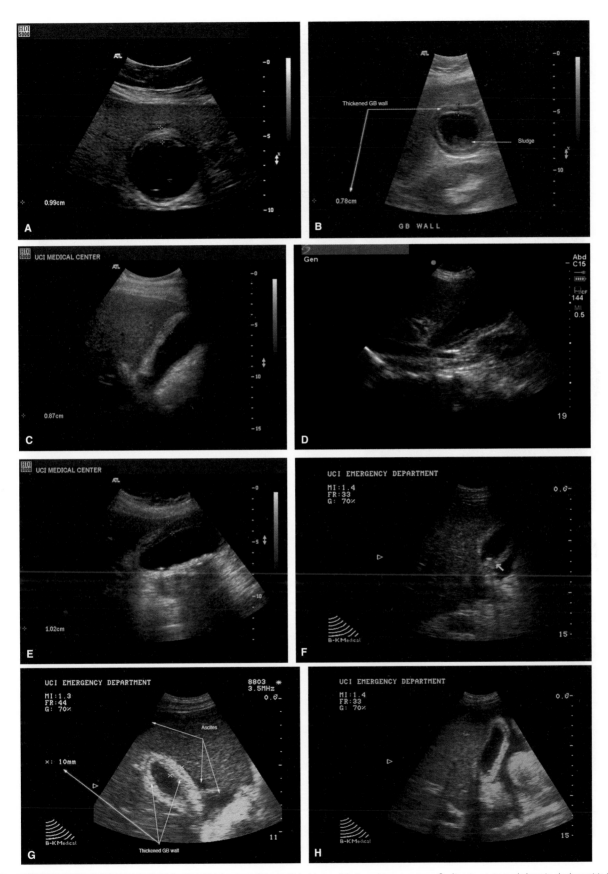

Figure 14.10. Gallbladder wall thickening: Thickening of the gallbladder wall (>3 mm) is a common finding in acute and chronic cholecystitis (A–E). Ascites and congestive heart failure are two common causes of wall thickening caused by systemic disease (F–H).

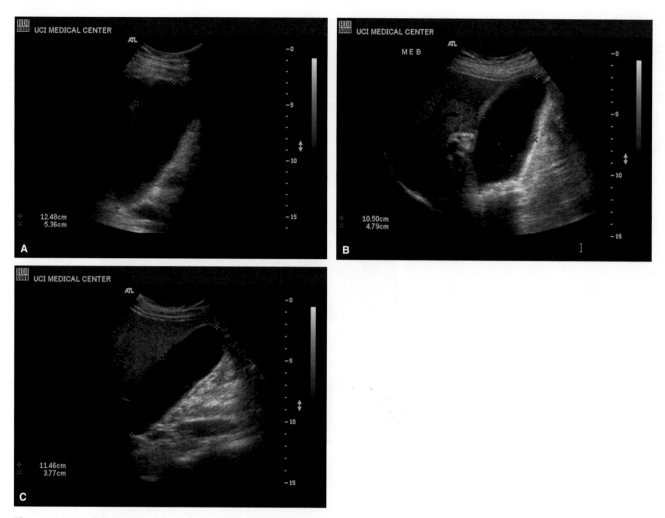

Figure 14.11. Gallbladder distension: Distention of the gallbladder beyond its normal limits (10 cm in length, 4 cm in width) may indicate increased intraluminal pressure from a distal obstruction that can lead to wall ischemia and inflammation (A, B).

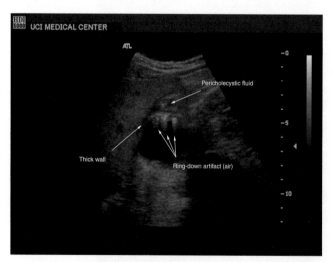

Figure 14.12. Emphysematous cholecystitis: While cholecystitis is not a sensitive finding, there are several findings of advanced cholecystitis that indicate greater morbidity/mortality. Emphysematous cholecystitis occurs with an anaerobic infection and ischemia/infarction of the gallbladder. Air is found within the gallbladder wall, as noted by ring-down artifacts (A). Perforation and mucosal sloughing also signify advanced disease (B). These complications generally are limited to the elderly and diabetic patients.

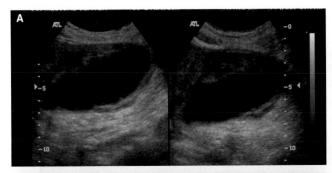

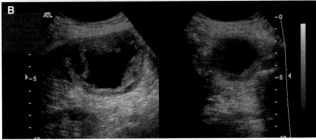

Figure 14.13. Gallbladder carcinoma: A rare cancer with a poor 5-year survival rate, carcinoma of the gallbladder often appears as irregular thickening of the gallbladder wall. Its appearance can mimic the echogenicity of sludge, but a neoplasm will demonstrate Doppler flow while sludge will not. Gallbladder carcinomas can take the form of a polyp. Polyps >1 cm are much more likely to be cancerous.

Porcelain gallbladder (not pictured) may also be the presenting finding of gallbladder carcinoma. The term is used when extensive calcification occurs within the gallbladder wall. The process is also related to chronic cholecystitis, but referral for prophylactic cholecystectomy and thorough evaluation for metastases are indicated.

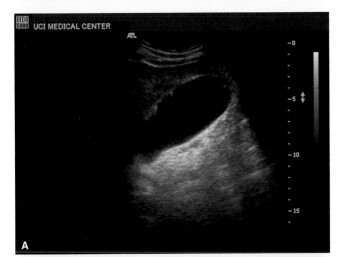

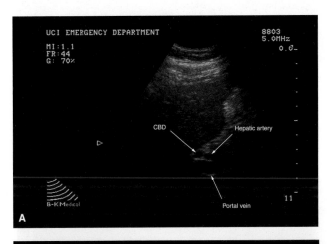

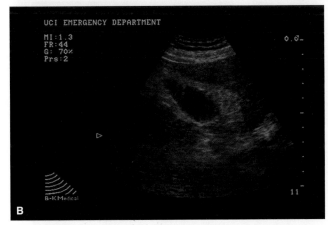

Figure 14.14. Adenomyomatosis is a disease of hypertrophy of the gallbladder wall. The mucosal layer of the wall can push into the muscular layer, creating small sinuses, which may fill with cholesterol crystals. These are called Rokitansky–Aschoff sinuses, and when they accumulate cholesterol crystals, they create bright reflections within the anterior wall of the gallbladder that demonstrate ring-down artifacts. The gallbladder wall will likely be thickened as well. The thickening may be localized or diffuse. Adenomyomatosis is most often benign and asymptomatic. However, it can cause abdominal pain and may require cholecystectomy.

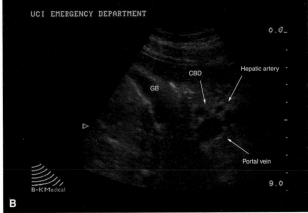

Figure 14.15. At its origin, the CBD runs anterior to the portal vein along with the right hepatic artery. In the short axis, the three have the appearance of a Mickey Mouse drawing (A, B). The right ear is the CBD, the left is the hepatic artery, and Mickey's head is the portal vein.

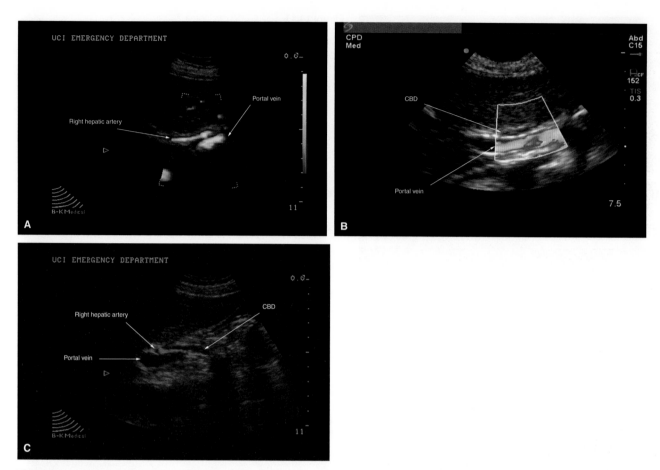

Figure 14.16. Both the right hepatic artery and the CBD run anterior to the portal vein. Either may be visualized anterior to the vein in the long axis. It is important to specifically differentiate the two. This is done in one of two ways. First, Doppler can be used to identify flow within the artery in the long axis as it runs parallel to the portal vein (A, B). The CBD will not show Doppler flow. Second, the right hepatic artery can turn perpendicular to the CBD and portal vein deeper within the liver parenchyma. It can often be identified in the short axis versus the long axis of the other two structures (C). There are variants to the normal appearance of the right hepatic arteries, including an anterior course to the CBD and duplicated arteries.

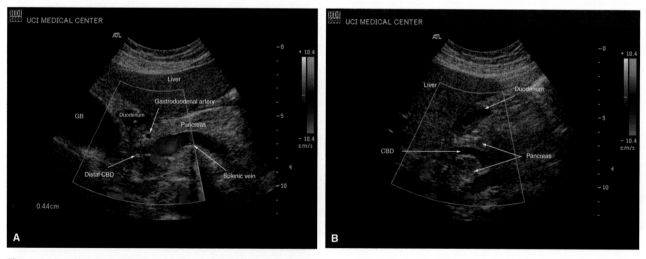

Figure 14.17. The distal CBD is found within the head of the pancreas. Image (A) demonstrates the distal CBD in the short axis. Image (B) finds it in the long axis.

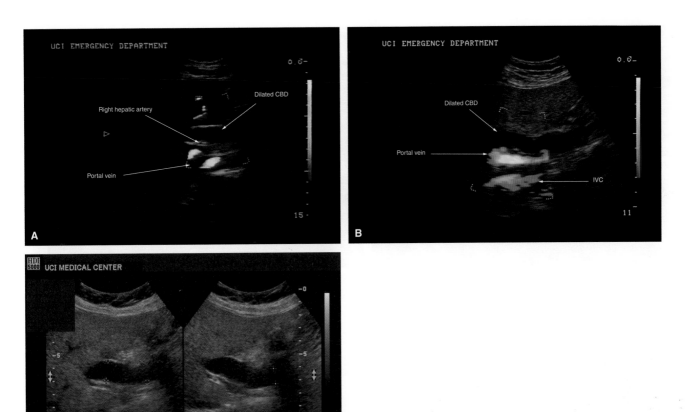

Figure 14.18. CBD measurement: The CBD is correctly measured inner wall to inner wall. With obstruction of the CBD, intraluminal pressure builds and dilates the duct (A–C). There are intrabiliary and extrabiliary causes of CBD dilation, as illustrated by Table 14.3.

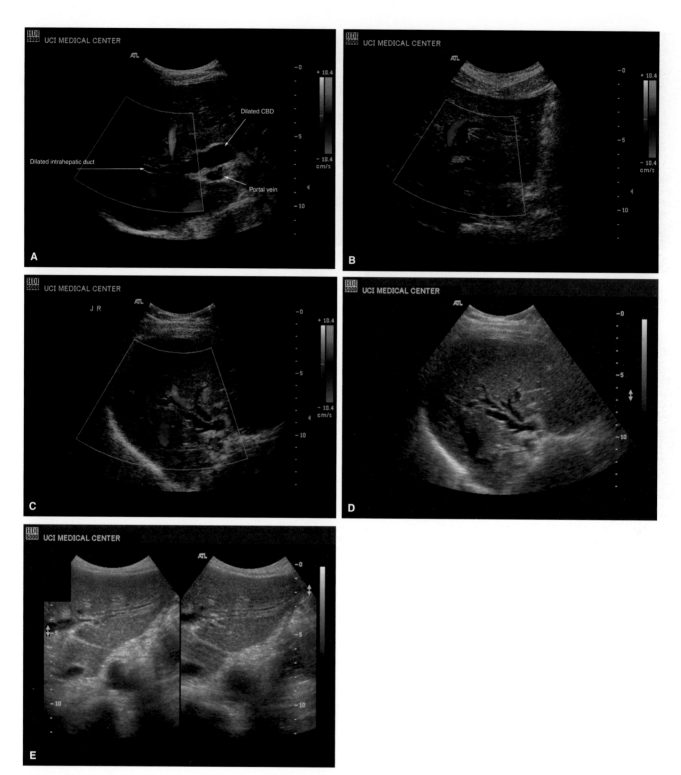

Figure 14.19. The intrahepatic biliary ducts are not normally visualized due to their small size. Duct obstruction leads to dilation (A, B). It is important to use Doppler when evaluating the ducts, as it can be difficult to distinguish vasculature from ducts (C, D). In the periphery of the liver, dilated biliary ducts running with their associate vessels may show a classic "shotgun" appearance (E).

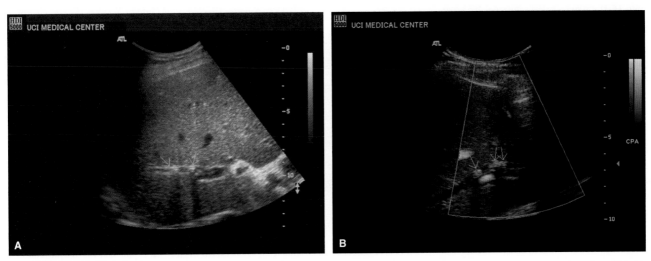

Figure 14.20. Choledocholithiasis: Stones within the biliary ducts are a rare finding (A, B). Those within the CBD almost always originate from the gallbladder but may form de novo within the duct.

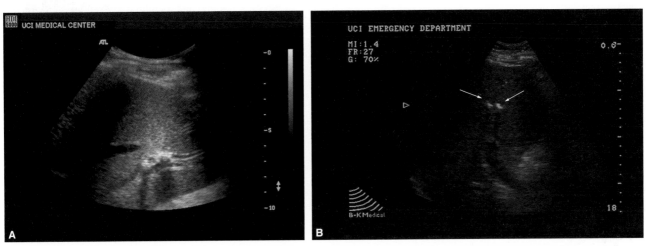

Figure 14.21. Pneumobilia: Air within the biliary tree is due to severe infection or procedure such as stent placement or ERCP. The appearance of air is variable but generally appears with a comet-tail artifact with indistinct shadowing (A). The patient in image A recently underwent an ERCP procedure. Within the biliary tract, we find the "dirty" shadowing produced by air. Image (B) demonstrates pneumobilia well into the intrahepatic ducts.

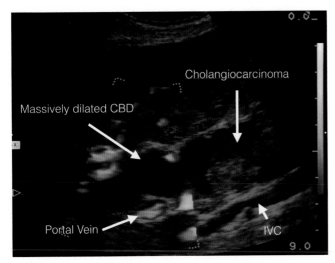

Figure 14.22. Cholangiocarcinoma is a cancer of the bile ducts and is an uncommon cause of obstruction.

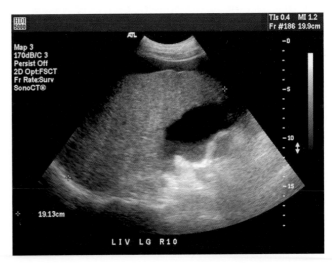

Figure 14.23. Cirrhosis: Cirrhotic livers lose their homogenous ultrasonic texture. The surface of the liver becomes nodular and the texture heterogenous and coarse, as this image of the cirrhotic liver surrounded by ascites demonstrates.

225

Table 14.1: Etiology of gallbladder wall thickening

Primary Biliary Disease
Acute cholecystitis
Chronic cholecystitis
Adenomyomatosis
Non-Biliary Disease
Congestive heart failure
Hepatic cirrhosis
Hypoproteinemia
Renal failure
Hepatitis
Pancreatitis

Table 14.2: Sonographic signs of acute cholecystitis

Gallstones
Impacted stone (in the neck of the gallbladder)
Thickened gallbladder wall (>3mm)
Pericholecystic fluid
Distended gallbladder (>10 cm length, >4 cm width)

Table 14.3: Causes of biliary obstruction

Intrahepatic
De novo stones
Parasitic infection
Neoplasm
Extrahepatic
Choledocolithiasis
Mirizzi syndrome
Cholangitis
Cholangiocarcinoma
Pancreatic neoplasm

References

1. Everhart JE, Khare M, Hill M, Maurer KR: Prevalence and ethnic differences in gallbladder disease in the United States. *Gastroenterology* 1999;**117**(3):632–9.

2. Go V, Everhart JE. Gallstones: In: Everhart JE (ed.), *Digestive diseases in the United States: epidemiology and impact.* *US Department of Health and Human Services, Public Health Service, National Institutes of Health, National Institute of Diabetes and Digestive and Kidney Diseases.* Washington, DC: US Government Printing Office, 1994.

3. Bree RL, Ralls PW, Balfe DM, et al.: Evaluation of patients with acute right upper quadrant pain. American College of Radiology. ACR appropriateness criteria. *Radiology* 2000;**215** Suppl:153–7.

4. Trowbridge RL, Rutkowski NK, Shojania KG: Does this patient have acute cholecystitis? *JAMA* 2003;**289**(1):80–6.

5. Spence SC, Teichgraeber D, Chandrasekhar C: Emergent right upper quadrant sonography. *J Ultrasound Med* 2009;**28**(4):479–96.

6. Shea JA, Berlin JA, Escarce JJ, et al.: Revised estimates of diagnostic test sensitivity and specificity in suspected biliary tract disease. *Arch Intern Med* 1994;**154**(22):2573–81.

7. Kiewiet JJS, Leeuwenburgh MM, Bipat S, et al.: A systematic review and meta-analysis of diagnostic performance of imaging in acute cholecystitis. *Radiology* 2012;**264**(3):708–20.

8. Fidler J, Paulson EK, Layfield L: CT evaluation of acute cholecystitis: findings and usefulness in diagnosis. *AJR Am J Roentgenol* 1996;**166**(5):1085–8.

9. Harvey RT, Miller WT: Acute biliary disease: initial CT and follow-up US versus initial US and follow-up CT. *Radiology* 1999;**213**(3):831–6.

10. Ross M, Brown M, McLaughlin K, et al.: Emergency physician-performed ultrasound to diagnose cholelithiasis: a systematic review. *Acad Emerg Med* 2011;**18**(3):227–35.

11. Summers SM, Scruggs W, Menchine MD, et al.: A prospective evaluation of emergency department bedside ultrasonography for the detection of acute cholecystitis. *Ann Emerg Med* 2010;**56**(2):114–22.

12. Bree RL, Greene FL, Ralls PW, et al.: Suspected liver metastases. American College of Radiology. ACR appropriateness criteria. *Radiology* 2000;**215** Suppl:213–24.

13. Saini S, Ralls PW, Balfe DM, et al.: Suspected abdominal abscess. American College of Radiology. ACR appropriateness criteria. *Radiology* 2000;**215** Suppl:173–9.

14. Nelson M, Ash A, Raio C, Zimmerman M: Stone-in-neck phenomenon: a new sign of cholecystitis. *Crit Ultrasound J* 2011;**3**(2):115–7.

15. Ralls PW, Colletti PM, Lapin SA, et al.: Real-time sonography in suspected acute cholecystitis. Prospective evaluation of primary and secondary signs. *Radiology* 1985;**155**(3):767–71.

Chapter 15

Trauma Ultrasound

Bret Nelson

Indications

The use of ultrasound in acute trauma has increased dramatically over the past 30 years. In the 1970s, ultrasound was first used to diagnose hemoperitoneum in the setting of blunt abdominal trauma. Since then, advances in ultrasound technology have led to portable machines that are smaller, are easier to use, and boast image quality comparable to their much larger counterparts. Thus, the range of traumatic conditions amenable to assessment with bedside sonography has increased dramatically. Bedside ultrasound is indicated in any patient with penetrating or blunt thoracoabdominal trauma and may be useful in the assessment of cranial trauma, ocular trauma, and long bone fractures as well.

The oldest and most established indication for ultrasound in the ED is blunt abdominal trauma. The focused assessment with sonography in trauma (FAST) exam has become a standard imaging modality in the setting of acute trauma and has been incorporated into the American College of Surgeons' Advanced Trauma Life Support guidelines. Ultrasound can be used to assess for free intraperitoneal fluid, and many decision rules support early operative intervention in patients with hemodynamic instability and hemoperitoneum. Hemoperitoneum can also be demonstrated in the setting of penetrating abdominal trauma.

When the FAST exam was first employed, a brief cardiac exam was performed to assess for hemopericardium and tamponade. Although this assessment is more useful in penetrating thoracic trauma than in blunt thoracic trauma, positive findings can rapidly alter management. A more thorough assessment of the thorax in both blunt and penetrating thoracic trauma has recently been advocated, with evaluation for pneumothorax and hemothorax incorporated into an extended FAST exam. Thus, most life-threatening thoracoabdominal injuries (hemoperitoneum, hemopericardium, cardiac tamponade, pneumothorax, and hemothorax) can be diagnosed noninvasively at the bedside with ultrasound.

In the setting of acute cranial trauma, ultrasound may be useful in the detection of elevated intracranial pressure. By measuring the diameter of the optic nerve sheath, a quantitative assessment of papilledema can be made, which can serve as a marker of intracranial pressure. Ocular ultrasound can also be used to evaluate for traumatic retinal detachment, globe rupture, foreign body, and assessment of extraocular movements and pupillary light reflex.

The diagnosis of long bone fractures can be made at the bedside by assessing for a break in the normal cortical contour of bones. This technique has been employed in fractures of the sternum, ribs, and extremities, and it has even been used to guide the reduction of fractures.

Diagnostic capabilities

In the setting of blunt abdominal trauma, rapidly ruling out hemoperitoneum is critical. Ultrasound has demonstrated a high negative predictive value (94%–100%) (1–3), with sensitivities ranging from 86% to 94%. One study noted much lower accuracy (false-negative rate of 78%) in the setting of seat belt markings in blunt trauma (4); care should be taken in this setting to place the FAST exam result in the appropriate clinical context. The specificity for detecting injury has been reported as high as 98%, with positive predictive values for hemoperitoneum ranging from 78% to 95% (1–3). Recently, intravenous contrast (in the form of stabilized microbubbles) has been studied in the setting of blunt abdominal trauma to better detect solid organ injury. Specifically, it may improve the visualization and characterization of hepatic, renal, and splenic injuries as compared with conventional ultrasound. This technique has demonstrated a sensitivity of 96.4%, a specificity of 98%, and positive and negative predictive values of 98.8% and 94.1%, respectively (5, 6).

The FAST exam is less reliable in detecting hemoperitoneum in penetrating abdominal injuries, with sensitivity between 28% and 100% and negative predictive value of 60% (7, 8). Thus, additional imaging is recommended in the setting of a negative FAST exam with penetrating injury. However, a positive FAST exam in the setting of penetrating trauma has specificity of 94% to 100% and a positive predictive value of 90%. Thus, there is a high incidence of intraabdominal injury in those with penetrating trauma and a positive FAST exam.

The detection of hemopericardium in penetrating thoracic injury has a high sensitivity (100%) and specificity (97%), and has been shown to allow faster disposition to surgery (9, 10). This reinforces that ultrasound should be the initial screening modality for penetrating trauma, especially precordial thoracic trauma.

As part of the extended FAST exam, evaluation of the thorax for hemothorax has a sensitivity of 97.5% and a specificity of 99.7% (11). Also, it can be performed faster than chest radiography. When compared with chest radiography, both modalities were 96.2% sensitive, 100% specific, and 99.6% accurate for detection of traumatic hemothorax (12). In cases of traumatic pneumothorax, ultrasound has a sensitivity of 98%, specificity of 99%, and negative and positive predictive values of 98% and 99% (13). A recent literature review suggests that ultrasound is a more sensitive screening test than supine AP chest radiography for the detection of pneumothorax with the US sensitivity from 86% to 98% and a sensitivity of 28% to 75% by chest radiograph (14).

In the evaluation of patients with suspected elevations in intracranial pressure, bedside measurement of increased optic nerve sheath diameter had a pooled sensitivity of 90%, a pooled specificity of 85%, and a pooled odds ratio of 51 in a systematic review of the data (15).

Although bedside ultrasound is 83% to 92% sensitive in the detection of long bone fractures, the exam is highly specific (100%) (16). Some have now used the technology to diagnose and aid in the reduction of distal forearm fractures with a sensitivity of 94% and specificity of 56% for identifying a successful reduction on post-reduction radiographs (17, 18). Also, imaging for elbow fractures in pediatric populations can be done easily with ultrasound and is highly sensitive for the presence of fractures. It may reduce the need for radiographs in this population (19).

Ultrasound for ocular trauma can be used to diagnose lens dislocation, retinal or choroidal detachment, vitreous hemorrhage, and intraocular foreign bodies. Ultrasound evaluation has been proposed also as an adjunct to physical exam in the trauma patient by assessing extraocular movements and pupillary light reflex without manual manipulation of eyelids (20).

Imaging pitfalls and limitations

Thoracoabdominal sonography can be limited by patient body habitus. Patients with larger girth necessitate longer distances for the ultrasound beam to travel, and significant attenuation of signal strength can occur. In the abdomen, bowel gas, subcutaneous emphysema, pneumoperitoneum, and rib shadows can hinder evaluation of deeper structures. Evaluation of the pelvis for free fluid is optimal with a full bladder – a patient who has recently voided or in whom a urethral catheter has been placed will not image optimally. Because the FAST exam relies on free-flowing fluid tracking to dependent areas within the peritoneum, patients who are not lying flat or in Trendelenburg position may yield false-negative results.

Evaluation of the heart and thorax can be limited by rib shadows, emphysematous lungs, pneumothorax, or subcutaneous emphysema. The subxiphoid cardiac view is more difficult in patients with large or tender abdomens, and many operators will forgo this approach in favor of a parasternal view to evaluate for a pericardial effusion.

Imaging the orbit should be done with care; no pressure should be applied to the eye, which could worsen pathology, causing retinal detachment or a ruptured globe. Be sure to fill the entire orbit with chilled gel prior to performing ultrasound.

Prehospital and tactical medicine

Parametics' use of ultrasound and, more specifically, the FAST exam have been examined in the prehospital setting. These images could potentially be transferred wirelessly for interpretation by a physician after image acquisition training by EMTs, or the images could be interpreted on scene by the prehospital care provider (21, 22). There is a growing body of literature that supports its use in this setting, especially with the introduction of more portable laptop and handheld devices.

Also, there is potential for point-of-care FAST examinations to be helpful in tactical medicine. These teams are often approaching austere environments and could use these data to assist in triage for retrieving patients with identifiable and treatable conditions. It could assist in personnel evacuation decision making by alerting the provider to patient acuity.

Trauma evaluation in pregnancy

Pregnant trauma patients are a particularly vulnerable population of patients where two lives are potentially at risk. Ultrasound in this population has the obvious benefit of rapid detection of abdominal free fluid but also has the added benefit of sparing the developing fetus from ionizing radiation. The FAST exam in trauma has a similar sensitivity in pregnant and nonpregnant patients and is suggested as the initial imaging modality of choice (23). Also, fetal heartbeat and viability can be detected by imaging the uterine contents by ultrasound exam. In the rare occurrence of traumatic uterine rupture, an empty uterus with a free intraabdominal uterus has been described (24).

It should be noted that a common cause of fetal demise in trauma patients is from placental abruption. Ultrasound is not highly sensitive for this diagnosis, and with clinical concern, further evaluation should be pursued (25). The most frequent cause of fetal death is maternal loss of life, so all efforts should be made initially to stabilize the mother.

Clinical images

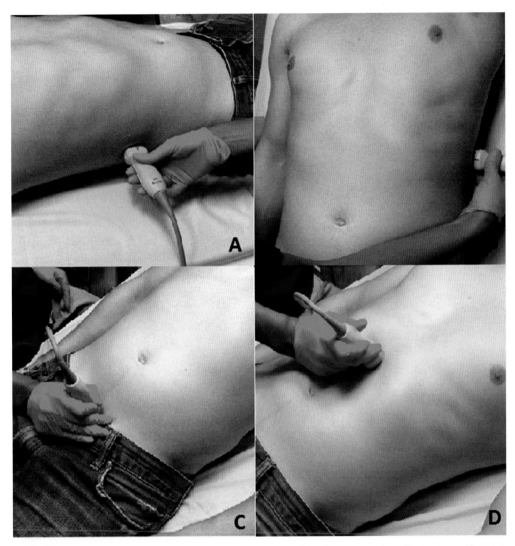

Figure 15.1. Probe positioning for FAST exam views demonstrating (A) right upper quadrant (Morison's pouch), (B) left upper quadrant (splenorenal recess), (C) pelvic, and (D) subxiphoid cardiac view.

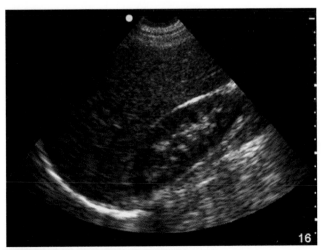

Figure 15.2. Normal FAST exam, Morison's pouch.

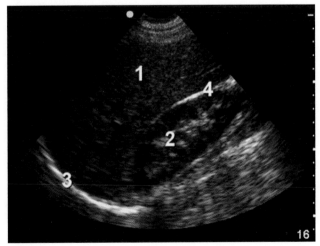

Figure 15.3. Schematic representation of Morison's pouch, demonstrating (1) liver, (2) kidney, (3) diaphragm, and (4) Morison's pouch.

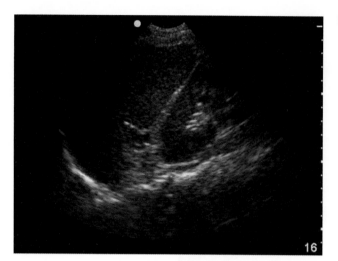

Figure 15.4. Normal FAST exam, splenorenal recess.

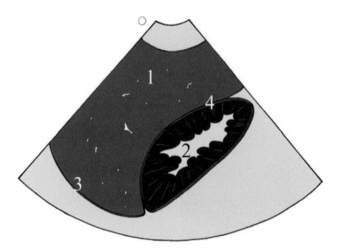

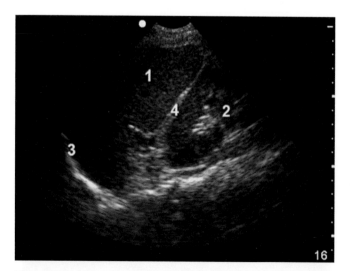

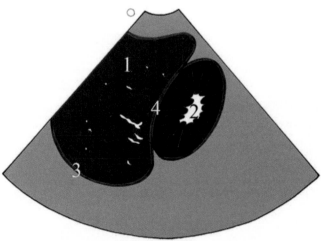

Figure 15.5. Schematic representation of the splenorenal recess, demonstrating (1) spleen, (2) kidney, (3) diaphragm, and (4) splenorenal recess.

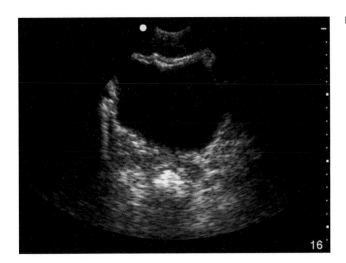

Figure 15.6. Normal FAST exam, pelvis.

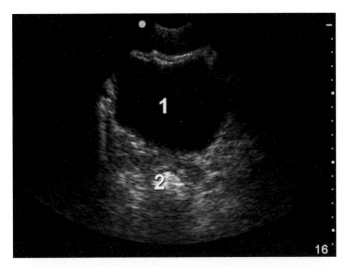
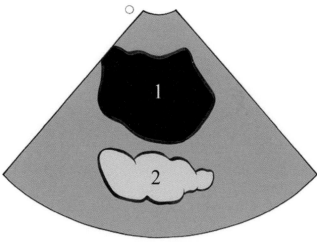

Figure 15.7. Schematic representation of the pelvis, demonstrating (1) bladder and (2) rectum.

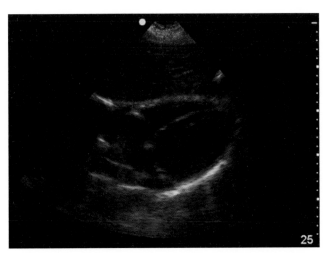

Figure 15.8. Normal FAST exam, subxiphoid cardiac view.

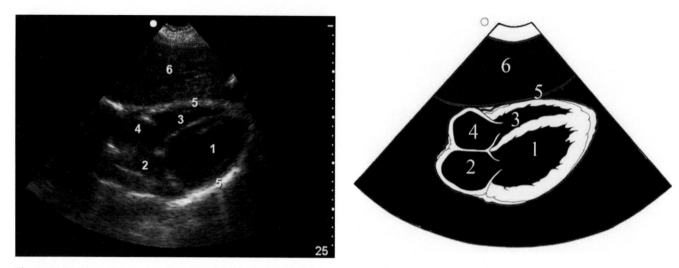

Figure 15.9. Schematic representation of subxiphoid cardiac view, demonstrating (1) left ventricle, (2) left atrium, (3) right ventricle, (4) right atrium, (5) pericardium, and (6) liver.

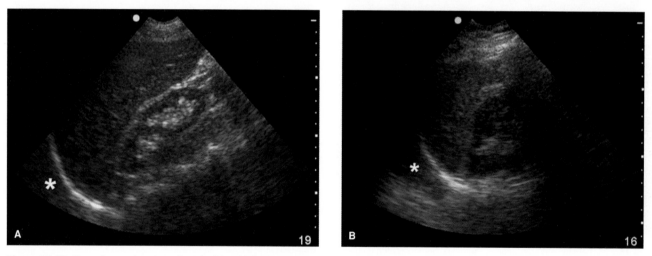

Figure 15.10. Normal costophrenic angle, right (A) and left (B). Note that the hemithorax above the diaphragm (*asterisk*) has a similar echotexture to the liver below the diaphragm. This mirror image artifact is normal and suggests no free fluid in the thorax.

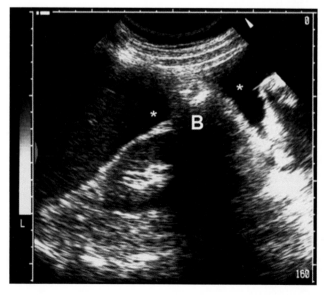

Figure 15.11. Hemoperitoneum visualized in Morison's pouch. Note a significant amount of fluid in the peritoneum (*asterisks*) as well as shadowing from overlying bowel gas (B).

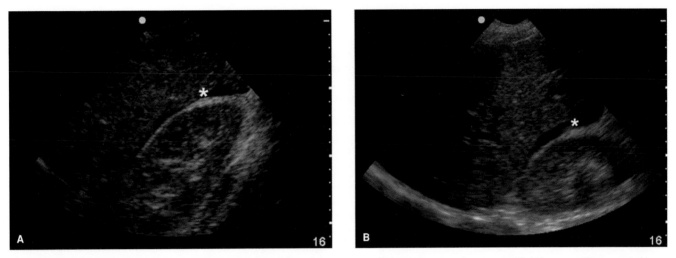

Figures 15.12A and B. Hemoperitoneum (*asterisks*) in Morison's pouch, demonstrating findings when a smaller amount of fluid is present. Note a much thinner anechoic stripe.

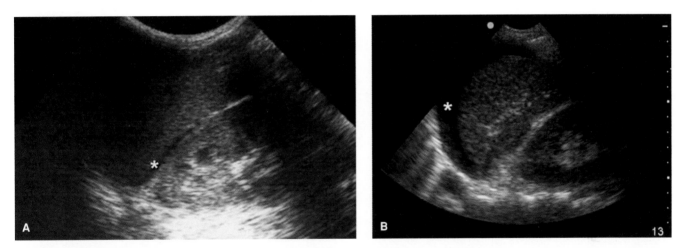

Figure 15.13. Hemoperitoneum (*asterisks*) visualized in the splenorenal recess (A) and surrounding spleen (B).

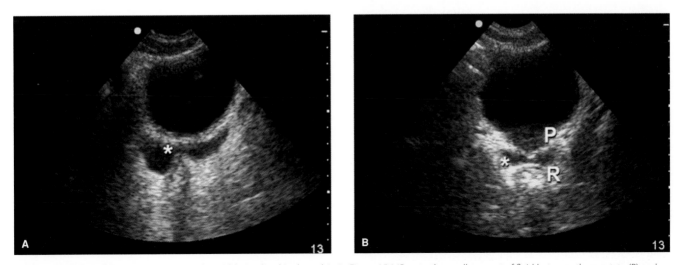

Figures 15.14A and B. Hemoperitoneum (*asterisks*) visualized in the pelvis. In Figure 15.14B, note the small amount of fluid between the prostate (P) and rectum (R).

233

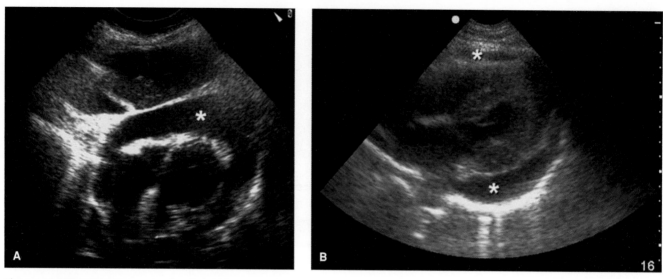

Figures 15.15A and B. Hemopericardium (*asterisks*).

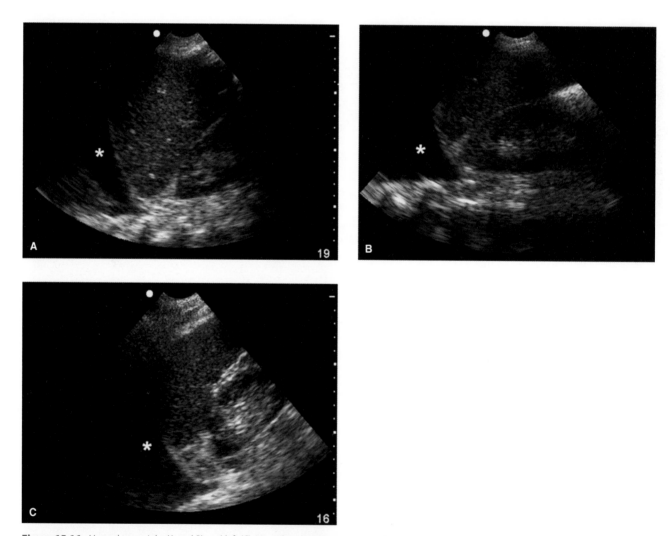

Figure 15.16. Hemothorax, right (A and B) and left (C). Note that the mirror-image artifact is no longer present, and a clear anechoic area is visible above the diaphragm (*asterisk*).

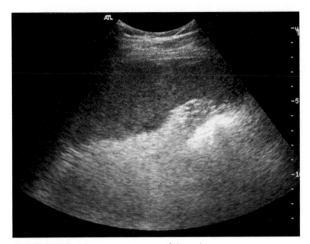

Figure 15.17. Noncontrast image of the spleen.
Image courtesy of Dr. Gianni Zironi, S. Orsola-Malpighi Hospital, University of Bologna, Italy.

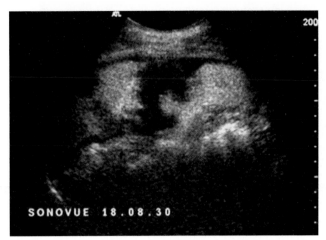

Figure 15.18. Contrast image of the spleen, demonstrating rupture of cortex.
Image courtesy of Dr. Gianni Zironi, S. Orsola-Malpighi Hospital, University of Bologna, Italy.

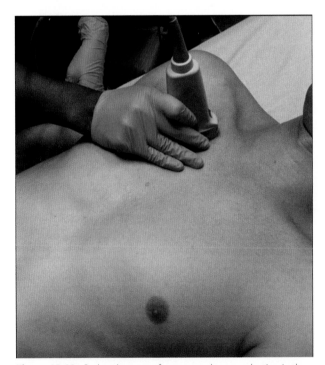

Figure 15.19. Probe placement for pneumothorax evaluation in the midclavicular line at the second to third intercostal space with the probe marker pointed caudally. The same position would be used on the left anterior chest wall.

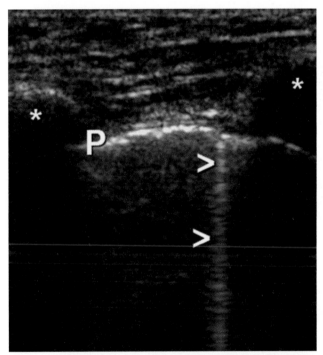

Figure 15.20. Normal pleura, demonstrating rib shadows (*asterisks*), pleural line (P), and comet tail artifact (*arrows*). In real time, the pleura would demonstrate a sliding motion back and forth (lung slide) with each respiration.

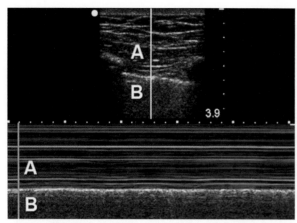

Figure 15.21. Normal pleura, demonstrating lung slide with M-mode. Note the smooth lines above the bright pleural line where no motion is occurring during respiration (A). Below the pleural line, sliding motion causes the M-mode tracing to be grainier (B).

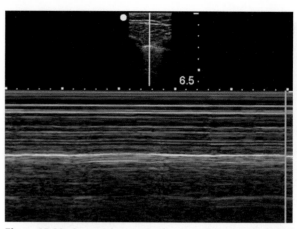

Figure 15.22. Pneumothorax. Note the pleura demonstrating lack of lung slide with M-mode. This image indicates a pneumothorax. Note the smooth lines above and below the bright pleural line; no motion is occurring during respiration.

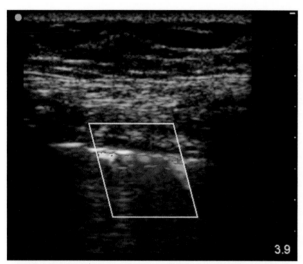

Figure 15.23. Normal pleura, demonstrating lung slide with power Doppler. Note the color demonstrating motion at the pleura.

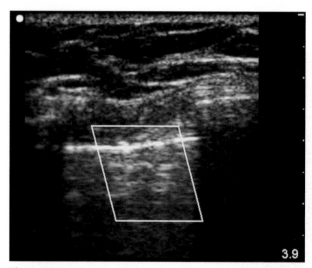

Figure 15.24. Pneumothorax. No lung slide is detected by power Doppler.

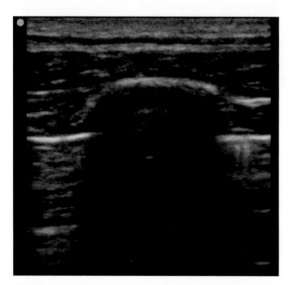

Figure 15.25. Pneumothorax: Lung point, in real time, no sliding would be visible on the left side (superior) and comet tails with sliding visible on the right (inferior). This is the exact point at which apposition of the pleura is lost.

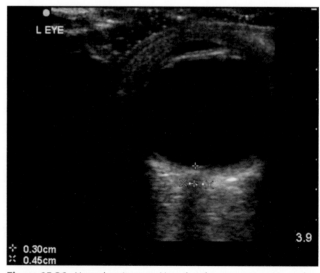

Figure 15.26. Normal optic nerve. Note that the measurement is made perpendicular to the long axis of the nerve sheath, 3 mm from the fundus.

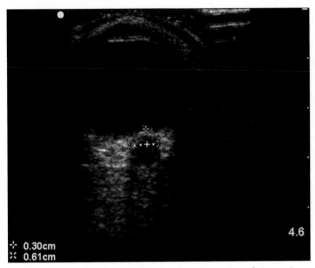

Figure 15.27. Dilated optic nerve sheath in the setting of elevated intracranial pressure.

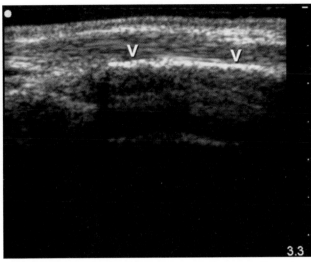

Figure 15.28. Distal radius, demonstrating normal contour of bone.

Figure 15.29. Distal radius fracture, demonstrating disruption in cortical line.

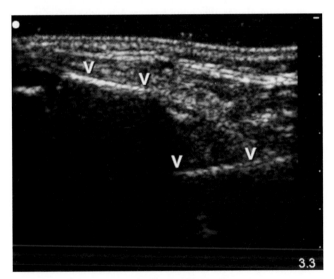

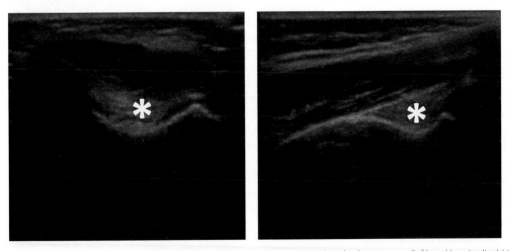

Figure 15.30. Olecranon with normal, flat fat pad (*asterisks*) seen posteriorly in both transverse (left) and longitudinal (right) views.

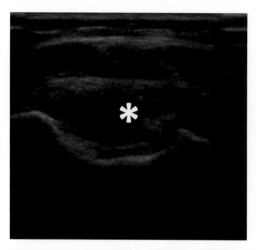 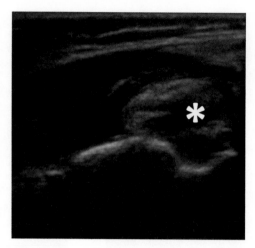

Figure 15.31. Olecranon with elevated fat pad (*asterisks*) seen in both transverse (left) and longitudinal (right) views, which signifies an elbow fracture.

References

1. Dolich MO, McKenney MG, Varela JE, et al.: 2,576 ultrasounds for blunt abdominal trauma. *J Trauma* 2001;**50**(1):108–12.

2. Lingawi SS, Buckley AR: Focused abdominal US in patients with trauma. *Radiology* 2000;**217**(2):426–9.

3. Natarajan B, Gupta PK, Cemaj S, et al.: FAST scan: is it worth doing in hemodynamically stable blunt trauma patients? *Surgery* 2010;**148**(4):695–700; discussion 700–1.

4. Stassen NA, Lukan JK, Carrillo EH, et al.: Abdominal seat belt marks in the era of focused abdominal sonography for trauma. *Arch Surg* 2002;**137**:718–23.

5. Valentino M, Serra C, Zironi G, et al.: Blunt abdominal trauma: emergency contrast-enhanced sonography for detection of solid organ injuries. *AJR Am J Roentgenol* 2006;**186**(5):1361–7.

6. Valentino M, Ansaloni L, Catena F, et al.: Contrast-enhanced ultrasonography in blunt abdominal trauma: considerations after 5 years of experience. *Radiol Med* 2009;**114**(7):1080–93.

7. Udobi KF, Rodriguez A, Chiu WC, Scalea TM: Role of ultrasonography in penetrating abdominal trauma: a prospective clinical study. *J Trauma* 2001;**50**(3):475–9.

8. Quinn AC, Sinert R: What is the utility of the focused assessment with sonography in trauma (FAST) exam in penetrating torso trauma? *Injury* 2011;**42**(5):482–7.

9. Meyer DM, Jessen ME, Grayburn PA: Use of echocardiography to detect occult cardiac injury after penetrating thoracic trauma: a prospective study. *J Trauma* 1995;**39**(5):902–7.

10. Rozycki GS, Feliciano DV, Ochsner MG, et al.: The role of ultrasound in patients with possible penetrating cardiac wounds: a prospective multicenter study. *J Trauma* 1999;**46**(4):543–51.

11. Sisley AC, Rozycki GS, Ballard RB, et al.: Rapid detection of traumatic effusion using surgeon-performed ultrasonography. *J Trauma* 1998;**44**(2):291–6.

12. Ma OJ, Mateer JR: Trauma ultrasound examination versus chest radiography in the detection of hemothorax. *Ann Emerg Med* 1997;**29**(3):312–5; discussion 315–6.

13. Blaivas M, Lyon M, Duggal S: A prospective comparison of supine chest radiography and bedside ultrasound for the diagnosis of traumatic pneumothorax. *Acad Emerg Med* 2005;**12**(9):844–9.

14. Wilkerson RG, Stone MB: Sensitivity of bedside ultrasound and supine anteroposterior chest radiographs for the identification of pneumothorax after blunt trauma. *Acad Emerg Med* 2010;**17**(1):11–7.

15. Dubourg J, Javouhey E, Geeraerts T, et al.: Ultrasonography of optic nerve sheath diameter for detection of raised intracranial pressure: a systematic review and meta-analysis. *Intensive Care Med* 2011;**37**(7):1059–68.

16. Dulchavsky SA, Henry SE, Moed BR, et al.: Advanced ultrasonic diagnosis of extremity trauma: the FASTER examination. *J Trauma* 2002;**53**(1):28–32.

17. Chinnock B, Khaletskiy A, Kuo K, Hendey GW: Ultrasound-guided reduction of distal radius fractures. *J Emerg Med* 2011;**40**(3):308–12.

18. Chern TC, Jou IM, Lai KA, et al.: Sonography for monitoring closed reduction of displaced extra-articular distal radial fractures. *J Bone Joint Surg Am* 2002;**84A**(2):194–203.

19. Rabiner JE, Khine H, Avner JR, et al.: Accuracy of point-of-care ultrasonography for diagnosis of elbow fractures in children. *Ann Emerg Med* 2013;**61**(1):9–17.

20. Harries A, Shah S, Teismann N, et al.: Ultrasound assessment of extraocular movements and pupillary light reflex in ocular trauma. *Am J Emerg Med* 2010;**28**(8):956–9.

21. Song KJ, Shin SD, Hong KJ, et al.: Clinical applicability of real-time, prehospital image transmission for FAST (focused assessment with sonography for trauma). *J Telemed Telecare* 2013;**19**(8)450–5.

22. Heegaard W, Hildebrandt D, Spear D, et al.: Prehospital ultrasound by paramedics: results of field trial. *Acad Emerg Med* 2010;**17**(6):624–30.

23. Goodwin H, Holmes JF, Wisner DH: Abdominal ultrasound examination in pregnant blunt trauma patients. *J Trauma-Injury Infect Crit Care* 2001;**50**:689–93.

24. Ma OJ, Mateer JR, DeBehnke DJ: Use of ultrasonography for the evaluation of pregnant trauma patients. *J Trauma* 1996;**40**(4):665–8.

25. Mirza FG, Devine PC, Gaddipati S: Trauma in pregnancy: a systematic approach. *Am J Perinatol* 2010;**27**(7):579–86.

Chapter 16

Deep Venous Thrombosis

Eitan Dickman, David Blehar, and Romolo Gaspari

Deep venous thrombosis (DVT) is an extremely common disorder estimated to occur in more than 300,000 patients in the United States per year (1). A significant number of patients with DVT will subsequently develop a pulmonary embolism, thereby emphasizing the importance of timely diagnosis and initiation of treatment. While there are numerous methods to diagnose a DVT, ultrasonography is the imaging modality of choice. Current diagnostic pathways include imaging performed by an ultrasound technician and interpreted by a physician, and imaging performed and interpreted by the clinician. Studies have shown that emergency physicians can accurately and efficiently employ point-of-care ultrasonography in the diagnosis of an acute proximal DVT (2–5).

A complete lower extremity vascular study images the veins of the leg from the groin to the ankle. Point-of-care ultrasonography does not usually involve a complete vascular exam, in that only the proximal vessels, the femoral and the popliteal veins, are imaged, without imaging the calf veins. Controversy remains regarding the clinical importance of diagnosing and treating calf DVTs (6, 7). Most calf vein DVTs spontaneously resolve, and even if they do embolize, they tend to be small and do not usually cause large pulmonary embolisms (8). However, many experts believe that an isolated calf DVT requires anticoagulation, as patients are at risk of clot propagation, pulmonary embolism, and development of post-thrombotic pain syndrome (7).

Indications

Ultrasonography of an extremity to check for the presence of a DVT is a commonly requested examination. Certain symptoms – such as unilateral swelling, pain, or erythema of an extremity – are classically associated with the presence of thrombus. However, a patient with a DVT may also be asymptomatic. Risk factors for the presence of a DVT include a hypercoagulable state and conditions of venous stasis (Table 16.1). A variety of clinical decision rules use a combination of history, physical exam findings, and a D-dimer test to determine if imaging is necessary. Although nonspecific, an elevated D-dimer is associated with thrombosis, and an ultrasonographic examination of the extremities may be warranted in this setting. In addition, patients with a superficial vein thrombosis may also be at risk for clot propagation, and consideration should be given to evaluating these patients for the presence of a DVT (9).

Table 16.1: Risk factors for DVT

Previous DVT
Recent surgery
Trauma
Active malignancy
Elderly
Long-distance travel
Prolonged bed rest
Pregnancy
Oral contraceptives
Hormone replacement therapy
Indwelling central venous catheter
Protein S deficiency
Protein C deficiency
Antithrombin deficiency
Factor V Leiden
Antiphospholipid syndrome

Diagnostic capabilities

Interestingly, only 25% of patients with signs and symptoms consistent with an acute DVT are ultimately diagnosed with the disease (10). Because physical exam findings are neither sensitive nor specific, a diagnostic test is necessary. Compression ultrasonography is the test of choice in symptomatic patients when there is concern of a possible DVT. The test has been shown in multiple studies to be both highly sensitive (97%–100%) and specific (98%–99%) in the assessment for proximal DVT (11, 12). In patients who prove not to have a DVT, an additional benefit of using ultrasonography is in detecting other pathology that may be causing the patient's symptoms, including cellulitis, abscess, seroma, lymphadenopathy, ruptured Baker's cyst, muscle tear, hematoma, superficial phlebitis, fasciitis, and edema (2).

Although ultrasonography is an excellent test for detection of a proximal DVT, it is not as reliable in detecting a distal thrombosis. Sensitivity and specificity ranges between 70%–93%, and 60%–99%, respectively, have been reported for the diagnosis of distal DVT (10, 13). Based on previous studies, it has been estimated that between 0% and 30% of untreated calf vein DVTs will propagate to a proximal vein (14–17). Because a proximal clot is at higher risk for embolization to the lungs, a prudent approach for a patient with a negative ultrasound of the proximal vessels is to have a follow-up ultrasound within 4 to 7 days. The repeat ultrasound will allow the sonographer to determine whether a potential distal DVT has propagated and become a proximal clot. This approach has been determined to be a safe practice in patients at risk for DVT (18).

Technique

The patient should be positioned so the veins of the leg are distended. In the acutely ill patient, this may involve raising the head of the bed to 30 degrees, or the patient may be supine with the stretcher then placed in the reverse Trendelenburg position. In a stable patient, the patient can sit with the legs hanging over the side of the stretcher. The leg should be externally rotated at the hip and flexed at the knee. Imaging with and without compression is the cornerstone of a lower extremity venous ultrasound and is accomplished by applying pressure with the probe to collapse the thin-walled veins. Lack of compressibility is the main determinant of a DVT.

Using a high-frequency linear transducer, imaging begins in the inguinal region in a transverse orientation (Fig. 16.1). The confluence of the common femoral vein (CFV) and the greater saphenous vein (GSV) is identified medial to the common femoral artery (CFA) (Fig. 16.2). Once these vessels are identified, pressure is applied with the transducer to collapse both of these veins. Coaptation of the venous vessel walls should easily occur with moderate pressure (Fig. 16.3). Although the GSV is a superficial vessel, if a thrombus is identified within two centimeters of the sapheno-femoral junction, the patient should be treated with anticoagulation due to the high risk of clot propagation and embolization (Fig. 16.2) (19).

Moving the probe distally, both the CFA and the CFV will bifurcate (Fig. 16.4). The deep femoral artery and vein dive deep into the proximal thigh musculature and quickly disappear. The superficial femoral artery and the femoral vein (FV) are actually the deep vascular structures that will be imaged. (Many experts have advocated referring to the "superficial femoral vein" as simply the "femoral vein" to eliminate confusion regarding the anatomy of this deep vessel [20, 21].) Examination of the FV continues from here, compressing the vessel every 1 to 2 cm as it courses distally. As scanning continues down the thigh, the femoral vein will transition from its position medial to the artery, to posterior to the artery, appearing below the artery on the ultrasound image (Fig. 16.5). Within Hunter's canal, because of the thigh muscles, it becomes easier to collapse venous structures by reverse compression. Rather than compressing the probe into the leg, the transducer is held steady and the nonscanning hand is used to compress the leg into the probe (Figs. 16.6 and 16.7).

Examination of the popliteal vein (PV) is performed with the patient's hip externally rotated and the knee in slight flexion (Fig. 16.8). The transducer is placed posteriorly in the popliteal fossa in a transverse orientation. This places the vein closer than the artery to the probe, creating the appearance of the vein being "on top" of the artery. The PV

is compressed at this location and then every 1 to 2 cm until it trifurcates into the anterior tibial, posterior tibial, and peroneal veins (Fig. 16.9). Although not routinely performed by most emergency physicians, the veins of the calf can be evaluated for evidence of thrombosis by assessing for non-compressibility. As described earlier, identification of vessels, particularly small veins in the calf, is facilitated by having the vessels distended. An alternative approach for evaluating distal veins is to localize the vessels at the level of the medial malleolus and then trace these vessels proximally.

Color and spectral Doppler can sometimes assist in the examination for DVT, although this is not a mandatory component of the exam. These modalities may be helpful in morbidly obese patients or in those with unusual anatomy. Both spectral and color Doppler can be used to differentiate venous from arterial flow. With color Doppler, arteries demonstrate pulsatile flow, and veins exhibit continuous flow. Using spectral Doppler, an arterial waveform can be differentiated from the respirophasic pattern seen in veins (Figs. 16.10 and 16.11). Augmentation, documented using either spectral or color Doppler, refers to increased blood flow in a proximal portion of a vein when a distal portion of that vein is squeezed and is a normal finding. Lack of augmentation is indirect evidence of a clot somewhere between the point of compression and the ultrasound probe. However, evidence suggests that only in rare cases does augmentation in the lower extremity add pertinent information that is not obtained from gray scale imaging (22).

When assessing the vessels of an upper extremity for the presence of thrombosis, the patient's head should be facing away from the arm being imaged. Similar to the lower extremity vessels, compressibility of the internal jugular, axillary, and brachial veins can be assessed. Evaluation of the brachiocephalic vein, the superior vena cava, and some segments of the subclavian vein can be more challenging due to difficulties in compressing these vessels because of the overlying bony thorax. For these specific vessels, color flow and augmentation can be assessed. Inspiratory collapse of the subclavian vein, which occurs due to the increased negative intrathoracic pressure, is another indicator of vein patency (23, 24).

See Figures 16.12 to 16.15 for examples of a variety of DVTs.

Imaging pitfalls and limitations

A study published in 2012 demonstrated that echogenic material could be visualized in a significant number of patients with a DVT (25). However, failure to sonographically visualize clot within the lumen of the vein does not exclude the presence of a DVT. Lack of vein compressibility is the main indicator of a thrombus.

Morbid obesity, significant edema, and lack of patient cooperation due to pain may all limit the ability of the sonographer to obtain technically adequate images. In a patient whose body habitus does not allow the sonographer to obtain the proper depth to visualize the venous structures using a high frequency transducer, one option is to switch to a lower frequency probe. Although some image quality may be lost, the added penetration may allow for determination of the presence of a DVT. As mentioned above, the vein must be completely compressed to evaluate for clot in that region (Fig. 16.16).

Lymphadenopathy may occasionally appear similar to a vascular structure. However, an enlarged lymph node has a characteristic appearance, with a hyperechoic center and a hypoechoic rim (Fig. 16.17). In addition, as opposed to a blood vessel, when moving the probe either cephalad or caudad, a lymph node will abruptly disappear from the screen.

Differentiating an acute from a chronic DVT can be challenging. A chronic clot tends to be more echogenic, and recanalization may be noted. Color Doppler may be helpful in visualizing flow through the organized clot. However, these findings may be difficult to appreciate (Fig. 16.18).

In the popliteal fossa, the PV is quite superficial. It is easily collapsed with mild compression. When imaging this area, if only one vessel is seen, the sonographer should attempt to reduce the force with which the probe is placed against the patient's skin because the PV may have been unintentionally compressed.

A potential pitfall occurs when a superficial vein is mistaken for a deep vein. Proximal deep vessels are paired structures. Verify that the vein being imaged is adjacent to an artery.

In a patient with an acutely swollen extremity, a limited bedside ultrasound does not exclude the presence of a DVT in the inferior vena cava, iliac, or pelvic veins. Spectral Doppler may demonstrate the loss of respirophasic flow in the CFV if a thrombus is located in one or more of these veins. If a clot is suspected in these abdominal vessels, further imaging should also be considered.

Although the sensitivity and specificity of ultrasonography for detecting DVT is quite high, it is not 100%, particularly for distal thrombosis. If there is persistent concern for an acute DVT, even if the ultrasound does not reveal the presence of thrombus, further testing may be warranted. This may include CT, MRI, venography, or a repeat ultrasound in 4 to 7 days, depending on the clinical scenario.

A Baker's cyst occurs when fluid from the knee joint enters the gastrocnemius-semimembranosus bursa. Patients can present with pain in the popliteal fossa and calf, as well as swelling of the distal extremity. Ultrasonography is extremely helpful in differentiating this entity from a DVT (Fig. 16.19).

Patients who have cellulitis in an extremity may present with swelling, pain, and erythema of the affected area. Due to the overlap of symptoms with that of DVT, clinical differentiation can be challenging (26). Sonography of the affected area reveals interstitial fluid, which manifests as hypoechoic or anechoic areas within the soft tissue (Fig. 16.20). A patient with an abscess may also present with swelling, pain, and redness. Sonographically, an abscess tends to have an ovoid appearance, with posterior acoustic enhancement. Internally, the abscess may be anechoic, hypoechoic, or hyperechoic (Fig. 16.21).

Summary

The use of bedside sonography in patients with a painful swollen extremity is helpful in diagnosing a deep venous thrombosis. The most important component of this examination is determining the compressibility of the veins. Bedside ultrasonography of the lower extremity generally only involves the proximal veins but may include imaging of the entire lower extremity in some patients.

Clinical images

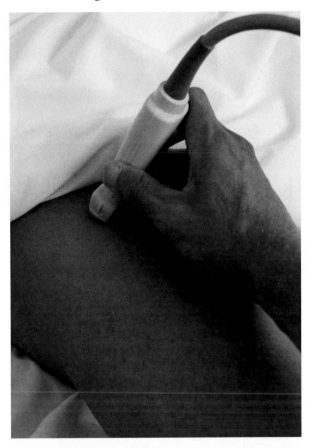

Figure 16.1. Inguinal probe placement. After appropriate draping, the probe is positioned just inferior to the inguinal ligament. Ultrasound gel is liberally applied to the medial aspect of the leg from the thigh to the knee.

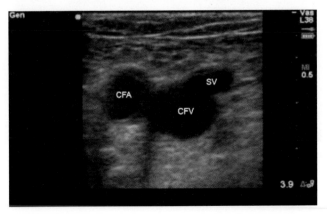

Figure 16.2. Inguinal view. The common femoral vein (CFV) is seen here in its relation to the common femoral artery (CFA) and greater saphenous vein (SV).

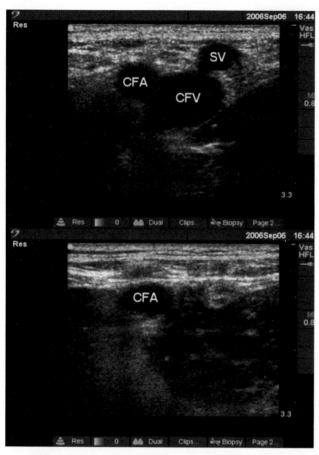

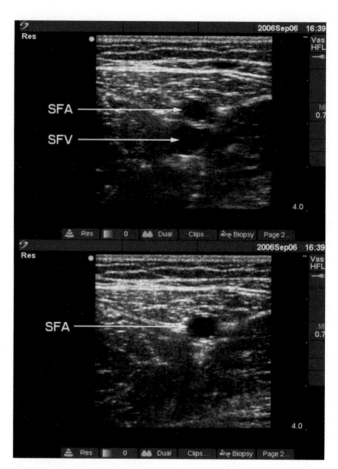

Figure 16.3. Inguinal view, noncompressed (*top*) and compressed (*bottom*). Pressure applied to the probe causes collapse of the SV and CFV. Because of a thicker wall and higher pressure, the artery remains patent.

Figure 16.5. SFA and FV. The probe is over the middle thigh, with the FV deep to the SFA. *Top*: noncompressed, the two vessels are visualized. *Bottom*: compression causes collapse of the vein, leaving only the SFA visible.

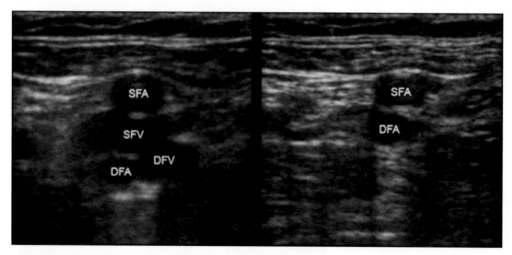

Figure 16.4. Femoral vessels. *Left*: the CFA bifurcates into the deep femoral artery (DFA) and the superficial femoral artery (SFA), whereas the CFV splits into the deep femoral vein (DFV) and the femoral vein (FV). *Right*: with compression, only the arteries remain patent.

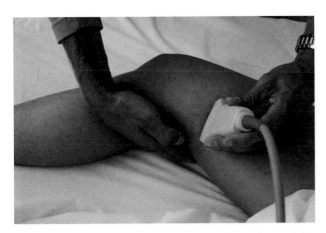

Figure 16.6. Reverse compression. The probe is held in place, and the nonscanning hand is placed behind the thigh and then compressed into the probe.

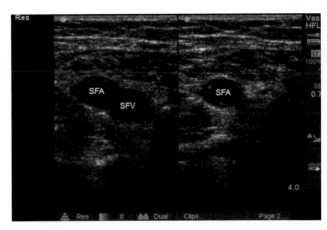

Figure 16.7. SFA and FV with and without compression. A split screen shows the SFA and FV without compression on the left side of the screen. The image on the right is with compression, with only the SFA remaining patent.

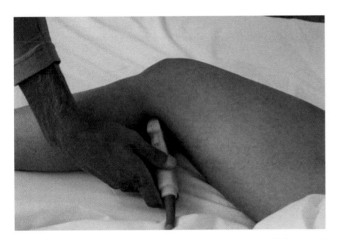

Figure 16.8. Popliteal fossa probe placement. The leg is slightly flexed at the knee and externally rotated at the hip.

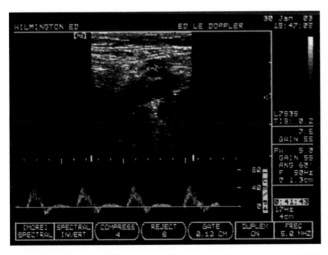

Figure 16.10. Spectral Doppler arterial waveform. The classic arterial high-resistance waveform has a triphasic appearance. The initial sharp upstroke in systole is followed by a brief period of retrograde flow in early diastole, followed by a period of antegrade flow.

Image courtesy of Dr. Paul Sierzenski.

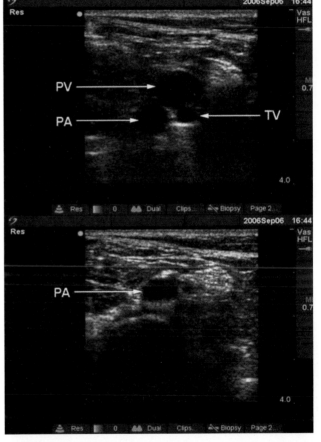

Figure 16.9. Popliteal vessels. *Top*: popliteal artery (PA) and popliteal vein (PV) are seen in addition to the anterior tibial vein (TV). *Bottom*: with compression, only the PA is visible.

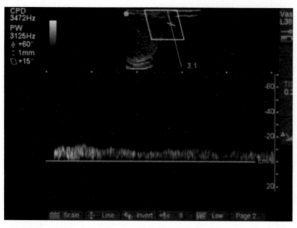

Figure 16.11. Spectral Doppler venous waveform. The veins of the proximal leg have continuous flow with a gently undulating respiratory pattern.

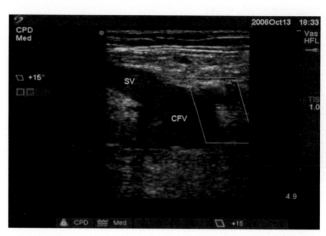

Figure 16.12. Proximal DVT. Echogenic thrombus is seen at the level of the saphenofemoral junction. Even with compression, the veins do not collapse. Flow is noted within the arterial system.

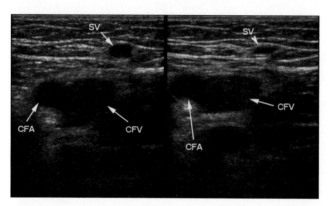

Figure 16.13. Right common femoral vein and greater saphenous vein DVT. *Left*: without compression, the CFA, CFV, and SV are all noted. *Right*: lack of compressibility of the CFV and SV.

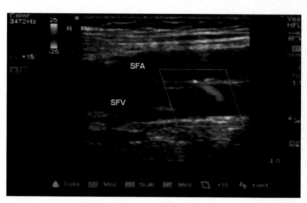

Figure 16.14. Longitudinal axis DVT. Longitudinal view of the femoral artery and vein, with a clot visible within the vein. "Rim flow" is demonstrated around the DVT.

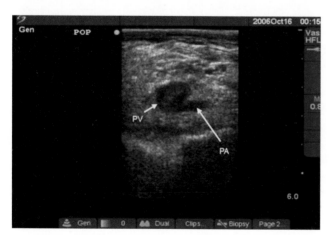

Figure 16.15. Popliteal DVT. Echogenic thrombus is noted within the PV. With compression, the PA has begun to collapse, but the PV has not.

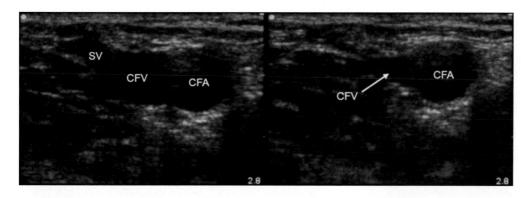

Figure 16.16. Incomplete compression. To exclude the presence of a DVT, the lumen of the vein must be completely compressed. Incomplete compression indicates either the presence of a DVT or a technically limited study.

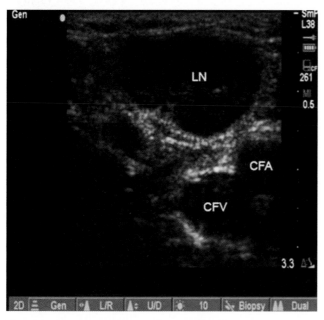

Figure 16.17. Lymph node. Typically, an enlarged lymph node will have a hyperechoic center and a hypoechoic rim.

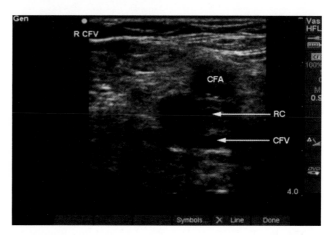

Figure 16.18. Chronic femoral DVT. Note the recanalization (RC) that has begun, visualized as an anechoic channel within the clot.

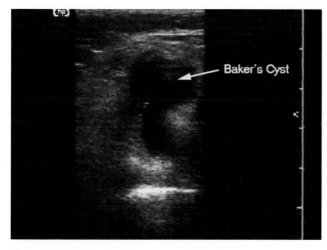

Figure 16.19. Baker's cyst. Found in the popliteal fossa, a Baker's cyst may be entirely anechoic. Alternatively, it may contain internal echoes or septations, or have irregular walls.

Image courtesy of Dr. Paul Sierzenski.

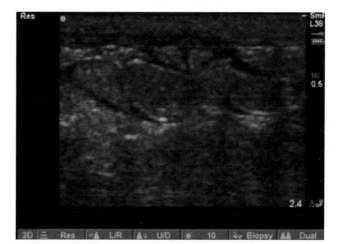

Figure 16.20. Cellulitis. This image demonstrates the classic "marbled" appearance of interstitial fluid within the soft tissue. Interstitial fluid secondary to congestive heart failure or pregnancy would have a similar gray scale appearance.

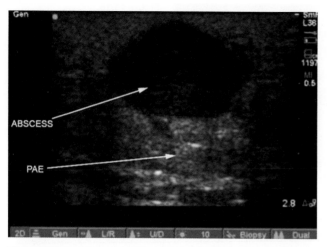

Figure 16.21. Abscess. Echogenic debris is located within the ovoid-shaped abscess. Note the posterior acoustic enhancement (PAE).

References

1. Centers for Disease Control and Prevention: Venous thromboembolism (blood clots): data & statistics. 2015. Available at: www.cdc.gov/ncbddd/dvt/data.html

2. Blaivas M, Lambert MJ, Harwood RA, et al.: Lower-extremity Doppler for deep venous thrombosis—can emergency physicians be accurate and fast? *Acad Emerg Med* 2000;**7**(2): 120–6.

3. Theodoro D, Blaivas M, Duggal S, et al.: Real-time B-mode ultrasound in the ED saves time in the diagnosis of deep vein thrombosis (DVT). *Am J Emerg Med* 2004;**22**(3):197–200.

4. Crisp JG, Lovato LM, Jang TB: Compression ultrasonography of the lower extremity with portable vascular ultrasonography can accurately detect deep venous thrombosis in the emergency department. *Ann Emerg Med* 2010 Dec;**56**(6):601–10.

5. Pomero F, Dentali F, Borretta V, et al.: Accuracy of emergency physician-performed ultrasonography in the diagnosis of deep-vein thrombosis: a systematic review and meta-analysis. *Thromb Haemost* 2013 Jan;**109**(1):137–45.

6. Righini M: Is it worth diagnosing and treating distal deep vein thrombosis? No. *J Thromb Haemost* 2007;**5**(suppl. 1):55–9.

7. Masuda EM, Kistner RL, Musikasinthorn C, et al.: The controversy of managing calf vein thrombosis. *J Vasc Surg* 2012 Feb;**55**(2):550–61.

8. Hirsh J, Hoak J: Management of deep vein thrombosis and pulmonary embolism. *Circulation* 1996;**93**:2212–45.

9. Binder B, Lackner HK, Salmhofer W, et al.: Association between superficial vein thrombosis and deep vein thrombosis of the lower extremities. *Arch Dermatol* 2009 Jul;**145**(7):753–7.

10. Patel RK, Lambie J, Bonner L, Arya R: Venous thromboembolism in the black population. *Arch Intern Med* 2004;**164**:1348–9.

11. Lensing AW, Prandoni P, Brandjes D, et al.: Detection of deep-vein thrombosis by real-time B-mode ultrasonography. *N Engl J Med* 1989;**320**:342–5.

12. Quintavalla R, Larini P, Miselli A, et al.: Duplex ultrasound diagnosis of symptomatic proximal deep vein thrombosis of lower limbs. *Eur J Radiol* 1992;**15**:32–6.

13. Gottlieb RH, Widjaja J, Tian L, et al.: Calf sonography for detecting deep venous thrombosis in symptomatic patients: experience and review of the literature. *J Clin Ultrasound* 1999 Oct;**27**(8):415–20.

14. Macdonald PS, Kahn SR, Miller N, Obrand D: Short-term natural history of isolated gastrocnemius and soleal vein thrombosis. *J Vasc Surg* 2003;**37**(3):523–7.

15. Lohr JM, Kerr TM, Lutter KS, et al.: Lower extremity calf thrombosis: to treat or not to treat? *J Vasc Surg* 1991;**14**(5): 618–23.

16. Deitcher SR, Caprini JA: Calf deep venous thrombosis should be treated with anticoagulation. *Med Clin North Am* 2003;**87**: 1157–64.

17. Wang CJ, Wang JW, Weng LH, et al.: Outcome of calf deep-vein thrombosis after total knee arthroplasty. *J Bone Joint Surg Br* 2003;**85B**(6):841–4.

18. Bernardi E, Camporese G, Büller HR, et al.: Serial 2-point ultrasonography plus D-dimer vs whole-leg color-coded Doppler ultrasonography for diagnosing suspected symptomatic deep vein thrombosis: a randomized controlled trial. *JAMA* 2008 Oct 8;**300**(14):1653–9.

19. Chengelis DL, Bendick PJ, Glover JL, et al.: Progression of superficial venous thrombosis to deep venous thrombosis. *J Vasc Surg* 1996 Nov;**24**(5):745–9.

20. Thiagarajah R, Venkatanarasimha N, Freeman S: Use of the term "superficial femoral vein" in ultrasound. *J Clin Ultrasound* 2011 Jan;**39**(1):32–4.

21. Caggiati A, Bergan JJ, Gloviczki P, et al.: International Interdisciplinary Consensus Committee on Venous Anatomical Terminology. Nomenclature of the veins of the lower limbs: an international interdisciplinary consensus statement. *J Vasc Surg* 2002 Aug;**36**(2):416–22.

22. McQueen AS, Elliott ST, Keir MJ: Ultrasonography for suspected deep vein thrombosis: how useful is single-point augmentation? *Clin Radiol* 2009 Feb;**64**(2):148–55.

23. Grant JD, Stevens SM, Woller SC, et al.: Diagnosis and management of upper extremity deep-vein thrombosis in adults. *Thromb Haemost* 2012;**108**:1097–1108.

24. Rumack C, Wilson SR, Charboneau JW, Levine D: *Diagnostic Ultrasound*, 4th ed. Philadelphia: Elsevier, 2011, 1034–7.

25. Mehta N, Schecter J, Stone M: Identification of intraluminal thrombus in emergency department patients with acute deep venous thrombosis. *J Emerg Med* 2012 May;**42**(5):566–8.

26. Rabuka CE, Azoulay LY, Kahn S: Predictors of a positive duplex scan in patients with a clinical presentation compatible with deep vein thrombosis or cellulitis. *Can J Infect Des* 2003 Jul–Aug;**14**(4):210–4.

Cardiac Ultrasound

Chris Moore and James Hwang

Indications

Cardiac ultrasound, or echocardiography, can be one of the most powerful noninvasive diagnostic tools available to the clinician in emergency situations involving critically ill or potentially critically ill patients (1–4).

The most dramatic indication for echo is the "code" or "near-code" situation, when a patient presents with pulseless electrical activity or severe hypotension (5, 6). Echo may quickly establish whether there is significant left ventricular (LV) dysfunction, marked volume depletion, cardiac tamponade, or severe right ventricular (RV) outflow obstruction. Echo may also confirm cardiac standstill or reveal evidence of fibrillation when the tracing appears to show asystole (7, 8). Echo is an integral part of the focused assessment with sonography in trauma (FAST) examination and is particularly important in the setting of penetrating chest trauma (9).

Echo should be considered in any medical patient with signs or symptoms of a significant pericardial effusion. Effusion may present with isolated chest pain, tachycardia, hypotension, or dyspnea (10, 11). Echo should be strongly considered in patients presenting with acute complaints and particular risk factors for effusion, such as malignancy or renal failure.

In many emergent conditions, echo may be a useful tool, but it should not be used in isolation to rule out the condition. Echo is not sensitive for acute coronary syndrome, pulmonary embolism, or thoracic aortic aneurysm or dissection, but it may be fairly specific for these conditions in the right clinical scenario (12–14). Thus, visualizing these entities on echo may quickly make the diagnosis, but not seeing them does not adequately rule out the diagnosis.

Acute valvular emergencies are uncommon, but echo is essential in diagnosing them. Bedside echo can augment cardiac auscultation and has been shown, in some instances, to be more accurate than physical examination (15). Detection of severe regurgitant or stenotic lesions can provide key information to the management of patients presenting with syncope, chest pain, or dyspnea. Although blood cultures and physical examination remain the mainstay of diagnosing endocarditis, valvular vegetations seen on transthoracic or transesophageal echo are diagnostic in the right clinical setting.

Emerging research suggests using echo as an aid in the noninvasive evaluation of sepsis, specifically in assessing preload and LV function (LVF) to help guide fluid resuscitation and choice of vasopressors (16, 17). In patients diagnosed with pulmonary embolism, echo helps risk-stratify patients, provides prognostic information, and aids in the decision to administer thrombolytic therapy (12, 18–21). Information about LVF may also provide overall prognostic information (22).

In general, the use of emergency ultrasound (and emergency echo) at the bedside is shifting from isolated, consultant-performed tests to goal-directed ultrasound intended to answer several symptom-specific questions. For example, in a patient presenting with unexplained hypotension, bedside ultrasound may be integrated with the physical examination as key interventions are pursued. While access is being obtained, the clinician may examine the heart for evidence of cardiac tamponade, LV failure, RV outflow obstruction, and decreased preload in the inferior vena cava (IVC), as well as examining the abdomen for evidence of intraperitoneal hemorrhage or abdominal aortic aneurysm (23, 24). Similarly, an evaluation of the patient with unexplained dyspnea could include echo, evaluation of both hemithoraces, and lower extremity ultrasound for proximal deep venous thrombosis (25). With practice, these integrated examinations may be performed accurately and rapidly (16, 24, 26).

In addition to diagnostic uses, echo is useful in bedside cardiac procedures, particularly pericardiocentesis and placing and confirming capture with transcutaneous or transvenous pacing (27–29).

Diagnostic capabilities

It is important to differentiate clinician-performed bedside echo from consultant-performed echo (typically performed by a sonographer and interpreted by a cardiologist). There are three major differences that separate these entities:

1. Experience with obtaining images and interpreting imaging pathology
2. Time available to perform the examination
3. Equipment capabilities and performance

Although there are exceptions, a consultant-performed study typically has the advantage of greater time for the consultant to perform the examination, more extensive experience of the consultant with echo, and higher-end equipment specifically devoted to echo. Patients are often removed from the immediate patient care area, as opposed to bedside clinician-performed echo. In addition, the clinician may have the advantage of more extensive historical and ancillary information about the patient.

In theory, a consultant-performed echo could be performed in every patient with a potential cardiovascular complaint, but in practice this is not feasible. In 2004, less than one-third of community ED directors reported that consultant-performed echo was "easily available," with more than one-fourth reporting that it was not available at all (30). Even if consultant-performed echo were constantly available, it would be impossible to provide it immediately in a patient with penetrating chest trauma or in code situations. For these reasons, it is essential that emergency practitioners understand the basics of obtaining and interpreting bedside echo. This is in no way meant to diminish the role of appropriately obtained consultant-performed echo, which will often be obtained once immediate life threats have been ruled out.

Different specialty societies have different recommendations regarding the amount of experience required to perform cardiac echo, from as little as 25 to more than 450 examinations. Note that the numbers should be different for goal-directed assessment of certain conditions (e.g., any effusion) than they would be for comprehensive echo (31–35). It is important that practitioners obtaining and interpreting cardiac images be aware of both their capabilities and their limitations and that this is appropriately reflected in documentation of the exam and communications with both the patient and subsequent care providers.

This chapter deals with transthoracic echocardiography, as differentiated from transesophageal echocardiography (TEE). Although TEE inevitably provides superior images and improved diagnostic capability, it requires more advanced equipment, more skilled operators, patient sedation, and the potential need for airway management. This is typically outside the scope of the emergency practitioner, although it may play a role in the diagnosis of endocarditis or aortic dissection.

When teaching bedside clinician-performed ultrasound, we recommend focusing primarily on three findings:

1. Presence and extent of pericardial effusion
2. Global LV function
3. Presence of RV strain

Determining the presence of a significant pericardial effusion is potentially the most straightforward application of echo, although this is not without pitfalls, as discussed later in the chapter. Effusions should generally be graded by size and measured as the largest pocket of fluid in end diastole. Small effusions are generally considered to be <1 cm; moderate, 1 to 2 cm; and large, >2 cm. Tamponade occurs when the right side of the heart cannot fill due to extrinsic compression. Although tamponade is a clinical diagnosis, echo may show diastolic collapse of the right atrium or ventricle, as well as increased respiratory variation in the Doppler signal of mitral inflow (the echo equivalent of pulsus paradoxus).

Global LVF is typically measured in terms of ejection fraction (EF). The gold standard for EF is nuclear studies or cardiac catheterization. Although formulas exist for calculating EF based on echo measurements, most cardiologists use a visual estimation of EF. We recommend classification of LVF into one of three categories: normal/hyperdynamic (EF >50%), mild to moderately depressed (EF 30%–50%), and severely depressed (EF <30%). With goal-directed training, physicians can reliably categorize LVF (17, 36).

RV strain is of importance in the critically ill patient because it may suggest a massive pulmonary embolism (12, 19, 21). Signs of RV strain include RV dilatation, RV hypokinesis, paradoxical septal motion, and tricuspid regurgitation. The normal RV:LV ratio is less than 0.7:1 when measured in an apical view across the tips of the atrioventricular valves. With acute outflow obstruction, the RV will dilate and may exceed the size of the LV. We recommend using a cutoff of 1:1 or greater. In other words, if the size of the RV exceeds that of the LV, it indicates significant RV strain. In the right clinical scenario, this may suggest pulmonary embolism. There are, however, many chronic conditions that cause RV dilatation, often with associated RV hypertrophy (i.e., pulmonary hypertension, chronic obstructive pulmonary disease [COPD]).

There are numerous other findings that may be of importance in emergent cardiac ultrasound, and the clinical images will detail many of the diagnostic capabilities of both clinician- and consultant-performed echo.

Imaging considerations

In contrast to imaging modalities such as plain radiographs or CT, it may be necessary for the clinician to obtain images using an ultrasound machine. Although a comprehensive review of the use of ultrasound imaging equipment is beyond the scope of this chapter, there are certain considerations that are specific to echo.

First, it is important to consider the positioning of the examiner and scanner relative to the patient. When a cardiologist or sonographer performs an echo, it is typically done from the left side of the patient, with the probe held in the examiner's left hand. Although this makes some sense (because the heart is on the patient's left side), it is opposite to the side from which other emergency ultrasound examinations are performed, and, frequently, we are performing both cardiac and abdominal imaging on the same patient (e.g., in the FAST exam). We found that it is easier to learn both ultrasound and echo when a consistent orientation is used and typically recommend that all ultrasound (including echo) be performed from the patient's right side, recognizing that sometimes space and patient care issues may require an exam to be done from a different side.

Second, it is important to understand the imaging conventions used in cardiology compared to other ultrasound. When you pick up a probe to begin imaging, you should find the "indicator" (typically, a bump or groove) and correlate this with the side of the screen as it is viewed. In abdominal and other emergency ultrasound applications, the indicator corresponds to the left side of the screen as it is viewed, with this side of the screen being marked by an indicator or logo. When a cardiology application is chosen, the indicator will typically switch to correspond to the right side of the screen as it is viewed. For physicians who are doing both abdominal and cardiac imaging, we recommend a consistent approach and teach our cardiac imaging in an abdominal orientation, with the indicator corresponding to the left side of the screen as it is viewed. Although the imaging convention used may differ from institution to institution, it is important to understand which convention is being used. The text and images in this chapter use an abdominal or emergency medicine orientation.

Probe selection and equipment are important in obtaining quality images. A phased array transducer – where the scan lines emanate from a single point and the beam is electronically steered – allows for the best imaging between ribs. If this is not available, a small footprint or microconvex curvilinear transducer may be the best choice. When available, tissue harmonic imaging will further improve the image by enhancing contrast, allowing more accurate identification of the endocardial border.

There are three basic views that are the most useful to the clinician performing echo: parasternal (long and short axis), subxiphoid or subcostal, and apical. When obtaining these images, the "axes" of the heart should be understood: the long axis runs from the base (valves) to apex, essentially from the patient's right shoulder to the left costal margin. The short axis is 90 degrees perpendicular to this, from the left shoulder to the right costal margin. Thus, when the probe is oriented toward the patient's right shoulder, it is along the long axis of the heart.

The parasternal long axis in an abdominal orientation is obtained by placing the probe lateral to the sternum and directing the indicator to the patient's right shoulder (37). This view will provide an image with the apex at the right of the screen and the base of the heart at the left. Note that this is reversed from a typical cardiology orientation, which may be obtained either by reversing the screen orientation on the machine or by directing the probe to the patient's left costal margin. The parasternal long axis should show the left atrium, mitral valve, LV and LV outflow tract, RV, and interventricular septum. The short axis is obtained by rotating the probe 90 degrees counterclockwise, providing a "donut" view of the LV.

The subcostal four-chamber view is obtained by placing the probe below the costal margin and directing the indicator to the patient's right. Images will be improved by flattening the probe on the abdomen and having the patient inhale. The IVC should be followed into the right atrium, and the view should include the RA, RV, LA, and LV, with the apex to the right of the screen. Note that this orientation is similar to the parasternal long axis, although lower (aortic root is not typically seen).

The apical four-chamber view is obtained by placing the probe at the point of maximal impulse, typically just lateral and inferior to the nipple in males or underneath the breast in females, with the indicator directed to the patient's right. Images will be improved by placing the patient in the left lateral decubitus position. The apex should be seen at the top of the screen with the interventricular septum running vertically. The LV, LA, RV, and RA should be visualized.

There are numerous other ancillary views, some of which are shown in the "Clinical images" section.

Imaging pitfalls and limitations

Patient body habitus and comorbid conditions may limit imaging. Having patients lie on their left sides allows the heart to rest more laterally against the chest wall and may provide improved images. In patients with obesity, abdominal trauma, or abdominal distension, a parasternal image may be most effective, whereas in patients with hyperexpanded lungs (COPD or intubated), the subxiphoid window may be the only view available. Although it is rare for a patient to have three quality views (parasternal, subxiphoid, or apical), most patients will have at least one adequate window.

The most common echo pitfall is that physiological pericardial fluid or epicardial fat may be misinterpreted as a pericardial effusion. A large percentage of patients will have some hypoechoic (dark) space around the heart. This is often most prominent in the anterior portion of the parasternal long-axis image and should not be mistaken for an effusion. Keys to identifying this correctly are the presence of internal echoes and obliteration of the space in cardiac diastole. There is unlikely to be a significant pericardial effusion if no fluid is seen *posteriorly* on the parasternal long-axis view because most fluid will be found posteriorly and inferiorly. It is important to regularly examine normal patients and to notice the presence of this space so it is not misinterpreted, particularly in a penetrating trauma situation (38). Pericardial fluid should not be confused with pleural fluid, which may appear adjacent to the heart in a patient with a left pleural effusion. If fluid around the heart is seen, a left lateral (coronal) view of the thorax should be obtained to assess for the presence of a left pleural effusion. The position of the fluid relative to the descending aorta may help further differentiate pericardial from pleural fluid.

Focal wall motion abnormalities may cause the heart to appear more normal in some views than others. Obtaining as many views as possible, specifically by adding a parasternal short-axis view, may help avoid this. Although focal wall motion abnormalities may occasionally be blatant, subtle abnormalities are often difficult to discern, and there is often significant interobserver variability, even among highly trained observers.

When identifying RV dilatation relative to the LV, it is important to maximize the LV size in your view because certain oblique cuts may make the LV appear much smaller, even in a normal heart. In particular, the subcostal view may overemphasize the size of the RV as it cuts across the heart from below. Attempt to obtain further images in both the parasternal and apical views.

Artifacts are common in ultrasound and may be seen in cardiac echo. Often a "side-lobe" artifact may appear as a hyperechoic space in the atria or ventricles. These may be attenuated by decreasing the gain or by obtaining alternate views to determine whether the artifact persists. Papillary muscles should also be identified because these may be misinterpreted as intracardiac masses or vegetations.

Clinical images

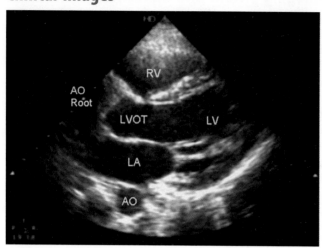
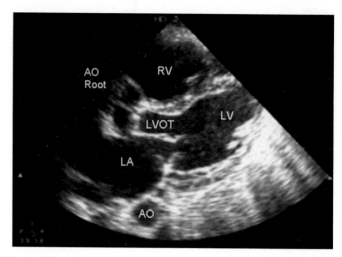

Figures 17.1A and B. Parasternal long-axis view demonstrating the RV, LA, MV, LV, LVOT, AO root, and descending AO. Note that this is in the abdominal orientation, with the apex of the heart pointing toward the right of the screen (reversed from a cardiology parasternal long-axis view).

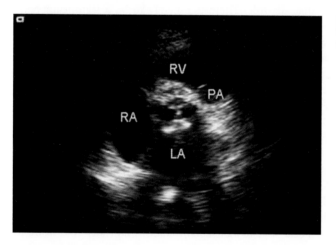

Figure 17.2. Parasternal short-axis view at the level of the aortic valve (reversed from a cardiology parasternal short-axis view). The aortic valve is trileaflet and demonstrates the "Mercedes Benz" sign.

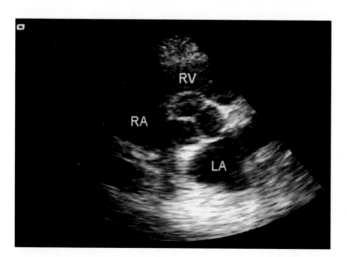
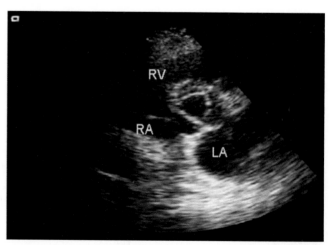

Figures 17.3A and B. Parasternal short-axis views at the level of the aortic valve – closed and open. Surrounding the AO valve at this level (clockwise) are the LA, RA, and RV (the pulmonary artery is not visualized).

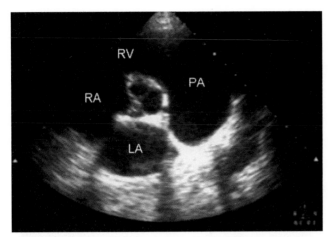

Figure 17.4. Parasternal short-axis view at the level of the aortic valve (closed). Note the dilated pulmonary artery (measured 5 cm on CT), which was pathologically enlarged due to pulmonary hypertension.

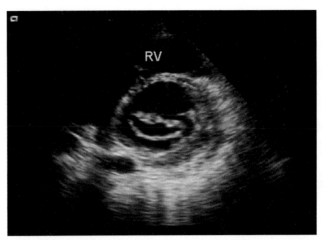

Figure 17.5. Parasternal short-axis view at the level of the mitral valve (reversed from a cardiology parasternal short-axis view). When the mitral valve is open, it yields a "fish mouth" appearance.

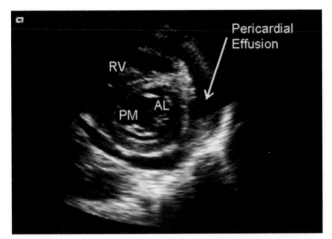

Figure 17.6. Parasternal short-axis view at the level of the papillary muscles. The anterolateral (AL) and posteromedial (PM) papillary muscles are identified. This view visualizes the concentric myocardium at the mid-ventricle level and thus is helpful in assessing LV function. A circumferential pericardial effusion is also identified.

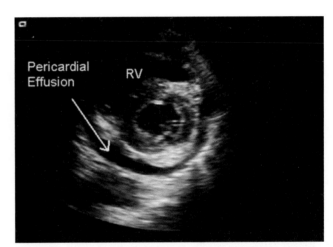

Figure 17.7. Parasternal short-axis view at the level of the apex. This is the typical "donut" view of the LV but is smaller at the apex as the LV cavity tapers down. A circumferential pericardial effusion is also identified.

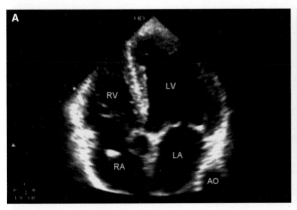
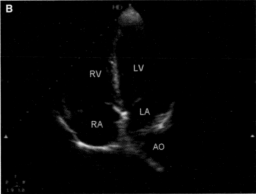

Figure 17.8. A: Apical four-chamber view. Leaflets of mitral valve are seen between the LA and LV. A portion of the descending aorta (AO) is visualized. B: Apical four-chamber view. Leaflets of the mitral valve and tricuspid valve are seen between the LA/LV and RA/RV, respectively. The descending AO is also visualized.

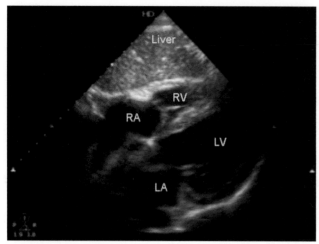

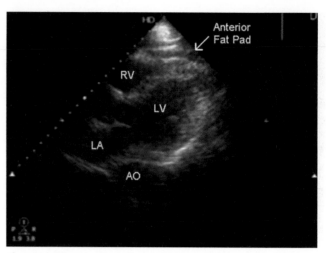

Figure 17.9. Subxiphoid view demonstrating all four chambers: RA, RV, LA, and LV. The tricuspid and mitral valves are also seen. This is an excellent view for patients with chronic obstructive pulmonary disease because hyperexpanded lungs shift the heart downward. The subxiphoid view, however, may overemphasize the relative size of the RV if it cuts across the RV in an oblique plane.

Figure 17.10. Parasternal long-axis view demonstrating an anterior fat pad. Anterior fat pads are normal variants and typically possess internal echoes. Note that there is no posterior pericardial fluid. Loculated anterior effusions are uncommon but can occur after cardiac surgery.

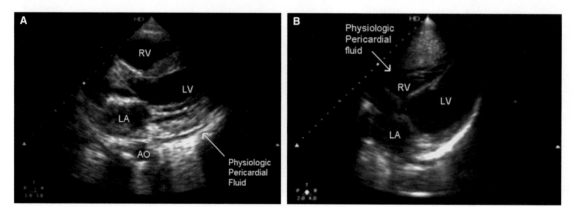

Figure 17.11. A: Parasternal long-axis view demonstrating physiological pericardial fluid. Pericardial effusions are characterized as small, moderate, or large. An effusion is considered small if the effusion along the posterior wall is <10 mm, moderate if 10 to 15 mm, and large if >15 mm. B: Subxiphoid view demonstrating physiological pericardial fluid. The RV is seen as a small wedge up against the liver.

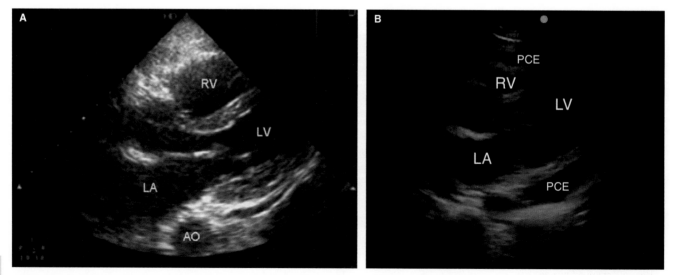

Figure 17.12. A: Parasternal long-axis view demonstrating a small pericardial effusion (measures <10 mm along the posterior LV wall). B: Parasternal long-axis view demonstrating a moderate pericardial effusion (measures between 10 and 15 mm along the posterior LV wall).

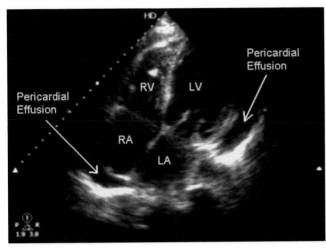
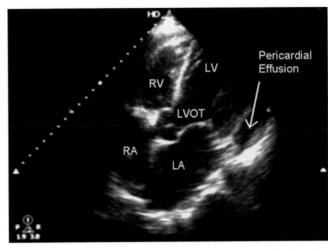

Figure 17.13. A: Apical four-chamber view (probe is somewhat medial to apex) with moderate-size circumferential pericardial effusion. B: Apical five-chamber view including the left ventricular outflow tract (LVOT). A moderate-size pericardial effusion is also visualized.

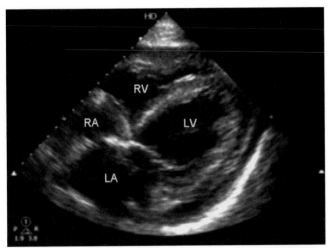

Figure 17.14. Subxiphoid view revealing a moderate-size pericardial effusion. The subxiphoid view is an excellent view for effusions because fluid around the heart tends to collect inferiorly. Also seen is a pacer wire traveling through the RA and tricuspid valve and toward the apex of the RV.

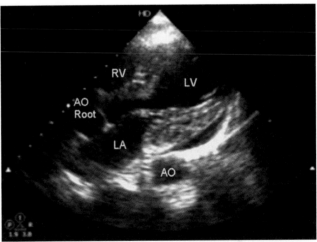

Figure 17.15. Parasternal long-axis view demonstrating a moderate-size pericardial effusion. To differentiate pericardial and pleural effusions, identify the position of the effusion relative to the descending thoracic aorta. Pericardial effusions occur anterior to the descending AO, whereas pleural effusions extend posterior to the descending AO.

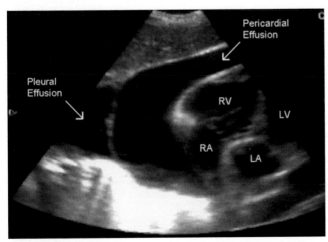

Figure 17.16. Subxiphoid view revealing both a pleural effusion and a pericardial effusion. The pericardium is clearly seen between the right pleural effusion and the large pericardial effusion.

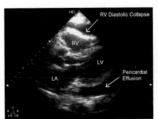
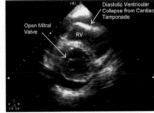

Figure 17.17. A: Parasternal long-axis view with a large circumferential pericardial effusion and RV free wall inversion during ventricular diastole. This finding is evidence of cardiac tamponade. Note the open mitral valve, which correlates with ventricular diastole. B: Parasternal short-axis view at the level of the mitral valve (reversed from a cardiology parasternal short-axis view). Note the RV free wall inversion due to the large circumferential pericardial effusion. This finding is consistent with cardiac tamponade.

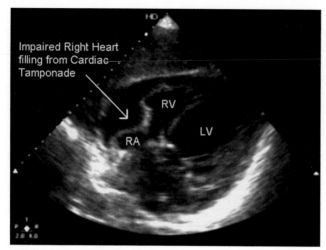

Figure 17.18. Subxiphoid view demonstrating a moderate to large pericardial effusion with evidence of right atrial inversion. It is important not to confuse atrial contraction, which occurs during atrial systole, with diastolic collapse.

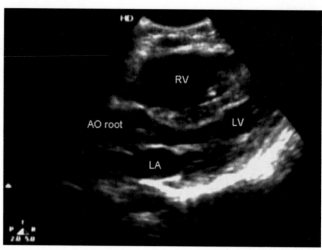

Figure 17.19. Parasternal long-axis view showing RV dilatation. The ratio of the RV to the LV is greater than 0.7 to 1 and exceeds 1:1 in this patient (incidentally found to have a large atrial septal defect).

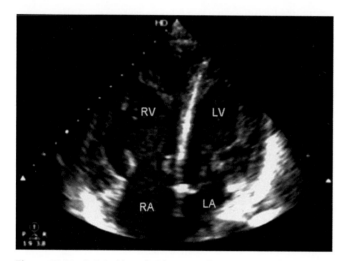

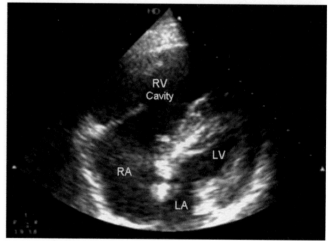

Figure 17.20. A: Apical four-chamber view of a patient with RV dilatation. The RV is larger than the LV. This patient had chronic pulmonary hypertension. Note the hypertrophy of the RV free wall. RV free wall thickness in excess of 5 mm suggests hypertrophy and a chronic etiology to the RV strain. B: Apical four-chamber view of a patient with RV dilatation. The RV is larger than the LV. This view is slightly medial – the septum is not vertical, and the apex of the heart is not visualized.

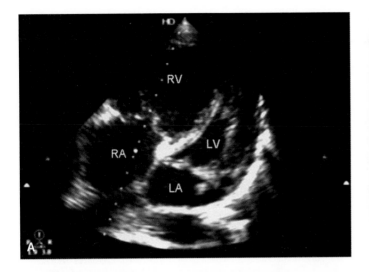

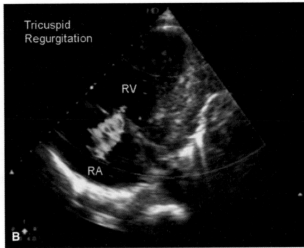

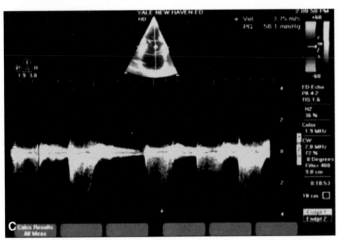

Figure 17.21. A: Apical four-chamber view (slightly medial – septum is not vertical) demonstrating a dilated RV. Color Doppler imaging can be used to assess for tricuspid regurgitation (TR). If TR is present, continuous wave spectral Doppler can then be used to estimate the pulmonary artery pressure. B: Color Doppler imaging demonstrating tricuspid regurgitation. Once the TR jet is identified by color Doppler, continuous wave spectral Doppler can then be used to calculate the maximal velocity of the TR jet. C: Measuring the maximal velocity of a TR jet. Velocities greater than 2.7 m/s are significant. Using the modified Bernoulli equation ($\Delta P = 4*V^2$), an estimate of the pulmonary artery pressure is then calculated. In this case, the pressure in the RV exceeds that of the RA by 56 mmHg, as calculated by software on the machine using the modified Bernoulli equation. An accurate RV pressure could be obtained by adding an estimate of RA pressure (often assumed to be 10 mmHg).

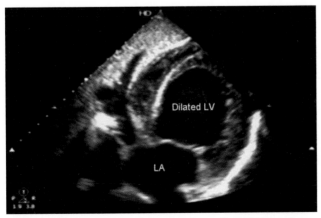

Figure 17.22. Subxiphoid view demonstrating a dilated LV. LV cavity diameters greater than 3.9 cm in systole or 5.2 cm in diastole are abnormal and consistent with left ventricular enlargement.

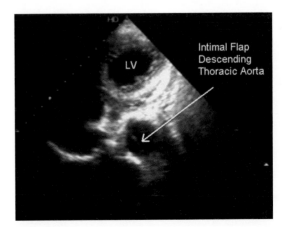

Figure 17.23. Parasternal view demonstrating the descending aorta with an intimal flap (dissection). Although visualized on this transthoracic echo, transesophageal echo is much more sensitive for the evaluation of aortic dissection.

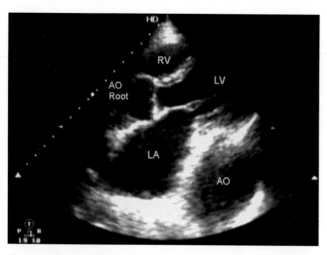
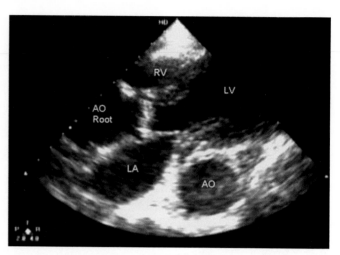

Figures 17.24A and B. Parasternal long-axis view demonstrating a thoracic aortic aneurysm. The aortic root is dilated (>4 cm) in (B). In both figures, the enlarged descending thoracic aorta can be seen behind the heart.

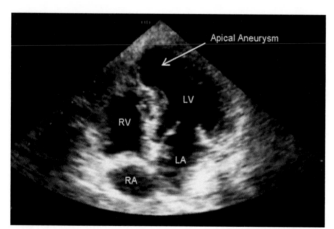

Figure 17.25. Apical four-chamber view demonstrating a left apical ventricular aneurysm. When seen in real time, this thin-walled portion of the apex was noted to be dyskinetic during ventricular systole.

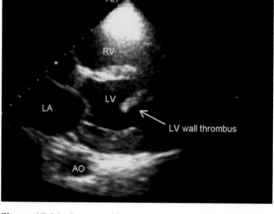

Figure 17.26. Parasternal long-axis view revealing a left ventricular wall thrombus. Patients with a recent myocardial infarct, wall motion abnormality, or ventricular aneurysm are at risk for developing a ventricular thrombus. Be careful not to confuse the papillary muscles with a thrombus. In this case, the structure was seen to be waving back and forth during cardiac activity. It was initially believed to be a ruptured papillary muscle, but the chordae tendinea and the valvular motion were intact.

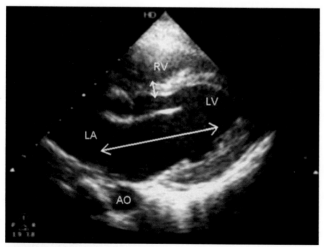

Figure 17.27. Parasternal long-axis view. To accurately assess for left ventricular hypertrophy (LVH), the measurement should be made in diastole (with the mitral valve open). The measurement should be made perpendicular to the LV long axis (*long arrow*) to avoid overestimation of wall thickness.

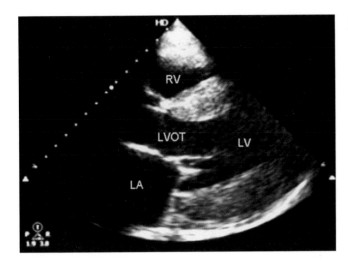

Figure 17.28. Parasternal long-axis view of a patient with LVH. A septal thickness greater than 1.1 cm during ventricular diastole is consistent with LVH.

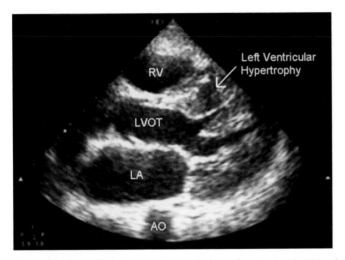
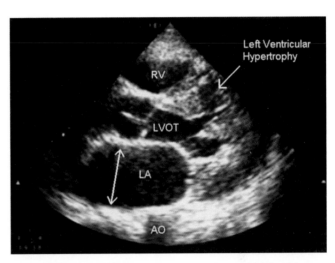

Figure 17.29A and B. Parasternal long-axis views of a patient with LVH and a prominent left atrium. LA diameters >4 cm are consistent with left atrial enlargement (LAE).

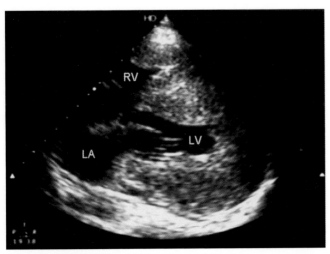
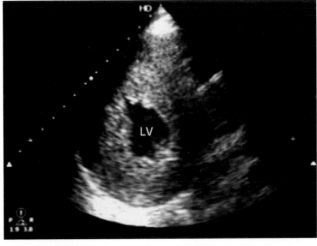

Figures 17.30A and B. Parasternal long- and short-axis views of a patient with Noonan syndrome. Note the marked LVH. Hypertrophic cardiomyopathy (obstructive and nonobstructive types) is present in up to 30% of patients.

257

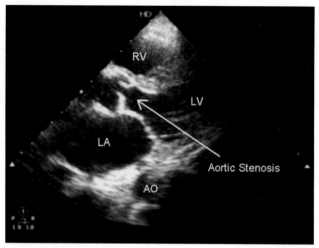

Figure 17.31. Parasternal long-axis view showing a reduced aortic outflow diameter. This patient had aortic stenosis.

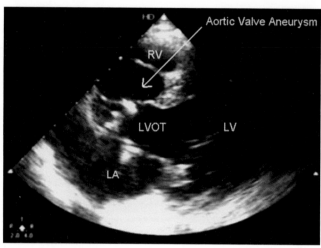

Figure 17.32. Parasternal long-axis view demonstrating an aortic valve aneurysm. This patient had a history of aortic valve replacement.

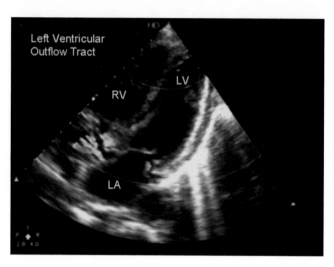

Figure 17.33. Color Doppler imaging outlining the left ventricular outflow tract. Evidence of mitral regurgitation is also noted.

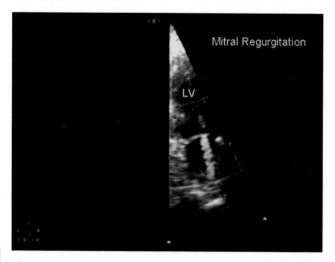

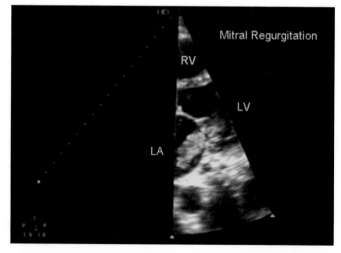

Figures 17.34A and B. Color Doppler imaging demonstrating mitral regurgitation. With the MR jet identified by color Doppler, continuous wave spectral Doppler is then used to characterize and quantify the severity of MR.

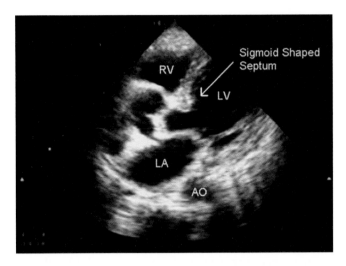

Figure 17.35. Parasternal long-axis view of an elderly heart. Elderly patients can develop a sigmoid-shaped septum (septal bulge) that can lead to an overestimation of LVH. Another common finding revealed in this image is aortic valve sclerosis. Other common findings (not seen here) include mitral annular calcification, mild aortic insufficiency, mild mitral regurgitation, and aortic root enlargement (secondary to prolonged hypertension).

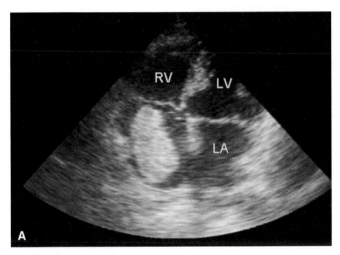
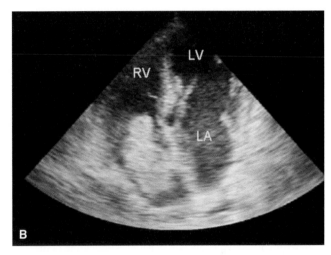

Figures 17.36A and B. Apical four-chamber views of a patient with a right atrial mass. Tricuspid and mitral valves seen closed and then open.

References

1. Cardenas E: Limited bedside ultrasound imaging by emergency medicine physicians. *West J Med* 1998;**168**(3):188–9.

2. Chizner MA: The diagnosis of heart disease by clinical assessment alone. *Curr Prob Cardiol* 2001;**26**(5):285–379.

3. Hauser AM: The emerging role of echocardiography in the emergency department. *Ann Emerg Med* 1989;**18**(12):1298–303.

4. Kimura BJ, Bocchicchio M, Willis CL, Demaria AN: Screening cardiac ultrasonographic examination in patients with suspected cardiac disease in the emergency department. *Am Heart J* 2001;**142**(2):324–30.

5. Bocka JJ, Overton DT, Hauser A: Electromechanical dissociation in human beings: an echocardiographic evaluation. *Ann Emerg Med* 1988;**17**(5):450–2.

6. Tayal VS, Kline JA: Emergency echocardiography to detect pericardial effusion in patients in PEA and near-PEA states. *Resuscitation* 2003;**59**(3):315–18.

7. Amaya SC, Langsam A: Ultrasound detection of ventricular fibrillation disguised as asystole. *Ann Emerg Med* 1999;**33**(3):344–6.

8. Blaivas M, Fox JC: Outcome in cardiac arrest patients found to have cardiac standstill on the bedside emergency department echocardiogram [comment]. *Acad Emerg Med* 2001;**8**(6):616–21.

9. Plummer D, Brunette D, Asinger R, Ruiz E: Emergency department echocardiography improves outcome in penetrating cardiac injury. *Ann Emerg Med* 1992;**21**(6):709–12.

10. Blaivas M: Incidence of pericardial effusion in patients presenting to the emergency department with unexplained dyspnea. *Acad Emerg Med* 2001;**8**(12):1143–6.

11. Shabetai R: Pericardial effusion: hemodynamic spectrum. *Heart* 2004;**90**(3):255–6.

12. Nazeyrollas P, Metz D, Jolly D, et al.: Use of transthoracic Doppler echocardiography combined with clinical and electrocardiographic data to predict acute pulmonary embolism. *Eur Heart J* 1996;**17**:779–86.

13. Peels CH, Visser CA, Kupper AJ, et al.: Usefulness of two-dimensional echocardiography for immediate detection of myocardial ischemia in the emergency room. *Am J Cardiol* 1990;**65**(11):687–91.

14. Roudaut RP, Billes MA, Gosse P, et al.: Accuracy of M-mode and two-dimensional echocardiography in the diagnosis of aortic dissection: an experience with 128 cases. *Clin Cardiol* 1988;**11**:553–62.

15. Kobal SL, et al: *Am J Card* 2005;**96**(7):1002.

16. Jones AET, Vivek S, Sullivan MD, Kline JA: Randomized controlled trial of immediate vs. delayed goal-directed ultrasound to identify the etiology of nontraumatic hypotension in emergency department patients. *Acad Emerg Med* 2004;**11**(5): 445–6.

17. Moore CL, Rose GA, Tayal VS, et al.: Determination of left ventricular function by emergency physician echocardiography of hypotensive patients. *Acad Emerg Med* 2002;**9**(3):186–93.

18. Grifoni S, Olivotto I, Cecchini P, et al.: Utility of an integrated clinical, echocardiographic, and venous ultrasonographic approach for triage of patients with suspected pulmonary embolism. *Am J Cardiol* 1998;**82**:1230–5.

19. Johnson ME, Furlong R, Schrank K: Diagnostic use of emergency department echocardiogram in massive pulmonary emboli. *Ann Emerg Med* 1992;**21**(6):760–3.

20. Kasper W, Konstantinides S, Geibel A, et al.: Prognostic significance of right ventricular afterload stress detected by echocardiography in patients with clinically suspected pulmonary embolism. *Heart* 1997;**77**:346–9.

21. Ribiero A, Lindmarker P, Juhlin-Dannfelt A, et al.: Echocardiography Doppler in pulmonary embolism: right ventricular dysfunction as a predictor of mortality rate. *Am Heart J* 1997;**134**(3):479–87.

22. Sabia P, Abbott RD, Afrookteh A, et al.: Importance of two-dimensional echocardiographic assessment of left ventricular systolic function in patients presenting to the emergency room with cardiac-related symptoms. *Circulation* 1991;**84**(4):1615–24.

23. Jones AET, Vivek S, Sullivan MD, Kline JA: Randomized controlled trial of immediate vs. delayed goal-directed ultrasound to identify the etiology of nontraumatic hypotension in emergency department patients. *Crit Care Med* 2004;**32**:1703–8.

24. Rose JS, Pershad J, Tayal V, et al.: The UHP ultrasound protocol: a novel ultrasound approach to the empiric evaluation of the undifferentiated hypotensive patient [comment]. *Am J Emerg Med* 2001;**19**(4):299–302.

25. Moore CL, Chen J, Lynch KA, et al.: Utility of focused chest ultrasound in the diagnosis of patients with unexplained dyspnea. *Acad Emerg Med* 2006;**13**(5):S201.

26. Pearson AC: Noninvasive evaluation of the hemodynamically unstable patient: the advantages of seeing clearly. *Mayo Clin Proc* 1995;**70**:1012–14.

27. Aguilera PA, Durham BA, Riley DA: Emergency transvenous cardiac pacing placement using ultrasound guidance. *Ann Emerg Med* 2000;**36**(3):224–7.

28. Callahan JA, Seward JB, Nishimura RA, et al.: Two-dimensional echocardiographically guided pericardiocentesis: experience in 117 consecutive patients. *Am J Cardiol* 1985;**55**(4):476–9.

29. Ettin D, Cook T: Using ultrasound to determine external pacer capture. *J Emerg Med* 1999;**17**(6):1007–9.

30. Moore CL, Molina AA, Lin H: Ultrasonography in community emergency departments in the United States: access to ultrasonography performed by consultants and status of emergency physician-performed ultrasonography. *Ann Emerg Med* 2006;**47**(2):147–53.

31. Stahmer SA: Correspondence: the ASE position statement on echocardiography in the emergency department. *Acad Emerg Med* 2000;**7**:306–7.

32. American Medical Association (AMA): H-230.960 Privileging for ultrasound imaging. Chicago: AMA, 2000. Available at: www.ama-assn.org/apps/pf_new/pf_online?f_n=browse& doc=policyfiles/HnE/H-230.960.HTM

33. DeMaria AN, Crawford MH, Feigenbaum H, et al.: Task force: training in echocardiography. *J Am Coll Cardiol* 1986;**7**(6): 1207–8.

34. Mateer J, Plummer D, Heller M, et al.: Model curriculum for physician training in emergency ultrasonography. *Ann Emerg Med* 1994;**23**(1):95–102.

35. American College of Emergency Physicians (ACEP). ACEP policy statement: emergency ultrasound guidelines. Available at: acep.org/webportal/PracticeResources/PolicyStatements/

36. Jones AE, Tayal VS, Kline JA: Focused training of emergency medicine residents in goal-directed echocardiography: a prospective study. *Acad Emerg Med* 2003;**10**(10):1054–8.

37. Moore C: Current issues with emergency cardiac ultrasound probe and image conventions. *Acad Emerg Med* 2008;**15**:278–84.

38. Blaivas M, DeBehnke D, Phelan MB: Potential errors in the diagnosis of pericardial effusion on trauma ultrasound for penetrating injuries. *Acad Emerg Med* 2000;**7**(11):1261–6.

Chapter 18

Emergency Ultrasonography of the Kidneys and Urinary Tract

Anthony J. Dean and Ross Kessler

Indications

The principal indication for renal ultrasound is in the diagnosis of ureteral calculi, which will give rise to hydronephrosis if they cause obstruction. Less commonly, retroperitoneal processes (tumors, fibrosis) or pelvic pathology originating in the prostate, ovaries, or urethra may give rise to hydronephrosis. The indications for most emergency ultrasound evaluations of the urinary tract are one or more of the following:

1. Acute flank or back pain
2. Hematuria
3. Urinary retention
4. Acute renal failure

Renal ultrasound can identify calculi larger than 5 mm in diameter within the kidney. However, these stones do not cause symptoms of obstruction and are clinically important only if they become a nidus of infection or pass into the ureter. The ureter from the renal pelvis to the iliac crest is rarely visualized unless dilated, and from that point to within a few centimeters of the ureterovesical junction (UVJ) is sonographically occult. Therefore, ureteral stones are usually diagnosed by inference from the presence of hydronephrosis. They are rarely seen per se, except when at the UVJ. Because some stones do not cause complete ureteral obstruction, they may not cause hydronephrosis, leading to a sensitivity and specificity of 83% and 92%, respectively, for emergency ultrasound alone in the detection of kidney stones (1). Some investigators have improved accuracy and attained sensitivities of greater than 90% by combining ultrasonography with an abdominal plain film. This approach will diagnose 95% of all stones larger than 3 mm (by the presence of hydronephrosis, identification of the stone on radiograph, or both). This approach has dual advantages. It identifies the stones that are very unlikely to pass spontaneously (those >6 mm, easily identified on plain film), and it "deprioritizes" patients who have hydronephrosis but no identifiable stone on plain film (either the sonogram is a false positive, or the stone is small and very likely to pass spontaneously).

Despite these considerations, the increasing availability of CT, its ability to give information about other abdominal pathology, and patient expectations of a definitive diagnosis have significantly increased the use of CT and reduced the use of sonography in the emergency evaluation of ureteral stones.

Interestingly, this trend toward CT has not changed the proportion of patients diagnosed with kidney stones, the proportion diagnosed with a significant alternative diagnosis, or the proportion admitted to the hospital for renal colic (2). These findings suggest that the increased use of CT has not had a significant effect on diagnosis or management of urolithiasis. More recently, a study comparing patients with renal colic evaluated in the ED by either CT, radiology ultrasound, or emergency bedside ultrasound with a six-month follow-up period has demonstrated similar outcomes for each group with respect to complications and interventions – but indicating significantly lower radiation exposure among those initially evaluated with ultrasound. These findings, combined with an increasing awareness of the oncogenic risk associated with increased lifetime radiation exposure, are prompting renewed interest in the role of ultrasound in the ED evaluation of renal colic. The argument for sonographic evaluation is particularly compelling in the evaluation of patients with a history of ureterolithiasis and (often multiple) previous CT scans.

Diagnostic capabilities

Technique and normal sonoanatomy

The kidneys lie almost parallel to the ribs lateral to the psoas muscles between the midscapular line and the posterior axillary line and between the eighth and twelfth ribs, although the location is subject to respiratory and individual variation. The right kidney is usually displaced caudally by the liver with respect to the left. The kidneys can be imaged directly through the flank – or, on the right, a more lateral or anterior approach may be used with the liver as a window. Patients may be scanned supine, although lateral decubitus, prone, or sitting positions may also be used. To widen the intercostal spaces, the patient can be asked to place the ipsilateral arm above his or her head and laterally bend the thorax to the opposite side (e.g., while examining the left kidney, the patient is told to "lower your right shoulder to your right hip"). When placed in the decubitus position, this may be augmented by placing a bolster under the patient. Respiratory maneuvers may be helpful: "take a deep breath and hold it" to obtain views below the ribs, or "take slow, deep breaths in and out" to scan from top to bottom of the kidney from within a single rib space.

The normal kidney is 10 to 12 cm long. A large or small size, as well as an irregular contour, can be congenital or pathological. The renal capsule is highly reflective and thus is echogenic on ultrasound. Some patients have a surrounding rim of perinephric fat with a stippled heterogeneous appearance of intermediate echogenicity. The renal "cortex" is less echogenic than the adjacent liver or spleen. The renal "medulla" is a region comprising renal pyramids (more hypoechoic than the cortex) and the columns of Bertini (extensions of the cortex between the pyramids). It is inside the cortex and surrounding renal sinus. The latter is composed of the collecting system, renal vasculature, and fatty tissue. Renal sinus fat is highly echogenic. In normal conditions, the collecting system contains no urine because of frequent and regular ureteral peristalsis and is therefore not visible on ultrasound. Therefore, hypoechoic structures in the renal sinus are vascular. These can be distinguished from hydronephrosis with color flow Doppler in cases of doubt.

Patients being evaluated for hydronephrosis should be adequately hydrated but not overhydrated (the latter can cause hydronephrosis), with a bladder that is filled without overdistension. A probe with a frequency range between 2.0 and 5.0 MHz is appropriate; a small sonographic footprint may be helpful. The evaluation of unilateral flank pain usually includes sonography of the contralateral kidney and bladder to exclude bilateral hydronephrosis or congenital absence, ectopic kidney, or other urinary tract pathology.

Hydronephrosis and ureteral stones

Hydronephrosis appears as an anechoic area within the renal sinus fat that is not vascular. It may be graded as absent, mild (grade I), moderate (grade II), or severe (grade III). These designations correspond to the degree of calyceal dilation. In mild (grade I) hydronephrosis, the calyces are fluid filled while maintaining normal anatomical structure. They can be seen to be connected in real-time scanning (unlike renal cysts). Hydronephrosis is seen in 60% of normal volunteers after vigorous hydration with ensuing bladder distension; one-fifth of the volunteers demonstrate grade II hydronephrosis (3). Interestingly in this study, 8% of normal volunteers had mild hydronephrosis at baseline, before voiding. Also of note, in those who had hydronephrosis with bladder distension after hydration, it did not resolve immediately after voiding. In moderate (grade II) hydronephrosis, the calyceal system becomes distended and appears confluent on single ultrasound images with a "bear's paw" appearance. Severe (grade III) hydronephrosis is characterized by effacement of the renal medulla and cortex due to extreme calyceal distension. Occasionally the passage of a stone disrupts the integrity of the renal pelvis resulting in an urinoma, which is seen sonographically as a layer of anechoic fluid surrounding the kidney.

In pooled studies, the sensitivity of ultrasound to identify ureteral stones is 45% (4). Visualization of the ureter from the renal pelvis to the iliac crest is technically difficult, and from that point to the UVJ, sound waves are obstructed from the ureter by the boney pelvis posteriorly, and many layers of bowel anteriorly. However, if hydronephrosis is identified, the sonologist should try to identify an offending ureteral stone because it will allow it to be assessed for size, which has prognostic consequences for stone passage. In one large series, stones of <4 mm passed spontaneously 80% of the time; those 4–6 mm, 60% of the time; and those >6 mm, only 20% of the time (5). If hydronephrosis is seen, the anechoic collecting system should be followed in real time into the proximal ureter. The ureteropelvic junction is a common site for ureteral stones to become lodged. The ureter should be followed caudally as far as possible in the flank.

If no stone is identified in the lumbar region, the UVJ (the most common site for a lodged ureteral stone) should be evaluated. The bladder is scanned in real time in the transverse plane from the level of the prostate. The UVJs are a few centimeters posterior and lateral. Continuing to fan superiorly, a dilated ureter will appear as an anechoic circular structure that travels laterally behind the bladder. Color flow Doppler can be used to confirm that the structure is not a blood vessel. Scanning the ureter in the reverse direction, it will be seen to terminate abruptly at the UVJ. The obstructing stone might be identifiable *per se*, although in many cases, it is revealed only by shadowing. Color flow Doppler may reveal the presence of the stone by "twinkle artifact" as well as color flow comet-tail artifact behind the stone. Because stones of <4 mm are at the threshold for sonographic resolution, the highest penetrating frequency possible should be used, and gain should be adjusted so that the urine in the bladder appears truly black. Far gain may also need to be adjusted down because of posterior acoustic enhancement. The focal zone should be placed at, or just below, the level of the area of interest. As usual, orthogonal views showing a longitudinal view of the dilated ureter and obstruction should be obtained.

Evaluation of ureteral jets is of uncertain utility in the diagnosis of ureteral stones. Their evaluation requires a small to moderate volume of urine in the bladder. A color flow Doppler window is placed in the transverse plane of the UVJs using a low flow scale (low pulse repetition frequency) and with color flow gain adjusted so that it is just below the threshold of spontaneous color gain artifact within the bladder. Various times have been used for this assessment; however, two minutes seems to be an appropriate compromise because ureters typically peristalse several times per minute. In some patients, especially those who are not well hydrated, jets may not be seen despite unobstructed ureters even within this timeframe. Jets should be of approximately symmetrical forcefulness and volume. Frequently a slow, continually dribbling jet is seen on the side of a partial obstruction.

The presence of any flow on the side of identified hydronephrosis gives some degree of reassurance to the clinician that the patient is not completely obstructed. Conversely, unilateral absence of flow on the side of hydronephrosis might prompt a more conservative approach or more urgent consultation with urology.

Renal cysts and masses

Simple renal cysts are quite common. The incidence ranges from around 5% in patients younger than 30 years to around 25% to 50% in patients older than 50 years, with two-thirds noted to be 2 cm or less in diameter. The relative sensitivity of ultrasound in the detection of parenchymal renal masses (including cysts and carcinomas) is around 80%. The sonographic appearance of renal cell carcinoma is extremely varied and can appear as an echogenic mass or a complex cyst with internal septations and irregular margins. Angiomyolipoma, notable for its echogenicity on ultrasound, may also occasionally be identified, but the sonographic appearance may be similar to that of renal cell carcinoma. The definitive distinction between various kinds of renal cysts and masses is beyond the scope of emergency ultrasound; however, benign renal cysts tend to be smooth with a well-defined margin, round or oval shaped, and without demonstrable internal echoes. They demonstrate the ultrasound artifact of posterior echo enhancement. Cysts that meet these criteria require no specific follow-up. Complex cysts and other renal masses should be followed up with further imaging studies or referral.

Urinary retention and evaluation of the bladder

Ultrasound can identify or confirm a distended bladder in suspected urinary retention and can also be used to estimate post-void residual. In both settings, ultrasound obviates the more time-consuming and invasive test of catheterization. Many techniques have been assessed for estimating bladder volume, but the simplest (which has been shown to be no less accurate than any of the others) is to measure it in three orthogonal planes (length × width × height) to obtain a rough estimate. Some advocate multiplying this product by 0.75. In general, because of bladder shape variability, there is an error range of 15% to 35%. Normally, the bladder is completely emptied in micturition, so any post-void residual urine represents some degree of outlet obstruction or detrusor dysfunction. Residual volumes of up to 250 cc in the adult are unlikely to generate significant retrograde pressure, but they do constitute increased risk of infection due to the failure of the defense mechanism of complete and regular bladder emptying.

The bladder walls should be scanned for irregularities. A diffusely hypertrophied wall suggests chronic cystitis, spastic bladder, or chronic outlet obstruction, depending on the clinical scenario. Other bladder findings include calculi, diverticula, cysts, clot, sediment, fungus balls (in the immunocompromised), and tumors. As described earlier in this chapter, in cases of hydronephrosis or unexplained renal failure, the region of the UVJ can be assessed by color flow Doppler for ureteral jets, which exclude complete obstruction.

Prostatic hypertrophy and carcinoma

The prostate is normally up to 4 cm in maximal dimension. Prostatic abnormalities may be incidentally identified in the evaluation of urinary retention or in the evaluation of flank pain or trauma. Diffuse enlargement of the prostate with maintenance of margins and normal anatomy is likely to be due to benign hypertrophy, whereas malignancy is likely to cause gross deformity. However, because sonography cannot exclude early carcinoma or isoechoic malignancy within a hypertrophic gland, identified abnormalities of the prostate should be referred for further evaluation.

Pitfalls and limitations

Renal ultrasonography may be limited by technical challenges in obtaining the images or by inherent characteristics of the test itself. Anatomy, body habitus, areas of injury or tenderness, patient positioning, and operator skill may restrict the quality of the study.

In addition to the nonobstructive causes of hydronephrosis already noted, calyceal distention may arise from diuretic use, previous obstruction, reflux, and pregnancy. In pregnancy, maximal dilation occurs around 38 weeks' gestation, with the right kidney more affected than the left. The dilatation may persist after delivery.

Multiple simple cysts may be mistaken for hydronephrosis, although real-time scanning should distinguish the two, and the cysts will lack surrounding sinus fat, which is seen as a thin echogenic band even in cases of severe hydronephrosis. Hydronephrosis affects the entire collecting system equally, whereas in polycystic kidney disease or acquired renal cystic disease, the cysts tend to be of many sizes.

False-negative exams for hydronephrosis occur when there is actual obstruction without calyceal dilation, which is rare unless the kidney was already nonfunctioning. However, false-negative exams for ureteral stones are more common because many are nonobstructing or only partially obstructing. Ultrasonography frequently fails to identify renal stones, as noted previously. The diagnosis of renal tumors is not within the standard purview of the emergency ultrasonographer. Ultrasound is limited in the identification of renal masses by both their size and sonographic appearance. Tumors of <5 mm cannot be seen, and larger lesions are easily overlooked, especially if they are of similar echotexture to the surrounding renal parenchyma. Expertise and sonographic skill play an important role in accurate identification of renal masses. For these reasons, the emergency sonographer is unlikely to exclude renal neoplasm, although it may be "ruled in" if it is seen.

Clinical images

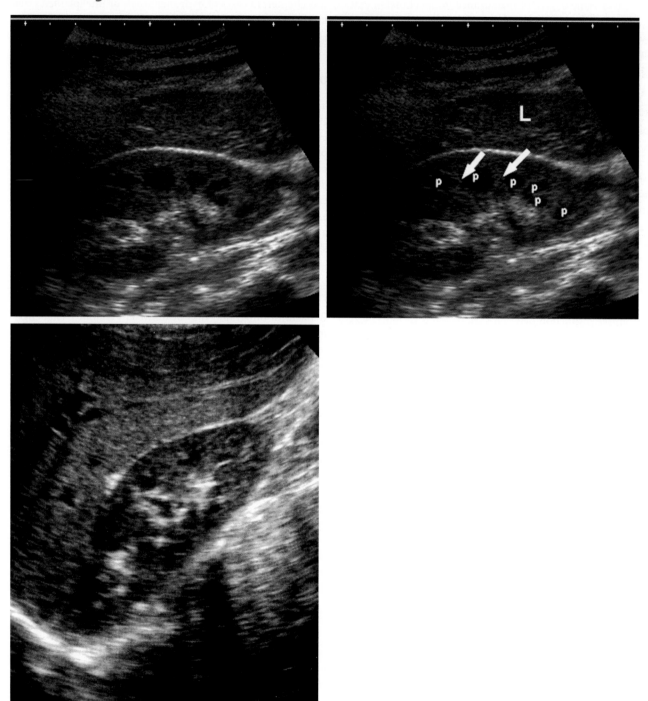

Figure 18.1. Here are several examples of normal kidneys. Figure 18.1A to D shows longitudinal views of the right kidney. The capsule surrounding the kidney (Glisson's) is strongly echogenic. The renal cortex is slightly hypoechoic relative to adjacent liver (L) (or spleen on the left). The renal pyramids (p) are much more hypoechoic, especially in the young, and, except for their anatomically predictable location, can be mistaken for cysts. An imaginary line along the outside of the pyramids defines the border between the cortex and medulla. The columns of Bertini (*arrows*) are extensions of cortical tissue between the pyramids. Figure 18.1E shows a transverse view with the renal artery (RA) and renal vein (RV) entering the renal hilum. Figure 18.1C shows the appearance of renal vessels within the renal sinus, as well as the psoas muscle (Ps) that lies medial to both kidneys. The hyperechoic renal sinus is seen in all of the images and indicated in some (*arrowheads*).

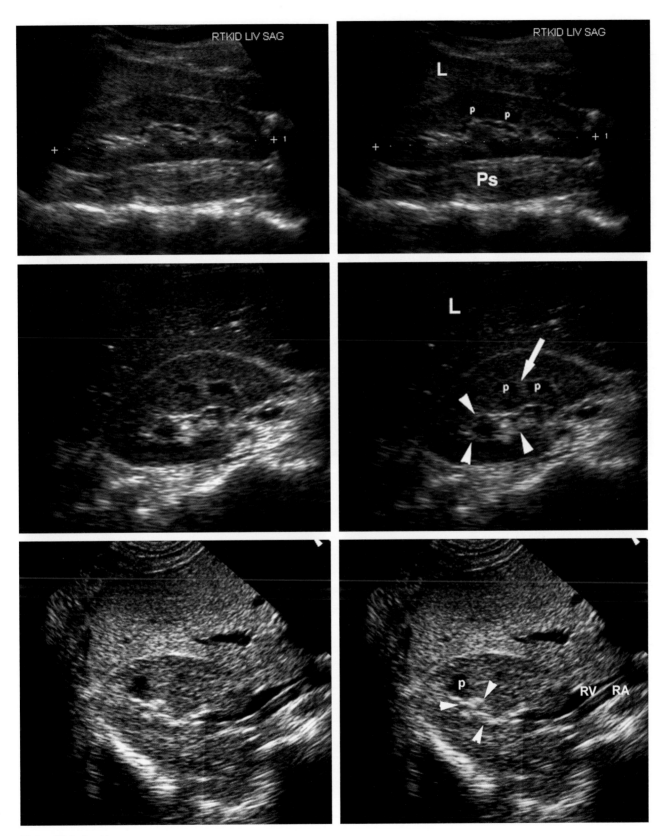

Figure 18.1. (cont.)

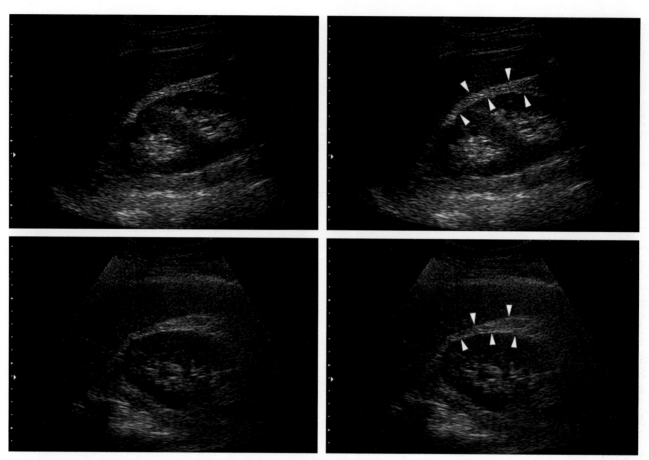

Figure 18.2. Perinephric fat and trauma. A 35-year-old male presents with right flank pain after a fall from a ladder. Figures 18.2A1 and A2 show his renal ultrasound demonstrating a normal-appearing right kidney, except for a small simple cyst. The hyperechoic perinephric fat may be mistaken for clotted intraperitoneal blood. It is differentiated by its even thickness (not "pointy" like free fluid), its symmetry with the opposite kidney, its diffuse finely heterogeneous sonoarchitecture typical of fat, and the fact that it will not be affected by repositioning the patient. Figures 18.2B1 and B2 show another example of perinephric fat. Renal sonography is not a sensitive tool for the detection of renal parenchymal injury.

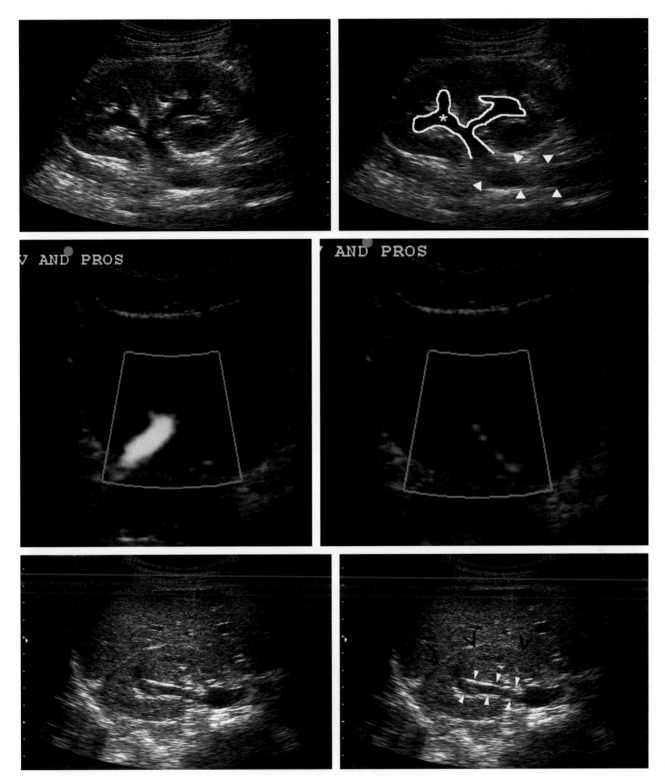

Figure 18.3. Mild hydronephrosis. A 46-year-old male presents with acute onset left flank/suprapubic pain. Urinalysis shows large blood, no leukocyte esterase or nitrites. Bedside ultrasound (Fig. 18.3A1 and A2) demonstrates mild (grade I) hydronephrosis of the left kidney, with proximal hydroureter (*arrowheads*). Color flow evaluation of the bladder shows a strong urinary jet from the right ureteral orifice (Fig. 18.3B1) and a dribbling continuous jet from the left UVJ (Fig. 18.3B2). Noncontrast CT of the patient's abdomen/pelvis demonstrated a 4 mm left ureteral calculus. Another example of grade I hydronephrosis is shown in a transverse view of a kidney (Fig. 18.3C, *white arrowheads*). The capsule of the kidney is unusually difficult to appreciate in this ultrasound (*black arrowheads*).

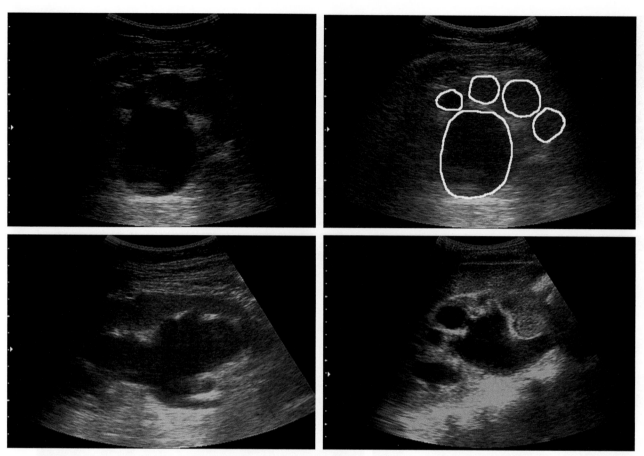

Figure 18.4. Moderate hydronephrosis. A 44-year-old female presents with 1 week of worsening left flank pain. The patient's primary physician diagnosed her with a urinary tract infection 3 days ago and started her on levofloxacin. Bedside ultrasonography demonstrates moderate (grade II) hydronephrosis. Note the central lucency marked in Figures 18.4A1 and A2, reminiscent of a bear's paw. There is no effacement of the renal cortex to suggest severe hydronephrosis. The patient was admitted to urology for intravenous antibiotics and operative management of an infected stone. Figures 18.4B and C also show examples of moderate hydronephrosis.

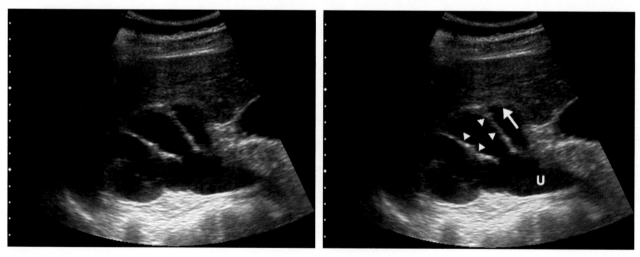

Figure 18.5. Severe hydronephrosis. A 43-year-old male presents with 3 days of intermittent right flank pain with hematuria. He carries a history of multiple renal stones with multiple CT scan evaluations. An emergency bedside ultrasound demonstrates severe hydronephrosis of the right kidney. There is extensive calyceal dilatation (*arrowheads*) and sonolucence of the entire renal sinus. There is effacement of the renal cortex (*arrow*), defining this as severe (grade III) hydronephrosis. There is posterior acoustic enhancement from the fluid-filled areas of the sinus. Marked proximal ureteral dilatation (U) is also evident. With such marked hydronephrosis, a noncontrast CT was obtained. An obstructing 7 mm stone was identified. Urology was consulted, the ureter was stented, and then the stone was removed cystoscopically.

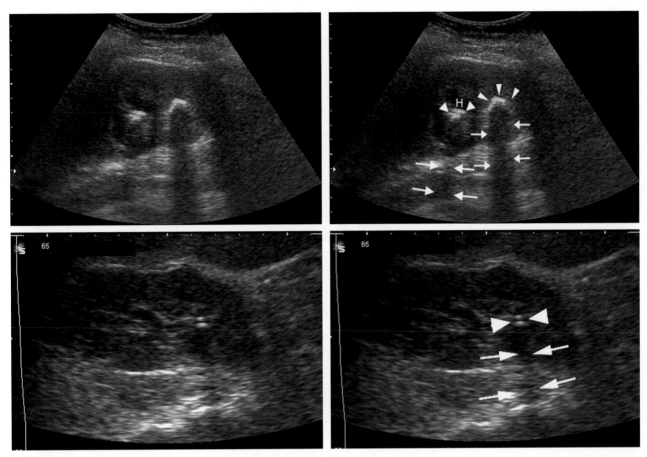

Figure 18.6. Renal stones. A 32-year-old patient presents with symptoms "just like my kidney stones." He has a urinalysis without blood or evidence of infection. Emergency medicine bedside ultrasound (Fig. 18.6A) shows two echogenic stones (*arrowheads*) with shadowing (*arrows*). Hydronephrosis (H) can also be seen. The renal stones have the same intense echogenicity as the renal sinus fat, so their presence can often be inferred only by the shadowing that they cause. Another example can be seen in Figure 18.6B, which shows a lower-quality renal ultrasound image with a subtle but definite echogenic stone (*arrowheads*) with shadowing (*arrows*) in the renal sinus. Renal stones do not cause pain (unless they pass into the ureter). Therefore, acute symptoms should prompt a search for pyelonephritis or a stone in the ureter.

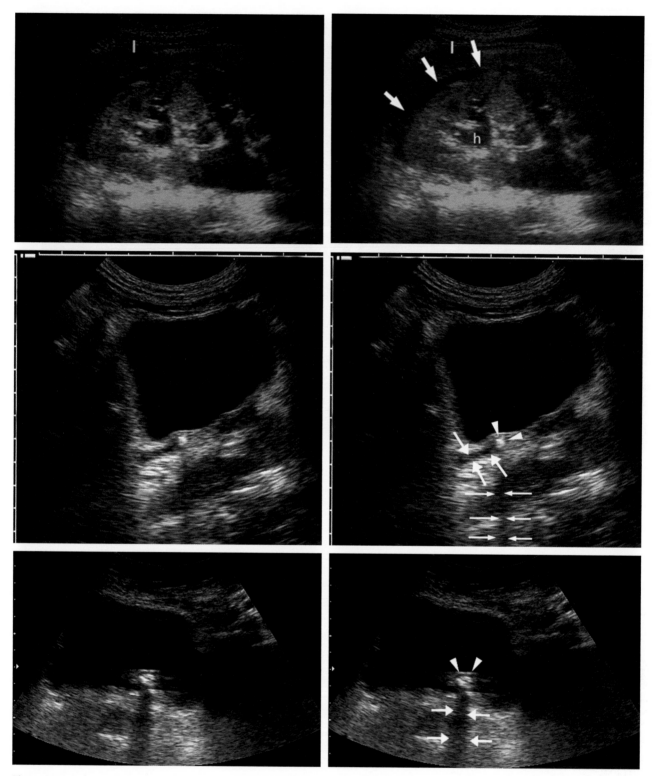

Figure 18.7. Left UVJ stone. A 54-year-old male presents with 1 day of intermittent left flank pain with nausea. While an IV is established and analgesics are given, a bedside ultrasound is performed. The left kidney (Figs. 18.7A1 and A2) demonstrates mild hydronephrosis (*h*) with an urinoma (*white arrows*). Bladder scans in the parasagittal (Figs. 18.7B1 and B2) and transverse (Figs. 18.7C1 and C2) planes are significant for a stone (*arrowheads*) with shadowing (*horizontal arrows*) in the UVJ with associated hydroureter (*larger arrows*). No further imaging was indicated. Stones <3 mm are usually not detected by ultrasound. In this case, the stone is not measured but is approximately 6 mm (using the on-screen centimeter scale).

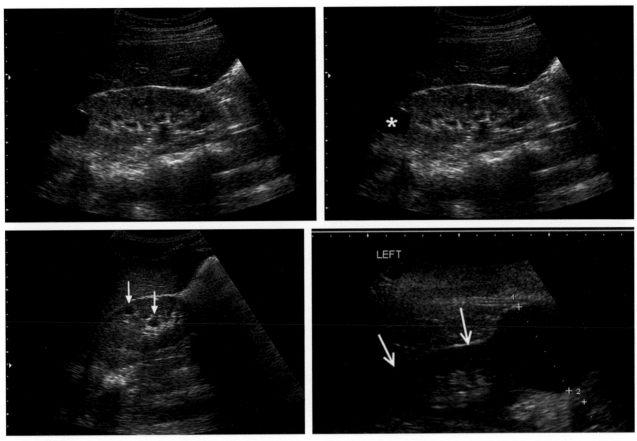

Figure 18.8. Simple renal cysts. A 17-year-old female presents with 3 days of right upper quadrant (RUQ) pain, nausea, and vomiting. She has no urinary symptoms. On emergency bedside ultrasonography of the RUQ, the incidental finding of a simple cyst in the right kidney is made (Fig. 18.8A, *asterisk*). Note that the cyst is round and well defined, with regular margins, and is entirely anechoic. Atypically, and of slight concern, no posterior acoustic enhancement is seen. This cyst is not related to the patient's symptoms. Two simple renal cysts from another patient are seen in Figure 18.8B (*arrows*). Figure 18.8C shows an example of a large subserosal cyst (*calipers*) associated with the inferior pole of the kidney (*arrows*). Such cysts can grow to 10 cm or more in diameter.

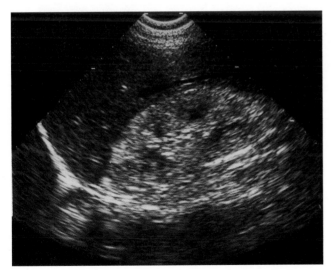

Figure 18.9. Renal disease. A 52-year-old female on dialysis with the brightly echogenic kidney typical of medical renal disease. In healthy patients, the kidneys are hypoechoic relative to the liver or spleen (right and left kidney, respectively). Kidneys may also be small in the setting of chronic disease, which is not evident in this case.

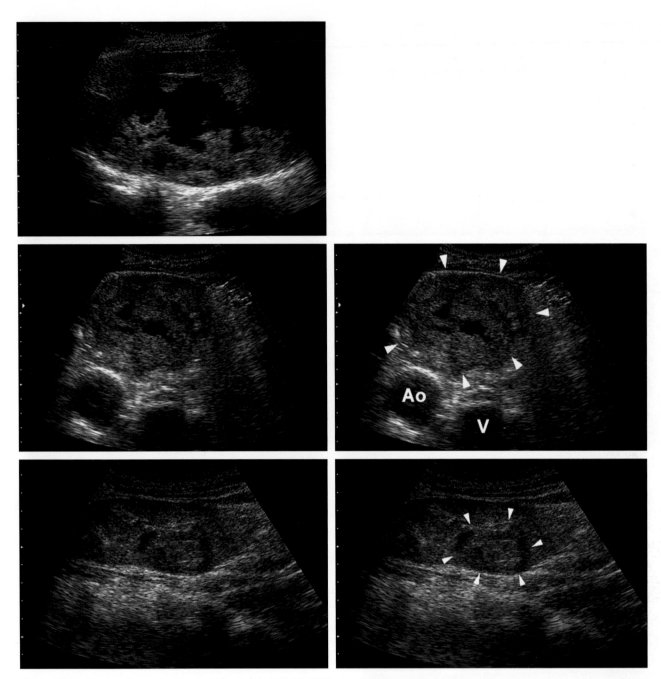

Figure 18.10. Renal carcinoma. An 83-year-old female presents with mild back pain and hematuria. An ultrasound reveals a massively enlarged left kidney with a large irregular cystic mass (Figs. 18.10A, B1, and B2). In contrast to a benign renal cyst (Figs. 18.8A–C), this mass has irregular poorly defined margins with internal echoes. Scanning of the contralateral kidney revealed a smaller, subtler 3 × 4 × 5 cm mass (Figs. 18.10C1 and C2). The patient was admitted, and biopsy of the left kidney revealed renal cell carcinoma. A CT of the chest and abdomen also revealed pulmonary metastases. The patient declined further treatment.

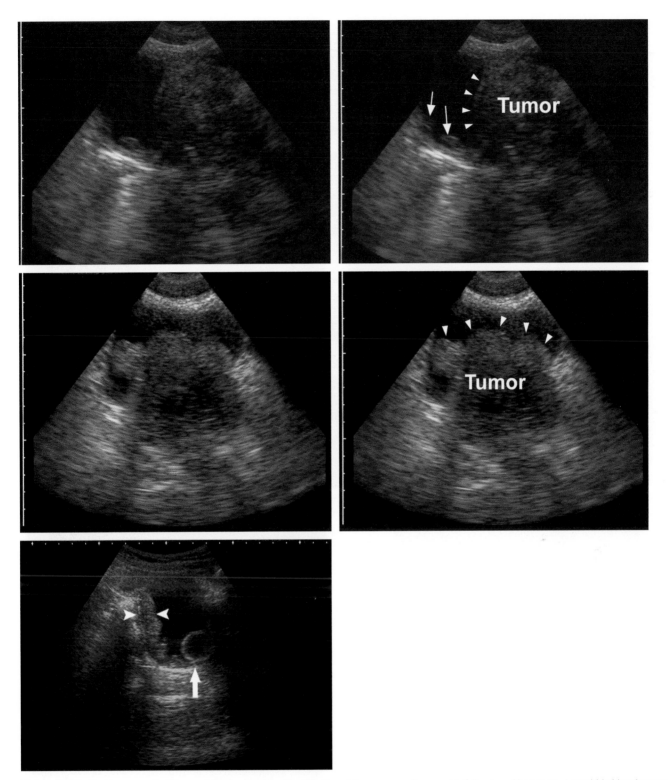

Figure 18.11. Bladder tumor. An 84-year-old male presents with difficulty voiding, a sense of suprapubic fullness, and hematuria. A renal/bladder ultrasound reveals a large echogenic mass that projects into the bladder (Figs. 18.11A and B). The location of this mass is consistent with either a prostatic or cystic source, although irregularities of the bladder wall might suggest the latter (Figs. 18.11A2, *arrows*). In this case, biopsy revealed a transitional cell tumor. Patients with chronic urinary retention develop hypertrophy of the bladder walls (*arrowheads*), which may appear as tumor, especially after Foley (*arrows*) decompression (Fig. 18.11C). These diagnoses cannot be reliably differentiated by emergency bedside ultrasonography, and such patients should be referred for urologic follow-up.

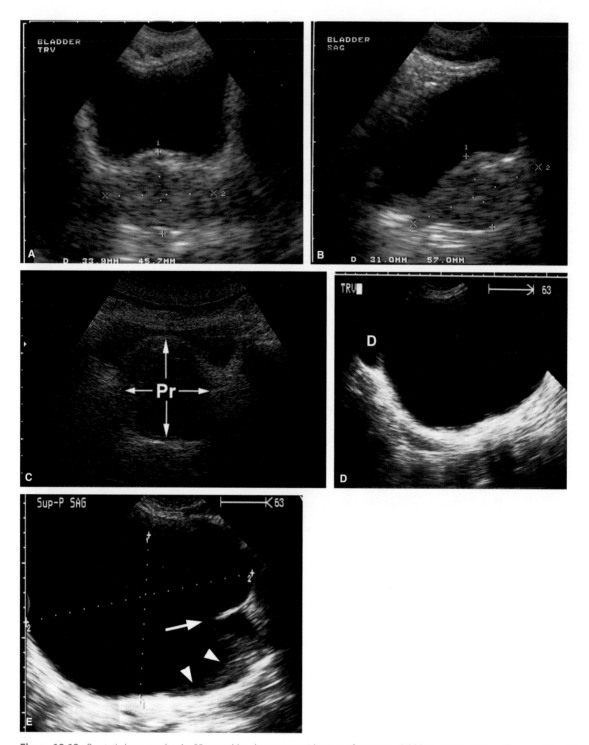

Figure 18.12. Prostatic hypertrophy. An 85-year-old male presents with urinary frequency, dribbling, and sensation of incomplete voiding. His creatinine is 1.3, unchanged from previously. The bladder dimensions are 6.0 × 8.3 × 7.5 cm (corresponding to estimated bladder volume of about 350 mL). The enlarged prostate is marked by calipers in Figure 18.12A (transverse) and B (sagittal). The normal prostate is typically a walnut-size organ, with maximal dimension less than 4 cm and a volume of less than 30 cc (estimated by orthogonal dimensions [a × b × c]/2) Benign prostate hypertrophy appears on ultrasound as a homogeneous mass with smooth margins arising from the floor of the bladder (compare with Figs. 18.11A–C). Another case of an enlarged prostate is shown in Figure 18.12C. Chronic bladder distension can result in the formation of diverticula (Fig. 18.12D, D) and trabeculae (Fig. 18.12E, *arrow*) in a patient with an extremely distended bladder containing urinary sediment (Fig. 18.12E, *arrowheads*). The patient had a Foley catheter placed with return of 1300 mL of urine. He was discharged with a leg-bag and instructions for urology referral.

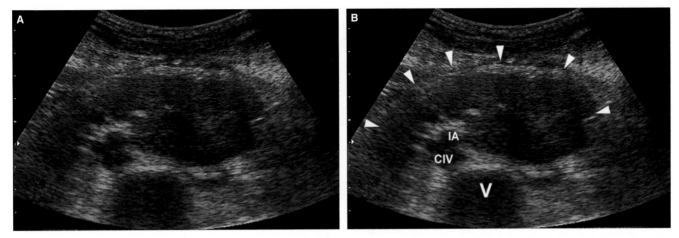

Figure 18.13. Horseshoe kidney. A "horseshoe kidney" was an incidental finding in this 65-year-old patient with abdominal pain who was being evaluated by ultrasound to exclude aortic aneurysm. The structure with recognizable renal morphology (*arrowheads*) was seen anterior to a sacral vertebra (V). The right common iliac artery (IA) and common iliac vein (CIV) can be seen. The vessels on the left were compressed, laterally displaced, and not seen on this image. The patient should be advised of the abnormally located kidney because it predisposes to complications, including recurrent infections and increased risk of trauma.

References

1. Gaspari RJ, Horst K: Emergency ultrasound and urinalysis in the evaluation of flank pain. *Acad Emerg Med* 2005;**12**(12):1180–4.

2. Westphalen AC, Hsia RY, Maselli JH, et al.: Radiological imaging of patients with suspected urinary tract stones: national trends, diagnoses, and predictors. *Acad Emerg Med* 2011;**18**(7):699–707.

3. Morse JW, Hill R, Greissinger WP, et al.: Rapid oral hydration results in hydronephrosis as demonstrated by bedside ultrasound. *Ann of Emerg Med* 1999;**34**(2):134–40.

4. Ray AA, Ghiculete D, Pace KT, Honey RJ: Limitations to ultrasound in the detection and measurement of urinary tract calculi. *Urology* 2010;**76**(2):295–300.

5. Ueno A, Kawamura T, Ogawa A, Takayasu H: Relation of spontaneous passage of ureteral calculi to size. *Urology* 1977;**10**: 544–6.

Chapter 19

Ultrasonography of the Abdominal Aorta

Deepak Chandwani

Indications

The primary indication for emergent ultrasonography of the aorta is to identify an abdominal aortic aneurysm (AAA). AAAs develop slowly and may be asymptomatic or present with life-threatening rupture. AAA rupture accounts for more than 10,000 deaths per year in the United States (1). Initial misdiagnosis is common because AAAs may present in a myriad of ways. In the words of Sir William Osler, "There is no disease more conducive to clinical humility than aneurysm of the aorta" (2). Ruptured AAAs can present with abdominal pain, flank pain, syncope, lower extremity paresthesias, or peripheral emboli (3, 4). Because physical examination is only moderately sensitive in the detection of AAAs, further evaluation with imaging is usually indicated (5).

Diagnostic capabilities

When ruptured or leaking AAA is suspected, ultrasound has many appealing qualities. Particularly for the hemodynamically unstable patient, bedside ultrasonography offers a prompt, accurate diagnosis. In even modestly experienced hands, ultrasound of the aorta can be performed rapidly and can detect the presence of an aneurysm in 95% to 98% of cases (6–8). In addition, it can be performed at the bedside, setting it apart from other modalities such as CT, MRI, and angiography, whereby the patient has to leave the emergency department. Lastly, it has the added advantage of not requiring radiation or exposure to contrast material.

Anatomy

The abdominal aorta is a retroperitoneal structure that lies anterior and to the left of the vertebral column. It enters the abdominal cavity at the level of the 12th thoracic vertebrae, which corresponds to the xyphoid anteriorly. As the aorta descends, it gives off five main branches and slightly tapers in size. The first branch is the celiac trunk, followed by the superior mesenteric artery, then the two renal arteries, and lastly the inferior mesenteric artery. The abdominal aorta then bifurcates into the common iliac arteries at the level of the fourth lumbar vertebrae, which corresponds to the umbilicus anteriorly (9, 10).

Aneurysms are abnormal dilatations of all three layers of the blood vessel wall – the intima, media, and adventitia. A normal aortic diameter is less than 2 cm. The aorta is considered aneurysmal when it is greater than 3 cm or 1.5 times greater in diameter than a proximal uninvolved segment (9). Of note, aneurysms may affect any portion of the aorta including its smaller branches as well as the iliac arteries.

Technique

Using a curvilinear or phased array probe, the abdominal aorta should be imaged in its entirety, both in longitudinal and transverse planes. The probe is initially placed just below the xyphoid process in the transverse orientation. The anterior portion of the vertebral body should be identified first. This is an excellent landmark, both for noting the location of the aorta and for making image optimization adjustments on the machine (e.g., depth and gain). The aorta will be seen as a circular, thick, hyperechoic walled structure anterior to the spinal column. To the right of the aorta lies the inferior vena cava, which is more thinly walled, ovoid in shape, collapsible, and shows variation with respiration. The aorta should be imaged completely from the diaphragm through the bifurcation with visualization of the common iliac arteries. This scan should be repeated in the longitudinal orientation. Measurements of the aorta should be taken from outer wall to outer wall and performed in two planes (10).

An aortic dissection may be encountered during bedside aortic ultrasound, as one-third of aortic dissections may extend into the abdominal aorta (11). A dissection is a tear in the intima, which causes blood to track within the media creating a true and false lumen. Sonographically, this is appreciated as a thin, hyperechoic structure within the lumen of the vessel that may move with pulsations.

Commonly, the aorta may be difficult to visualize secondary to bowel gas and may lead to poor-quality ultrasound imaging. In approximately 10% of emergency department cases, more than one-third of the aorta may be obscured (12). Gentle pressure may be applied to the ultrasound probe to displace gas to facilitate imaging. At times, body habitus or bowel gas may make obtaining appropriate images extremely difficult. In such cases, oblique coronal views may be used. This is achieved by placing the patient in the left lateral decubitus position. Scanning from the right flank, in a longitudinal orientation, the liver is used as an acoustic window. Probe position may be adjusted anteriorly or posteriorly to optimize imaging. This coronal oblique view may be similarly obtained from the left flank with the patient in the right lateral decubitus position (13).

Imaging pitfalls and limitations

Although ultrasound is an excellent modality for identifying AAA, it is not effective in identifying whether rupture or leaking has occurred. The diagnosis of a ruptured AAA is based on the sonographic presence of an aneurysm in conjunction with the patient's clinical presentation. Infrequently, findings of rupture, such as a retroperitoneal hematoma (which may displace the ipsilateral kidney) or free fluid in the peritoneum (if leaking has occurred in the peritoneal space), can be seen with ultrasound (6, 9). If the patient is stable, further imaging with CT is usually indicated (see Chapter 33).

Clinical images

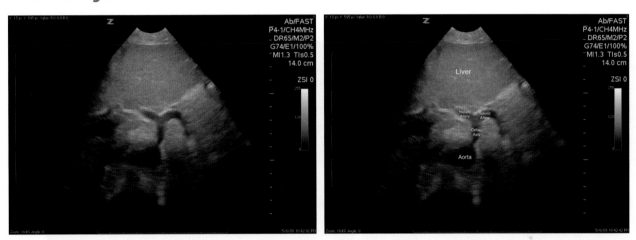

Figure 19.1. A: Normal abdominal aorta, transverse view at the level of the celiac artery showing the "seagull sign," which corresponds to the common hepatic and splenic arteries. B: Schematic.

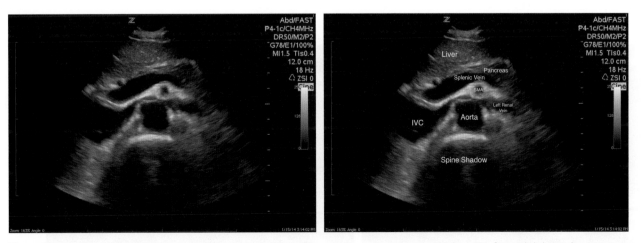

Figure 19.2. A: Normal abdominal aorta, transverse view at the level of the superior mesenteric artery. B: Schematic of normal abdominal aorta, transverse view.

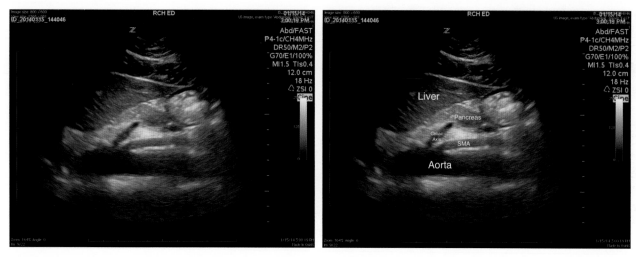

Figure 19.3. A: Normal abdominal aorta, longitudinal view, displaying the origins of the celiac artery and superior mesenteric artery. B: Schematic of aorta, longitudinal view.

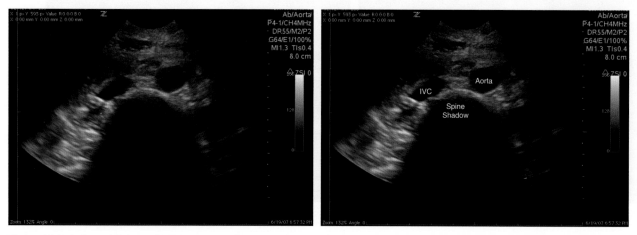

Figure 19.4. A: Normal abdominal aorta, transverse view, proximal to the bifurcation. B: Schematic of aorta, transverse view.

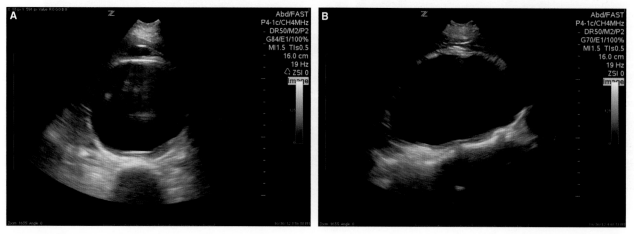

Figure 19.5. A: AAA transverse view. B: Longitudinal view.

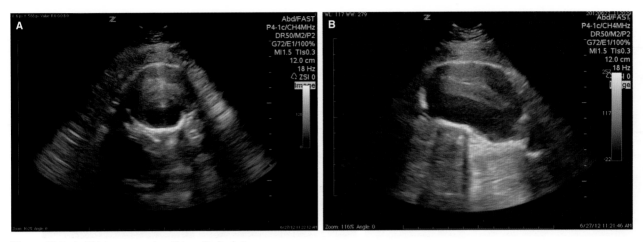

Figure 19.6. A: AAA transverse view. B: Longitudinal view.

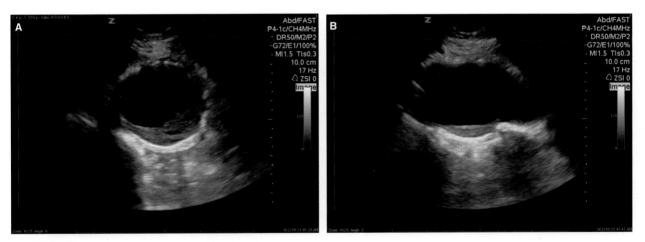

Figure 19.7. A: AAA transverse view. B: Longitudinal view.

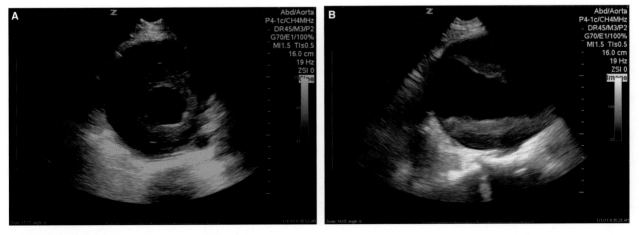

Figure 19.8. A: AAA transverse view. B: Longitudinal view.

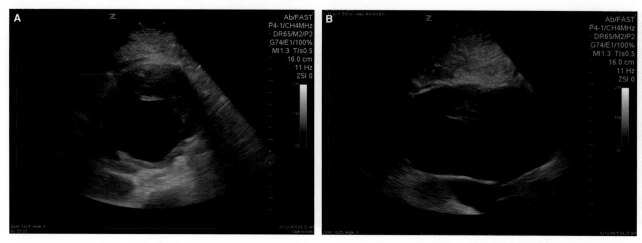

Figure 19.9. A: AAA transverse view. B: Longitudinal view.

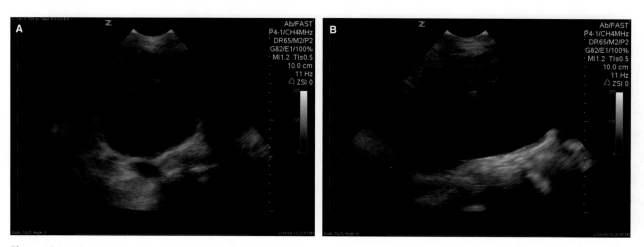

Figure 19.10. A: AAA transverse view. B: Longitudinal view.

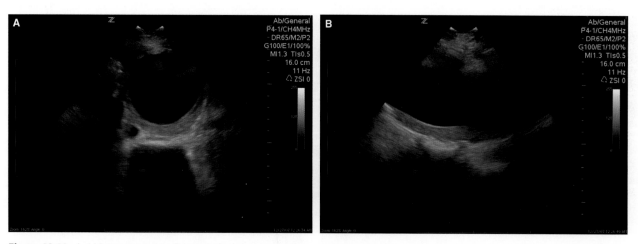

Figure 19.11. A: AAA transverse view. B: Longitudinal view.

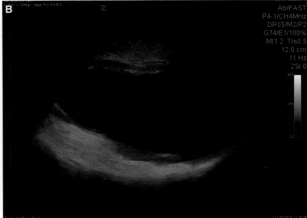

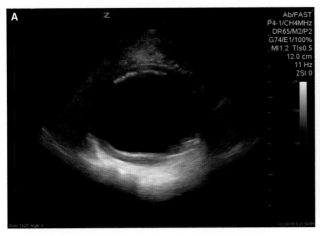

Figure 19.12. A: AAA transverse view. B: Longitudinal view.

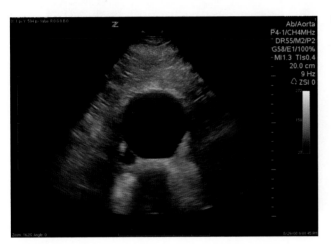

Figure 19.13. AAA, transverse view.

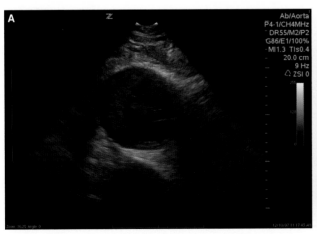

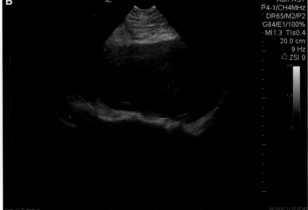

Figure 19.14. A: AAA transverse view. B: Longitudinal view.

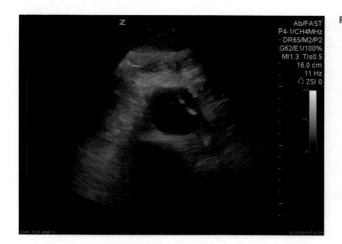

Figure 19.15. Aortic dissection, transverse view.

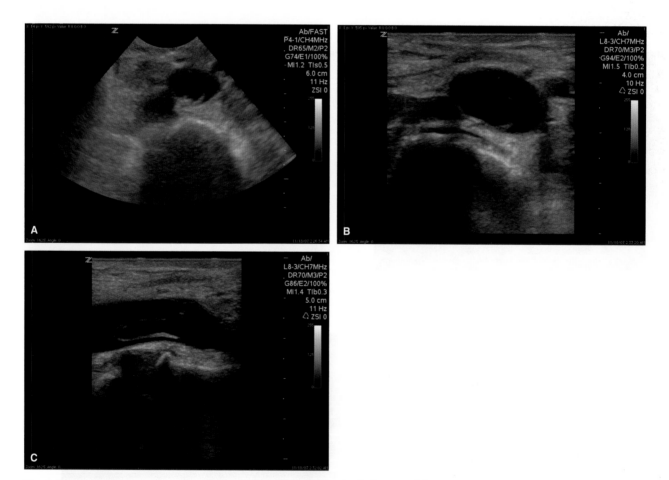

Figure 19.16. A: Aortic dissection, transverse view. B, C: Transverse and longitudinal images of the same patient using a high-frequency vascular probe.

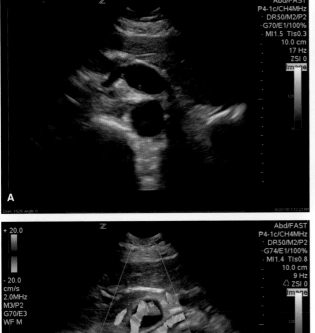

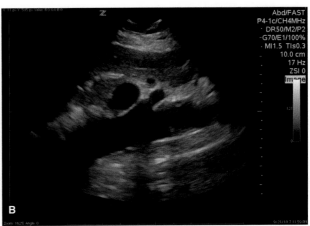

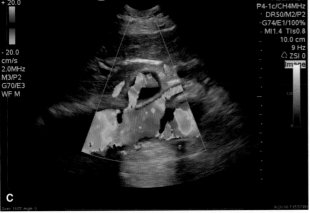

Figure 19.17. A: Celiac artery aneurysm, transverse view. B: Longitudinal view. C: Longitudinal view with color Doppler.

References

1. Gillum RF: Epidemiology of aortic aneurysm in the United States. *J Clin Epidemiol* 1995;**48**:1289–98.

2. Verma S, Lindsay T: Regression of aortic aneurysms through pharmacologic therapy? *N Engl J Med* 2006;**354**:2067–8.

3. Rogers RL, McCormack R: Aortic disasters. *Emerg Med Clin North Am* 2004;**22**(4):887–908.

4. Marston WA, Ahlquist R, Johnson G, Meyer A: Misdiagnosis of ruptured abdominal aortic aneurysms. *J Vasc Surg* 1992;**16**:17–22.

5. Fink HA, Lederle FA, Roth CS, et al.: The accuracy of physical examination to detect abdominal aortic aneurysm. *Arch Intern Med* 2000;**160**:833–6.

6. Miller J, Grimes P: Case report of an intraperitoneal ruptured abdominal aortic aneurysm diagnosed with bedside ultrasonography. *Acad Emerg Med* 1999;**6**:662–3.

7. Johansen K, Kohler RT, Nicholls SC, et al.: Ruptured abdominal aortic aneurysms: the Harborview experience. *J Vasc Surg* 1991;**13**:240–7.

8. Shuman WP, Hastrup W Jr, Kohler TR, Nyberg KY: Suspected leaking abdominal aortic aneurysm: use of sonography in the emergency room. *Radiology* 1988;**168**:117–9.

9. Zwiebel WJ, Sohaey R: *Introduction to ultrasound*. Philadelphia: Saunders, 1998.

10. Simon BC, Snoey ER: *Ultrasound in Emergency and Ambulatory Medicine*. Mosby, 1997.

11. Fojtik JP, Costantino TG, Dean AJ: The diagnosis of aortic dissection by emergency medicine ultrasound. *J Emer Med* 2007;**32**:191–6.

12. Blaivas M, Theodoro D: Frequency of incomplete abdominal aorta visualization by emergency department bedside ultrasound. *Acad Emerg Med* 2004;**11**:103–5.

13. Pardes JC, Aum YH, Kneeland JB, et al.: The oblique coronal view in sonography of the retroperitoneum. *Am J Roentgenol* 1985;**144**:1241–7.

Chapter 20

Ultrasound-Guided Procedures

Daniel D. Price and Sharon R. Wilson

Suprapubic bladder catheterization

Indications

Urinalysis is critical in evaluating and treating patients with suspected urinary tract infections or complex urosepsis. Urethral catheterization is a standard method for obtaining urine samples, but it is not always possible or successful. Ultrasound evaluation of bladder volume has been shown to significantly improve catheterization success rates in children when compared to blind catheterization (1, 2). Urethral catheterization may not be possible secondary to obstruction (e.g., prostatic hypertrophy, urethral stricture), or it may be contraindicated secondary to trauma (e.g., suspected urethral injury). Placement of a suprapubic catheter for bladder decompression is indicated in such cases. Ultrasound guidance for suprapubic bladder catheterization has been shown to improve success rates, decrease number of attempts, and decrease complications (3–9).

Anatomical considerations

The urinary bladder is protected by the pelvis in adults and older children. In younger children, the bladder may extend into the abdomen. Anechoic urine provides an excellent acoustic window, and the bladder, with rounded walls surrounding dark urine, is usually easy to visualize (Fig. 20.1). An empty bladder is more difficult to visualize, and sonographers should look for collapsed walls containing small amounts of urine (Fig. 20.2) similar to a collapsed gallbladder (see Chapter 14). Bowel gas may impede a clear view of the bladder. The inferior epigastric vessels should be avoided, as when performing a paracentesis (Figs. 20.3 and 20.4).

Procedure

Ultrasound is used to confirm the presence of fluid in the bladder and mark the optimal site for needle puncture. A 2 to 5 MHz abdominal or phased array transducer should provide excellent images of the urinary bladder. A setting of 5 MHz will provide better images in most children and lean adults. A lower setting, such as 3.5 or 2 MHz, may be needed to achieve adequate penetration in obese children or adults. The transducer should abut the symphysis pubis, and the ultrasound beam should be directed into the pelvis and abdomen as needed to obtain an optimal view of the bladder. Although a sagittal view (Fig. 20.5) should be obtained to fully survey the bladder, the transverse view is more accurate in estimating the volume of urine. Dimensions of the bladder can be measured with calipers or estimated using tics along the right side of the screen (Fig. 20.6).

A randomized control trial assessed the volume of urine required for successful urethral catheterization. Patients with a transverse bladder diameter less than 2 cm on ultrasound were directed to wait an additional 30 minutes prior to catheterization. Sufficient urine was obtained in 94% of patients using ultrasound guidance compared with 68% in the conventional blind catheterization group (2).

Success rates for suprapubic bladder catheterization have been demonstrated to be lower if the transverse bladder diameter is less than 2 cm. These patients should be fluid resuscitated and the procedure performed in 30 minutes, or when the bladder diameter is at least 3.5 cm. Guidance for suprapubic bladder catheterization can be done by marking the optimal site for aspiration or performing the procedure under direct visualization in real time. The optimal site is the largest area of fluid closest to the transducer while avoiding important structures, such as loops of bowel (Fig. 20.7) and the inferior epigastric artery (Figs. 20.3 and 20.4). After marking this site, the procedure is performed as usual.

Direct guidance is most helpful when bladder volumes are low. Following an ultrasound survey of the bladder to identify an optimal region, anesthetic is injected into the skin and abdominal wall. Sterile preparation of the area is performed, and the transducer is placed in a sterile cover. An 18- or 21-gauge needle connected to a syringe is used. The transducer should be in transverse orientation with respect to the patient, but the needle is advanced directly under the transducer in its long axis (Fig. 20.8) to maintain the needle within the ultrasound beam and allow visualization of the needle throughout the procedure. The needle tip can be immediately identified in the near field at the top of the screen (Fig. 20.9), and the angle and depth of the needle can be adjusted to guide insertion into the bladder. Urine obtained in the syringe may be sent for analysis. If bladder decompression is needed, a stopcock or tubing setup similar to those used for paracentesis or thoracentesis can be employed.

Imaging pitfalls and limitations

- Avoid performing bladder aspiration if only small pockets of fluid are visible unless diagnostic evaluation of the fluid is crucial to management of the patient. Fluid resuscitation and waiting 30 minutes is strongly recommended.
- Use real-time guidance and a longitudinal approach of the needle to the transducer (Figs. 20.8 and 20.9) when accessing small fluid collections to avoid puncturing important structures.
- Fluid-filled loops of bowel can be distinguished from the bladder by the presence of peristalsis and hyperechoic

bubbles (Fig. 20.10). Urine should be uniformly anechoic.
- Hematuria can be avoided if the first syringe of urine is discarded and the sample in a second syringe is sent for urinalysis.

Clinical images

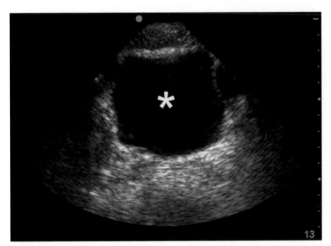

Figure 20.1. Ultrasound image of a transverse view of a normal urinary bladder with homogenous, anechoic urine (*asterisk*) contained within rounded walls.

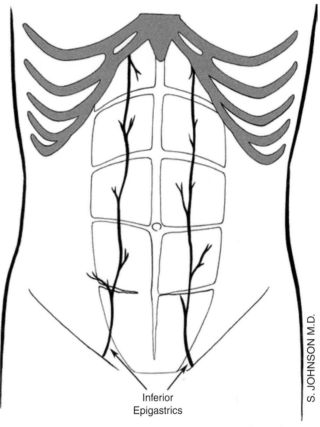

S. JOHNSON M.D.

Inferior
Epigastrics

Figure 20.3. Abdomen demonstrating the typical course of the inferior epigastric vessels.

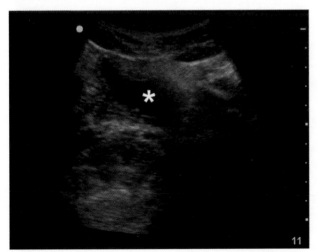

Figure 20.2. Ultrasound image of a transverse view of an empty urinary bladder with collapsed walls containing a small stripe of anechoic urine (*asterisk*).

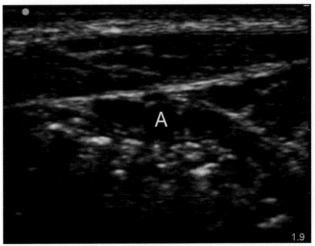

Figure 20.4. Ultrasound image of a transverse view of the inferior epigastric artery (A).

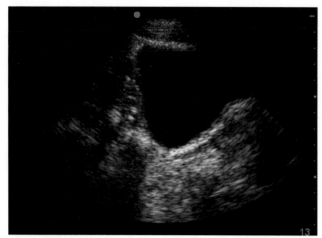

Figure 20.5. Ultrasound image of a sagittal view of the urinary bladder. This view should be used to complete a 3D survey of the bladder.

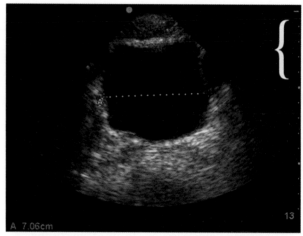

Figure 20.6. Ultrasound image of a transverse view of the urinary bladder with calipers measuring the bladder width and bracket-identifying ticks along the right side of the screen, indicating depth.

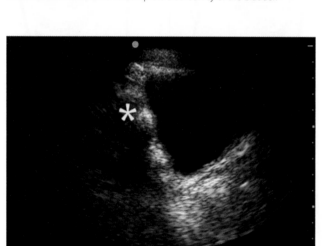

Figure 20.7. Ultrasound image of a longitudinal view of the urinary bladder showing adjacent loops of bowel, casting characteristic nebulous gray shadows (*asterisk*), impeding a clear image.

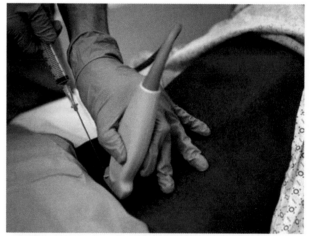

Figure 20.8. Needle advancing under the transducer in the longitudinal axis of the probe. The transducer is in transverse orientation with respect to the patient. This approach allows continuous visualization of the needle throughout its course, including the depth of the needle tip.

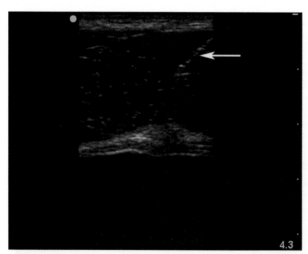

Figure 20.9. Ultrasound image of a transverse view of the urinary bladder with the superficial needle tip in the near field at the top right of the screen (*arrow*).

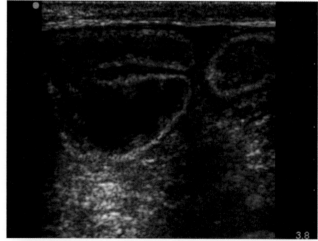

Figure 20.10. Ultrasound image of fluid-filled loops of bowel with small echogenic bubbles. Urine within the bladder is uniformly anechoic (except for the turbulence of ureteral jets, which appear differently) and does not demonstrate peristalsis, as seen in bowel.

Central venous catheter placement

Background

Ultrasound guidance for placement of central venous catheters (CVCs) is one of the most important uses of ultrasound in the clinical setting. More than 5 million CVCs are placed by physicians in the United States each year (10), often in situations in which vascular access is critical. Relying solely on anatomical landmarks can be difficult and risky, particularly in patients who are obese, hypovolemic, in shock, or have local scarring from injection drug use, surgery, or radiation. Ultrasound guidance allows the physician to clearly visualize the vein, guide the catheter into its lumen, and avoid adjacent neurovascular structures.

Ultrasound guidance can dramatically improve the likelihood of success and decrease the risk of complications. Complications have been reported in more than 15% of CVC placements (11). Serious complications include pneumothorax, nerve injury, arterial puncture with potential arteriovenous malformation, and hemorrhage. Risk of complication is higher for patients with pathological or therapeutic coagulopathies (12). Treatment of these complications may delay therapeutic interventions.

In a recent meta-analysis of seven randomized controlled trials of internal jugular vein (IJV) CVC placements in adults, the addition of ultrasound guidance resulted in an 86% reduction in the relative risk of failed catheter placement, a 57% reduction in the risk of complications, and a 41% reduction in the risk of failure on the first attempt (13). Results of three trials in pediatric patients are even more dramatic. The relative risk of complications was reduced by 73%, and the average number of attempts was reduced by two. Successful cannulation was achieved an average of 349 seconds more quickly with ultrasound guidance (13).

These results have led national organizations to recommend the use of ultrasound to guide CVC placement whenever possible. In its landmark report on iatrogenic errors, the Institute of Medicine advocates ultrasound guidance as an important modality to decrease complications (14). The Agency for Healthcare Research and Quality reviewed 79 patient safety practices. The authors list ultrasound guidance for CVC placement as a top 10 patient safety recommendation (15). In its extensive appraisal, the British National Institute for Clinical Excellence describes ultrasound guidance as the preferred method for insertion of CVCs into the IJV in adults and children (16). Finally, in a study of closed malpractice claims related to CVCs, almost half of the claims were judged to be possibly preventable with ultrasound guidance (17).

Anatomical considerations

The internal jugular vein lies deep to the sternocleidomastoid muscle at the level of the bifurcation of its sternal and clavicular heads (Fig. 20.11). The carotid artery generally lies deep and medial to the IJV (Fig. 20.12). The relationship of these vessels can change, depending on head position. Turning the patient's head 30 degrees to the opposite side of the intended CVC placement is recommended. In addition to position, the IJV can be distinguished from the carotid artery by its compressibility, less uniformly round shape, less pulsatility, and characteristic Doppler wave form (Fig. 20.13). The right IJV is usually preferred because of its more direct path to the superior vena cava.

Procedure

This section focuses on the use of ultrasound to guide IJV-CVC placement and presumes experience with standard techniques of CVC placement. The reader is referred to a recent *New England Journal of Medicine* review of central venous catheterization (18). Although techniques for ultrasound guidance of subclavian vein CVC placement have been described, they are more difficult, rarely used, and have less supporting evidence (19). Ultrasound guidance for femoral vein catheterization has been shown to be helpful in code situations in which the femoral pulse may not be present (20). Femoral vein CVC placement is similar to the IJV and follows the same principles discussed herein (Fig. 20.14).

A 6 to 13 MHz linear transducer is used to provide a high-resolution image of the superficial IJV. The lower frequency setting (e.g., 7.5 MHz) on the linear transducer may be needed to adequately image the deeper femoral vessels. Ultrasound can guide CVC placement in either a static or dynamic manner. In the static approach, ultrasound is used to verify vascular anatomy in preparation for an otherwise standard anatomical landmark technique. If desired, the path of the IJV can be marked with a sterile surgical pen (Fig. 20.15) or with indentations in the skin. This approach is easily performed by a single provider and does not require a sterile cover for the transducer. However, the anatomy of the neck can change dramatically if the patient moves his head.

The dynamic approach can be performed by one or two providers (Figs. 20.16 and 20.17). In the two-provider technique, the assisting physician or nurse operates the ultrasound machine. A sterile transducer sleeve and coupling gel are required. The assistant positions the IJV in the center of the screen, which correlates with the center of the transducer, and directs the physician as she advances the needle. In the single-provider technique, the physician controls the ultrasound transducer with her nondominant hand and advances the needle with the dominant hand. It is important for the physician to pass the needle through the plane of the ultrasound beam to detect the needle on the screen (Fig. 20.18). The echodense needle brightly reflects the sound waves and may produce a characteristic "ring-down" artifact (Fig. 20.19). Although following the hyperechoic needle tip is advised, evidence of the needle may be indirect in the form of soft tissue movement and deformation of the vessel wall. This view is usually adequate to guide CVC placement.

Once a flash of blood confirms the needle is in the IJV, the transducer is removed from the field, and catheterization proceeds by standard technique. The advantage of the

287

dynamic approach is that it is more reliable and allows real-time guidance.

As in other ultrasound applications, examining the structure of interest in two perpendicular planes can be helpful. The transverse plane is used the majority of the time for CVC placement because it allows the physician to direct the needle laterally or medially to intersect the IJV and avoid the carotid artery (Fig. 20.20). In a longitudinal view, the needle remains within the ultrasound beam and is therefore visualized on the screen throughout its trajectory (Fig. 20.21). The longitudinal plane contributes a view of the depth of the needle. This can be helpful if the needle has advanced through the IJV but does not reveal whether the needle passes to the side of the vessel. The longitudinal view can also be helpful in mapping the course of the IJV for a static approach (Figs. 20.15 and 20.22).

Avoiding imaging pitfalls

- *Index marker* – When the physician stands at the head of the patient's bed to place the IJV catheter, the index marker on the transducer facing the patient's left will correlate with the index marker on the left side of the ultrasound screen. So, when one identifies the need to move the needle to the left or right on the screen, one can naturally move in the same direction with respect to the patient.

- *Depth* – Decrease the depth setting on the ultrasound machine so the target IJV and adjacent carotid artery fill the screen.
- *Maneuvers* – Multiple studies have analyzed the effect of Trendelenburg position, positive-pressure ventilation, hepatic compression, and the Valsalva maneuver on IJV size (21–23). These maneuvers produce an increase in the cross-sectional diameter of the IJV, with Valsalva having the largest independent effect (24). A correlation between IJV dimension and successful first-pass catheterization has also been shown (25).
- *Pressing too hard* – The IJV may easily collapse from excessive pressure on the transducer, particularly in hypovolemic patients. This can lead to the needle passing through the flattened IJV and into the underlying carotid artery. Pressure on the vessels can be minimized by bracing the operator's hypothenar eminence or fingers on the patient's clavicle.
- *Failure to locate the needle* – To be seen on the screen, the needle must pass through the plane of the transducer. Movement of tissue can also provide evidence of the needle's location.
- *Failure to distinguish artery from vein* – The target IJV must be identified with certainty prior to advancing the needle (see "Anatomical considerations" earlier in this section).

Clinical images

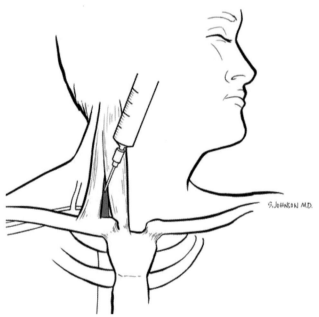

Figure 20.11. Neck anatomy and typical location of right internal jugular central venous catheterization at the bifurcation of the sternal and clavicular heads of the sternocleidomastoid muscle.

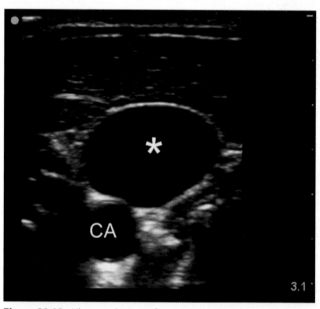

Figure 20.12. Ultrasound image of a transverse view of the right neck at the bifurcation of the sternal and clavicular heads of the sternocleidomastoid muscle showing the IJV (*asterisk*) and the carotid artery (CA).

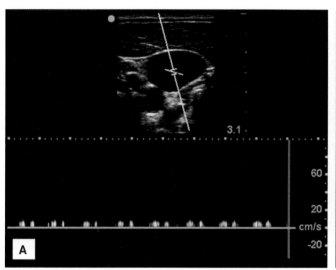

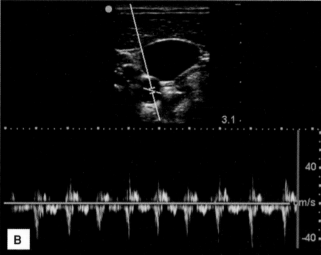

Figure 20.13. Ultrasound images of Doppler wave forms of IJV (A) and CA (B) in two panels.

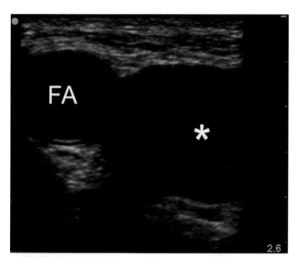

Figure 20.14. Ultrasound image of a transverse view of the femoral artery (FA) and vein (*asterisk*).

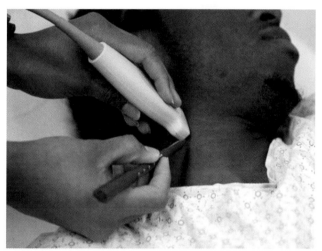

Figure 20.15. Surgical pen delineating the path of the right IJV.

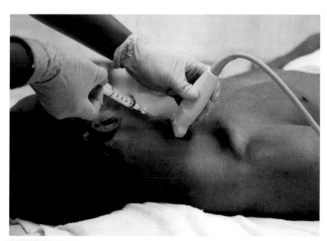

Figure 20.16. One-provider technique of central venous catheterization of the right IJV.

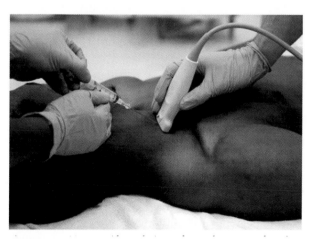

Figure 20.17. Two-provider technique of central venous catheterization of the right IJV.

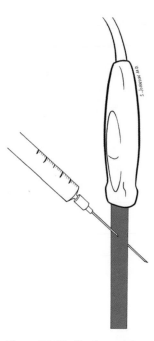

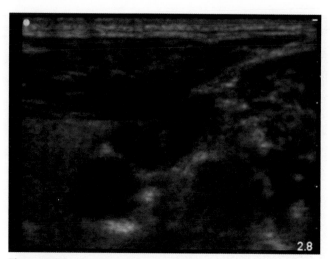

Figure 20.19. Ultrasound image of a transverse view of the right neck with the needle producing a characteristic ring-down artifact.

Figure 20.18. Needle passing transversely through the ultrasound beam. The needle will only be visible on the screen where it passes through the ultrasound beam.

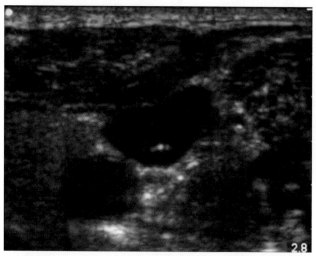

Figure 20.20. Ultrasound image of a transverse view of the neck, showing the needle within the right IJV.

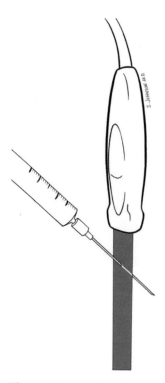

Figure 20.21. Needle within the ultrasound beam throughout its trajectory. This view adds the dimension of depth, but it cannot determine whether the needle passes to the side of the vein.

Foreign body detection and retrieval

Indications

Undetected foreign bodies during initial ED visits may lead to complications, including inflammatory reaction, infection, delayed wound healing, poor cosmetic outcome, and, less often, life-threatening illness (26–31). They are one of the leading causes of lawsuits against emergency physicians (32, 33).

Plain radiographs have historically proven beneficial in the detection and removal of radiopaque foreign bodies. Ultrasound accurately detects soft tissue foreign bodies as small as 1 mm and enables better localization than other imaging techniques (27–30, 34–42). Metals, plastics, wood, cactus, thorns, fish bones, sea urchin spines, gravel, and grit are all detectable and retrievable with ultrasound guidance but may be missed on x-ray.

The object's size, location, depth, 3D orientation, and relationship to surrounding anatomical structures can be demonstrated (28, 32). Ultrasonography should be considered the imaging modality of choice for ED detection and retrieval of soft tissue foreign bodies, particularly in the hands and feet (28, 36, 38, 43, 44).

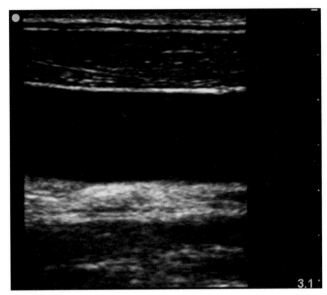

Figure 20.22. Ultrasound image of a longitudinal view of the right IJV.

Anatomical considerations

Ultrasound-guided detection, localization, and retrieval of foreign bodies require familiarity with the anatomy of the area being scanned. The ultrasonographic appearance of muscle is characterized by a uniformly hypoechoic texture with internal striations, whereas its fascia is brightly echogenic and thin. Tendons appear as echogenic ovoid structures when scanned transversely. Scanned longitudinally, they appear linear with a characteristic internal fibrillar appearance (45). The surface of bone is characteristically brightly echogenic with far-field acoustic shadows (Fig. 20.23).

All soft tissue foreign bodies are echogenic, and most produce characteristic patterns (27, 34, 36, 46–49). The degree of echogenicity is proportional to the difference in acoustic impedance at the interface of the foreign body and surrounding tissue (27, 34–36, 44). Reverberation artifact or shadowing deep to the foreign body is due to proximity to anatomical structures and surface quality.

Several foreign bodies produce unique echographic patterns. Glass and metal will leave characteristic comet tail effects (Fig. 20.24). Wood, plastic, and cactus spines are hyperechoic with nondistinct distal shadowing (Fig. 20.25). Sand and pebbles have strong distinct acoustic shadows (29, 32, 40, 47, 50). A hypoechoic rim surrounding a foreign body is often secondary to an inflammatory soft tissue reaction and is often seen when a foreign body has been present for more than 24 hours (Fig. 20.26) (27, 28, 30, 38).

Procedure

Optimal transducer frequency and type may vary, depending on location and character of the foreign body. High-frequency 6 to 13 MHz linear transducers offer excellent resolution and a shallow focal zone, and they have been recommended for imaging small superficial foreign bodies. Lower frequency 2 to 5 MHz transducers have been recommended for imaging soft tissue foreign bodies embedded in deeper tissue planes (27–32, 34–40, 42–47, 50–56).

The probe is held perpendicular to the skin surface as it scans for the foreign body in multiple planes. The frequency, depth, and gain may be adjusted to search various soft tissue depths. Once detected, the foreign body is centered in relation to the probe, and its position marked with a pen (27, 32). The foreign body is evaluated in both longitudinal and transverse planes. The sonographer should note depth and proximity to anatomical structures. An important benefit of ultrasound localization is the opportunity to identify existing abnormalities, such as neurovascular injury, tendon rupture, fractures, or fluid collections (27). Once localized, whether retrieval of the foreign body is appropriate should be addressed. Inert, nonreactive, and asymptomatic objects do not require removal (31).

Anesthesia may be achieved with local infiltration or nerve block. If the foreign body is positioned near an existing wound and can be retrieved without traversing a long distance, retrieval through the wound is recommended. The wound opening may be extended as needed.

Although often not necessary, the foreign body may be retrieved with real-time ultrasound guidance using careful blunt dissection. Alligator forceps are easiest to maneuver and are recommended for retrieval (Fig. 20.27). Absence of a substantial entry wound, inaccessibility of the foreign body through the wound, or the existence of a missile tract may necessitate a direct incision over the foreign body for retrieval. Sterile technique using a probe cover with coupling gel on both sides of the barrier has been recommended if a new incision is made to facilitate retrieval or when scanning open wounds.

Adjuncts to direct incision and retrieval have proven beneficial. A 20-gauge needle inserted over the foreign body can be advanced with ultrasound guidance until the tip contacts the object (Figs. 20.28, 20.29, and 20.30). An incision is made down to the needle tip. The soft tissue is bluntly dissected, and the foreign body removed (32). Deeply embedded foreign bodies can be retrieved with needle localization and open retrieval (35, 38, 57, 58). Using ultrasound guidance, two sterile needles are directed under the foreign body at a 90-degree angle to each other (Figs. 20.31 and 20.32) (57). Using the two needles as landmarks, real-time ultrasonography is used to guide the incision and blunt dissection down to the intersection of the needles.

Imaging pitfalls and limitations

- Foreign bodies embedded under bone may go undetected.
- Hyperechoic objects may be mistaken for bone or tendon.
- Smaller objects may exceed the limit of a transducer's resolution, and low-frequency transducers may not detect superficial objects.
- Rare false-positive results may be secondary to scar tissue formation, cartilage ossification, soft tissue calcifications, sesamoid bones, calcified vasculature, or hemorrhage. Scanning contralateral structures may help identify normal anatomy.

291

Clinical images

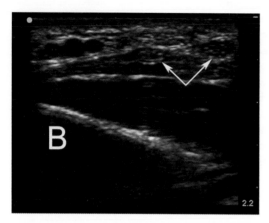

Figure 20.23. Ultrasound image of a transverse view of the wrist, demonstrating bone (B) and tendons (*arrows*).

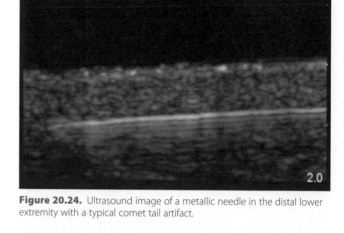

Figure 20.24. Ultrasound image of a metallic needle in the distal lower extremity with a typical comet tail artifact.

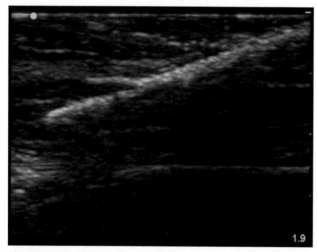

Figure 20.25. Ultrasound image of a wooden foreign body with nondistinct distal shadowing.

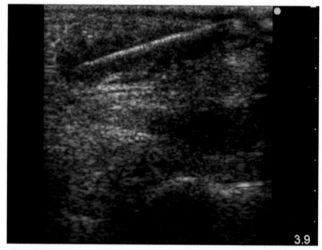

Figure 20.26. Ultrasound image of a foreign body with hypoechoic rim of surrounding inflammatory reaction.

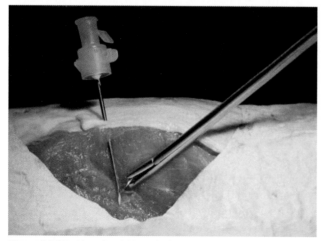

Figure 20.27. Blunt dissection with alligator forceps clasping a glass foreign body in a marinated leg of lamb.

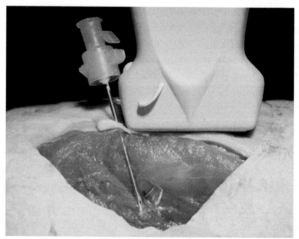

Figure 20.28. Needle contacting a glass foreign body with ultrasound guidance of the localization in a leg of lamb.

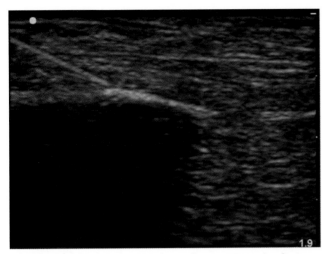

Figure 20.29. Ultrasound image of a needle contacting a glass foreign body in a leg of lamb.

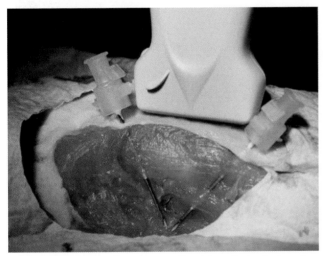

Figure 20.31. Two-needle technique of localizing a foreign body under ultrasound guidance in a leg of lamb.

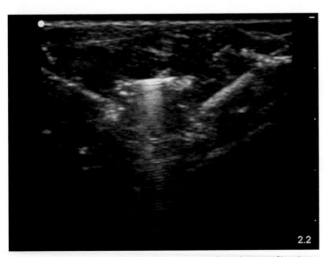

Figure 20.32. Ultrasound image of the two-needle technique of localizing a foreign body under ultrasound guidance in a leg of lamb.

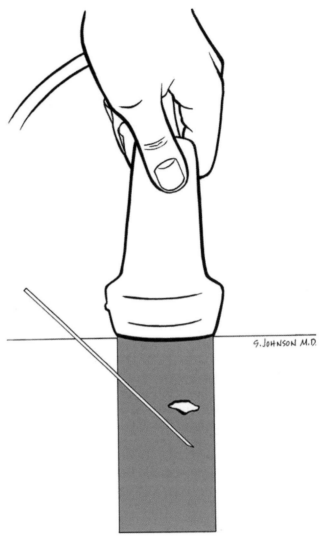

Figure 20.30. One-needle technique of localizing a foreign body under ultrasound guidance.

Thoracentesis

Indications

Diagnostic thoracentesis is performed when the etiology of a pleural effusion is unknown. Therapeutic thoracentesis is performed when patients are symptomatic due to an effusion. Ultrasound has been shown to be helpful in identifying pleural effusions and guiding management decisions (59). It is also beneficial in selecting an optimal site to insert a thoracentesis needle (60).

Pneumothorax is the major complication associated with thoracentesis. Performed without ultrasound guidance, thoracentesis has yielded pneumothorax rates of 4% to 30% (61–64). Under ultrasound guidance, rates of pneumothorax during thoracentesis have been reported as low as 1.3% to 2.5% (65, 66). Ultrasound has been used to rule out pneumothorax with a sensitivity higher than chest x-ray when compared with CT (67).

293

Anatomical considerations

Pleural effusions respond to gravity by collecting above the diaphragm in the upright patient or when the head of the bed is slightly elevated. The liver and spleen provide excellent acoustic windows, allowing better visualization of pleural effusions. The standard focused assessment with sonography for trauma (FAST) exam views of the right (Fig. 20.33) and left (Fig. 20.34) upper quadrants provide familiar anatomical landmarks (Figs. 20.35 and 20.36). During expiration, the diaphragm rises into the chest; therefore, respiratory changes should be considered when choosing a site for thoracentesis. The neurovascular bundle runs along the inferior aspect of each rib and should be avoided (Fig. 20.37). The location of the heart contraindicates left anterior and lateral approaches.

Procedure

The patient is positioned sitting forward. The head of the bed can be raised slightly, if the patient is unable to sit upright. A 2 to 5 MHz abdominal or phased array transducer in a longitudinal orientation can be used to identify the pleural effusion in the left or right upper quadrant views with the ultrasound beam directed cephalad into the chest (Figs. 20.33 and 20.34). The probe can then be moved to the patient's back and changed to a transverse orientation to fit between the ribs. The effusion is mapped by marking the level of the diaphragm inferiorly and the edge of the lung superiorly (Fig. 20.38). Identifying the deepest pocket of fluid between these two landmarks is the goal. Pleural fluid overlies the brightly echogenic diaphragm and will be darkly anechoic (Fig. 20.39). Hyperechoic collections of proteinaceous debris may be present (Fig. 20.40). Air scatters sound waves, and the lung will appear gray and nebulous (Fig. 20.41). Bone of the scapula and ribs will be brightly echogenic in the near field with typical underlying shadows (Fig. 20.42). Once the ideal location is identified, the area should be observed during respiration to determine if the lung, liver, or spleen moves into the selected space.

The optimal area in the midscapular line should be marked with a sterile pen, and the thoracentesis should proceed as usual under sterile conditions using local anesthesia or an intercostal nerve block. The depth of the fluid pocket should be kept in mind, and the needle should only be advanced deeply enough to obtain fluid. The needle should pass directly over the adjacent rib to avoid the neurovascular bundle. Use of a plastic catheter is recommended to minimize the risk of pneumothorax.

Although real-time ultrasound guidance can be used, it is technically difficult and rarely necessary. If the pleural effusion is small (Fig. 20.43), the physician should strongly reconsider the importance of obtaining the fluid sample.

Imaging pitfalls and limitations

- Map the pleural effusion and observe changes with respiration.
- Choose a thoracentesis site well above the level of the liver or spleen.
- Insert the needle over the rib to avoid the neurovascular bundle.
- Carefully avoid the lung because pneumothorax is the most common and serious complication.
- Avoid attempting to tap a small pleural effusion.

Clinical images

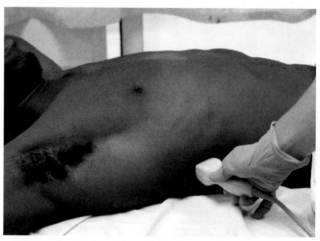

Figure 20.33. Ultrasound exam of the right upper quadrant with the transducer in longitudinal orientation and the sound beam directed into the chest.

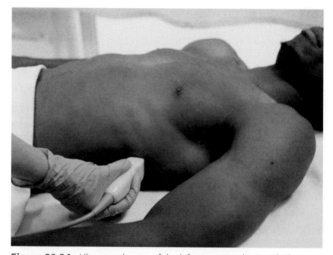

Figure 20.34. Ultrasound exam of the left upper quadrant with the transducer in longitudinal orientation and the sound beam directed into the chest.

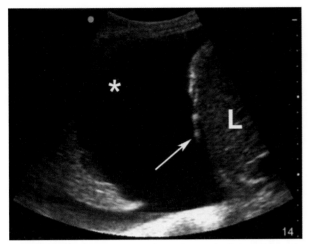

Figure 20.35. Ultrasound image from a longitudinal view of the right upper quadrant showing a right pleural effusion (*asterisk*) overlying the diaphragm (*arrow*) and liver (L).

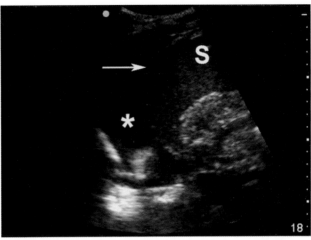

Figure 20.36. Ultrasound image from a longitudinal view of the left upper quadrant showing a left pleural effusion (*asterisk*) overlying the diaphragm (*arrow*) and spleen (S).

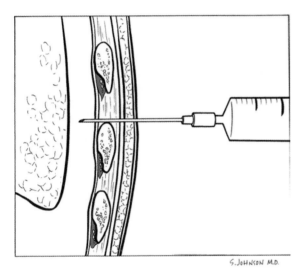

Figure 20.37. Longitudinal view through the bony chest showing a thoracentesis needle advancing over a rib to avoid the neurovascular bundle running along the inferior aspect of the ribs.

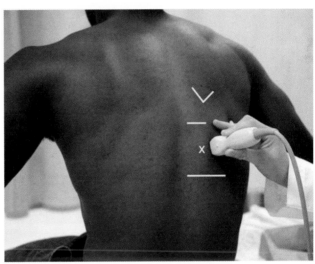

Figure 20.38. Ultrasound exam of a patient's back, mapping the level of the scapula and lung superiorly and the diaphragm inferiorly. The transducer is oriented transversely, and an optimal location for thoracentesis is indicated by an X.

Lumbar puncture

Indications

Lumbar puncture (LP) is one of the most frequently performed procedures in the acute care setting. Obtaining a sample of cerebrospinal fluid (CSF) is crucial to diagnosing central nervous system infection or subarachnoid hemorrhage. This procedure is successfully performed using anatomical landmarks. In obese patients or when multiple attempts have been unsuccessful, ultrasound may help identify an appropriate site for puncture. Emergency physicians, radiologists, and anesthesiologists have reported ultrasound to be helpful in identifying spinal anatomy (68–73). A recent randomized controlled trial found that the use of ultrasound significantly reduced the number of LP failures and improved the ease of the procedure in obese patients (74).

Anatomical considerations

Ultrasound is used to identify the optimal location for passing the LP needle between the posterior spinous processes and into the dural space (Fig. 20.44). When anatomical landmarks cannot be accurately palpated, ultrasound allows visualization of the spinous processes, enabling identification of the midline and the interspaces. As is typical for dense structures with

295

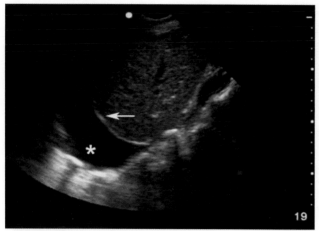

Figure 20.39. Ultrasound image from a longitudinal view of the right upper quadrant, showing anechoic pleural fluid (*asterisk*) overly the brightly echogenic diaphragm (*arrow*).

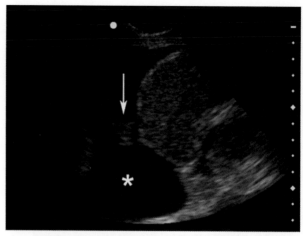

Figure 20.40. Ultrasound image from a longitudinal view of the right upper quadrant, showing anechoic pleural fluid (*asterisk*) containing hyperechoic collections of proteinaceous debris (*arrow*).

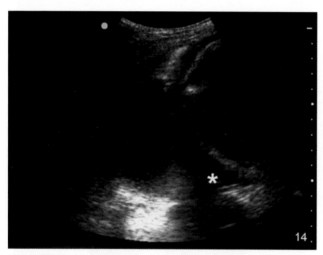

Figure 20.41. Ultrasound image from a longitudinal view of the right upper quadrant, demonstrating nebulous gray lung overlying a small anechoic pleural effusion (*asterisk*).

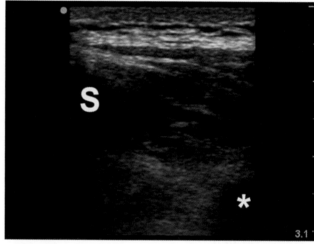

Figure 20.42. Ultrasound image from a longitudinal view of the back, demonstrating bone of the scapula (S) and rib (*asterisk*). Bone appears brightly echoic in the near field with hypoechoic underlying shadows.

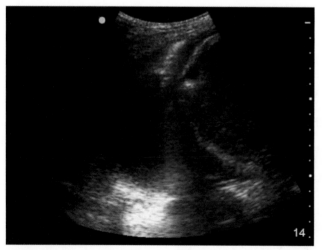

Figure 20.43. Ultrasound image of a longitudinal view of a small pleural effusion overlying the right hemidiaphragm. Performing a thoracentesis on an effusion this small is not recommended.

high acoustic impedance, the boney spinous processes reflect most of the sound waves and appear echogenic in the near field. Few sound waves are conducted deeply, so shadows appear below the superficial surface of the bone (Fig. 20.45).

Procedure

In children and nonobese adults, a 7.5 MHz linear transducer will provide a more detailed image. However, ultrasound guidance is more often required in obese patients. An abdominal, microconvex, or phased array transducer in the range of 3.5 to 5 MHz may be needed to penetrate more deeply. The patient should be positioned on his side so an accurate opening pressure can be measured.

The transducer can be placed in transverse or longitudinal orientation based on image quality and physician preference. In a longitudinal view with the index marker toward the head, two adjacent spinous processes are identified. The probe is positioned so the interspace (usually L4–5) is in the center of the screen (Fig. 20.45). The midline is marked at both ends of the transducer. The interspace is marked on both sides of the center of the transducer (Fig. 20.46). With the transducer in transverse orientation, the probe is moved up and down the spine to identify adjacent spinous processes (Fig. 20.47). The interspace is marked at the ends of the transducer, and the midline is marked on both sides of the center of the transducer (Fig. 20.48).

Once the optimal location is marked, the LP can be performed as usual under sterile conditions. Ultrasound should be used to estimate the depth the needle will need to advance to reach the dural space. Real-time guidance is technically difficult and not recommended because of the small

interspinous space and the angle of the spinous processes. Other details of spinal anatomy can be seen in some patients, but they can be difficult to identify and add little to basic identification of the midline and interspinous spaces.

Imaging pitfalls and limitations

- Do not mark the interspace with the patient sitting and then perform the LP with the patient on her side because the overlying skin and soft tissue may shift.
- Based on depth estimated by ultrasound, a longer spinal needle may be needed.

Clinical images

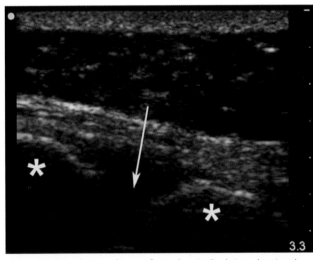

Figure 20.45. Ultrasound image from a longitudinal view, showing the spinous processes (*asterisk*) of lumbar vertebrae and an arrow indicating the target spinal interspace.

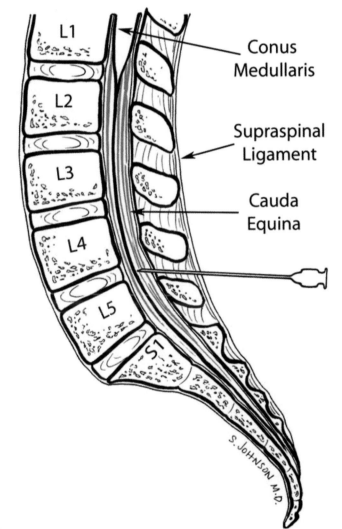

Figure 20.44. Sagittal view of the lumbosacral spine, demonstrating a spinal needle advancing between the spinous processes of L4 and L5 into the dural space.

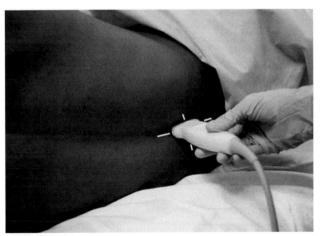

Figure 20.46. Ultrasound used to identify and mark the L4–5 interspace with the transducer in a longitudinal orientation. Marks are made on the skin at the ends and middle of the transducer.

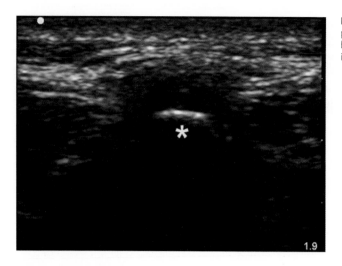

Figure 20.47. Ultrasound image from a transverse view showing the spinous process (*asterisk*) of a lumbar vertebra with acoustic shadowing. The probe should be advanced cephalad and caudad to confirm midline and identify the intervertebral space between spinous processes.

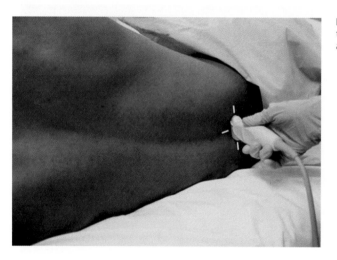

Figure 20.48. Ultrasound used to identify and mark the L4–5 interspace with the transducer in a transverse orientation. Marks are made on the skin at the ends and middle of the transducer.

Paracentesis

Indications

The amount of peritoneal fluid in patients requiring therapeutic paracentesis may be large enough that ultrasound is not necessary. However, physical examination of the abdomen for detecting ascites is often inaccurate with a sensitivity as low as 50% and an overall accuracy of 58% (75). In a recent study, 25% of patients suspected of having ascites did not have adequate amounts of peritoneal fluid to be safely drained by needle puncture (76). In these cases, ultrasound would allow the physician to quantify the amount of peritoneal fluid and, if necessary, guide the needle puncture to avoid complications such as bowel or bladder perforation. Ultrasound-guided paracentesis is especially beneficial in coagulopathic patients who are at increased risk for bleeding from punctures of the abdominal wall or intraabdominal structures.

A randomized controlled trial of 100 patients with suspected ascites compared ultrasound-guided paracentesis with the traditional blind technique. Ultrasound guidance significantly improved the success rate of paracentesis (95% vs. 61%). When the blind technique initially failed, the procedure was repeated using ultrasound guidance. Peritoneal fluid was successfully obtained in 87% of the repeated procedures (76).

Anatomical considerations

In addition to confirming the presence of peritoneal fluid, ultrasound is most commonly used to determine the optimal site for needle puncture. This use of ultrasound is important when peritoneal fluid has not adequately accumulated in the left lower quadrant of the abdomen as traditionally taught. A study examining the pattern of ascitic fluid accumulation found the largest pockets of fluid in the perihepatic region. The next most common sites of fluid collection were around the bladder, the right paracolic gutter, and then in the left flank. In six of eight patients with peritoneal fluid in the left flank, loops of bowel were identified between the abdominal wall and the fluid collection in the expected path of a blind puncture (77).

Traditionally, the risk of bladder perforation was minimized by requesting patients to void or by catheter drainage of urine. Ultrasound guidance allows the bladder to be distinguished and avoided. Other anatomical structures to avoid, especially in coagulopathic patients, are the inferior epigastric vessels (Figs. 20.49 and 20.51). The authors are currently studying the use of ultrasound to identify this vascular structure.

Procedure

An abdominal 2 to 5 MHz transducer is typically used to identify intraabdominal fluid. Elevating the head of the bed will help fluid drain into the dependent lower quadrants and create larger pockets. Sterile preparation and probe covers are unnecessary for the initial ultrasound survey of the abdomen.

Once an optimal anatomical site is identified, it can be marked with a sterile surgical pen. The site should access a significant collection of fluid while avoiding important anatomical structures such as bowel, bladder, and inferior epigastric vessels (Fig. 20.52). If the patient does not change position, the ultrasound probe can be set aside and the procedure performed as usual (Fig. 20.53). If the patient does move, the optimal puncture site should be reconfirmed.

Paracentesis can also be performed under real-time ultrasound guidance, but this is only necessary if pockets of fluid are small or vulnerable anatomical structures are present (Fig. 20.54). Ultrasound guidance is especially important in these cases, and the need for paracentesis should be carefully weighed against the risks of complications. A linear 6 to 13 MHz transducer with probe cover can be used for real-time guidance under sterile conditions. The linear transducer is also best for identifying the inferior epigastric artery, which can be further elucidated with color and pulse wave Doppler (Fig. 20.51).

As with any needle-guided procedure, the needle will only be seen on the screen as it passes through the plane of the ultrasound beam. In the transverse plane (see Fig. 20.18 in the "Central venous catheter placement" section), the transducer should be centered over the optimal site for puncture. The needle should then be passed directly under the center of the transducer at a steep angle. It will appear in the near field at the top of the screen and can be redirected medially or laterally as needed. In a transverse view, the probe should be advanced to maintain a constant view of the needle tip to avoid penetrating too deeply (Fig. 20.55). Characteristic ringdown artifact can help confirm the presence of the needle (Fig. 20.56).

In the longitudinal plane, the needle is viewed throughout its course into the peritoneal cavity (Fig. 20.57). However, because the sound beam is thin, it can be difficult to keep the needle within the image and on the screen. The sonologist's ability to maintain visualization improves with experience, and in anatomically difficult circumstances, this is the recommended technique. Real-time ultrasound-guided paracentesis is typically performed as a one-person procedure (Fig. 20.58), although a second person can operate the ultrasound machine, freeing the other provider to concentrate on the paracentesis.

Imaging pitfalls and limitations

- Avoid performing paracentesis if only small pockets of fluid are visible unless diagnostic evaluation of the fluid is crucial to management of the patient.
- Use real-time guidance and a longitudinal view of the needle when accessing small fluid collections to avoid puncturing important structures.
- A full bladder extending into an otherwise attractive area of collected fluid can be avoided if the patient is able to void or a catheter is placed to drain the bladder.

Clinical images

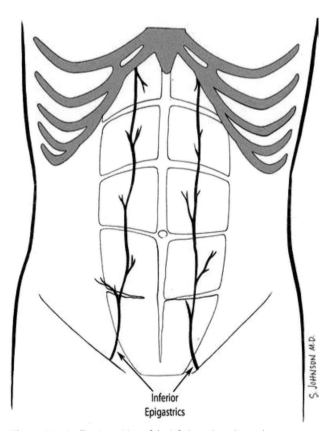

Figure 20.49. Classic position of the inferior epigastric arteries.

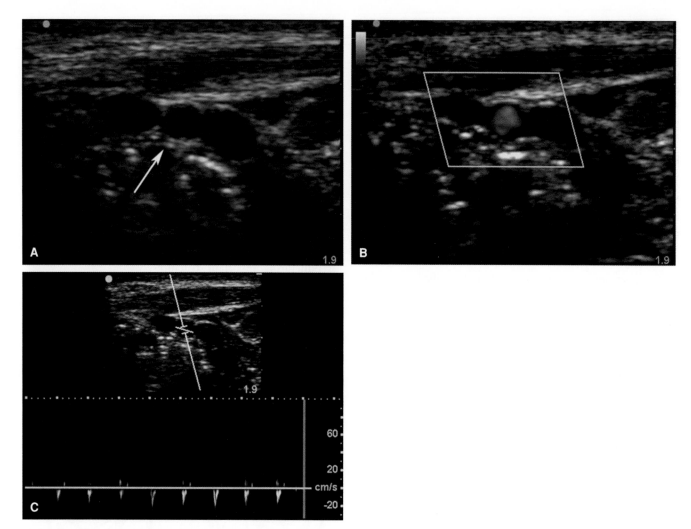

Figure 20.50. Ultrasound images with an arrow indicating the hypogastric vessels in B mode (A), with color power Doppler (B) and pulse wave Doppler (C).

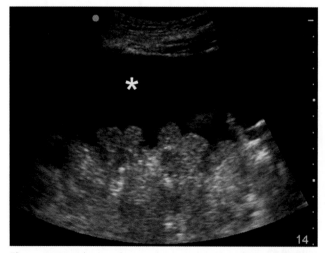

Figure 20.51. Ultrasound image showing optimal site for paracentesis with a significant fluid collection (*asterisk*), while avoiding important anatomical structures such as bowel, bladder, and inferior epigastric vessels.

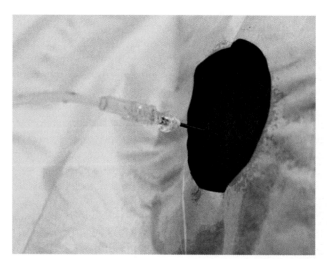

Figure 20.52. Paracentesis needle draining clear ascitic fluid.

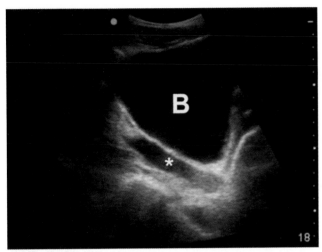

Figure 20.53. Ultrasound image of a longitudinal view showing the bladder (B) and a small fluid collection (*asterisk*).

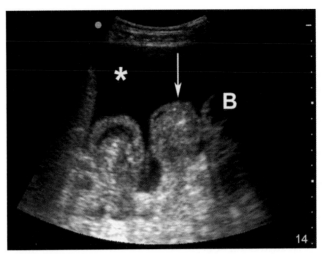

Figure 20.54. Ultrasound image of a longitudinal view of the bladder (B) and ascitic fluid (*asterisk*) with vulnerable loops of bowel (*arrow*).

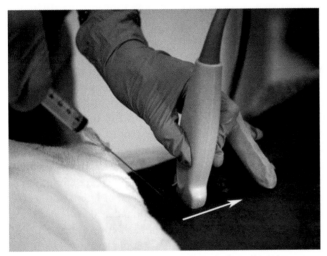

Figure 20.55. Transversely oriented transducer and needle with arrow indicating advancement of transducer performed to maintain the needle tip within view.

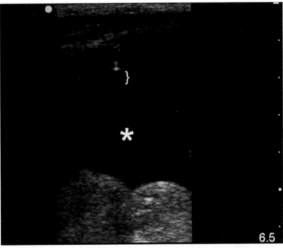

Figure 20.56. Ultrasound image of transverse view of needle passing into peritoneal cavity filled with ascites (*asterisk*). Characteristic ring-down artifact from the needle is indicated by the bracket.

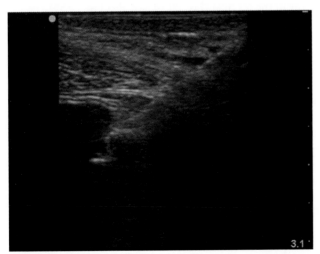

Figure 20.57. Ultrasound image of a longitudinal view showing the needle passing into the peritoneal cavity. This is the safest technique of real-time ultrasound guidance if quantities of peritoneal fluid are small and a sample is crucial to patient management because the needle is visualized throughout its course.

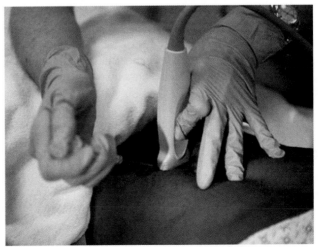

Figure 20.58. Single-person paracentesis technique with the needle in the longitudinal axis of transducer.

Pericardiocentesis

Indications

Unrecognized pericardial tamponade is one of the most quickly fatal pathological entities in medicine. Fortunately, ultrasound can accurately make this diagnosis within seconds and guide pericardiocentesis, a lifesaving intervention. Ultrasound has been regarded as the gold standard for diagnosis of pericardial tamponade since the mid-1960s (78). Accurate scanning for tamponade by noncardiologists has been demonstrated (79) and led to its inclusion in the FAST exam (see Chapter 15) and Advanced Trauma Life Support (80).

Traumatic pericardial tamponade is typically treated surgically with an open thoracotomy or pericardial window. The acute treatment of nontraumatic pericardial tamponade is needle pericardiocentesis. Pericardiocentesis is indicated when a pericardial effusion is identified on ultrasound (Fig. 20.59) and when the patient is hypotensive or at risk for soon becoming hypotensive.

Traditional blind pericardiocentesis entails needle insertion using a longer subxiphoid approach (Fig. 20.60). The subxiphoid ultrasound view (Fig. 20.61) demonstrates that this approach traverses the liver. In addition, the needle has the potential to inadvertently puncture the right atrium, the right ventricle, or a coronary artery more than 100 times per minute as the heart rapidly contracts. Pneumothorax is another known complication of the blind subxiphoid approach (81, 82).

Studies of the blind subxiphoid technique have yielded morbidity and mortality rates as high as 50% and 6%, respectively (82–89). A series of 1,127 pericardiocenteses demonstrated that the addition of ultrasound guidance reduced the morbidity and mortality rates to less than 4.3% and 0.1%, respectively. The overall success rate in this large series was 97%, with success on the first attempt in 89% of cases (90). In pediatric patients, ultrasound-guided pericardiocentesis was even more consistently successful and safer (91).

Ultrasound also provides new and safer approaches to pericardiocentesis by allowing the offending fluid to be accessed from positions on the body surface where the effusion is closest to the transducer and vital structures are avoided (92, 93). In the series of 1,127 ultrasound-guided pericardiocenteses, the apical (Fig. 20.62) or parasternal approaches (Figs. 20.63 and 20.64) were the preferred entry sites in 79% of cases, with the subcostal approach chosen in only 15% (90).

Anatomical considerations

Tamponade occurs when a sufficient volume of fluid accumulates in the pericardial space to inhibit the heart's ability to relax and fill with blood during diastole. This is indicated on ultrasound by bowing or collapse of the right atrial or ventricular wall during diastole (Fig. 20.59). These patients are usually hypotensive, and the continued fluid accumulation will lead to further hemodynamic instability and death (94–98).

The pericardiocentesis needle must avoid multiple vital structures. The liver, which appears gray and homogenous under the echogenic diaphragm, is especially vulnerable if the subxiphoid approach is chosen (Figs. 20.60 and 20.61). The gray myocardium may be highlighted by surrounding anechoic (black) fluid within the hyperechoic pericardium (Fig. 20.65). Air scatters ultrasound waves, causing the lung to appear characteristically gray and nebulous (Fig. 20.66). The physician should choose an approach that avoids the left internal mammary artery running longitudinally 3 to 5 cm lateral to the sternal border (Fig. 20.64) and the intercostal neurovascular bundle inferior to each rib (see Fig. 20.37 in the "Thoracentesis" section).

Chapter 17 fully reviews the basic cardiac views. Using a 1 to 5 MHz phased array or microconvex transducer to minimize rib shadow (an abdominal probe can also be used), a pericardial effusion should be examined in the subxiphoid, parasternal long-axis, parasternal short-axis, and apical four-chamber views to determine the most appropriate path for the pericardiocentesis needle.

In the subxiphoid view, the transducer is placed directly subjacent to the xiphoid with the index marker pointing to the patient's right (Fig. 20.67). To obtain the proper coronal view of the heart (Fig. 20.61), the angle of the probe should be shallow with the sound beam directed cephalad and slightly to the patient's left. This view can be difficult to obtain in obese patients or when the abdomen is tender. The sound beam should fan through the heart from anterior to posterior to identify an early dependent posterior effusion. However, most pericardial effusions leading to tamponade are circumferential, filling the pericardial space (Fig. 20.65). Smaller, acutely acquired effusions can lead to tamponade.

In the parasternal long-axis view, the transducer is placed perpendicular to the chest wall at nipple level with the index marker pointing to the patient's right shoulder (Fig. 20.68). The transducer is fanned to the left and right to view the entire heart (Fig. 20.69). A dependent pericardial effusion will first appear in the far field (Fig. 20.70, see also Fig. 20.59).

The parasternal short-axis view is obtained by rotating the transducer 90 degrees clockwise from the parasternal long-axis view, so the index marker is pointed to the patient's left shoulder (Fig. 20.71). The transducer is fanned through the heart in a cross-sectional orientation (Fig. 20.72). An effusion will initially be seen in the dependent far field (Fig. 20.73).

In the apical four-chamber view, the transducer is placed at the point of maximum impulse, with the index marker to the patient's right (Fig. 20.74). The sound beam is directed cephalad and slightly to the patient's right at a shallow angle similar to the subxiphoid view (Fig. 20.75). The sound beam should fan through the heart from anterior to posterior to identify a dependent posterior effusion (Fig. 20.76).

Procedure

The goal of the ultrasound exam is to determine the insertion point and course of the pericardiocentesis needle. All four views should be used to determine the largest collection of fluid closest to the skin surface and away from vital structures. Using real-time ultrasound guidance for pericardiocentesis can be difficult. Marking the best needle insertion site with a surgical pen and noting the best angle for insertion based on the angle of the sound beam is generally the best approach. Depth of insertion should be noted by measuring the distance or estimating the depth based on the 1-cm ticks along the right side of the screen. Once the site and angle are determined, the patient should not move, or the anatomical position of the heart will change.

Once the patient has been prepped and draped, the transducer should be placed in a sterile sheath and the needle's insertion site, angle, and depth reconfirmed prior to the procedure to secure the needle trajectory in the operator's mind. If time permits, the insertion site should be anesthetized. Commercially available pericardiocentesis kits contain the necessary supplies. A saline-filled syringe is attached to a 16- or 18-gauge sheathed needle, which is advanced along the predetermined trajectory into the pericardial effusion. A flash of fluid suggests placement within the pericardium. If the location is unclear, the needle tip may be visualized by ultrasound. Injection of saline from the syringe will create turbulence that can be seen on B-mode ultrasound and with color Doppler (Figs. 20.77 and 20.78).

Saline echo-contrast medium can be created by connecting a 5 mL syringe loaded with normal saline and an empty 5 mL syringe to a three-way stopcock, and rapidly injecting back and forth between the two syringes (Fig. 20.79). The agitated saline is quickly injected into the needle and observed on B-mode ultrasound (Fig. 20.80). If the needle is in the pericardial sac, the procedure may continue. If the needle is not in the pericardial sac, it should be repositioned by slight withdrawal, or it may need to be withdrawn

completely and pericardiocentesis reattempted with reassessment of the needle trajectory by ultrasound (93).

Once the pericardial location of the needle is confirmed, the needle is advanced approximately 2 mm, and the catheter is advanced over the needle. The steel needle core is withdrawn. Fluid can be removed until cardiac function is adequate to provide hemodynamic stability. The catheter can be sutured in place and a secure dressing applied. The catheter should be left in place, even during transport, to allow drainage of reaccumulated fluid. Fluid that reaccumulates should be aspirated intermittently rather than continuously and the sheath flushed with normal saline to avoid catheter obstruction (93). A pigtail catheter has been recommended for malignant effusions (99) or postoperative pericardial effusions (100).

Imaging pitfalls and limitations

- Pneumothorax is a significant risk with the blind technique and can be avoided when ultrasound is used. The air within the lung scatters the sound waves, producing a characteristic nebulous gray appearance (Fig. 20.66).
- Laceration of the intercostal vessels can result if the needle passes along the inferior aspect of a rib (see Fig. 20.37 in the "Thoracentesis" section).
- Coronary arteries can be avoided by keeping the needle within the pocket of fluid and away from the heart.
- The left internal mammary awrtery runs longitudinally, 3 to 5 cm lateral to the sternum, and should be avoided (Fig. 20.64). Injury of this vessel is an extremely rare complication.

Clinical images

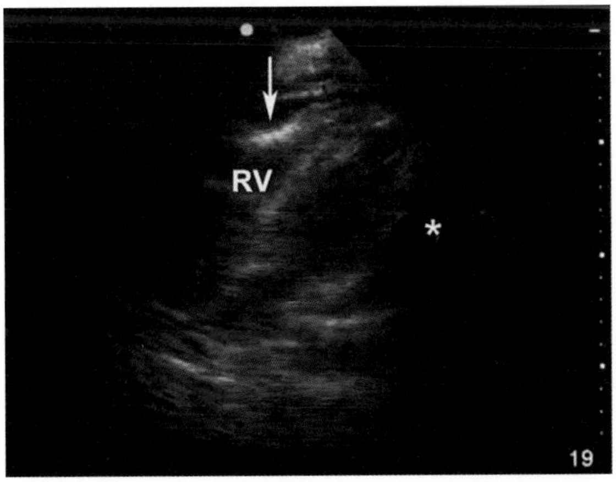

Figure 20.59. Ultrasound image from a parasternal long-axis view showing a large pericardial effusion (*asterisk*) with diastolic collapse (*arrow*) of the right ventricle (RV), indicating tamponade.

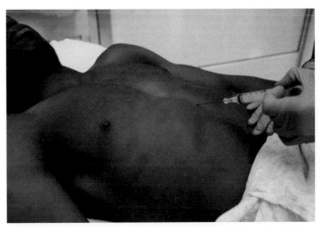

Figure 20.60. Subxiphoid pericardiocentesis approach.

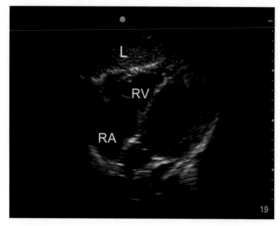

Figure 20.61. Ultrasound image from a normal subxiphoid view showing the liver (L) in the near field within the typical pericardiocentesis needle trajectory toward the heart (RA, right atrium; RV, right ventricle).

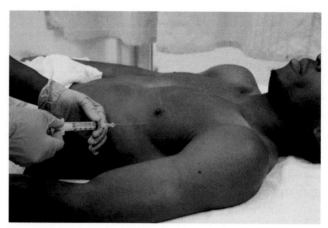

Figure 20.62. Apical pericardiocentesis approach.

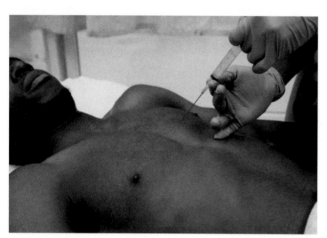

Figure 20.63. Parasternal pericardiocentesis approach.

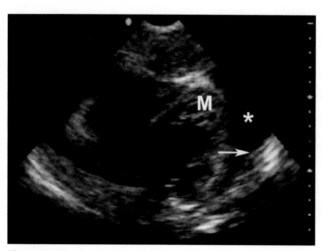

Figure 20.65. Ultrasound image from a subxiphoid view, demonstrating a circumferential pericardial effusion (*asterisk*) between the hyperechoic pericardium (*arrow*) and the gray myocardium (M).

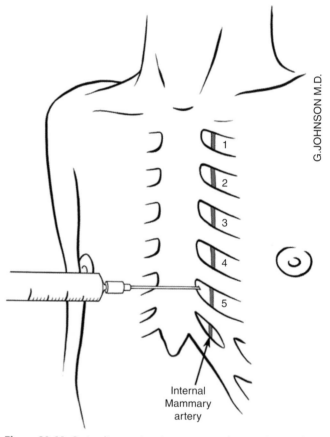

Figure 20.64. Pericardiocentesis, using a parasternal approach. Note the path of the left internal mammary artery (LIMA).

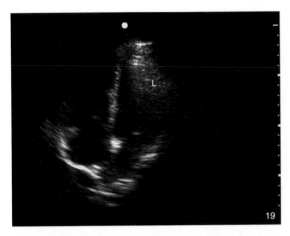

Figure 20.66. Ultrasound image from an apical four-chamber view showing the characteristic nebulous gray pattern of air within the lung (L).

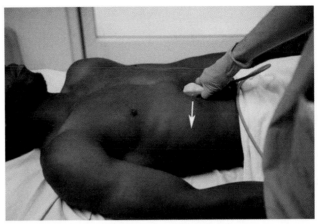

Figure 20.67. Proper placement of the ultrasound transducer to obtain a subxiphoid view. The index marker is pointed to the patient's right (*arrow*).

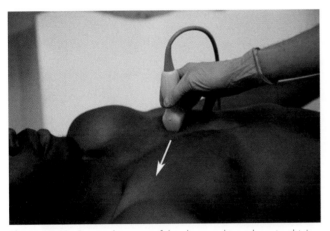

Figure 20.68. Proper placement of the ultrasound transducer to obtain a parasternal long-axis view. The index marker is pointed to the patient's right shoulder (*arrow*).

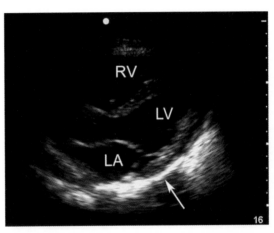

Figure 20.69. Ultrasound image from a normal parasternal long-axis view showing the left atrium (LA), left ventricle (LV), right ventricle (RV), and hyperechoic pericardium (*arrow*).

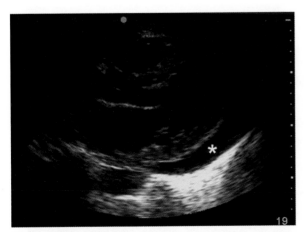

Figure 20.70. Ultrasound image from a parasternal long-axis view, showing a small pericardial effusion (*asterisk*). Although small, if acquired acutely and enlarging, this effusion could lead to tamponade.

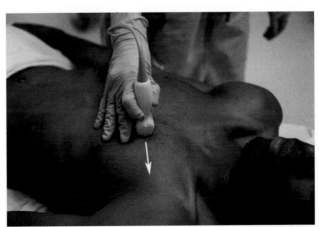

Figure 20.71. Proper placement of the ultrasound transducer to obtain a parasternal short-axis view. The index marker is pointed to the patient's left shoulder (*arrow*).

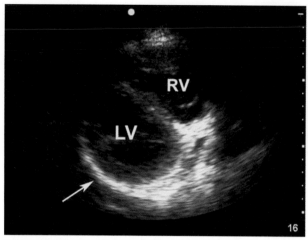

Figure 20.72. Ultrasound image from a normal parasternal short-axis view, showing the left ventricle (LV), right ventricle (RV), and hyperechoic pericardium (*arrow*).

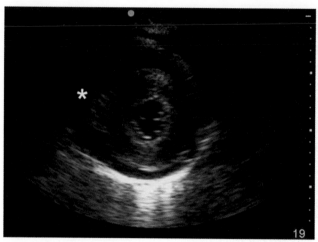

Figure 20.73. Ultrasound image from a parasternal short-axis view demonstrating a circumferential pericardial effusion (*asterisk*).

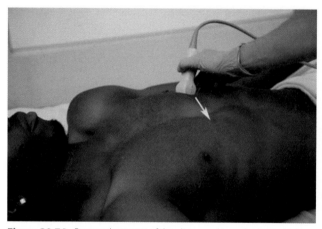

Figure 20.74. Proper placement of the ultrasound transducer to obtain an apical four-chamber view. The index marker is pointed to the patient's right (*arrow*).

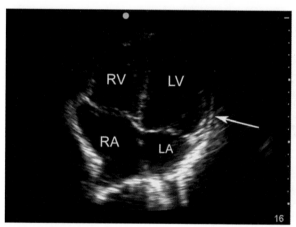

Figure 20.75. Ultrasound image from a normal apical four-chamber view, showing the left atrium (LA), left ventricle (LV), right atrium (RA), right ventricle (RV), and hyperechoic pericardium (*arrow*).

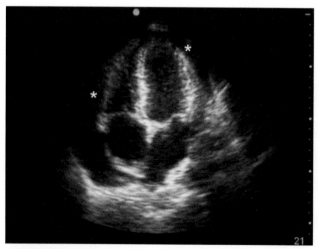

Figure 20.76. Ultrasound image from an apical four-chamber view demonstrating a circumferential pericardial effusion (*asterisk*).

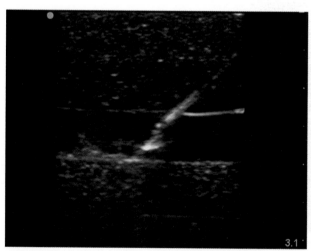

Figure 20.77. Ultrasound image showing turbulence within a phantom vessel.

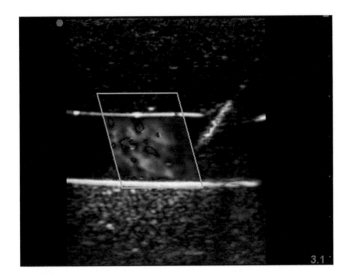

Figure 20.78. Ultrasound image showing turbulence within a phantom vessel highlighted by color Doppler.

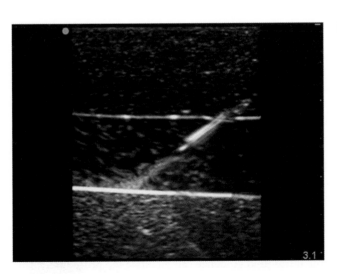

Figure 20.79. Process of agitating saline ultrasound contrast.

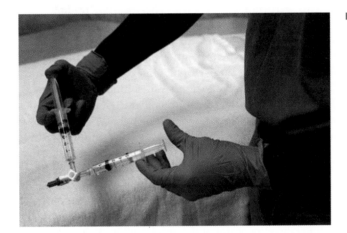

Figure 20.80. Ultrasound image of agitated saline within a phantom vessel.

Arthrocentesis

Indications

The indications for arthrocentesis may be divided into two categories: (1) removing fluid from a joint and (2) instilling fluid into a joint. Ultrasound-guided arthrocentesis has been shown to improve success rates and decrease complications for each of these indications.

In the case of a warm erythematous joint, a diagnostic arthrocentesis is indicated. Fluid should be removed and analyzed to differentiate a septic joint requiring antibiotics and likely surgical washout, as opposed to a joint plagued by gout. A diagnostic arthrocentesis may be difficult in these cases because of severe pain and tenderness of the joint. Ultrasound-guided arthrocentesis has been shown to improve accuracy (101–103), increase aspirated fluid volume (104–106), produce less procedural pain (104–106), shorten procedure time (105), and improve clinical outcome (102, 104, 106, 107) when compared with traditional techniques based on anatomic landmarks. Arthrocentesis to remove fluid may be therapeutic if the effusion is causing pain due to increased pressure within the joint. In addition to symptomatic improvement, removal of blood from a joint, such as the shoulder, may facilitate rehabilitation by increasing mobility and preventing an adhesive capsulitis.

Arthrocentesis that stills fluid into a joint may be diagnostic. For example, a saline arthrogram can demonstrate joint integrity or traumatic disruption. Instilling medication into an inflamed or injured joint may be therapeutic. For example, an injection of steroids into an inflamed arthritic joint has proven to be therapeutic. The synovial lining contains opiate receptors. The intra-articular injection of a combination of an opiate and local anesthetic (e.g., bupivicaine or lidocaine) may provide prolonged analgesia sufficient to allow for successful reduction of a dislocated joint.

Anatomical considerations

Knowledge of the ultrasound appearance of normal anatomy is crucial to facilitate successful penetration of the joint space and avoid injury to important structures. Bone reflects most sound waves and demonstrates a bright reflection with underlying shadow. The joint capsule appears echogenic, similar to the pericardium, and is often highlighted by an effusion. Blood vessels have round or ovoid walls with central anechoic lumens that demonstrate blood flow with Doppler (see Fig. 20.50, earlier in this chapter). Nerves have a honeycomb appearance and may be hyperechoic or hypoechoic depending on anatomic location. Tendons resemble both nerve and muscle with a laminated slippery appearance. Bursas, filled with fluid or gel, are generally hypoechoic. Bursas are ovoid and self-contained, which may be demonstrated by scanning in two orthogonal planes.

In cases of bursitis, they will light up with Doppler showing inflammatory hyperemia.

Abnormal joint anatomy is primarily fluid detected within the joint space. Fluid appears anechoic and black or dark gray depending on the density of the effusion.

Procedure

Most joints are superficial, and, therefore, a high-frequency linear transducer will provide the best ultrasound image for arthrocentesis. The main exception would be the hip joint, in which case a lower frequency curvilinear transducer may be most appropriate. Adjust gain settings to optimize the image quality. Fluid within blood vessels and effusions appear black, and cortex of bone appears white. Depth should be adjusted to maximize the size of the joint on the screen while allowing important deep structures to be visible in the far field.

To appreciate the 3D anatomy, scan the area of interest in two perpendicular planes. The location of important structures, such as nerves, tendons, and blood vessels, should be noted as the path of the needle is plotted. Doppler flow may help identify blood vessels, though this is usually unnecessary. Doppler may be used to identify flow of an obscure effusion as the joint is compressed. This is similar to the flow of pus identifying an abscess as it is compressed. Note the depth of the effusion, and estimate the distance the needle will travel during the arthrocentesis. In general, the trajectory of the needle should aim for the largest pocket of the effusion while avoiding important adjacent structures.

In most cases, arthrocentesis is performed without real-time ultrasound guidance. Ultrasound is used to identify the optimal insertion point of the needle and its path to the joint. The transducer should be moved so the insertion point is in the middle of the screen, which corresponds to the middle of the transducer. A surgical pen can then be used to mark the skin adjacent to the center of the transducer. Marking the ends of the transducer as well allows the insertion point to be triangulated and marked at the intersection of the lines drawn through these points. Prep and drape the area in the usual sterile fashion. Pass the needle through the skin at the marked insertion point and advance until the tip lies within the joint and synovial fluid is withdrawn. Send a sample of the fluid to the laboratory for analysis. To alleviate pain from joint pressure and improve range of motion, aspirate as much fluid as possible. When aspiration is completed, a syringe containing analgesics or a steroid may be attached to the needle and injected into the joint to provide additional symptomatic relief.

In cases where the effusion is small and a diagnostic arthrocentesis is crucial, such as ruling out a septic joint, real-time ultrasound guidance can facilitate the procedure. Using a sterile probe cover, insert the needle at the end of the transducer. The needle should be maintained within the plane of the sound beam throughout the procedure. This allows the sonographer to visualize the needle at all times and make adjustments to guide the needle into the joint space. Once the tip of the needle is within the joint space, the transducer may be set aside and the procedure continued as usual.

Imaging pitfalls and limitations

- In the management of trauma patients, complete primary and secondary trauma surveys prior to focusing on joint injuries.
- The in-plane technique for real-time guidance may offer improved safety.
- Careful attention to sterile technique during arthrocentesis decreases the risk of introducing infection.
- Review joint anatomy prior to procedure to reduce risk of injury to surrounding structures.
- Aspirate before all injections.
- Failure to adhere to sterile technique may result in the introduction of infection into the joint.
- Avoiding a dry tap by demonstrating a joint or bursa absent of fluid.
- Be careful to prevent instillation of medication into a vascular or neurologic structure.
- Injury to surrounding structure may occur as a result of lack of knowledge or sonographic appearance of surrounding anatomy.
- One may introduce discomfort and decreased mobility by overfilling joints during instillation of medication.

Acknowledgements

The authors would like to thank David E. LaTouche, the model for this chapter, and Alfredo Tirado, MD; Arun Nagdev, MD; and Michael Stone, MD, RDMS, for providing images.

References

1. Chen L, Hsiao AL, Moore CL, et al.: Utility of bedside bladder ultrasound before urethral catheterization in young children. *Pediatrics* 2005;**115**(1):108–11.

2. Witt M, Baumann BM, McCans K: Bladder ultrasound increases catheterization success in pediatric patients. *Acad Emerg Med* 2005;**12**(4):371–4.

3. Chu RW, Wong YC, Luk SH, Wong SN: Comparing suprapubic urine aspiration under real-time ultrasound guidance with conventional blind aspiration. *Acta Paediatr* 2002;**91**(5):512–16.

4. Garcia-Nieto V, Navarro JF, Sanchez-Almeida E, Garcia-Garcia M: Standards for ultrasound guidance of suprapubic bladder aspiration. *Pediatr Nephrol* 1997;**11**(5):607–9.

5. Gochman RF, Karasic RB, Heller MB: Use of portable ultrasound to assist urine collection by suprapubic aspiration. *Ann Emerg Med* 1991;**20**(6):631–5.

6. Goldberg BB, Meyer H: Ultrasonically guided suprapubic urinary bladder aspiration. *Pediatrics* 1973;**51**(1):70–4.

7. Kiernan SC, Pinckert TL, Keszler M: Ultrasound guidance of suprapubic bladder aspiration in neonates. *J Pediatr* 1993;**123** (5):789–91.

8. Ozkan B, Kaya O, Akdag R, et al.: Suprapubic bladder aspiration with or without ultrasound guidance. *Clin Pediatr (Phila)* 2000;**39**(10):625–6.

9. Sagi EF, Alpan G, Eyal FG, et al.: Ultrasonic guidance of suprapubic aspiration in infants. *J Clin Ultrasound* 1983;**11**(6): 347–8.

10. Raad I: Intravascular-catheter–related infections. *Lancet* 1998;**351**(9106):893–8.

11. Merrer J, De Jonghe B, Golliot F, et al.: Complications of femoral and subclavian venous catheterization in critically ill patients: a randomized controlled trial. *JAMA* 2001;**286**(6): 700–7.

12. Gallieni M, Cozzolino M: Uncomplicated central vein catheterization of high risk patients with real time ultrasound guidance. *Int J Artif Organs* 1995;**18**(3):117–21.

13. Hind D, Calvert N, McWilliams R, et al: Ultrasonic locating devices for central venous cannulation: meta-analysis. *BMJ* 2003;**327**(7411):361.

14. Kohn L, Corrigan J, Molla S, Donaldson M: *To err is human: building a safer health system.* Washington, DC: Committee on Quality of Health Care in America, Institute of Medicine, 1999.

15. Shojania KG, Duncan BW, McDonald KM, Wachter R, eds: *Making health care safer: a critical analysis of patient safety practices. Evidence report/technology assessment no. 43.* Rockville, MD: Agency for Healthcare Research and Quality, 2001. AHRQ Publication No. 01-E058.

16. Grebenik CR, Boyce A, Sinclair ME, et al.: NICE guidelines for central venous catheterization in children: is the evidence base sufficient? *Br J Anaesth* 2004;**92**(6):827–30.

17. Domino KB, Bowdle TA, Posner KL, et al.: Injuries and liability related to central vascular catheters: a closed claims analysis. *Anesthesiology* 2004;**100**(6):1411–18.

18. McGee DC, Gould MK: Preventing complications of central venous catheterization. *N Engl J Med* 2003;**348**(12):1123–33.

19. Terai C, Anada H, Matsushima S, et al.: Effects of mild Trendelenburg on central hemodynamics and internal jugular vein velocity, cross-sectional area, and flow. *Am J Emerg Med* 1995;**13**(3):255–8.

20. Lobato EB, Florete OG Jr, Paige GB, Morey TE: Cross-sectional area and intravascular pressure of the right internal jugular vein during anesthesia: effects of Trendelenburg position, positive intrathoracic pressure, and hepatic compression. *J Clin Anesth* 1998;**10**(1):1–5.

21. Mallory DL, Shawker T, Evans RG, et al.: Effects of clinical maneuvers on sonographically determined internal jugular vein size during venous cannulation. *Crit Care Med* 1990;**18**(11): 1269–73.

22. Armstrong PJ, Sutherland R, Scott DH: The effect of position and different manoeuvres on internal jugular vein diameter size. *Acta Anaesthesiol Scand* 1994;**38**(3):229–31.

23. Gordon AC, Saliken JC, Johns D, et al.: US-guided puncture of the internal jugular vein: complications and anatomic considerations. *J Vasc Interv Radiol* 1998;**9**(2):333–8.

24. Gualtieri E, Deppe SA, Sipperly ME, Thompson DR: Subclavian venous catheterization: greater success rate for less experienced operators using ultrasound guidance. *Crit Care Med* 1995;**23**(4):692–7.

25. Hilty WM, Hudson PA, Levitt MA, Hall JB: Real-time ultrasound-guided femoral vein catheterization during cardiopulmonary resuscitation. *Ann Emerg Med* 1997;**29**(3): 331–6.

26. Yanay O, Vaughan DJ, Diab M, et al.: Retained wooden foreign body in a child's thigh complicated by severe necrotizing fasciitis: a case report and discussion of imaging modalities for early diagnosis. *Pediatr Emerg Care* 2001;**17**(4): 354–5.

27. Boyse TD, Fessell DP, Jacobson JA, et al.: Ultrasound of soft-tissue foreign bodies and associated complications with surgical correlation. *Radiographics* 2001;**21**(5):1251–6.

28. Hung YT, Hung LK, Griffith JF, et al.: Ultrasound for the detection of vegetative foreign body in the hand – a case report. *Hand Surg* 2004;**9**(1):83–7.

29. Graham DD: Ultrasound in the emergency department: detection of wooden foreign bodies in the soft tissues. *J Emerg Med* 2002;**22**(1):75–9.

30. Soudack M, Nachtigal A, Gaitini D: Clinically unsuspected foreign bodies: the importance of sonography. *J Ultrasound Med* 2003;**22**(12):1381–5.

31. Lammers RL, Magill T: Detection and management of foreign bodies in soft tissue. *Emerg Med Clin North Am* 1992;**10**(4): 767–81.

32. Schlager D: Ultrasound detection of foreign bodies and procedure guidance. *Emerg Med Clin North Am* 1997;**15** (15):895–912.

33. Trautlein JJ, Lambert RL, Miller J: Malpractice in the emergency department – review of 200 cases. *Ann Emerg Med* 1984;**13**(9 pt 1):709–11.

34. Gilbert FJ, Campbell RS, Bayliss AP: The role of ultrasound in the detection on non-radiopaque foreign bodies. *Clin Radiol* 1990;**41**(2):109–12.

35. Shiels WE, Babcock D, Wilson J, Burch R: Localization and guided removal of soft-tissue foreign bodies with sonography. *AJR Am J Roentgenol* 1990;**155**(6):1277–81.

36. Rockett MS, Gentile SC, Gudas CJ, et al.: The use of ultrasonography for the detection of retained wooden foreign bodies in the foot. *J Foot Ankle Surg* 1995;**34**(5):478–84; discussion 510–11.

37. Crawford R, Matheson AB: Clinical value of ultrasonography in the detection and removal of radiolucent foreign bodies. *Injury* 1989;**20**(6):341–3.

38. Blankstein A, Cohen I, Heiman Z, et al.: Localization, detection and guided removal of soft tissue in the hands using sonography. *Arch Orthop Trauma Surg* 2000;**120**(9):514–17.

39. Jacobson JA, Powell A, Craig JG, et al.: Wooden foreign bodies in soft tissue: detection with ultrasound. *Radiology* 1998;**206**(7): 45–8.

40. Bradley M, Kadzombe E, Simms P, Eyes B: Percutaneous ultrasound guided extraction of non-palpable soft tissue foreign bodies. *Arch Emerg Med* 1992;**9**:181–4.

41. Heller M, Jehle D: *Ultrasound in emergency medicine.* Oxford, UK: WB Saunders, 1995.

42. Lyon M, Brannam L, Johnson D, et al.: Detection of soft tissue foreign bodies in the presence of soft tissue gas. *J Ultrasound Med* 2004;**23**(5):677–81.

43. Gooding GA, Hardiman T, Sumers M, et al.: Sonography of the hand and foot in foreign body detection. *J Ultrasound Med* 1987;**6**(8):441–7.

44. Banerjee B, Das RK: Sonographic detection of foreign bodies of the extremities. *Br J Radiol* 1991;**64**(758):107–12.

45. Schlager D, Johnson T, Mcfall R: Safety of imaging exploding bullets with ultrasound. *Ann Emerg Med* 1996;**28** (13):183–7.

46. Turner J, Wilde CH, Hughes KC, et al.: Ultrasound-guided retrieval of small foreign objects in subcutaneous tissue. *Ann Emerg Med* 1997;**29**(5):731–4.

47. Schlager D: Ultrasound detection of foreign bodies and procedure guidance. *Emerg Med Clin North Am* 1997;**15** (15):895–912.

48. Oikarinen KS, Nieminen T, Makarainen H, Pyhtinen J: Visibility of foreign bodies in soft tissue in plain radiographs, computed tomography, magnetic resonance imaging, and ultrasound: an in vitro study. *Int J Oral Maxillofac Surg* 1993;**22** (2):119–24.

49. Scanlan KA: Sonographic artifacts and their origins. *AJR Am J Roentgenol* 1991;**156**(6):1267–72.

50. Hill R, Conron R, Greissinger P, Heller M: Ultrasound for the detection of foreign bodies in human tissue. *Ann Emerg Med* 1997;**29**(10):353–6.

51. Fornage BD: The hypoechoic normal tendon: a pitfall. *J Ultrasound Med* 1987;**6**(1):19–22.

52. Leung A, Patton A, Navoy J, Cummings RJ: Intraoperative sonography-guided removal of radiolucent foreign bodies. *J Pediatr Orthop* 1998;**18**(2):259–61.

53. Orlinsky M, Knittel P, Feit T, et al.: The comparative accuracy of radiolucent foreign body detection using ultrasonography. *Am J Emerg Med* 2000;**18**(6):401–3.

54. Nelson AL, Sinow RM: Real-time ultrasonographically guided removal of nonpalpable and intramuscular Norplant capsules. *Am J Obstet Gynecol* 1998;**78**(12):1185–93.

55. Frankel DA, Bargiela A, Bouffard JA: Synovial joints: evaluation of intraarticular bodies with US. *Radiology* 1998;**206**(16):41–4.

56. Manthey DE, Storrow AB, Milbourn JM, Wagner BJ: Ultrasound versus radiography in the detection of soft-tissue foreign bodies. *Ann Emerg Med* 1996;**28**(11):7–9.

57. Teisen HG, Torfing KF, Skjodt T: Ultrasound pinpointing of foreign bodies: an in vitro study. *Ultraschall Med* 1988;**9**(3):135–7.

58. Blankstein A, Cohen I, Heiman Z, et al.: Ultrasonography as a diagnostic modality and therapeutic adjuvant in the management of soft tissue foreign bodies in the lower extremities. *Isr Med Assoc J* 2001;**3**(6):411–13.

59. Tayal VS, Nicks BA, Norton HJ: Emergency ultrasound evaluation of symptomatic nontraumatic pleural effusions. *Am J Emerg Med* 2006;**24**(7):782–6.

60. Diacon AH, Brutsche MH, Soler M: Accuracy of pleural puncture sites: a prospective comparison of clinical examination with ultrasound. *Chest* 2003;**123**(2):436–41.

61. Bartter T, Mayo PD, Pratter MR, et al.: Lower risk and higher yield for thoracentesis when performed by experienced operators. *Chest* 1993;**103**(6):1873–6.

62. Collins TR, Sahn SA: Thoracocentesis: clinical value, complications, technical problems, and patient experience. *Chest* 1987;**91**(6):817–22.

63. Grogan DR, Irwin RS, Channick R, et al.: Complications associated with thoracentesis: a prospective, randomized study comparing three different methods. *Arch Intern Med* 1990;**150**(4):873–7.

64. Seneff MG, Corwin RW, Gold LH, Irwin RS: Complications associated with thoracocentesis. *Chest* 1986;**90**(1):97–100.

65. Jones PW, Moyers JP, Rogers JT, et al.: Ultrasound-guided thoracentesis: is it a safer method? *Chest* 2003;**123**(2):418–23.

66. Mayo PH, Goltz HR, Tafreshi M, Doelken P: Safety of ultrasound-guided thoracentesis in patients receiving mechanical ventilation. *Chest* 2004;**125**(3):1059–62.

67. Blaivas M, Lyon M, Duggal S: A prospective comparison of supine chest radiography and bedside ultrasound for the diagnosis of traumatic pneumothorax. *Acad Emerg Med* 2005;**12**(9):844–9.

68. Coley BD, Shiels WE II, Hogan MJ: Diagnostic and interventional ultrasonography in neonatal and infant lumbar puncture. *Pediatr Radiol* 2001;**31**(6):399–402.

69. Cork RC, Kryc JJ, Vaughan RW: Ultrasonic localization of the lumbar epidural space. *Anesthesiology* 1980;**52**(6):513–16.

70. Currie JM: Measurement of the depth to the extradural space using ultrasound. *Br J Anaesth* 1984;**56**(4):345–7.

71. Peterson MA, Abele J: Bedside ultrasound for difficult lumbar puncture. *J Emerg Med* 2005;**28**(2):197–200.

72. Sandoval M, Shestak W, Sturmann K, Hsu C: Optimal patient position for lumbar puncture, measured by ultrasonography. *Emerg Radiol* 2004;**10**(4):179–81.

73. Wallace DH, Currie JM, Gilstrap LC, Santos R: Indirect sonographic guidance for epidural anesthesia in obese pregnant patients. *Reg Anesth* 1992;**17**(4):233–6.

74. Nomura JT, Leech SJ, Shenbagamurthi S, et al.: A randomized controlled trial of ultrasound-assisted lumbar puncture. *J Ultrasound Med* 2007;**26**(10):1341–8.

75. Cattau EL Jr, Benjamin SB, Knuff TE, Castell DO: The accuracy of the physical examination in the diagnosis of suspected ascites. *JAMA* 1982;**247**(8):1164–6.

76. Nazeer SR, Dewbre H, Miller AH: Ultrasound-assisted paracentesis performed by emergency physicians vs the traditional technique: a prospective, randomized study. *Am J Emerg Med* 2005;**23**(3):363–7.

77. Bard C, Lafortune M, Breton G: Ascites: ultrasound guidance or blind paracentesis? *CMAJ* 1986;**135**(3):209–10.

78. Feigenbaum H, Waldhausen JA, Hyde LP: Ultrasound diagnosis of pericardial effusion. *JAMA* 1965;**191**:711–14.

79. Mazurek B, Jehle D, Martin M: Emergency department echocardiography in the diagnosis and therapy of cardiac tamponade. *J Emerg Med* 1991;**9**(1–2):27–31.

80. American College of Surgeons (ACS) Committee on Trauma: *Advanced trauma life support course for doctors: student course manual*, 7th ed. Chicago: ACS, 2004.

81. Guberman BA, Fowler NO, Engel PJ, et al.: Cardiac tamponade in medical patients. *Circulation* 1981;**64**(3):633–40.

82. Wong B, Murphy J, Chang CJ, et al.: The risk of pericardiocentesis. *Am J Cardiol* 1979;**44**(6):1110–14.

83. Vayre F, Lardoux H, Pezzano M, et al.: Subxiphoid pericardiocentesis guided by contrast two-dimensional echocardiography in cardiac tamponade: experience of 110 consecutive patients. *Eur J Echocardiogr* 2000;**1**(1):66–71.

84. Ball JB, Morrison WL: Cardiac tamponade. *Postgrad Med J* 1997;**73**(857):141–5.

85. Bishop LH Jr, Estes EH Jr, McIntosh HD: The electrocardiogram as a safeguard in pericardiocentesis. *JAMA* 1956;**162**(4):264–5.

86. Buzaid AC, Garewal HS, Greenberg BR: Managing malignant pericardial effusion. *West J Med* 1989;**150**(2):174–9.

87. Hingorani AD, Bloomberg TJ: Ultrasound-guided pigtail catheter drainage of malignant pericardial effusions. *Clin Radiol* 1995;**50**(1):15–19.

88. Krikorian JG, Hancock EW: Pericardiocentesis. *Am J Med* 1978;**65**(5):808–14.

89. Suehiro S, Hattori K, Shibata T, et al.: Echocardiography-guided pericardiocentesis with a needle attached to a probe. *Ann Thorac Surg* 1996;**61**(2):741–2.

90. Tsang TS, Enriquez-Sarano M, Freeman WK, et al.: Consecutive 1127 therapeutic echocardiographically guided pericardiocenteses: clinical profile, practice patterns, and outcomes spanning 21 years. *Mayo Clin Proc* 2002;**77**(5):429–36.

91. Tsang TS, El-Najdawi EK, Seward JB, et al.: Percutaneous echocardiographically guided pericardiocentesis in pediatric patients: evaluation of safety and efficacy. *J Am Soc Echocardiogr* 1998;**11**(11):1072–7.

92. Callahan JA, Seward JB, Tajik AJ: Cardiac tamponade: pericardiocentesis directed by two-dimensional echocardiography. *Mayo Clin Proc* 1985;**60**(5):344–7.

93. Tsang TS, Freeman WK, Sinak LJ, Seward JB: Echocardiographically guided pericardiocentesis: evolution and state-of-the-art technique. *Mayo Clin Proc* 1998;**73**(7):647–52.

94. Appleton CP, Hatle LK, Popp RL: Cardiac tamponade and pericardial effusion: respiratory variation in transvalvular flow velocities studied by Doppler echocardiography. *J Am Coll Cardiol* 1988;**11**(5):1020–30.

95. Armstrong WF, Schilt BF, Helper DJ, et al.: Diastolic collapse of the right ventricle with cardiac tamponade: an echocardiographic study. *Circulation* 1982;**65**(7):1491–6.

96. Burstow DJ, Oh JK, Bailey KR, et al.: Cardiac tamponade: characteristic Doppler observations. *Mayo Clin Proc* 1989;**64**(3):312–24.

97. Feigenbaum H, Zaky A, Grabhorn LL: Cardiac motion in patients with pericardial effusion: a study using reflected ultrasound. *Circulation* 1966;**34**(4):611–19.

98. Kronzon I, Cohen ML, Winer HE: Diastolic atrial compression: a sensitive echocardiographic sign of cardiac tamponade. *J Am Coll Cardiol* 1983;**2**(4):770–5.

99. Tsang TS, Seward JB, Barnes ME, et al.: Outcomes of primary and secondary treatment of pericardial effusion in patients with malignancy. *Mayo Clin Proc* 2000;**75**(3):248–53.

100. Tsang TS, Barnes ME, Hayes SN, et al.: Clinical and echocardiographic characteristics of significant pericardial effusions following cardiothoracic surgery and outcomes of echo-guided pericardiocentesis for

management: Mayo Clinic experience, 1979–1998. *Chest* 1999;**116**(2):322–31.

101. Im SH, Lee SC, Park YB, et al.: Feasibility of sonography for intra-articular injections in the knee through a medial patellar portal. *J Ultrasound Med* 2009;**23**(11):1465–70.

102. Cunnington J, Marshall N, Hide G, et al.: A randomized, double-blind, controlled study of ultrasound-guided corticosteroid injection into the joint of patients with inflammatory arthritis. *Arthritis Rheum* 2010;**62**(7): 1862–9.

103. Raza K, Lee CY, Pilling D, et al.: Ultrasound guidance allows accurate needle placement and aspiration from small joints in patients with early inflammatory arthritis. *Rheumatology* 2003;**42**(8):976–9.

104. Sibbitt W, Kettwich L, Band P, et al.: Does ultrasound guidance improve the outcomes of arthrocentesis and corticosteroid injections of the knee? *Scand J Rheumatol* 2012;**41**(1):66–72.

105. Wiler JL, Constantino TG, Filippone L, et al.: Comparison of ultrasound-guided and standard landmark techniques for knee arthrocentesis. *J Emerg Med* 2010;**39**(1):76–82.

106. Sibbitt WL, Peisajovich A, Michael AA, et al.: Does sonographic needle guidance affect the clinical outcome of intraarticular injections? *J Rheumatol* 2009;**36**(9):1892–1902.

107. Soh E, Li W, Ong KO, et al.: Image-guided versus blind corticosteroid injections in adults with shoulder pain: a systematic review. *BMC Musculoskelet Disord* 2011;**12**:137.

Chapter 21

Abdominal–Pelvic Ultrasound

Mike Lambert

Indications

Abdominal-pelvic ultrasounds ordered or performed in the ED are used to diagnose life-threatening obstetrical or gynecological diseases that may require emergent surgery. Any pregnant patient with lower abdominal pain with or without vaginal bleeding requires an ultrasound to rule out an extrauterine gestation (ectopic pregnancy). Nonpregnant patients with lower abdominal pain, pelvic pain, or tenderness on bimanual examination are also candidates for a pelvic ultrasound to rule out ovarian torsion or tuboovarian abscess. Pelvic ultrasound is also capable of helping guide the emergency physician in the management of other nonemergent obstetrical or gynecological disease processes, such as incarcerated uterus, abnormal intrauterine pregnancies, no definitive pregnancies, and ruptured ovarian cysts.

Diagnostic capabilities

The following entities are readily diagnosed using abdominal-pelvic ultrasound:

1. Extrauterine pregnancies
2. Incarcerated uterus
3. Live intrauterine pregnancies (LIUPs)
4. Intrauterine pregnancies (IUPs)
5. Abnormal intrauterine pregnancies (AbnIUPs)
6. No definitive intrauterine pregnancies (NDIUPs)
7. Ovarian torsion
8. Tuboovarian abscess
9. Ovarian cysts (OCs)
10. Uterine fibroids
11. Gynecological cancer

Imaging pitfalls and limitations

There are some potential limitations to abdominal-pelvic ultrasound:

- Transabdominal ultrasound imaging – Obesity can frequently interfere with the quality of the image displayed by providing further distance between the transducer and the area of interest. An unfilled or small bladder bowel allows bowel to become interposed between the peritoneum and the uterus, causing the sound beam to scatter and thus produce poor imaging of the pelvis.
- Endovaginal ultrasound imaging – A full bladder typically repositions the normally anteverted uterus farther away

from the transducer, limiting the imaging quality of this high-frequency probe. It also creates side lobe artifacts, which commonly distort the view of the uterine fundus and its contents.

Clinical images

This section is divided into three parts. Part 1 includes gynecological normal images of the uterus, ovaries, and bladder in sagittal and coronal planes. Part 2 includes obstetrical normal images of the uterus and ovaries in sagittal and coronal planes.

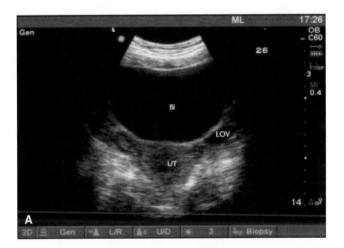

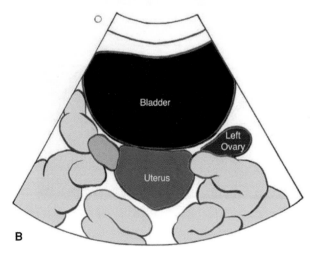

Figure 21.1. A: Transabdominal axial (transverse) view of the UT, OV, and Bl. B: Schematic of transabdominal axial (transverse) view of the UT, OV, and Bl.

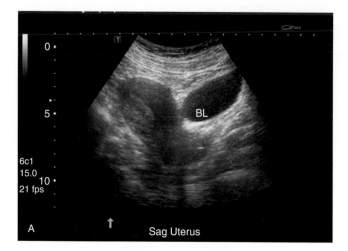

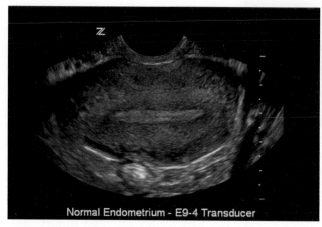

Figure 21.4. Endovaginal coronal view of the UT and EMS.

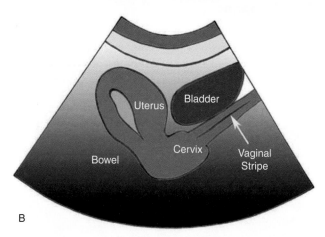

Figure 21.2. A: Transabdominal sagittal (longitudinal) view of the UT, vaginal stripe, and Bl. B: Schematic transabdominal sagittal view of the UT, vaginal stripe, and Bl.

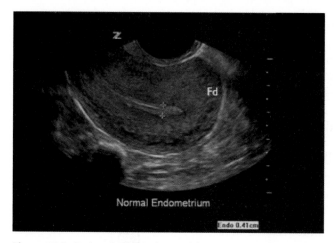

Figure 21.5. Endovaginal sagittal view of the retroverted UT. Notice the fundus (Fd) of the UT is oriented toward the right side of the image.

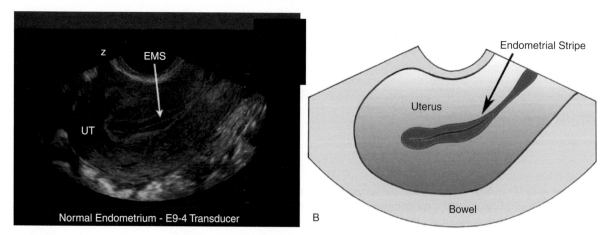

Figure 21.3. A: Endovaginal sagittal view of the UT and the three distinct layers of the endometrial stripe (EMS). B: Schematic endovaginal sagittal view of the UT and EMS.

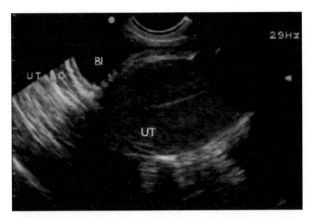

Figure 21.6. Endovaginal longitudinal view of the UT and Bl anterior and superior to the UT.

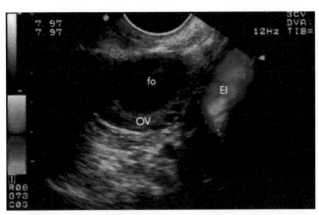

Figure 21.7. Endovaginal sagittal view of the left OV. There is a large follicle (fo) in the center of the OV with smaller follicles at the periphery. The external iliac (EI) vessel is visualized in its long axis just inferior to the ovary.

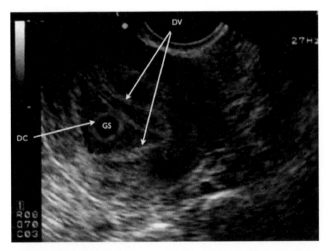

Figure 21.8. Endovaginal sagittal view of an IUP. The anechoic GS of ~8 mm has a thick concentric hyperechoic rim. During pregnancy, the hyperechoic endometrial lining of the UT (decidua vera = DV) also envelops the GS (referred to as the decidua capsularis = DC) to illustrate the "double bubble" (or DDS sign).

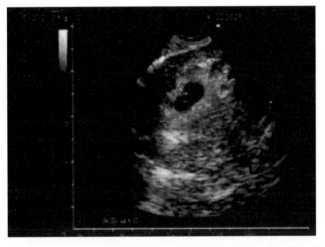

Figure 21.9. IUP. Transabdominal sagittal (longitudinal) view of the UT, with YS seen within the GS. A safe criterion for IUP is a GS with a mean sac diameter (MSD) greater than 5 mm and evidence of a YS or FP. Although a DDS is the earliest sign of pregnancy, it can be mistaken for a pseudogestational sac (PGS).

Part 3 includes interesting and pathological images of the uterus, ovaries, and adnexa in sagittal, coronal, and some oblique planes.

Part 1: The following images are normal gynecological ultrasound images or images with normal variants of the uterus (UT), ovaries (OV), and bladder (Bl) in sagittal and coronal planes.

Part 2: The following images are obstetrical ultrasound images of the UT, OV, and adnexa in sagittal and coronal planes. When pregnancy has been established by a urine or serum pregnancy test, an ultrasound documents where the pregnancy is located. There are three ultrasound categories commonly used to describe the location of a pregnancy: 1) within the endometrial echo of the UT, 2) outside the endometrial echo of the UT, and 3) the pregnancy cannot be clearly localized.

Section 1: Pregnancy localized within the endometrial echo of the UT. There are three distinct diagnostic criteria to pregnancies localized within the UT: IUP, LIUP, and AbnIUP. IUP documented by ultrasound using this label should clearly provide landmarks (LMs) of a gestational sac (GS) of at least 5 mm with a concentric echogenic rim *within* the endometrial echo of the UT with evidence of a double decidual sac (DDS) sign, a yolk sac (YS), or a fetal pole (FP).

Section 2: Pregnancy localized outside the endometrial echo of the UT. This extrauterine gestation (EUG) is commonly referred to as an ectopic pregnancy. To fulfill this criterion, we would need LMs of a GS of at least 5 mm MSD with an echogenic rim *outside* the endometrial echo of the UT with evidence of a YS or an FP.

Section 3: Pregnancy cannot be clearly localized. To fulfill this category, we would need LMs of an empty UT, or if there

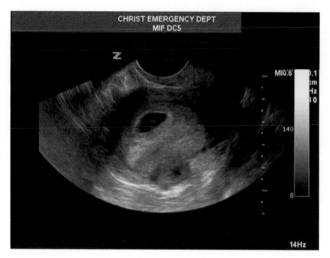

Figure 21.10. Endovaginal longitudinal view of the UT. A definitive sign of early pregnancy is the YS seen within the GS. LIUP documented by ultrasound using this label should clearly provide LM of a GS *within* the endometrial echo of the UT containing an FP with evidence of cardiac activity (CA).

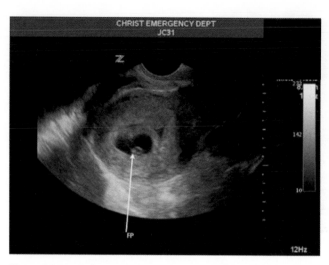

Figure 21.11. Endovaginal longitudinal view of the UT. A YS is seen within the GS, and on the left border, the hyperechoic sidecar is the FP with CA.

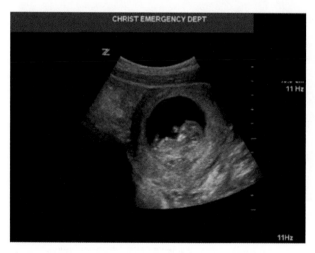

Figure 21.12. Transverse longitudinal view of the UT. An obvious FP with head, arm, and leg are visualized.

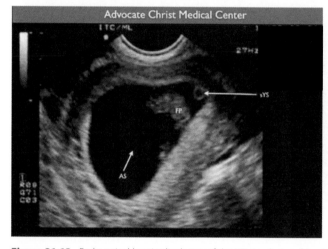

Figure 21.13. Endovaginal longitudinal view of the UT. An obvious fetus is visualized as well as the amniotic sac (AS), which is frequently seen between the ninth and twelfth gestational weeks. The secondary YS is also apparent posterior to the fetus.

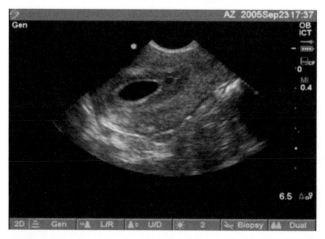

316

Figure 21.14. AbnIUP. Endovaginal sagittal view of the UT reveals a large empty GS. A GS with an MSD greater than 10 mm and no evidence of a YS.

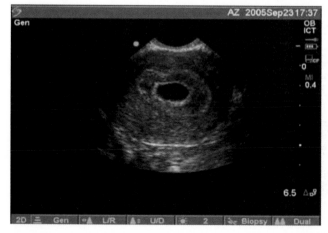

Figure 21.15. AbnIUP. Endovaginal coronal view of the UT reveals a large empty GS.

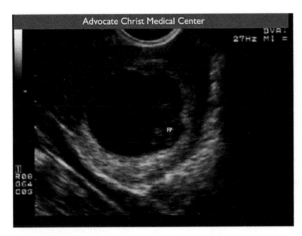

Figure 21.16. AbnIUP. Endovaginal coronal view of the UT reveals a large GS with an obvious FP and no evidence of CA.

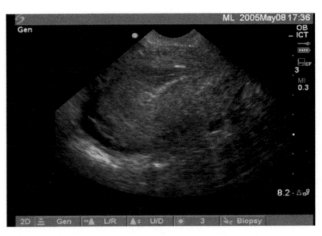

Figure 21.17. Endovaginal midline sagittal view of the UT without evidence of a GS within the endometrial echo of the UT.

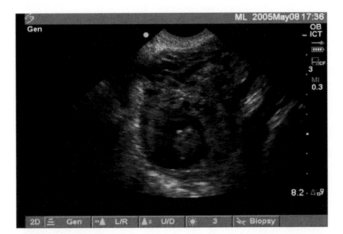

Figure 21.18. Endovaginal right sagittal view of the UT with a GS and FP outside the endometrial echo of the UT. Three hyperechoic extremity buds are visible.

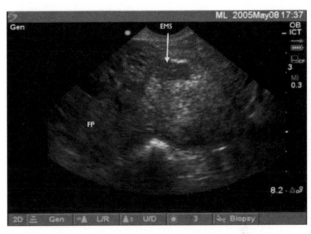

Figure 21.19. Endovaginal coronal view of the UT without evidence of a GS within the endometrial echo of the UT. The right adnexa reveals a poorly visible FP better seen in the more anterior coronal image in Figure 20.18.

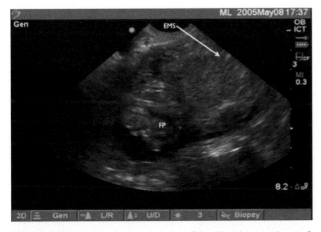

Figure 21.20. Endovaginal coronal view of the UT without evidence of a GS within the endometrial echo of the UT.

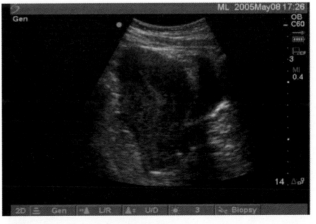

Figure 21.21. Transabdominal view of the UT without evidence of a GS within the endometrial echo of the UT.

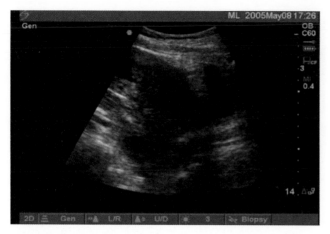

Figure 21.22. Same patient as in Figure 21.21. Transabdominal sagittal view left of the midline with suspicious mass superior and anterior to the UT.

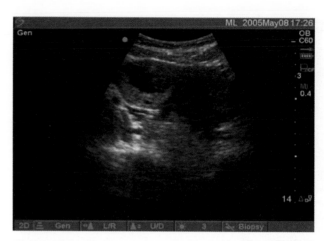

Figure 21.23. Same patient as in Figure 21.21. Transabdominal sagittal view left of the midline with GS and FP superior and slightly anterior to the UT.

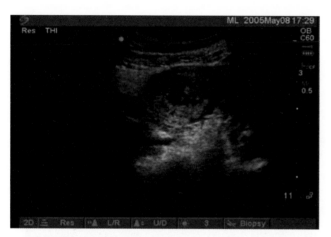

Figure 21.24. Same patient as in Figure 21.21. Transabdominal view of the UT without evidence of a GS within the endometrial echo of the UT.

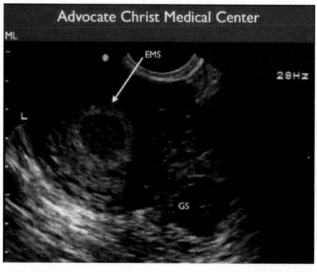

Figure 21.25. Endovaginal coronal view of the UT without evidence of a GS within the endometrial echo of the UT. Adjacent to the right border of the UT is a GS with FP.

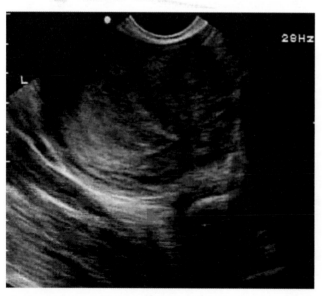

Figure 21.26. The EMS is pointing to the right side of the UT. This is commonly referred to as the "endometrial line sign."

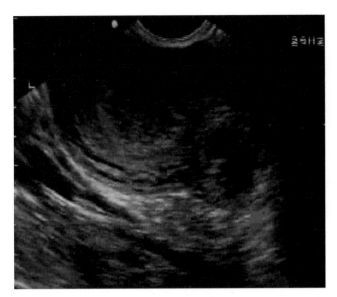

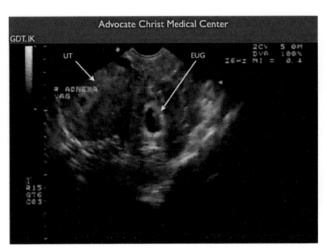

Figure 21.27. Same patient as in Figure 21.26. The EMS is pointing to the right adnexa. This is commonly referred to as the "endometrial line sign." Notice that the GS is partially within the myometrium of the UT. This pregnancy is within the fallopian tube as it passes through the myometrium. This is commonly referred to as a "cornuate" or "interstitial ectopic."

Figure 21.28. Endovaginal sagittal view of the pelvis with evidence of a live EUG posterior to the UT. The saclike structure within the UT has no DDS sign, nor does it meet criteria for an IUP. This is commonly referred to as a PGS.

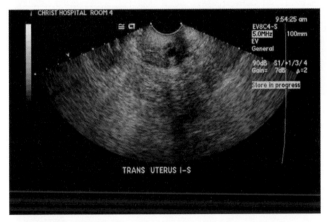

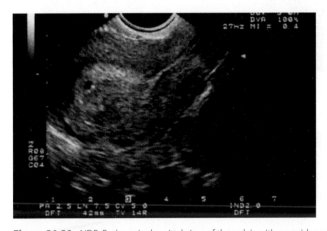

Figure 21.29. NDP. Endovaginal sagittal view of the pelvis with no evidence of a definitive IUP. Images through the pelvis revealed no EUG as well.

Figure 21.30. NDP. Endovaginal sagittal view of the pelvis with no evidence of a definitive IUP. Images through the pelvis revealed no EUG as well.

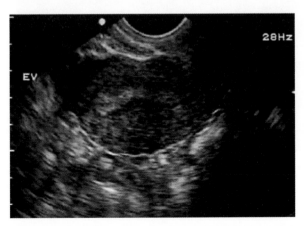

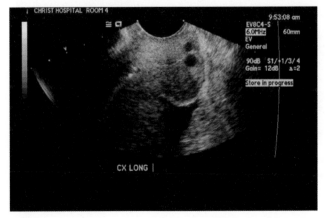

Figure 21.31. Nabothian cysts. Endovaginal longitudinal view of the UT at the level of the cervix. Two anechoic, circular structures near the endocervical canal. These are normal findings in women who have had children.

Figure 21.32. Nabothian cysts. Endovaginal transverse view of the UT at the level of the cervix, demonstrating one of the nabothian cysts in the same patient as in Figure 21.31.

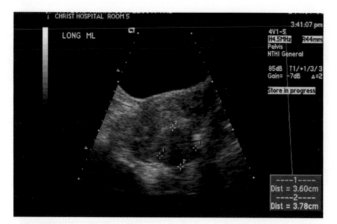

Figure 21.33. Fibroid. Transabdominal axial view of the UT. The concentric hypoechoic mass is the most frequent appearance by ultrasound.

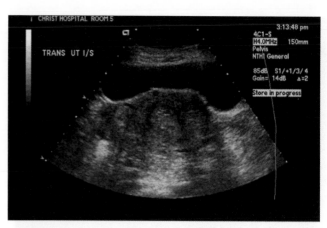

Figure 21.34. Fibroid. Transabdominal axial view of the UT. Fibroids may vary in their degree of echogenicity. In this image, the fibroids appear more hyperechoic.

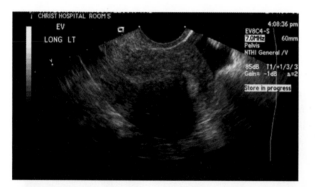

Figure 21.35. Sagittal endovaginal view of UT reveals acoustic shadowing posterior to a uterine fibroid.

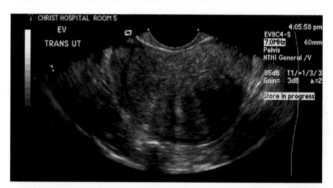

Figure 21.36. Coronal endovaginal view of the same patient as in Figure 21.35, which reveals acoustic shadowing posterior to a uterine fibroid.

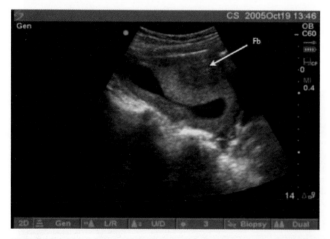

Figure 21.37. Submucosal fibroid. Relatively rare fibroid whose submucosal growth toward the endometrial canal can cause complications in pregnancy.

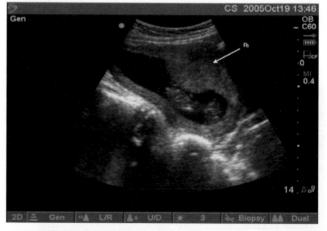

Figure 21.38. Submucosal fibroid. Relatively rare fibroid whose submucosal growth toward the endometrial canal can cause complications in pregnancy.

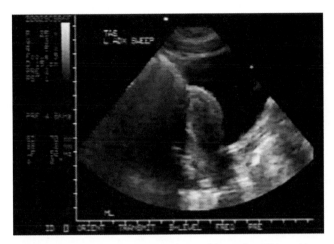

Figure 21.39. Transabdominal sagittal view of the midline UT in an 11-year-old girl with abdominal pain, hypotension, and severe anemia.

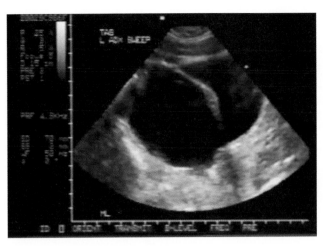

Figure 21.40. Transabdominal sagittal view of the left adnexa in the same patient as in Figure 21.39 reveals a large hemorrhagic OC.

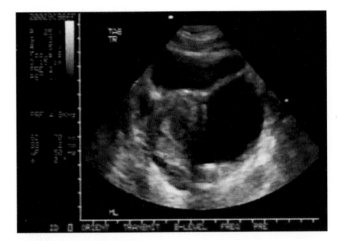

Figure 21.41. Transabdominal transverse view in same patient as in Figure 21.39 reveals a large hemorrhagic OC.

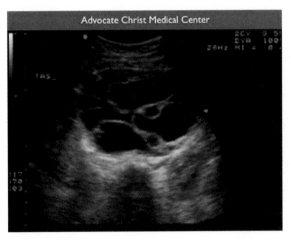

Figure 21.42. Transabdominal sagittal view of a massive OC in a patient with distended abdomen and abdominal pain.

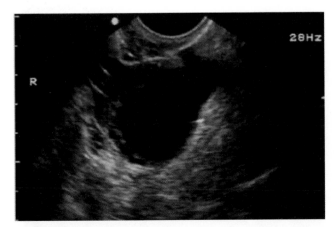

Figure 21.43. OC. Endovaginal sagittal view of the right ovary reveals a typical circular, anechoic OC with thin walls and posterior enhancement.

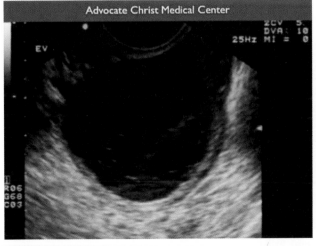

Figure 21.44. Hemorrhagic OC. Endovaginal sagittal view of the right ovary reveals a large OC with internal septation and posterior enhancement.

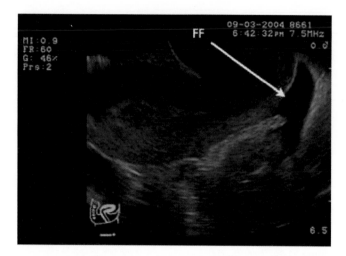

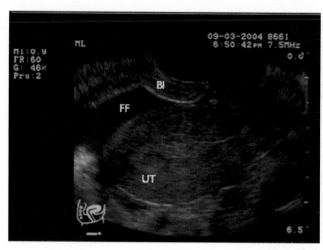

Figure 21.46. Endovaginal longitudinal view of the UT reveals FF in the uterovesicular pouch (anterior cul-de-sac). Notice the empty Bl anteriorly.

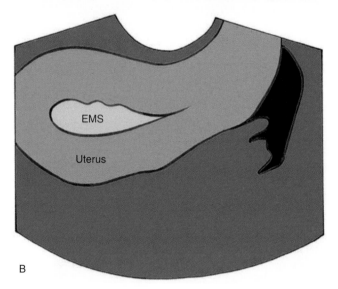

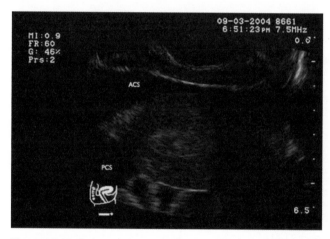

Figure 21.45. A: Endovaginal longitudinal view of the UT reveals free fluid (FF) in the pouch of Douglas (posterior cul-de-sac). Small amount of FF in the pouch of Douglas is a normal variant. B: Schematic of endovaginal longitudinal view of the uterus, revealing FF in the pouch of Douglas (posterior cul-de-sac).

Figure 21.47. Endovaginal coronal view of the UT reveals FF in the uterovesicular pouch (anterior cul-de-sac) and pouch of Douglas (posterior cul-de-sac).

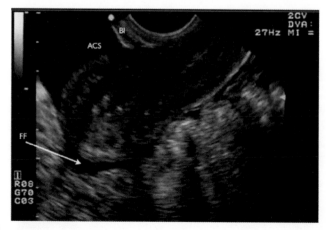

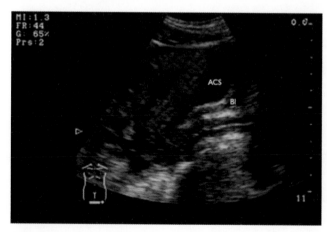

Figure 21.48. Endovaginal longitudinal view of the UT reveals FF in the anterior cul-de-sac (ACS) and surrounding the UT.

Figure 21.49. Transabdominal longitudinal view of the UT reveals FF in the ACS. Notice the empty Bl anteriorly.

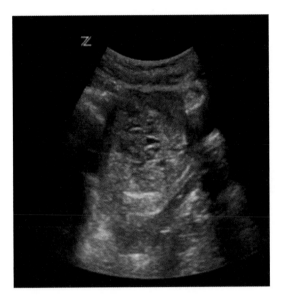

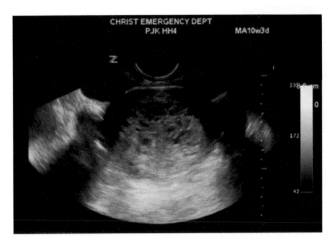

Figure 21.51. Molar pregnancy. Endovaginal coronal view of the UT shows the typical "clusters of grapes" or "snowstorm" appearance.

Figure 21.50. Molar pregnancy ("hydatidiform mole"). Transabdominal longitudinal view of the UT of a pregnant patient shows multiple atypical cystic structures within the endometrial echo of the UT.

appears to be a GS, it does not meet criteria for an IUP. Three diagnostic possibilities exist: 1) the pregnancy is in the correct location, but it is too early to definitively call an IUP; 2) the pregnancy is extrauterine, but there are no definitive LMs to be categorized as an EUG; or 3) spontaneous abortion has occurred. When we cannot clearly localize a pregnancy, it is commonly referred to as an NDIUP. A more concise term would be "no definitive pregnancy" (NDP).

Part 3: Interesting and pathological images of the UT, OV, and adnexa in sagittal, coronal, and some oblique planes.

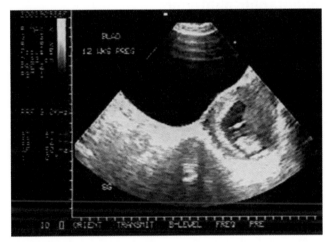

Figure 21.52. Incarcerated uterus. An uncommon pregnancy complication typically occurring around the beginning of the second trimester. Acute urinary retention is present post void in this patient ~12 weeks' gestation.

Ocular Ultrasound

Viet Tran and Zareth Irwin

Introduction

Ultrasound has long been an integral part of the ophthalmologist's evaluation of the eye and orbit. In fact, the use of ocular ultrasound was first published in 1956 (1) and has since come to be used extensively with A-scan, B-scan, Doppler, and, more recently, 3D approaches.

Many of these applications are proving to be useful for emergency medicine clinicians as well. Ocular ultrasound can be used in the outpatient ophthalmology setting for common ED complaints such as retinal detachment (2, 3), ocular foreign bodies (4–8), and optic neuritis (9), among many other applications. Recent studies indicate an even broader use of ocular ultrasound, such as in the early diagnosis of increased intracranial pressure (ICP) (10–17).

The implication, therefore, of an increased integration of ocular ultrasound in the ED is an improvement, not only of the triage of patients presenting with an acute ocular complaint, but also in the systems-based assessment and treatment of critically ill patients. The ophthalmic region is well suited for sonographic evaluation. The acoustically empty anterior chamber and vitreous cavity allow for good visualization of the ocular structures, and movement of the globe in conjunction with the ultrasound transducer facilitates visualization of nearly all parts of the eye. The need for depth penetration is small, allowing for use of high sonographic frequencies and superb resolution. In addition, ultrasound offers distinct advantages over traditionally employed imaging techniques, such as CT or MRI, which require patient transport out of the department. This is particularly important in cases of multiply injured or unstable patients.

Diagnostic capabilities

Although ultrasound machines found in ophthalmology settings typically use higher-frequency transducers and thus allow for better resolution than those in most EDs, the ophthalmology literature supports the use of standard ED machines with small parts probes for the diagnosis of many emergent conditions (18). Ultrasound is of great utility for conditions that may be hard to detect on physical exam, such as retinal detachment and optic neuritis, and may be the only means of bedside detection of posterior ocular pathology when the anterior segment is opacified, such as in the setting of hyphema or cataract. In addition, ultrasound is superior to x-ray examination for the recognition of nonmagnetic intraocular foreign bodies such as wood (4).

In a trauma setting, ultrasound provides a unique means of visualizing the globe and integrity of extraocular muscles when direct ophthalmoscopy may be prevented by palpebral edema or opacification of anterior structures. Recognition of increased ICP via evaluation of optic nerve sheath diameter is of further benefit in this setting, and the body of literature supporting its use for this indication is rapidly growing. This may be of particular benefit for rapid diagnosis and triage of patients in situations when patients are too unstable for CT scanning or where a CT scanner is not readily available, as in mass casualty settings or rural and wilderness medicine.

Sonographic anatomy

Normal sonographic anatomy of the eye consists of a clear anterior chamber, a hyperechoic lens, a clear posterior chamber, and a smooth retina indistinct from the underlying choroid (Figs. 22.1 and 22.2). The head of the optic nerve should be flush with the retina with no protrusion into the posterior chamber. The optic nerve sheath diameter, measured at a point 3 mm behind the globe, should not exceed 5.0 to 5.7 mm in the healthy adult (15, 16). The fovea and macula region lies slightly lateral (temporal) to where the optic nerve exits (optic disc) (Figs. 22.1 and 22.2).

Sonographic techniques

The use of ultrasound for evaluation of the eyes and orbits requires application of copious amount of lubricant gel to reduce signal loss to tissue-air interface. This can sometimes lead to patient discomfort as the gel may seep into their eyes. For this reason, some clinicians apply less ultrasound gel; however, this can lead to poor image quality or too much pressure applied to the globe. It has been shown that using transparent dressing (Tegaderm) can help reduce eye discomfort from ultrasound gel seepage (19). It also keeps the eyes clean and the cleanup process much more efficient. Ocular ultrasound evaluation in the ED is typically performed with the patient in the supine position and using a 7.5 MHz linear probe, which has a high frequency and better resolution than other probes (Fig. 22.3A and B).

The common approaches employed in ED ultrasound of the eyes and orbits are the transverse, axial, and longitudinal methods. With the transverse approach (the most commonly used), the probe is placed opposite to the examined meridian, and the plane of the probe is tangential to the limbus, with probe marker points cephalad for scans at the 3 o'clock and 9 o'clock positions and toward the nose for scans at the 6 o'clock and 12 o'clock positions. With the transverse approach, the sound beam bypasses the lens and is directed perpendicularly to the optic nerve. This is accomplished with the patient fixating slightly nasally, with the probe placed on the temporal horizontal meridian (i.e., transverse scan of the 3 o'clock meridian of the right orbit and the 9 o'clock meridian of the left orbit – Fig. 22.4). This method avoids diffraction by the lens and shadowing from the optic disc and, thus, may provide more accurate measurements of the optic nerve sheath diameter. However, to date there is little research correlating optic nerve sheath diameter between the two approaches (20), and there is currently no generally preferred method.

For the axial approach, the patient fixates in primary gaze, the probe is centered on the cornea, and the sound passes through the lens toward the optic nerve. This is typically performed with a linear probe placed directly on the closed eyelids in a horizontal plane with the probe indicator pointed nasally. This approach can be augmented with additional imaging in the vertical (sagittal) plane, where the probe indicator is pointing cephalad (Fig. 22.3). The cooperative patient may assist the sonographer in obtaining complete visualization of the ocular contents by moving the eye throughout its range of motion during the exam.

The longitudinal approach, more feasible with an ophthalmologic ultrasound probe, allows for detection of anterior-posterior extent of pathology. With this approach, the patient looks toward the area of interest, and the probe is placed opposite to the meridian of interest, with the plane of the probe perpendicular to the limbus and the probe indicator pointed toward the pupil. The shadow of the optic nerve is always at the bottom of the scan (Fig. 22.5). This approach allows for more detail interrogation and description of eye pathology (retinal detachment); therefore, it is often employed by the ophthalmologists for examination of small retinal detachment. This approach, however, is not as feasible with the bulky ultrasound probes available in the ED.

Specific applications

Perhaps the application of greatest initial utility for the novice sonographer is in the evaluation of suspected retinal detachment. Although retinal detachment may be difficult to appreciate with fundoscopy, it is easily recognized with ocular sonography. Whereas in the normal eye the retina is contiguous with the underlying choroid (Figs. 22.2 and 22.5), retinal detachment results in the appearance of a distinct hyperechoic line anterior to the choroid with an anechoic area of vitreous between the choroid and detached retina (Fig. 22.6A and B). In some instances, through detailed ocular sonographic evaluation, a clinician can delineate between a mac-on versus mac-off retinal detachment, which suggests different degrees of emergency. The macula is an oval-shaped area that lies just lateral (temporal) to the optic disc, specializing in

high-acuity vision. With careful examination, the clinician often can determine whether the retina is still tethered to the choroid at the macula region or if it has been separated (Fig. 22.6A and B). In the case of a mac-on detachment, a more emergent (surgical) treatment is warranted, within 24 hours, because most of the vision maybe salvageable. The mac-off retinal detachment also requires surgical intervention but with less urgency, within 7 to 10 days (21).

Because of the emphasis on recognizing acute life-threatening conditions in the ED, the application of ocular ultrasound most widely studied in the emergency medicine literature is in the recognition of ICP by evaluating optic nerve sheath diameter (10–17). Although it is widely accepted that increased ICP results in papilledema, this finding may be difficult to appreciate on fundoscopy. Sonographically, papilledema in the adult is defined as an optic nerve sheath diameter greater than 5.0 to 5.7 mm at a point 3 mm behind the globe when measured with the axial approach (Fig. 22.7A and B).

As mentioned previously, ultrasound may be of particular value in ocular trauma when direct visualization of the eye and its contents are hindered by the unwilling patient; palpebral edema; or opacification of the anterior chamber, lens, or vitreous cavity. In this setting, the possibility of globe rupture necessitates the use of copious amounts of sterile gel and a delicate exam to minimize the risk of further injury and extrusion of ocular contents.

Ultrasound easily allows identification of lens dislocation, foreign body retention, vitreous hemorrhage, and globe rupture, among other traumatic conditions (2). With lens dislocation, the lens is no longer centered in the anterior segment and may be found free floating within the vitreous or adjacent to the retina (Fig. 22.8). Similarly, a foreign body may also appear as a hyperechoic free-floating object (usually) in the vitreous body (Fig. 22.9). Vitreous hemorrhage appears as a hyperechoic area within the anechoic vitreous. The blood may layer out in the dependent portion of the globe or may be free floating within the vitreous (Fig. 22.10). Vitreous detachment, where the vitreous membrane separates from the retina, can appear very similar to retinal detachment on ultrasound exam (Fig. 22.11). Posterior globe rupture often presents with hemorrhagic chemosis and vitreous hemorrhage (22), but the rupture itself may be occult and the pressure may be normal (2). Ultrasound readily identifies the vitreous hemorrhage and may show a loss of ocular volume in addition to irregular contour, thickening, or a hypoechoic area of the sclera (23) (Fig. 22.12).

ED ultrasound may also prove to be useful in the evaluation of optic neuritis. Although this condition is rarely definitively diagnosed in the ED without the use of MRI, it may be readily visible with bedside ultrasound as seen by protrusion of the optic nerve head into the posterior segment (Fig. 22.13). This may be beneficial as a tool to aid the clinician in choosing additional diagnostic imaging modalities (CT vs. MRI) in patients with abnormal ocular and neurologic examinations.

Summary

Ocular ultrasound is a relatively new ED imaging modality that is rapidly gaining acceptance among emergency clinicians. As with other ultrasound applications, it is well suited to this environment due to its portability, ease of use, lack of ionizing radiation, and diagnostic capabilities. Although ED ocular ultrasound is not a substitute for evaluation by an ophthalmologist or CT scanning of the head, as new applications for ocular ultrasound are discovered and perfected, it is likely that this tool will become increasingly used in the ED for improved diagnosis of acute ocular complaints and evaluation of patients with head injury.

Clinical images

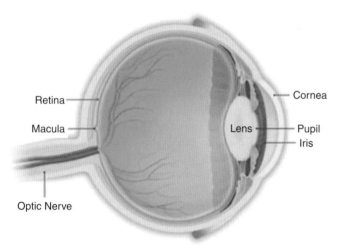

Figure 22.1. Diagram of a coronal section of a normal eye.

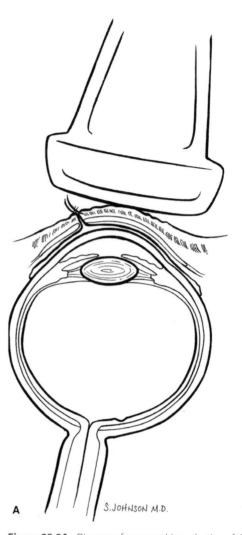

Figure 22.3A. Diagram of sonographic evaluation of the eye and optic nerve through a closed lid.

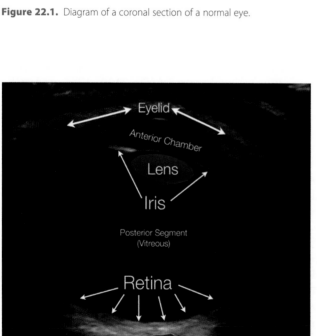

Figure 22.2. Sonographic image of a coronal section of a normal eye.

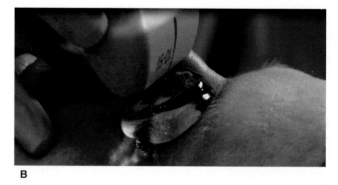

Figure 22.3B. Sonographic evaluation of the eye via ocular ultrasound using the high-frequency probe, through a closed lid and transparent dressing (tegaderm).

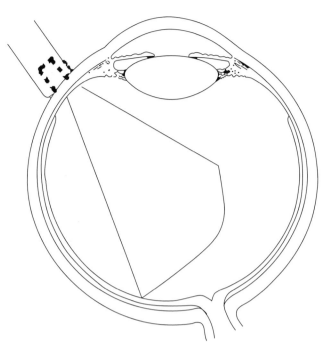

Figure 22.4. Diagram of sonographic evaluation of the eye and optic nerve using the transverse approach. Cross-sectional view of the right eye with caudal-cephalad orientation. Notice the probe indicator is pointing away from the page (toward the head), and the plane of the probe is tangential to the limbus of the eye.

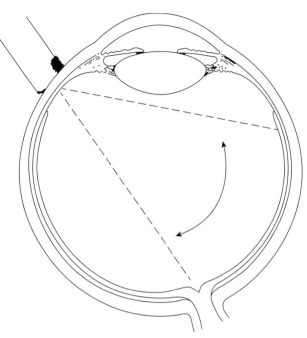

Figure 22.5. Diagram of sonographic evaluation of the eye and optic nerve with use of the longitudinal approach. The probe indicator is pointing toward the pupil with the resulting view of the optic nerve shadow at the opposite end of the indicator.

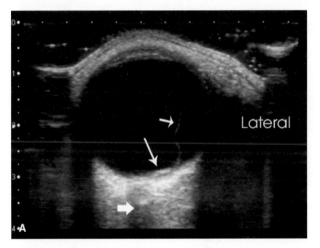

Figure 22.6A. Mac-on retinal detachment. Note the hyperechoic, detached retina separated by the anechoic vitreous from the underlying choroid in two patients with a retinal detachment. Also note the shadow of the optic nerve and the macula region just lateral to it, where the retina is still tethered to the choroid membrane.

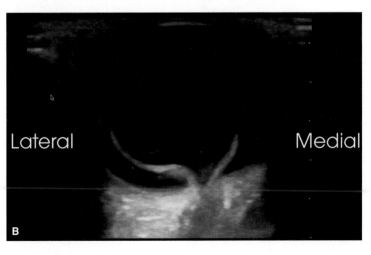

Figure 22.6B. Mac-off retinal detachment. Note the macula region just lateral to the optic disc (where the retina is still tethered), where the retina is completely detached from the choroid membrane.

A

B

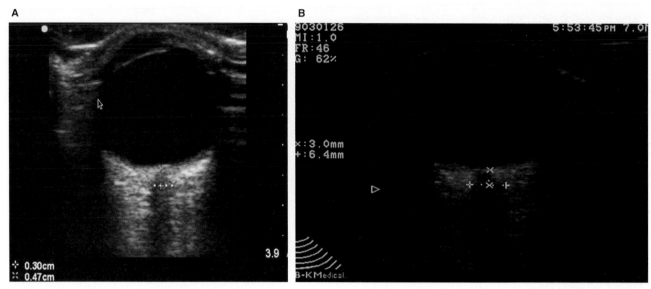

Figure 22.7. A: Measurement of the optic nerve sheath diameter in a normal patient. B: Measurement of an enlarged optic nerve sheath (6.5 mm) in a patient with increased ICP.

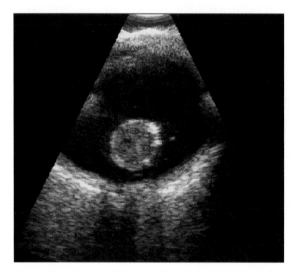

Figure 22.8. Sonographic image of lens dislocation. Note the lens within the vitreous in the posterior segment of the eye.

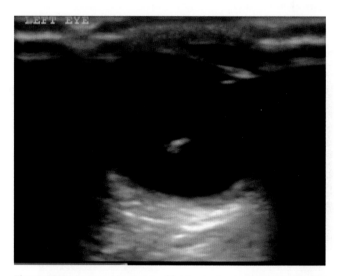

Figure 22.9. Sonographic image of foreign body retention in the eye. Note the hyperechoic FB floating within the vitreous in the posterior segment of the eye.

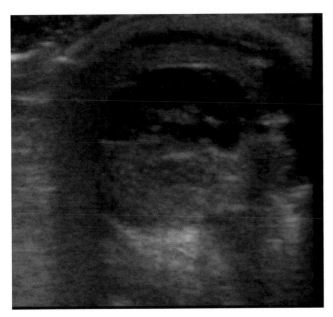

Figure 22.10. Vitreous hemorrhage. Note the hyperechoic layer of blood adjacent to the retina in the posterior segment of the eye in a patient found in the supine position after ocular trauma.

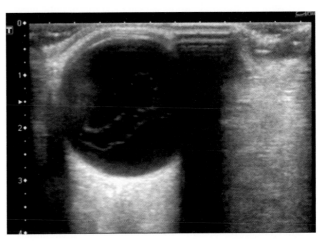

Figure 22.11. Sonographic image of vitreous detachment. Note how similar it can look to retinal detachment.

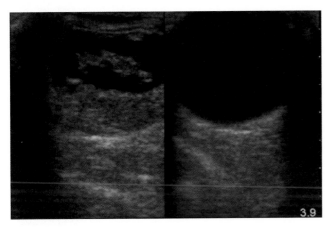

Figure 22.12. Sonographic images comparing a ruptured globe (left) with a normal globe (right). Note the abnormal contour and hemorrhage within the vitreous body of the left image.

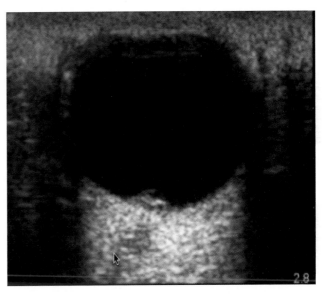

Figure 22.13. Optic neuritis. Note the protrusion of the optic nerve head into the posterior segment in the absence of increased optic nerve sheath diameter.

References

1. Mundt GH, Hughes WF: Ultrasonics in ocular diagnosis. *Am J Ophthalmol* 1956;**42**:488–98.

2. Byrne SF, Green RL: *Ultrasound of the eye and orbit*, 2nd ed. St. Louis, MO: Mosby, 2002.

3. Hughes JR, Byrne SF: Detection of posterior ruptures in opaque media. In: Ossoinig KC (ed.), *Ophthalmic echography*. Dordrecht, The Netherlands: Dr W Junk, 1987:333.

4. Fledelius HC: Ultrasound in ophthalmology. *Ultrasound Med Biol* 1997;**23**(3):365–75.

5. Green RL, Byrne SF: Diagnostic ophthalmic ultrasound. In: Ryan SJ (ed.), *Retina*. St. Louis, MO: Mosby, 1989:191.

6. Ossoinig KC, Bigar F, Kaefring SL, McNutt L: Echographic detection and localization of BB shots in the eye and orbit. *Bibl Ophthalmol* 1975;**83**:109.

7. Reshef DS, Ossoinig KC, Nerad JA: Diagnosis and intraoperative localization of a deep orbital organic foreign body. *Orbit* 1987;**6**:3.

8. Skalka HW: Ultrasonography in foreign body detection and localization. *Ophthalmic Surg* 1976;**7**(2):27.

9. Dutton JJ, Byrne SF, Proia AD: *Diagnostic atlas of orbital diseases*. Philadelphia: WB Saunders, 2000.

10. Blaivas M, Theodoro D, Sierzenski P: Elevated intracranial pressure detected by bedside emergency ultrasonography of the optic nerve sheath. *Acad Emerg Med* 2003;**10**(4):376–81.

11. Girisgin AS, Kalkan E, Kocak S, et al.: The role of optic nerve ultrasonography in the diagnosis of elevated intracranial pressure. *Emerg Med J* 2007;**24**:251–4.

12. Ahmad S, Kampondeni S, Molyneux E: An experience of emergency ultrasonography in children in a sub-Saharan setting. *Emerg Med J* 2006;**23**:335–40.

13. Ashkan AM, Bavarian S, Mehdizadeh M: Sonographic evaluation of optic nerve diameter in children with raised intracranial pressure. *J Ultrasound Med* 2005;**24**:143–7.

14. Newman WD, Hollman AS, Dutton GN, Carachi R: Measurement of optic nerve sheath diameter by ultrasound: a means of detecting acute raised intracranial pressure in hydrocephalus. *Br J Ophthalmol* 2002;**86**:1109–13.

15. Geeraerts T, Launey Y, Martin L, et al.: Ultrasonography of the optic nerve sheath may be useful for detecting raised intracranial pressure after severe brain injury [serial online]. *Intensive Care Med* 2007;**33**(10):1704–11.

16. Tayal VS, Neulander M, Norton HJ, et al.: Emergency department sonographic measurement of optic nerve sheath diameter to detect findings of increased intracranial pressure in adult head injury patients. *Ann Emerg Med* 2007;**49**:508–14.

17. Kimberly H, Shah S, Marill K, Noble V: Correlation of optic nerve sheath diameter with direct measurement of intracranial pressure. *Acad Emerg Med* 2007;**14**(5 Suppl 1):98.

18. Kwong JS, Munk PL, Lin DTC, et al.: Real-time sonography in ocular trauma. *AJR Am J Roentgenol* 1992;**158**:179–82.

19. Roth K, Gafni-Pappas G: Unique method of ocular ultrasound using transparent dressing. *J Emerg Med* 2011 Jun;**40**(6):658–60.

20. Shah S, Kimberly H, Marill K, Noble V: Measurement of optic nerve sheath diameter using ultrasound: is a specialized probe necessary? *Acad Emerg Med* 2007;**14**(5 Suppl 1):98.

21. Lang, GK: *Ophthalmology: a short textbook.* New York: Thieme Stuttgart, 2000.

22. Liggett PE, Mani N, Green RE, et al.: Management of traumatic rupture of the globe in aphakic patients. *Retina* 1990;**10**(Suppl 1):59.

23. Fielding JA: The assessment of ocular injury by ultrasound. *Clin Radiol* 2004;**59**:301–12.

24. Mowatt L: Macula off retinal detachments. How long can they wait before it is too late. *Eur J Ophthalmol* 2005;**15**(1):109–17.

Testicular Ultrasound

Paul R. Sierzenski and Gillian Baty

Testicular ultrasound has emerged as the imaging modality of choice for any patient with testicular or scrotal complaints (1). Triplex ultrasound – the combination of three ultrasound modes, including gray scale ultrasound, color Doppler imaging (CDI), and spectral Doppler imaging (SDI) – has proven highly sensitive, specific, and repeatable in the detection of acute and chronic testicular diseases (2).

Indications

The primary indication for testicular ultrasound is acute scrotal or testicular pain. The most common etiologies of acute scrotal pain are epididymitis, orchitis, testicular torsion, and scrotal trauma (1). Additional indications for urgent testicular ultrasound include, but are not limited to, hematuria, dysuria, and a palpable testicular or scrotal mass.

As with the diagnostic approach for any organ system or complaint, pertinent historical features aid the healthcare provider in creating a differential diagnosis based on patient age, risk factors, symptom onset, duration, and quality. Most disease states for the testicle present acutely, including epididymitis, orchitis, testicular torsion, and testicular trauma. The most time-critical diagnoses include testicular torsion and testicular rupture, because testicular salvage and fertility are inversely related to time to surgical repair from disease onset. In general, testicular function is recovered when surgery is performed within 6 hours of symptom onset (1). The incidence of testicular torsion is greatest in those 6 to 15 years of age and decreases significantly after 25 years of age.

Complications of testicular torsion include testicular infarction and testicular atrophy, both of which can be diagnosed by ultrasound.

Diagnostic capabilities

Testicular ultrasound is both the initial imaging modality of choice as well as the preferred diagnostic method for follow-up of patients with acute, recurrent, or chronic testicular and scrotal symptoms. Scrotal ultrasound is performed with a linear, high-frequency transducer with ultrasound frequencies ranging from 5 to 12 MHz. Occasionally, an abdominal transducer is used when significant edema and swelling are present.

Triplex ultrasound is 100% sensitive and up to 97% specific for acute inflammatory disease states (2). However, because the sensitivity for ultrasound detection of testicular torsion is 90%, surgical exploration remains the gold standard (3). Ultrasound is noninvasive, rapid, and inexpensive in comparison to other scrotal imaging modalities, and it does not require administration of contrast agents or exposure to ionizing radiation. Current-day testicular ultrasound has evolved to include gray scale imaging, CDI, and SDI, including waveform analysis. Waveform analysis is performed both to verify the presence of venous and arterial flow and to compare the resistive index of the arterial waveform from the affected and unaffected testicle.

Sonographic findings for testicular complaints can be divided into one of several categories: increased vascular flow, decreased vascular flow, and intratesticular or extratesticular abnormalities (fluid, collections, and masses). Epididymitis with or without orchitis represents a spectrum of testicular inflammation, which is the most common diagnosis in patients presenting with testicular pain, swelling, or mass (4). Radionucleotide imaging of the scrotum and testicles is still used today, but to a lesser extent than sonography, due to both the need for intravenous access and the avoidance of radiation exposure.

Sonographic anatomy

The scrotum has a dual-layer compartment that is further divided by the median raphe. Each scrotal side normally contains a testicle, epididymis, vas deferens, and spermatic cord. The ovoid testes measure approximately $3 \times 3 \times 5$ cm and lie vertically in the scrotum. Septations divide the testicle into lobules. The mediastinum testis is the dense band of connective tissue that provides internal support for vessels and ducts of the testicle. The tunica albuginea forms the outer capsule of the testicle, while the inner wall of the scrotum is lined by the tunica vaginalis (5).

The echotexture of the testicle is normally homogenous and similar to that of the thyroid. The epididymis runs posterolaterally along the length of the testicle and includes a head, body, and tail. A normal epididymal head measures less than 1 cm.

Basic technique

Ultrasound of the scrotum is best performed by immobilizing the scrotum using a towel "sling" between the patient's legs. The penis is placed on the abdomen and covered with a second towel (Fig. 23.1). Often the testicle must also be stabilized using the nondominant hand. Scanning should begin on the unaffected side, in gray scale, and then include CDI and pulsed Doppler imaging. Views should include sagittal and transverse planes, preferably with a transverse view of the testicles for comparison using dual image or with a larger footprint transducer. The length, height, and width of the testicle is measured, along with the epididymal head. The epididymal head can be difficult to delineate in some patients. CDI and PDI are cornerstones to testicular ultrasound. In a normal state, both intratesticular arterial and venous blood flow should be identified (6). Intratesticular arterial flow is normally "low resistance" with preserved flow in diastole (Fig. 23.3A).

This is in contrast to the high-resistance flow in extratesticular vessels such as those in the spermatic cord. CDI gain and frequency should be compared between the unaffected and affected sides. Venous flow in the testicle displays little or no phasicity (Fig. 23.3B). It is essential to identify both central venous and arterial waveforms in the exclusion of testicular torsion and ischemia. The Doppler settings should be initially set and baseline measurements obtained using the asymptomatic side.

Imaging pitfalls and limitations

Pitfalls in testicular ultrasound may be divided into several categories. It is essential that the physician or sonographer be familiar with these to avoid misdiagnosis or a delay in care.

The most critical scanning pitfall relates to a misunderstanding of the skill and knowledge required for using CDI, power Doppler imaging (PDI), or SDI. An understanding of Doppler physics and practical optimization of instrumentation are essential. Optimization of Doppler pulse repetition frequencies, filters, and scale must be emphasized and practiced.

Testicular ischemic states can present confusing sonographic findings. Torsion, as well as a compressive hydrocele, or

hematocele, or pyocele, can result in testicular ischemia. The presence of *peripheral* testicular blood flow (hyperemia) with a relative deficiency or absence of *central* testicular blood flow is an essential pitfall to recognize. The diagnosis of testicular torsion does not mandate an absence of any blood flow on ultrasound but rather an insufficiency in blood flow (7). To avoid this potential pitfall, the sonographer should initially scan the asymptomatic testicle. If peripheral blood vessels appear with increased flow, but central color and spectral signals are difficult to identify, this may represent torsion, intermittent torsion, or focal infarct.

Clinical images

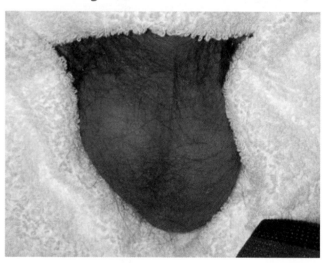

Figure 23.1. Patient draping.

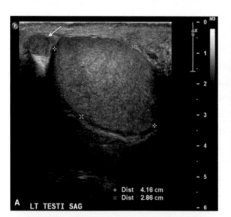

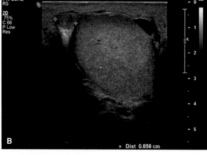

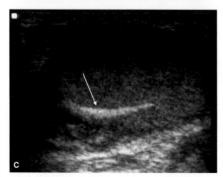

Figure 23.2. The normal testicle. A: Normal homogenous testicular echotexture. Measuring the epididymal head. Look for the "edge artifact," as noted in this image, to aid in differentiating the epididymis from the superior pole of the testicle. C: The echogenic curved line (*arrow*) seen in this image is the mediastinum testis.

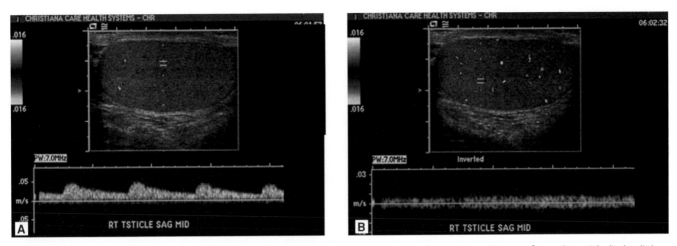

Figure 23.3. Doppler imaging. A: Low-resistance intratesticular arterial flow, demonstrating forward flow in diastole. B: Venous flow in the testicle displays little or no phasicity, as displayed in this image.

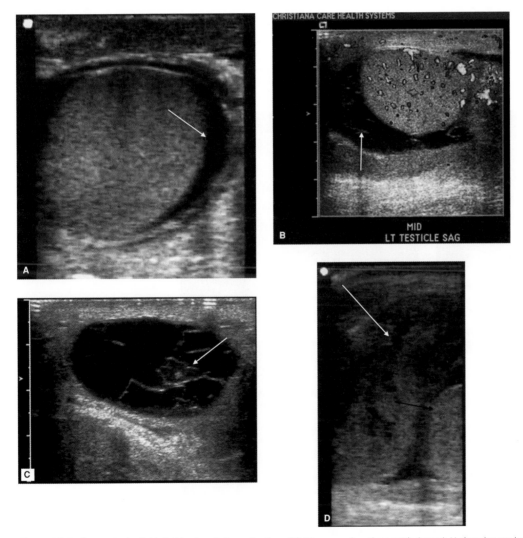

Figure 23.4. Extratesticular fluid. A: A hydrocele is a collection of fluid surrounding the testicle (*arrow*). Hydroceles can be congenital or acquired, the result of epididymitis, orchitis, testicular torsion, or tumor. Sonographically, it is anechoic. If small, it may be dependent and may not fully surround the testicle. B and C: If the fluid surrounding the testicle is infected, this is termed a "pyocele," which may demonstrate banding or septations (*arrows*). D: Blood that surrounds the testicle defines a hematocele. This can follow trauma or surgery, or be spontaneous. A hematocele in the setting of trauma increases the potential for testicular rupture, a surgical emergency. Often the hematocele (*white arrow*) is larger than the testicle (*black arrow*), as noted in this image (8).

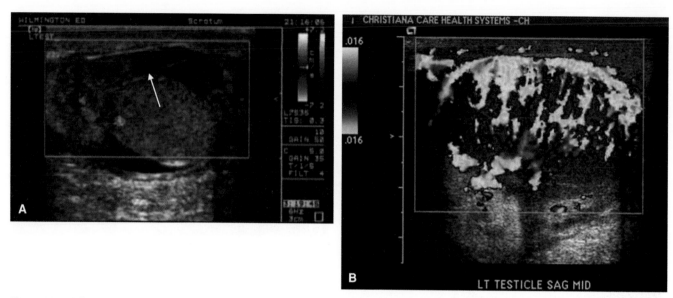

Figure 23.5. Inflammatory states. A: Epididymitis is often the result of an infection extending from the lower urinary tract. This is most commonly bacterial but can be of viral etiology (9). Sonographically, the epididymis is enlarged (most commonly the head or globus major), with increased color or power Doppler flow. The inflamed epididymis usually measures greater than 1 cm and is often associated with a reactive hydrocele (*arrow*), as noted in this image. B: Orchitis often follows an infection of the epididymis. Mumps remains the most common viral cause of orchitis. Increased testicular size and increased Doppler flow are the hallmarks of orchitis. As with epididymitis, a reactive hydrocele or pyocele is often identified. A decrease in the resistive index less than 0.5 is associated with inflammatory testicular states (7).

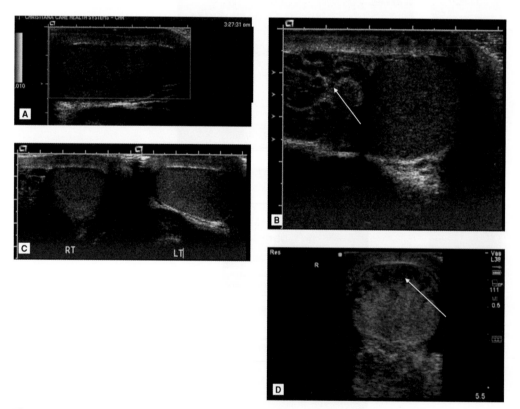

Figure 23.6. Testicular torsion. A: Testicular torsion represents the most time-sensitive, organ-threatening condition to identify with testicular ultrasound. Due to the low threshold for Doppler flow using nondirectional PDI, this ultrasound mode is very useful for torsion. The hallmark of torsion on ultrasound is represented by a decrease in blood flow of the affected testicle compared with the unaffected testicle. The degree of decreased flow depends on the degree of torsion of the spermatic cord and, thus, the testicular blood flow. Associated findings include testicular swelling, peripheral hyperemia, and decreased echogenicity. B: The spermatic cord (*arrow*) may appear twisted, as shown in this ultrasound. C: A clinical hallmark of testicular torsion includes an abnormal lie of the testicle; this may be difficult to assess due to pain and swelling. This dual-screen sagittal image demonstrates an abnormal lie of the right testicle, which is torsed. D: This patient presented 2 days after the onset of symptoms. Note the testicular atrophy and heterogeneous echogenicity (*arrow*) of the testicle. Delays in torsion treatment result in testicular infarction (10).

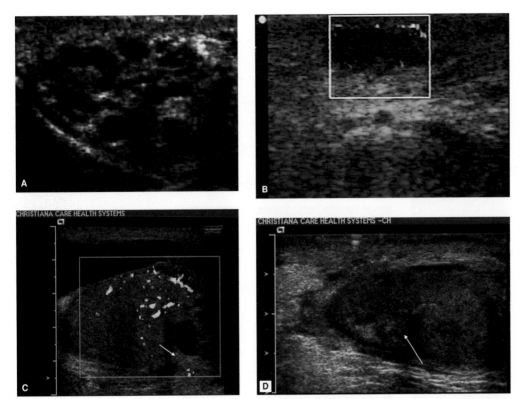

Figure 23.7. Benign testicular masses. Testicular masses are the second most frequent presenting complaint for patients. Both benign and malignant causes of testicular masses exist. Benign lesions such as cysts and abscesses are frequently encountered. A: A varicocele results from distention of the pampiniform plexus, which is more common for the left testicle based on anatomical variances from the left and right venous drainage (11). Sonographically, these dilated veins are frequently seen in the superior pole. CDI reflux is noted by having the patient perform a Valsalva maneuver. B: Scrotal abscesses have increased in incidence as the incidence of bacteria such as methicillin-resistant *Staphylococcus aureus* has also risen. Most "scrotal" abscesses occur outside the tunica vaginalis. Note the reactive hyperemia at the edge of the abscess. C: Testicular abscesses are often the complication of epididymoorchitis. On ultrasound, they are generally fluid filled, may have septations, and can be difficult to differentiate from a testicular tumor. As in this image, they usually display posterior acoustic enhancement (*arrow*) and have an associated reactive hydrocele. D: Testicular and scrotal hematomas are generally the result of scrotal trauma. Note the posttraumatic epididymitis with hematoma (*arrow*) in this patient. High suspicion for testicular rupture must exist in the setting of trauma with the presence of a testicular hematoma/hematocele (12–15).

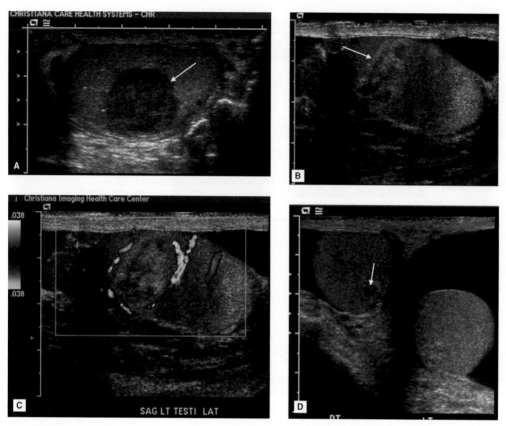

Figure 23.8. Malignant testicular masses. A: This patient presented with a testicular mass (*arrow*) noted on self-examination. The vast majority of malignant testicular tumors are echogenic, but hypoechoic compared to normal testicle echotexture. More than 90% of patients with testicular neoplasms present with a painless mass on one testicle (11). B: Note the increased echogenicity (*arrow*) and irregularity of this testicular mass. C: CDI aids in demarcation of the area of concern. Echogenicity is not a sensitive or specific characteristic to differentiate malignant from benign solid masses. Bleeding, autoinfarction ("burned-out tumors"), and infection can alter the appearance of a tumor; thus, malignancy remains a diagnosis of exclusion for the majority of solid testicular masses. D: Small masses, such as this mass (*arrow*) at the right posterior inferior pole, may represent a benign epidermoid cyst or, as in this case, a seminoma, the most common testicular tumor in adults.

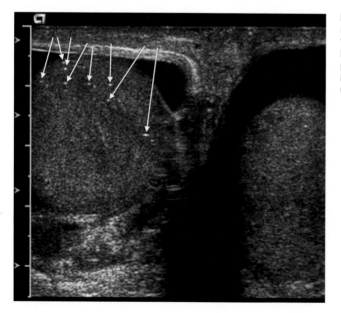

Figure 23.9. Calcifications. Multiple intratesticular calcifications (*arrows*) numbering more than five in this image are seen in this patient with "microlithiasis" calcifications within the seminiferous tubules. Several studies have followed patients with microlithiasis, resulting in the development of primary germ cell tumors in up to 40% of patients with this condition. Microlithiasis is graded based on the presence of more than five calcifications per ultrasound image and requires repeat ultrasounds every 6 months (4).

References

1. Patriquin HB, Yazbeck S, Trinh B, et al.: Testicular torsion in infants and children: diagnosis with Doppler sonography. *Radiology* 1993;**188**:781–5.

2. Baker LA, Sigman D, Mathers RI, et al.: An analysis of clinical outcomes using color Doppler testicular ultrasound for testicular torsion. *Pediatrics* 2000;**105**:604–7.

3. Burks DD, Markey BJ, Burkhard TK, et al.: Suspected testicular torsion and ischemia: evaluation with color Doppler sonography. *Radiology* 1990;**175**:815–21.

4. Ragheb D, Higgins JL: Ultrasonography of the scrotum: technique, anatomy, and pathologic entities. *J Ultrasound Med* 2002;**21**:171–85.

5. Dogra VS, Gottlieb RH, Oka M: Sonography of the scrotum. *Radiology* 2003;**227**:18–36.

6. Dogra VS, Rubens DJ, Gottlieb RH: Torsion and beyond: new twists in spectral Doppler evaluation of the scrotum. *J Ultrasound Med* 2004;**23**:979–81.

7. Yazbeck S, Patriquin HB: Accuracy of Doppler sonography in the evaluation of acute conditions of the scrotum in children. *J Pediatr Surg* 1994;**29**(9):1270–2.

8. Having K, Holtgrave R: Trauma induced testicular rupture. *J Ultrasound Med* 2003;**19**:379–81.

9. Dambro TJ, Stewart RR, Carroll BA: Scrotum. In: Rumack C, Wilson S, Charboneau J (eds), *Diagnostic ultrasound*, 2nd ed. St. Louis, MO: Mosby, 1998:791–821.

10. Rozauski T: Surgery of the scrotum and testis in children. In: Walsh PC, Retik AB, Vaughan ED, Wein AJ (eds), *Campbell's urology*, 7th ed. Philadelphia: WB Saunders, 1998:2200–2.

11. Sanders RC: Scrotum. In: *Exam preparation for diagnostic ultrasound: abdomen and OB/GYN*. Baltimore: Williams & Wilkins, 2002:32.

12. Hricak H, Lue T, Filly RA, et al.: Experimental study of the sonographic diagnosis of testicular torsion. *J Ultrasound Med* 1983;**2**:349–56.

13. Middleton WD, Middleton MA, Dierks M, et al.: Sonographic prediction of viability in testicular torsion: preliminary observations. *J Ultrasound Med* 1997;**16**:23–7.

14. Cohen HL, Shapiro ML, Haller JO, Glassberg K: Sonography of intrascrotal hematomas simulating testicular rupture in adolescents. *Pediatr Radiol* 1992;**22**:296–7.

15. Blaivas M, Batts M, Lambert M: Ultrasonographic diagnosis of testicular torsion by emergency physicians. *Am J Emerg Med* 2000;**18**(2):198–200.

Abdominal Ultrasound

Shane Arishenkoff

Indication

The applications of abdominal ultrasound in emergency medicine continue to evolve. Currently, the diagnostic characteristics of ultrasound are on par with or even exceed those of other imaging modalities, such as CT, for certain applications. In addition, ultrasound has many features that make it attractive for the environment and clinical situations encountered in the emergency department. First, ultrasound is portable, which makes bedside assessment of unstable patients possible. Second, it allows for interaction with the patient during the examination, thereby allowing the sonographer to incorporate clinical information to help guide image acquisition. Finally, it does not rely on potentially toxic contrast agents that can be harmful and time consuming to administer.

Many of the indications for abdominal ultrasound – including right upper quadrant pain, assessment of the abdominal aorta, and trauma – are covered in different chapters. This chapter focuses on a variety of other important areas not covered elsewhere.

Diagnostic capabilities

Gastrointestinal tract

Acute appendicitis

Ultrasound should be considered the initial imaging modality of choice for children suspected of appendicitis (1, 2). Based on a meta-analysis from 2004, a conservative estimate of the sensitivity and specificity of ultrasound in the diagnosis of appendicitis is 86% and 81%, respectively (3). This report, however, includes studies dating back to the 1960s. More modern literature reports the sensitivity and specificity of ultrasound to be as high as 91% and 98%, respectively (4). Given the favorable test characteristics, the American College of Radiology recommends ultrasound, followed by CT as needed (1). The American College of Emergency Physicians (ACEP) makes a similar recommendation, suggesting CT should be used if the diagnosis remains uncertain after ultrasound. Current evidence supports this staged approach in which ultrasound is performed first, followed by CT when results are equivocal (5, 6). Krishnamoorthi and colleagues found this approach accurately identified patients with

appendicitis and reduced the number of CT scans by more than 50% (5). And despite the decreased reliance on CT, it has been shown that when a staged ultrasound and CT protocol is established, the perforation and negative appendectomy rates are markedly reduced (7).

Figure 24.1 shows a normal-appearing appendix found in the right lower quadrant. ACEP reports the diagnostic criteria for appendicitis as an appendix greater than 6 mm in diameter, a noncompressible appendix, and appendiceal tenderness (2). Figures 24.2 and 24.3 show an enlarged non-compressible appendix in long and short axes consistent with a diagnosis of appendicitis. Additional associated features include a "ring of fire," whereby there is increased flow at the periphery of the appendix when viewed in short axis using Doppler (Fig. 24.4), free fluid in the right lower quadrant (Fig. 24.5), presence of an appendicolith (Figs. 24.6 and 24.7) and signs of a localized paralytic ileus (8). Furthermore, the shape of the appendix also seems to be helpful. It has been reported that appendicitis is associated with a round rather than ovoid shape when viewed in cross section with a negative predictive value of 100% (Fig. 24.3) (9).

Imaging pitfalls and limitations

It is important to consider the limitations of ultrasound when choosing the initial imaging modality. Limitations are related to level of sonographer expertise and underlying patient characteristics, including obesity, inability to tolerate the examination because of pain, and orientation of the appendix. The limitations associated with poorly controlled pain can often be mitigated by a proactive approach to analgesia. A retrocecal appendix may make it more difficult to visualize the appendix (2). However, it has been shown that in the absence of secondary features of appendicitis, an exam in which the appendix is not visualized is still associated with a favorable negative predictive value (10). Ultimately, if the body habitus is unfavorable or clinical suspicion remains high despite a non-diagnostic ultrasound, a CT scan is often recommended.

Infantile hypertrophic pyloric stenosis

Classically, infantile hypertrophic pyloric stenosis (IHPS) is suspected in a previously healthy infant presenting with nonbilious projectile vomiting between 2 and 8 weeks of age. Clinicians are becoming less successful at identifying the physical exam findings associated with IHPS and, thus, are more reliant on the use of imaging to make the diagnosis (11). Ultrasound should be pursued in infants if IHPS is suspected (11). Ultrasound is the most expedient diagnostic examination and has a sensitivity of 97% to 100% and a specificity approaching 100% for the detection of IHPS (12–14). Figure 24.8 shows a normal-appearing pylorus. The diagnosis of IHPS by ultrasound can be made by demonstrating an increase in pyloric length or muscle thickness. The particular number varies in the literature with a pyloric length greater than 15 to 18 mm or a pyloric muscle thickness greater than 3 to 4 mm considered in the diagnostic range (Figs. 24.8 and 24.9) (14–16). Additional findings include a pyloric lumen crowded by redundant mucosa and gastric peristaltic activity that fails to distend the pylorus (13).

Intussusception

Intussusception should be considered in children between the ages of 6 months and 2 years with intermittent, sudden onset abdominal pain. While some institutions continue to use fluoroscopy as the initial diagnostic procedure, ultrasound is now advocated by many as the primary imaging modality of choice (17). Ultrasound findings associated with intussusception include the "donut," "target," and "pseudokidney" signs (Fig. 24.10) (18). Sonography has a sensitivity of 98% to 100% and a specificity of 88% to 100% for the diagnosis of intussusception (18). In addition, ultrasound can identify pathologic lead points, including a Meckel's diverticulum, or mass such as lymphoma (18). Nonoperative pneumatic or hydrostatic reduction can be performed under fluoroscopic or sonographic guidance. Although direct comparisons are lacking, reduction success rates using sonographic guidance appear comparable to fluoroscopic methods (18). Ultrasound is attractive given the lack of radiation and benefits associated with repeated attempts at reduction if the initial attempt is unsuccessful (19).

Abdominal wall hernias

Ultrasound can be a useful imaging modality for abdominal wall hernias. Abdominal wall hernias can be classified by location and may result from defects secondary to previous surgeries or spontaneously as with groin hernias, the most common abdominal wall hernia. The history and physical exam is often sufficient for making the diagnosis. However, the physical exam does not provide details about the content of the hernia. Ultrasound can differentiate among fluid, mesenteric fat, and bowel. Imaging has also been found to be useful in situations where the history remains suggestive of a hernia and the physical exam is unhelpful. Occult hernias missed during physical exam can put the patient at risk for complications including strangulation and rupture (20). A recent meta-analysis from 2013 showed a pooled sensitivity of 96.6% and specificity of 84.4% for groin hernias (21). The authors concluded that ultrasound is helpful when the diagnosis remains unclear after clinical evaluation (21).

Ultrasound allows real-time imaging, both during dynamic maneuvers such as Valsalva and with the patient in the upright position, which can reveal a hernia that would have otherwise been reduced at rest (20). In addition, ultrasound is helpful in assessing for complications associated with abdominal wall hernias and identifying an alternative explanation for the patient's symptoms. Free fluid in the hernia sac has been identified as a sensitive and specific sign for incarceration (22). Other signs suggestive of incarceration include bowel wall thickness in hernia greater than or equal to 4 mm, fluid within the herniated bowel loop, and dilated bowel loops in the abdomen. One report showed that demonstrating two or more of these findings had a sensitivity and specificity of 100% each (22). Figures 24.11 and 24.12 show typical findings of intraabdominal contents connected by a stalk protruding through an abdominal wall defect.

Pancreas

Figures 24.13 and 24.14 demonstrate a normal pancreas as seen on ultrasound along with associated anatomy. Although a dedicated ultrasound examination of the pancreas is not routinely sought out in the ED, it does play a role in the workup of certain pancreatic diseases regularly encountered in the ED. For example, the American College of Gastroenterology guidelines on the management of acute pancreatitis strongly recommend that ultrasound be performed to evaluate for cholelithiasis (23). Unfortunately, pancreatitis is often associate with an adynamic ileus, making visualization of the entire pancreas difficult with ultrasound. Therefore, CT remains the diagnostic modality of choice for confirming the diagnosis of pancreatitis if not initially clear and for identifying the presence of early complications associated with acute pancreatitis.

Ultrasound is often used as the initial imaging modality in patients presenting with undifferentiated abdominal pain or suspicion for obstructive jaundice. Pancreatic pathology that may be identified under such circumstances includes evidence of acute and chronic pancreatitis (Figs. 24.15 and 24.16), pseudocysts (Figs. 24.17 and 24.18), pancreatic duct dilation (Fig. 24.19), and pancreatic tumors. The diagnostic accuracy of transabdominal ultrasound for diagnosing pancreatic tumors is 50% to 70% (24).

Spleen

Other than in trauma, emergency sonography of the spleen is not routinely ordered from the ED. However, as with the pancreas, incidental findings may be noted on routine imaging of the abdomen for other indications. A normal spleen is seen in Figure 24.20. Splenomegaly (Fig. 24.21), splenic masses (Fig. 24.22), cysts, infarcts, abscesses, accessory spleens (Fig. 24.23), and splenic artery aneurysms may be noted. The spleen is usually less than 12 cm in its longest dimension (25).

Clinical images

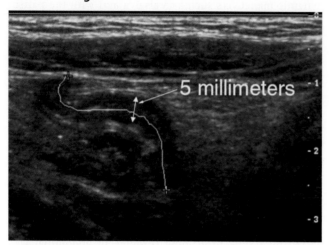

Figure 24.1. Normal-appearing appendix using a high-frequency linear transducer. Note that this is a blind-ended tubular structure in the right lower quadrant. In real time, there would be compressibility of this structure, and it would not demonstrate peristalsis. An artificial line has been drawn through the lumen of this normal appendix.

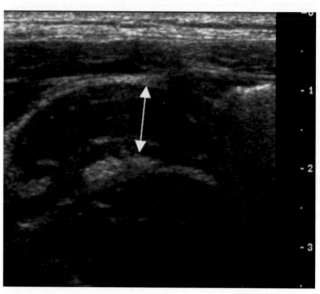

Figure 24.2. Appendicitis in the long-axis view demonstrates a 1.1 cm inflamed appendix. Note that it is a blind-ended tubular structure and, in real time, lacks compressibility and peristalsis.

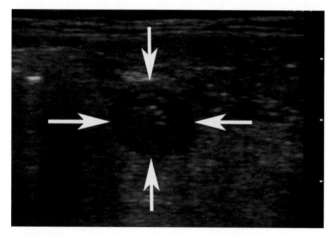

Figure 24.3. Acute appendicitis in short axis. The outer edges of the appendix are demonstrated by arrows. The hash marks are 1 cm increments.

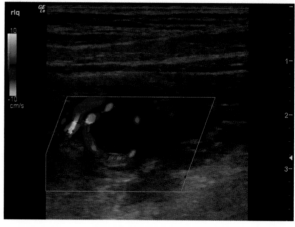

Figure 24.4. The "ring of fire" sign may be seen in acute appendicitis. Color Doppler or power Doppler is used to demonstrate hyperemia of the inflamed appendix.

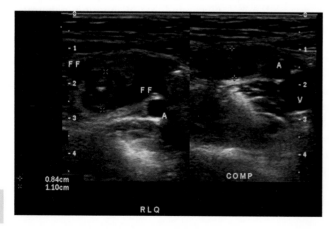

Figure 24.5. Young woman with right lower quadrant pain. The image on the left shows a 1.1 cm structure that is nonperistalsing. Note that the tubular structure is adjacent to a wedge of free fluid (FF). The image on the right is the same window; however, compression (COMP) is used. The structure changes from 11.0 mm to 8.4 mm, demonstrating noncompressibility of the inflamed appendix. Also noted are the iliac artery (A) and iliac vein (V).

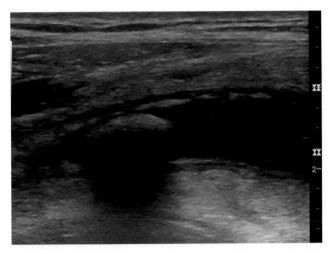

Figure 24.6. A fecalith may be seen in acute appendicitis. A longitudinal view of the appendix shows a rounded structure sitting in the appendiceal lumen. Note the shadow created by the fecalith.

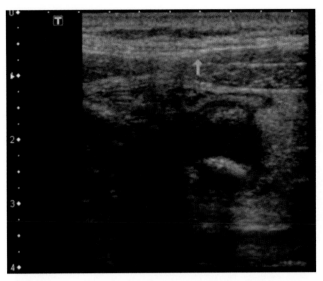

Figure 24.7. A fecalith seen the appendiceal lumen in short axis.

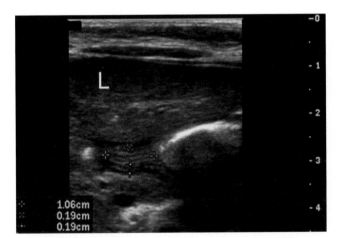

Figure 24.8. Normal pylorus. Note that the length, denoted by the (+) calipers, is less than 14 mm, while the wall thickness, denoted by the (x) calipers, is less than 2 mm. Total pylorus thickness is less than 10 mm. "L" is the adjacent liver.

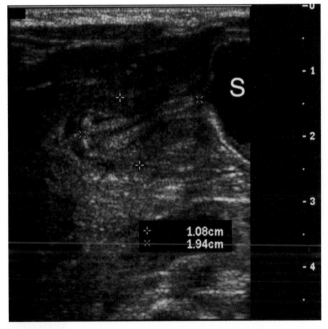

Figure 24.9. Infantile hypertrophic pyloric stenosis. The length, denoted by the (x) calipers, is greater than 14 mm. The diameter, denoted by the (+) calipers, is wider than 10 mm. The stomach, which is on the right side of the image, is noted by the "S" and demonstrates a fluid-filled distended stomach.

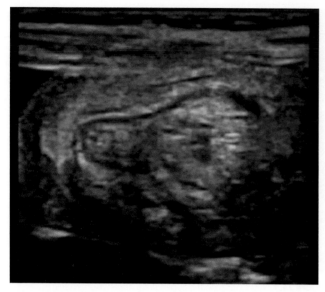

Figure 24.10. The "donut sign." The image demonstrates the characteristic multilayered appearance of intussusception.

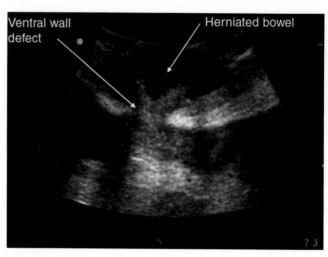

Figure 24.11. Ventral wall hernia with incarcerated bowel. Note the ventral wall defect with protrusion of fluid-filled bowel through the defect and adjacent free fluid within the herniated sac. In real-time ultrasound, there was a lack of peristalsis noted.

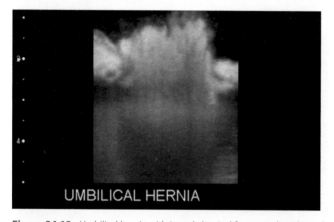

Figure 24.12. Umbilical hernia with intraabdominal fat protruding through the abdominal wall defect. Also note the anechoic fluid in the hernia sac.

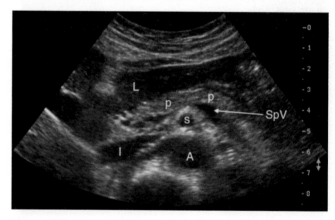

Figure 24.13. Transverse view of a normal pancreas (p). The echotexture of the pancreas is homogenous and slightly hyperechoic relative to the adjacent liver (L); however, it can also have very similar echogenicity to that of the liver. Also noted are the inferior vena cava (I), superior mesenteric artery (s), splenic vein (SpV), and Aorta (A).

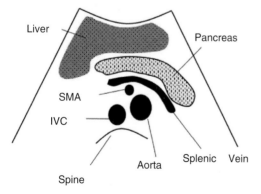
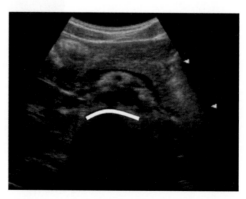

Figure 24.14. Ultrasound image of the pancreas on the right, with its corresponding schematic on the left. Note that the pancreas can be difficult to image, illustrating why knowledge of the surrounding anatomy is vital to the identification of this organ. Also noted are superior mesenteric artery (SMA) and IVC.

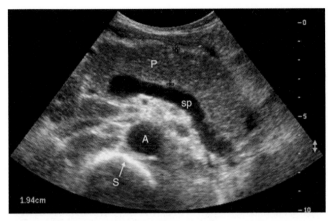

Figure 24.15. Acute pancreatitis. Note the enlarged and heterogenous pancreas (P), which is not as homogenous as the normal pancreas seen in Figure 24.13. Note also the splenic vein (sp), aorta (A), and spine shadow (S).

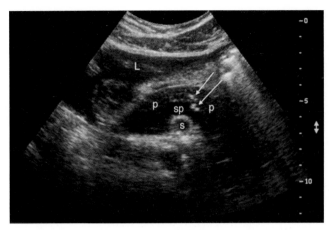

Figure 24.16. Chronic pancreastitis, indicated by hyperechoic structures (*arrows*) in the body of the pancreas (p). Note also the liver (L), superior mesenteric artery (s), and splenic vein (sp).

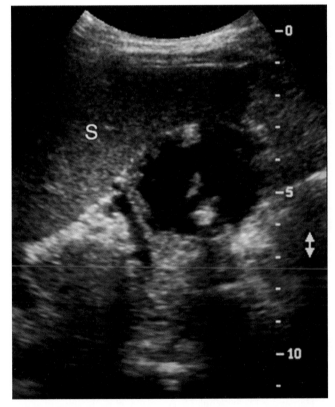

Figure 24.17. Pancreatic pseudocyst adjacent to the splenic hilum. Note that the spleen (S) is shown in the upper left corner of the image and that the pseudocyst is separate from the spleen.

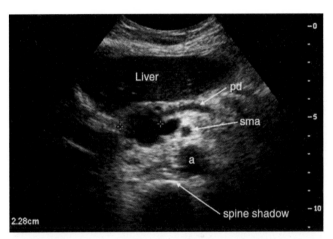

Figure 24.18. A 2.28 cm pancreatic pseudocyst in the head of the pancreas. Note that there may be dilatation of the pancreatic duct distally as well. The pancreatic tissue is not well visualized; however, identification of the pathology is aided by knowledge of the surrounding anatomy, including the pancreatic duct (pd), aorta (a), and superior mesenteric artery (sma).

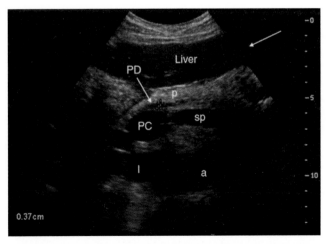

Figure 24.19. Pancreatic duct dilatation (PD). The normal pancreatic duct is generally 2 to 2.5 mm in diameter (25). Note the adjacent pancreas (p), portal confluence (PC), splenic vein (sp), inferior vena cava (I), and aorta (a).

343

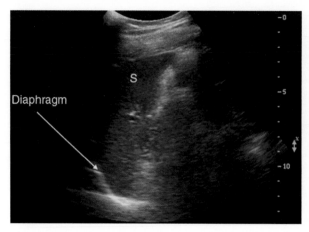

Figure 24.20. Normal spleen (S). Note that the echotexture of the spleen is similar to the liver.

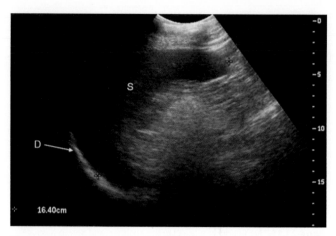

Figure 24.21. Splenomegaly, as indicated by a spleen (S) with a length of 16.5 cm. The spleen is generally less than 12 cm (25). "D" is the adjacent diaphragm.

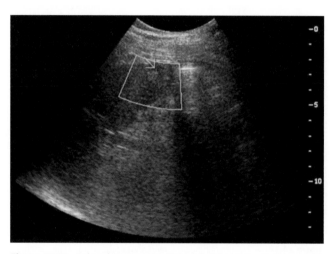

Figure 24.22. Spleen hemangioma. Note well-defined, circular lesion within the splenic parenchyma (*arrow*) that is hyperechoic relative to the surrounding tissue.

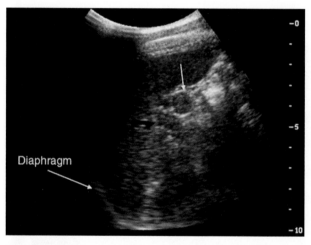

Figure 24.23. Accessory spleen (*arrow*). This is a common finding seen as a normal variant and also known as a splenunculus. They are small, rounded masses with similar echotexture to the spleen and are usually less than 5 cm (25).

References

1. Rosen MP, Ding A, Blake MA, et al.: ACR Appropriateness Criteria right lower quadrant pain – suspected appendicitis. *J Am Coll Radiol* 2011 Nov;**8**(11):749–55.

2. Howell J, Eddy O, Lukens T, et al.: ACEP clinical policy: critical issues in the evaluation and management of emergency department patients with suspected appendicitis. *Ann Emerg Med* 2010;**55**:71–116.

3. Terasawa T, Blackmore CC, Bent S, Kohlwes RJ: Systematic review: computed tomography and ultrasonography to detect acute appendicitis in adults and adolescents. *Ann Intern Med* 2004;**141**(7):537–46.

4. Toorenvliet B, Wiersma F, Bakker R, et al.: Routine ultrasound and limited computed tomography for the diagnosis of acute appendicitis. *World J Surg* 2010;**34**:2278–2285.

5. Krishnamoorthi R, Ramarajan N, Wang NE, et al.: Effectiveness of a staged US and CT protocol for the diagnosis of pediatric appendicitis: reducing radiation exposure in the age of ALARA. *Radiology* 2011 Apr;**259**(1):231–9.

6. Hernandez JA, Swischuk LE, Angel CA, et al.: Imaging of acute appendicitis: US as the primary imaging modality. *Pediatr Radiol* 2005;**35**(4):392.

7. Peña BM, Taylor GA, Fishman SJ, Mandl KD: Effect of an imaging protocol on clinical outcomes among pediatric patients with appendicitis. *Pediatric* 2002;**110**(6):1088.

8. Hahn H, Hoeppner F, Kalle T, et al.: Sonography of acute appendicitis in children: 7 years experience. *Pediatr Radiol* 1988;**28**:147–51.

9. Rettenbacher T, Hollerweger A, Macheiner P, et al.: Ovoid shape of the vermiform appendix: a criterion to exclude acute appendicitis-evaluation with US. *Radiology* 2003;**226**:95–100.

10. Pacharn P, Ying J, Linam L, et al.: Sonography in the evaluation of acute appendicitis: are negative sonographic findings good enough? *J Ultrasound Med* 2010;**29**:1749–55.

11. Hernanz-Schulman M: Infantile hypertrophic pyloric stenosis. *Radiology* 2003 May;**227**:319–31.

12. Godbole P, Sprigg A, Dickson J, Lin P: Ultrasound compared with clinical examination in infantile hypertrophic pyloric stenosis. *Arch Dis Chi* 1997;**75**(4):335–7.

13. Hernanz-Schulman M, Sells L, Ambrosino M, et al.: Hypertrophic pyloric stenosis in the infant without a palpable olive: accuracy of sonographic diagnosis. *Radiology* 1994;**193**(3):771–6.

14. Niedzielski J, Kobielski A, Sokal J, Krakós M: Accuracy of sonographic criteria in the decision for surgical treatment in infantile hypertrophic pyloric stenosis. *Arch Med Sci* 2011;**7**(3):508–11.

15. Rohrschneider WK, Mittnacht H, Darge K, Tröger J: Pyloric muscle in asymptomatic infants: sonographic evaluation and discrimination from idiopathic hypertrophic pyloric stenosis. *Pediatr Radiol* 1998;**28**(6):429.

16. Lund Kofoed PE, Høst A, Elle B, Larsen C: Hypertrophic pyloric stenosis: determination of muscle dimensions by ultrasound. *Br J Radiol* 1988;**61**(721):19.

17. Ko HS, Schenk JP, Tröger J, Rohrschneider WK: Current radiological management of intussusception in children. *Eur Radiol* 2007;**17**(9):2411.

18. Applegate KE: Intussusception in children: evidence-based diagnosis and treatment. *Pediatr Radiol* 2009;**39**(Suppl 2): S140–3.

19. Sanchez T, Potnick A, Graf J, et al.: Sonographically guided enema for intussusception reduction: a safer alternative to fluoroscopy. *J Ultrasound Med* 2012;**31**:1505–8.

20. Jamadar D, Jacobson J, Morag Y, et al.: Sonography of inguinal region hernias. *AJR* 2006;**187**:185–90.

21. Robinson A, Light D, Nice C: Meta-analysis of sonography in the diagnosis of inguinal hernias. *J Ultrasound Med* 2013;**32**(2):339.

22. Rettenbacher T, Hollerweger A, Macheiner P, et al.: Abdominal wall hernias: cross-sectional imaging signs of incarceration determined with sonography. *AJR* 2001 Nov;**177**(5):1061–6.

23. Tenner S, Baillie J, DeWitt J, Swaroop Vege S: American College of Gastroenterology guideline: management of acute pancreatitis. *Am J Gastroenterol* 2013 July;**108**:1400–15.

24. Tumala P, Junaidi O, Agarwal B: Imaging of pancreatic cancer: an overview. *J Gastrointest Oncol* 2011 Sep;**2**(3).

25. Rumack C: *Diagnostic ultrasound*, 2nd ed. St Louis, MO: Mosby, 1998.

Emergency Musculoskeletal Ultrasound

Tala Elia and JoAnne McDonough

The use of bedside ultrasound to address musculoskeletal injuries has a growing and useful role in the ED, with a range of applications. Diagnostic uses include the rapid imaging of a long bone fracture in an unstable trauma patient, the finding of a tendon rupture or joint effusion, or the confirmation of a rib fracture in a patient with a negative chest x-ray. Ultrasound is also useful to facilitate procedures such as joint aspirations or fracture reductions in children. This chapter discusses the techniques, pathology, and potential pitfalls involved in the use of musculoskeletal ultrasound in the ED.

Technical considerations

With a few exceptions, the structures under examination in musculoskeletal ultrasound are relatively superficial and sometimes subtle. This requires the use of a high-frequency (7 to 11 MHz) linear probe for almost all musculoskeletal applications. For some deeper structures, where resolution is not as crucial (e.g., femur fractures or the imaging of hip joints), a general abdominal probe with a frequency range of 2 to 5 MHz may be used.

Often the structure in question is within centimeters of the skin surface. Because image resolution is poor in the first 1 to 2 cm, a standoff pad or water bath should be used to distance the probe surface from the structure being evaluated, thereby placing that structure in an area of better resolution. There are commercially made standoff pads available that can be placed on the skin and elevate the probe from the skin surface while providing an acoustic window in place of gel. Other more readily available options also exist. For example, you could use a 250-cc saline bag between two layers of ultrasound gel as a makeshift standoff pad. Cold gel is also useful in that it has a firmer consistency that may allow for some distancing of the probe and for less pressure to be applied on a potentially painful area. Alternatively, a water bath may be used. In this technique, the area or interest is placed in a basin of water, with the probe suspended in the water 1 to 2 cm above the skin surface. The sonographer should be certain the cord of the probe is intact and not submerged with this method. This technique is especially useful for contoured areas, such as the hands and feet, where it is difficult to maintain good contact consistently between the probe surface and the skin.

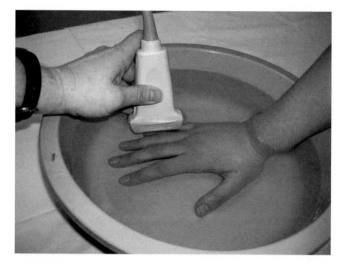

Figure 25.1. Performing ultrasound on a finger in a water bath.

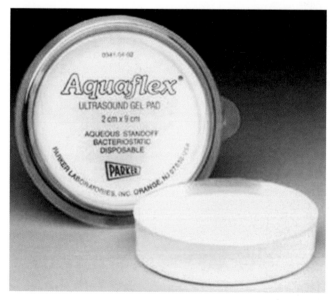

Figure 25.2. Ultrasound standoff pad.

Sonographic anatomy

Before discussing the uses of ultrasound for musculoskeletal disorders in the ED, it is helpful to review the sonography features of the relevant structures and specific imaging techniques.

Tendons

Normal tendons consist of multiple tight fiber bundles that, when viewed in the long axis, are hyperechoic with a linear fibular appearance. When scanned in a short axis, they appear as a clearly delineated cluster of hyperechoic dots. The evaluation of tendons involves a challenge particular to these structures. Tendon fibers need to be imaged with both the probe and transducer beam held at a 90-degree angle to the tendon fibers. When viewed perpendicular to the ultrasound beam, the fibers appear hyperechoic. However, if the ultrasound beam is oblique or less than 90 degrees to the tendon, the fibers appear hypoechoic. This phenomenon is called "anisotropy," and the sonographer must be aware of it because it can easily be misinterpreted as a tendon abnormality. Useful imaging of tendons requires that the ultrasound beam be held strictly perpendicular to the axis of the tendon (1).

Muscle

Like tendons, muscle also consists of multiple fibers. However, muscle fibers are less compact than those of tendons and are arranged in groupings called fasicles. These fasicles are hypoechoic but are encapsulated by a hyperechoic connective tissue. The muscle itself is composed of many of these fasicles, and the overall appearance will be as groups of hypoechoic fibers with hyperechoic septations.

Bone

The bony cortex is highly reflective and well visualized by ultrasound. Normal bone cortex appears as a smooth linear or curvilinear echogenic structure. Beyond the bony cortex, there is little penetration of the ultrasound beam, and the area appears hypoechoic. This is the result of a high-attenuation artifact, or posterior acoustic shadow, blocking the imaging of any structures deep to the bony cortex.

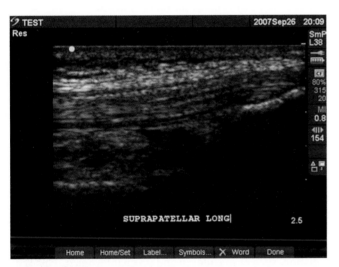

Figure 25.3. Ultrasound image of normal tendon in longitudinal axis.

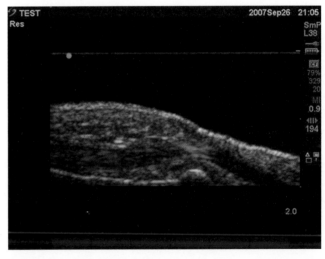

Figure 25.4. Ultrasound image of anisotropy.

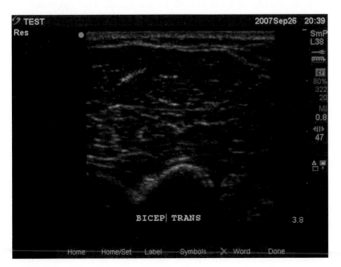

Figure 25.5. Ultrasound image of normal muscle in transverse axis.

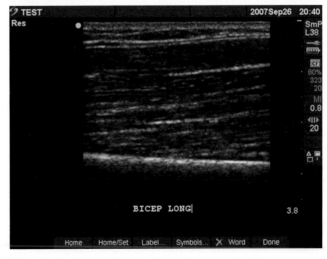

Figure 25.6. Ultrasound image of muscle in longitudinal axis.

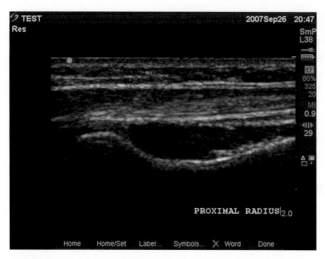

Figure 25.7. Ultrasound image of normal bone.

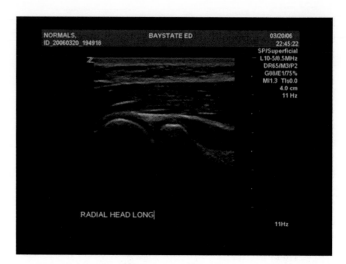

Figure 25.8. Ultrasound image of joint space.

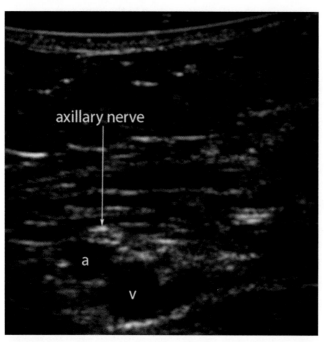

Figure 25.9. Ultrasound image of axillary nerve.

Joints

The important structures to identify when imaging the joint are the bone surfaces, tendons, and ligaments, as well as any fluid collections. A working knowledge of the basic anatomy of the joint in question is essential to allow the identification of tendons and bursa. The curvilinear surfaces of articulating bones make distancing techniques such as standoff pads particularly useful for properly visualizing joint spaces.

Ligament and nerves

Ligaments are similar in appearance and echogenicity to tendons, but the fibers within the ligaments tend to be more compact than those of tendons. Ligaments are also subject to anisotropy. Because of the varied angles that ligaments run, they tend to be difficult to see on ultrasound.

Nerves are less echogenic and more fascicular than tendons. They are often part of a neurovascular bundle, so they may be identified in close proximity of vascular structures.

Indications

Fractures

Although fractures are typically diagnosed in the ED by radiography, there is a role for ultrasound in diagnosing fractures. In rural or field settings, ultrasound is more portable and less expensive than radiography (2–4). Early bedside identification of fractures by ultrasound can guide decisions regarding early treatment and evacuation. There is also a role for sonography in patients where there is a desire to limit ionizing radiation, such as in children and pregnant women. This is of particular utility where multiple radiographs may be needed, such as during the reduction of fractures. The accuracy of ultrasound for fracture diagnosis is variable, depending on the skill of the sonographer, the body habitus of the patient, and the area under examination.

There may be a move toward ultrasound as opposed to radiography in simple fractures such as uncomplicated forearm fractures and clavicle fractures in children. In addition to limiting radiation, ultrasound can be effective in decreasing the length of stays and reducing cost in these cases (5–7). Ultrasound is also useful in diagnosing some fractures (e.g., rib, sternum) that are not readily discernible by plain radiography while also evaluating adjacent structures for injury.

To evaluate for a fracture, the bone should be identified, and then the probe should be aligned along its long axis. The probe should then be moved in the long axis along the bone. Obvious discontinuities and irregularities or fluid collections should be noted because they, too, can be subtle signs of a fracture. Once the fracture or area of suspicion is visualized, a transverse

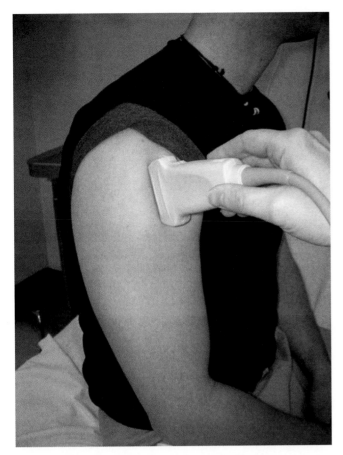

Figure 25.10. Probe on deltoid insonating proximal humerus.

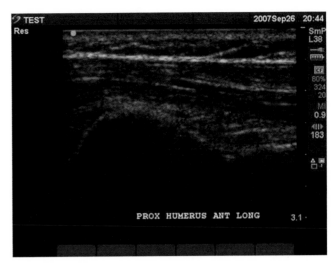

Figure 25.11. Ultrasound image of proximal humerus.

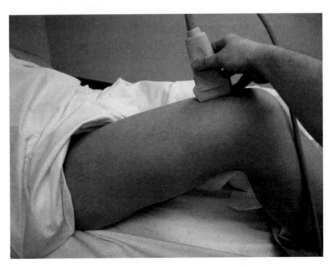

Figure 25.12. Probe on distal femur.

examination should also be done to confirm the fracture. The transverse view is important because a fracture line may not be visualized if it is parallel to the probe. In most cases, the contralateral extremity can be scanned for comparison and to verify an abnormality. Fractures are seen as an irregularity or step-off of the usually continuous echogenic cortical line and are most often associated with an anechoic hematoma.

Sonography is capable of detecting even very small fractures (8). In studies using cadaver bones, fractures as small as 1 mm are visualized by ultrasound (9). Very small fractures may be represented only by a disturbance in the dorsal acoustic shadow, whereas larger fractures, 2.7 mm or greater, are clearly visualized as a cortical step-off (9). One must be careful to have appropriate gain settings in the imaging of fractures because a small fracture can be obscured in an overgained image.

Long bone fractures

Sonography is very accurate in detecting fractures of the humerus, midshaft femur, radius/ulna, and tibia/fibula. One study showed ultrasound to be 100% sensitive in detecting humeral and midshaft femoral fractures (3). Another study had a sensitivity for detecting fractures of 92% in the upper extremity (humerus, radius, ulna) and 83% in the lower extremity (femur, tibia, fibula) (10). Sonography is least accurate for fractures of the femur proximal to the

intratrochanteric line (3, 10). But the specificity of all long bone examinations was 100% in one prospective study (3).

Humerus

To evaluate the humerus, the transducer should be placed over the distal humerus anteriorly. The bone is sometimes more easily identified in the transverse plane, and then the probe can be rotated 90 degrees. The probe should gradually be moved longitudinally along the humerus to the greater tuberosity. To view the humeral head, place the probe just distal to the acromial process of the scapula.

Femur

Imaging of the femur should begin at the distal femur by placing the probe superior to the patella over the thigh laterally. The femur should first be visualized in a transverse plane to ensure proper identification, and then the probe should be rotated 90 degrees and the length of the

349

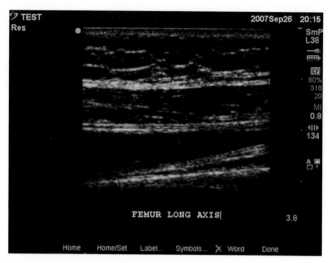

Figure 25.13. Ultrasound image of distal femur.

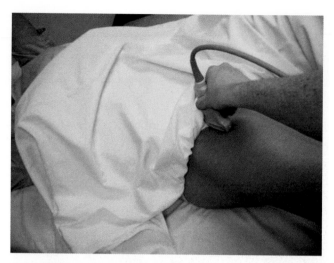

Figure 25.14. Probe position for femoral head.

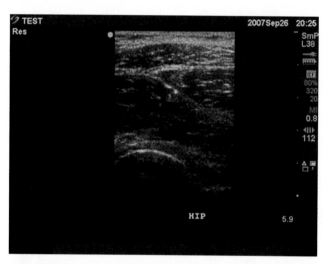

Figure 25.15. Ultrasound image of normal femoral head and acetabulum.

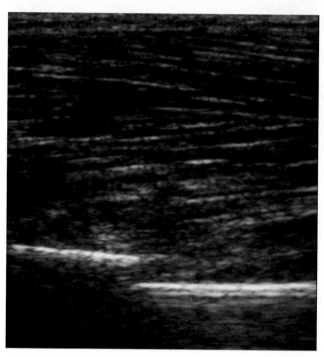

Figure 25.16. Longitudinal view of long bone fracture.

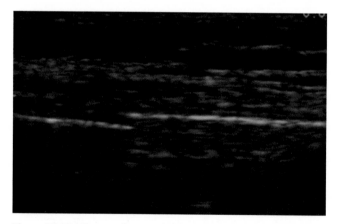

Figure 25.17. Ultrasound image of rib fracture.

femur scanned by moving the probe proximally. The probe should be angled at the femoral neck, with the indicator toward the pubic symphysis, to visualize the femoral neck, head, and pelvic acetabulum. This usually requires scanning up to the middle of the inguinal ligament, although this proximal portion of the femur exam may be limited due to body habitus.

Other long bones

The radius, ulna, tibia, and fibula are imaged in a similar fashion (11, 12). Beginning distally, the bone is first identified in cross section. The probe is then moved proximally over the long-itudinal plane of the bone to look for cortical irregularities. It is important to note that each bone should be scanned separately to more accurately evaluate for injury. Again, a transverse view at the site of injury will help confirm a fracture.

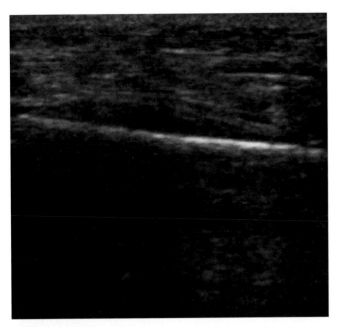

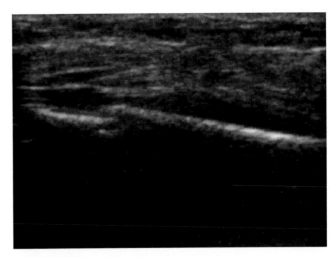

Figure 25.19. Sternal fracture.

Figure 25.18. Normal sternum.

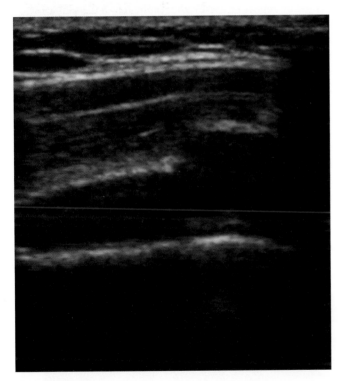

Figure 25.20. Clavicle fracture.

Rib and sternum

Rib fractures are often difficult to detect on radiographs. In the case of a suspected rib fracture, ultrasound can be used to confirm the diagnosis. Unlike plain films, where overlying lung, cardiac, and bowel shadows can obscure the rib shadows and hide a fracture, the ultrasound probe can be placed directly over the area of tenderness. One caveat is that the patient will need sufficient analgesia to tolerate the pressure of the probe on an acute fracture. Another technique is to use cooled ultrasound gel because the gel will have a firmer consistency and require less pressure to be applied. The identification of rib fractures by ultrasound can help accurately diagnose patients, in some cases eliminating an extensive workup to exclude other causes of pain (13).

Similarly, a sternum fracture, not always obvious on plain films, can also be identified by ultrasound (14). The evaluation of rib and sternum fractures by ultrasound also has the advantage of being able to simultaneously evaluate adjacent organs and identify associated injuries, such as a pneumothorax.

Clavicle

Clavicle fractures are easily identified by both radiography and ultrasound. In some cases, however, ultrasound may be more advantageous. Because many of these fractures occur in children, a quick bedside diagnosis without exposure to ionizing radiation is desirable. In fact, in one study of newborns with clinically suspected clavicle fracture, ultrasound was shown to be as accurate as x-ray and was recommended as the study of choice (6).

When suspecting a clavicle fracture, both clavicles should be imaged for comparison. A normal clavicle should appear as a continuous s-shaped echogenic line. A fracture will appear as a disruption of this line, and, in some cases, one may see movement of the fragments with respirations. Depending on the body habitus of the patient, a standoff pad may be needed.

Small bones

There is some evidence to support the use of ultrasound to detect fractures in the hands and feet. However, preliminary studies have found that ultrasound results in a decreased sensitivity in the hands and feet as compared with long bones (2, 15, 16). Because of the small surface areas and irregular contours of the hands and feet, a water bath or

351

standoff pad should be used. To evaluate the foot, the sonographer should scan the foot anteriorly, medially, laterally, and posteriorly, evaluating each bone for cortical deformities. This study is technically difficult, and preliminary data demonstrate a sensitivity of 50% in diagnosing hand and foot fractures (17). Despite this, there is evidence that ultrasound can be used to detect occult foot and ankle fractures not seen on initial radiograph (18). In these cases, a focused bedside ultrasound exam may be effective in that it allows the clinician to focus on the area of highest suspicion. Ultrasound can also detect secondary signs of fracture, such as hematoma

or callus formation, which may not be readily apparent on radiography. However, there was a high false-positive rate in one study, and more research is still needed in this area (19).

Facial fractures

In patients with suspected facial fractures, ultrasound can be used to detect factures, as well as assess for degree of displacement. In particular, nasal bone and zygomatic arch fractures can be readily imaged using ultrasound. This can provide a diagnosis and reassurance to patients without subjecting them to unnecessary radiation from x-ray or CT imaging.

Occult fractures

Although radiography is still the method of choice in the initial diagnosis of most fractures, there are some instances in which ultrasound can detect fractures in patients with pain and soft tissue swelling but who have negative radiographs. In most cases, bedside ultrasound should be used to rule in a suspected fracture with negative radiographs, rather than to rule out a fracture. Case reports of detection of occult fracture by ultrasound include a child with a spiral femur fracture and an infant with a clavicle fracture, both of which were confirmed by repeat delayed radiography 6 to 8 days later (8).

There has also been some research in the area of detecting scaphoid fractures by ultrasound in patients with negative x-rays. The diagnosis of scaphoid fracture by ultrasound is technically challenging, with only moderate sensitivity (17, 20). Given the high potential liability of scaphoid fractures, conventional management of suspected scaphoid fracture with a negative radiograph is unlikely to be altered by bedside ultrasound at this time.

Fracture reduction

Reducing a fracture in the ED may mean multiple trips to the radiography suite to assess the patient's bones for proper alignment. Bedside ultrasound can expedite fracture reduction and minimize the patient's exposure to ionizing radiation.

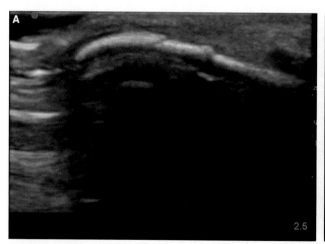

Figure 25.21. Ultrasound image of fracture prereduction.

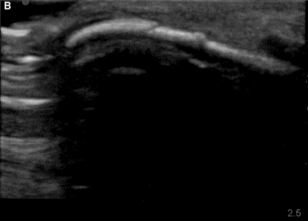

Figure 25.21A. Nasal bone fracture.

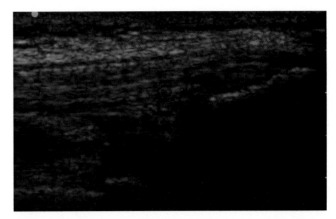

Figure 25.23. Normal knee joint.

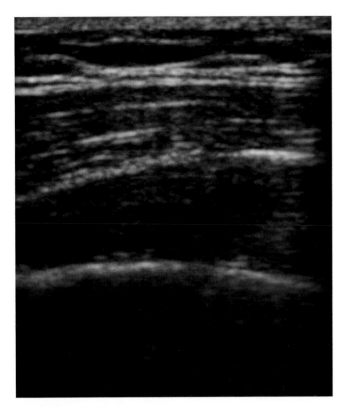

Figure 25.22. Ultrasound image of fracture postreduction.

The fracture should first be visualized using a high-frequency linear probe both in a long and short axis. It will appear as a break and displacement in the bright linear cortical surface, and both the degree of separation and displacement should be noted before reduction. After the first reduction attempt, the same area should be scanned to determine if the reduction was successful. The bright echogenic cortical line should be more closely aligned, with the step-off narrowed or missing. If there is still signification separation or displacement, another reduction attempt can be made immediately and reassessed for adequate alignment. Rather than placing a cast or splint and sending the patient for a postreduction x-ray, a bedside ultrasound can visualize the alignment of the fractured segments in real time and allow for adjustments before immobilization.

Joint effusions

Sonography also has a role in identifying and assisting with the aspiration of joint effusions. Although some joint effusions may be readily diagnosed clinically, some joints such as the hip are more difficult to assess. Also, patients with a difficult body habitus may not lend themselves to an easy clinical exam; sonography can facilitate diagnosis and aspiration in these cases (21). Ultrasound can only determine the presence or absence of an effusion; it cannot differentiate between infectious or inflammatory effusions. Although ultrasound cannot determine the nature of the effusion, it can assist in the aspiration of fluid for analysis. In one case

report, a successful ultrasound-guided hip arthrocentesis was performed by the emergency physician after multiple failed attempts at blind arthrocentesis by both the emergency physician and the orthopedist (22).

Appearance

Simple joint effusions appear as an anechoic area within the joint capsule. The fluid associated with an effusion is closely aligned with the bone cortex itself. Normal bursa are either not visualized or are seen as a thin hypoechoic space. However, in the case of bursitis, the increased fluid in the bursa may be anechoic, mimicking an effusion. By having knowledge of the anatomical location of bursas in the joint in question and by recognizing that an effusion typically lies directly adjacent to bone, the sonographer should be able to distinguish between the two processes (18). A complex effusion, such as a hemarthrosis in which the blood has begun to clot, may appear hypoechoic, or brighter than a simple effusion.

Arthrocentesis

Sonographically guided joint aspirations use similar approaches as traditional joint aspirations but allow for greater accuracy. The actual site of needle insertion will not differ from a traditional technique, but the ultrasound image can help more accurately guide that needle to the effusions. The probe should be held in a position that does not interfere with the needle insertion site yet allows for visualization of the needle tip. This is a different position for each joint. For example, if attempting to aspirate an elbow effusion, the probe can be held transversely in the antecubital fossa while a lateral approach at aspiration is attempted. The joint in question should first be imaged in multiple planes before the best approach is decided.

Hip effusions

Multiple studies and case reports have demonstrated the utility of ultrasound in identifying hip effusions and guiding arthrocentesis (22–28). Fluid around the hip joint is usually visualized in the anterior recess and is hypoechoic. To identify

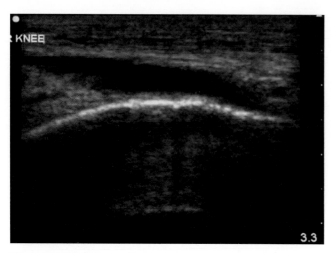

Figure 25.24. Knee joint effusion.

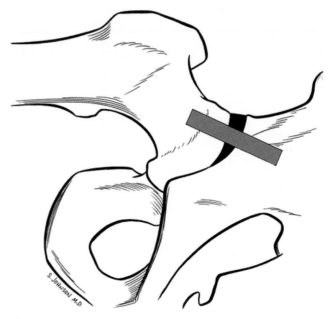

Figure 25.25. Schematic diagram of probe orientation to hip joint.

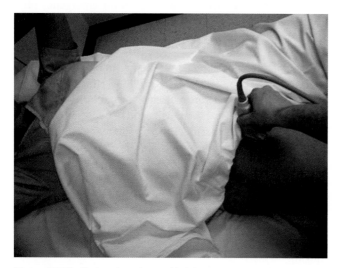

Figure 25.26. Probe orientation on hip joint.

typically more lateral and is not directly adjacent to the femoral cortex.

Knee effusions

Knee effusions can be imaged by ultrasound in cases where it is difficult to ascertain whether an effusion is present or if ultrasound guidance for an arthrocentesis is desired. The linear probe should be held in the sagittal plane, just superior to the patella, with the leg extended. This will allow for adequate visualization of the knee joint and for a lateral approach to arthrocentesis under ultrasound guidance if indicated. A transverse view can also be obtained to determine the extent of the effusion.

Elbow effusions

There are two approaches to imaging an elbow effusion. The transverse view is typically obtained by holding the elbow in 90 degrees of flexion and placing the linear probe in the antecubital fossa. The sagittal view is obtained by holding the probe on the lateral aspect of the joint, again with the elbow flexed at 90 degrees.

Tendon injury

There are several findings indicative of a tendon tear. In the case of a partial tear, there may be a hypoechoic irregularity in the usually hyperechoic organized linear structure of the tendon. Partial-thickness tears need to be differentiated from anisotropy by realigning the probe so the sound beam is perpendicular to the area of interest, to ascertain whether the irregularity is an artifact or true pathology. Ultrasound is more sensitive at detecting full-thickness tears, although their appearance can be more variable. Nonvisualization of the tendon, especially when compared to the normal side, is

an effusion and guide in hip aspiration, the probe should be placed in a sagittal position, with the indicator toward the pubic symphysis. A larger patient may require the use of a lower-frequency probe to achieve the appropriate depth. A normal fluid stripe does exist in the anterior recess and typically measures 3.5 to 5.5 mm in adults and 3.5 to 4.5 mm in children. When attempting to determine whether a clinically significant hip effusion is present, both hips should be scanned, comparing the symptomatic side to the contralateral joint. If the difference is greater than 1 to 3 mm, or if the stripe is greater than 6 mm in the symptomatic side, then an effusion is present. One useful landmark is the iliofemoral ligament, which appears as a hyperechoic structure in front of the femoral cortex. An effusion will displace the iliofemoral ligament from the femoral neck by a hypoechoic or anechoic band. One pitfall is the potential to mistake trochanteric bursitis for an intra-articular effusion. However, the hypoechoic fluid collection associated with trochanteric bursitis is

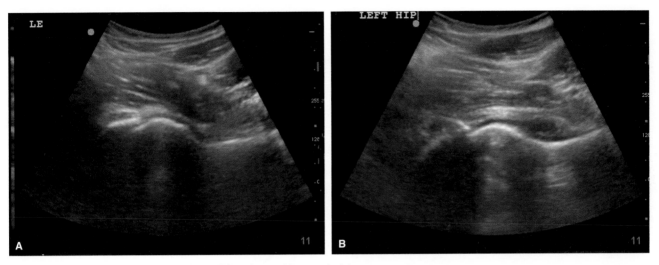

Figure 25.27. Ultrasound image of hip effusion (left) and normal hip joint (right).

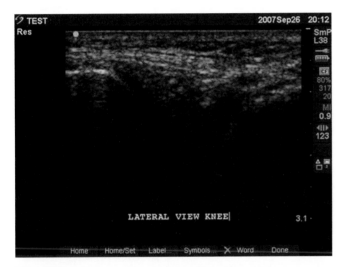

Figure 25.28. Ultrasound image of normal lateral knee joint.

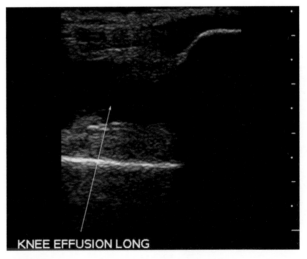

Figure 25.29. Ultrasound image of knee effusion.

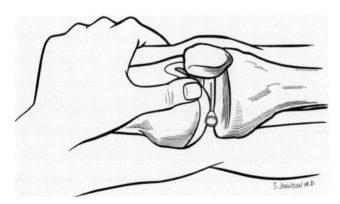

Figure 25.30. Schematic of knee arthrocentesis.

indicative of a complete tendon disruption. In some instances, the end of the retracted tendon may appear as a blunt or mass like structure. A fluid collection or hypoechoic shadowing may also be present at the site of injury and can help aid in the diagnosis. The diagnosis of subtle abnormalities may be aided by scanning the contralateral side and by scanning during motion of the joint.

Ultrasound has been found to identify tendon injuries in 97% of patients, as compared with physical exam, which identified 86% of injuries (29). Ultrasound can also be a useful adjunct when the physical exam is limited to swelling, pain, or patient cooperation (29–31).

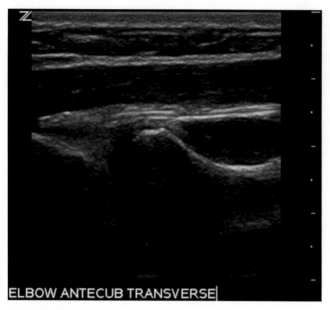

Figure 25.31. Ultrasound of normal elbow.

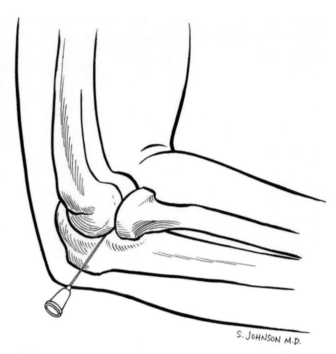

S. JOHNSON M.D.

Figure 25.32. Schematic of elbow arthrocentesis.

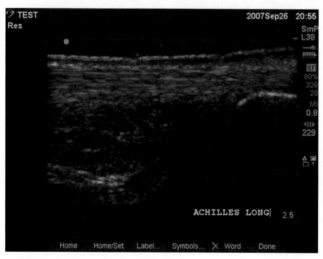

Figure 25.33. Long axis of Achilles tendon.

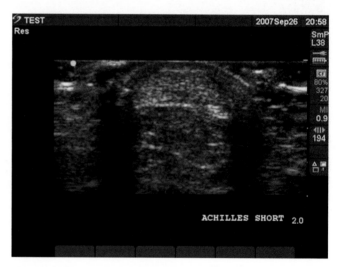

Figure 25.34. Short axis of Achilles tendon.

Tenosynovitis

The clinical findings of tenosynovitis can be confirmed by directly visualizing fluid surrounding the tendon sheath. When faced with a patient with a swollen painful finger, differentiating between cellulitis and infectious tenosynovitis can mean a significant difference in management. The clinical findings of infectious tenosynovitis, known as Kanavel's signs (fusiform swelling of the digit, finger held in flexion, pain with passive extension, and tenderness along the tendon sheath), may be equivocal or difficult to assess. Ultrasound can provide a direct look into the tendon sheath. In the setting of an infected finger, the ultrasound finding of fluid within the tendon sheath can help to aid the diagnosis. Fluid or pus in the tendon sheath appears anechoic and can clearly be seen outlining the tendon. Because of the irregular contours of the finger and because the tendons are very superficial, it is useful to emerge the patient's hand in a water bath and suspend the probe 3 to 4 cm above the surface of the finger to allow for optimal visualization of the tendon sheath. Asking the patient to flex and extend the finger and observing the movement of the tendons can also help to identify the tendon and any surrounding abnormalities (32).

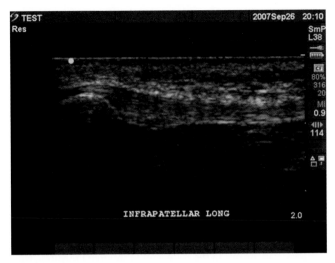

Figure 25.35. Ultrasound image of normal patellar tendon.

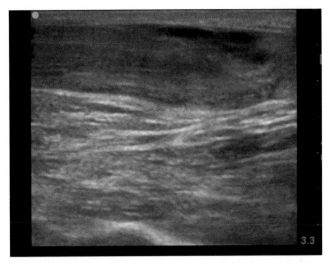

Figure 25.36. Achilles tendon rupture.

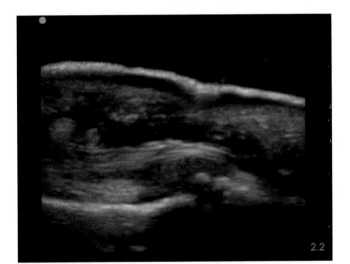

Figure 25.37. Tenosynovitis – long axis.

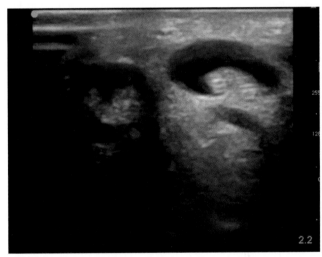

Figure 25.38. Tenosynovitis – short axis.

Imaging pitfalls and limitations

- As in all imaging, very large patients will be more difficult to image, especially when deeper structures such as the hip joint are involved.
- Be sure to use the highest frequency that will allow adequate penetration to the area of interest.
- Adjust the gain as needed; a subtle fracture can be missed if the image is overgained.
- When imaging tendons, be sure to orient the sound beam perpendicular to the axis of the tendon. Otherwise, a portion of the tendon may appear hypoechoic due to anisotropy and may be falsely interpreted as a tendon rupture.

References

1. Jacobson JA: Ultrasound in sports medicine. *Radiol Clin North Am* 2002;**40**:363–86.

2. Brooks AJ, Rice V, Simms M, et al.: Handheld ultrasound diagnosis of extremity fractures. *J R Army Med Corps* 2004;**150** (2):78–80.

3. Marshburn TH, Legome D, Sargsyan A, et al.: Goal-directed ultrasound in the detection of long-bone fractures. *J Trauma* 2004;**57**:329–32.

4. Legome E, Pancu D: Future application for emergency ultrasound. *Emerg Med Clin North Am* 2004;**22**:817–27.

5. Durston W: Ultrasound guided reduction of pediatric forearm fractures in the ED. *Am J Emerg Med* 2000;**18**(1):72–7.

6. Katz R, Landman J, Dulitzky F, Bar-Ziv J: Fracture of the clavicle in the newborn. An ultrasound diagnosis. *J Ultrasound Med* 1988;**7**:21–3.

7. Williamson D, Watura R, Cobby M: Ultrasound imaging of forearm fractures in children: a viable alternative? *J Accid Emerg Med* 2000;**17**:22–4.

8. Graif M, Stahl V, Ben Ami T: Sonographic detection of occult bone fractures. *Pediatr Radiol* 1988;**18**:383–7.

9. Grechenig W: Scope and limitations of ultrasonography in the documentation of fractures – an experimental study. *Arch Orthop Trauma Surg* 1998;**117**:368–71.

10. Dulchavsky SA: Advanced ultrasonic diagnosis of extremity trauma: the FASTER examination. *J Trauma* 2002;**53**:28–32.

11. Hunter JD, Mann CJ, Hughs PM: Fibular fracture: detection with high resolution diagnostic ultrasound. *J Accid Emerg Med* 1998;**15**:118–24.

12. Kilpatrick AW, Brown R, Diebel LN, et al.: Rapid diagnosis of an ulnar fracture with portable hand-held ultrasound. *Mil Med* 2003;**168**(4):312–3.

13. Mariacher-Gehler S, Michel BA: Sonography: a simple way to visualize rib fractures. *AJR Am J Roentgenol* 1994;**163**:1268.

14. Hendrich C, Finkewitz U, Berner W: Diagnostic value of ultrasonography and conventional radiography for the assessment of sternal fractures. *Injury* 1995;**26**:601–4.

15. Chau CLF, Griffith JF: Musculoskeletal infections: ultrasound appearances. *Clin Radiol* 2005;**60**:149–59.

16. Christiansen TG, Rude C, Lauridsen KK, Christensen OM: Diagnostic value of ultrasound in scaphoid fractures. *Injury* 2001;**22**(5):397–9.

17. Munk B, Boliva L, Kronier K, et al.: Ultrasound for the diagnosis of scaphoid fractures. *J Hand Surg* 2000;**25**(4):369–71.

18. Wang S, Chhem R, Cardinal E, Cho K: Musculoskeletal ultrasound: joint sonography. *Radiol Clin North Am* 1999;**3**(4):653–68.

19. Wang CL, Shieh JY, Wang TG, Hsieh FJ: Sonographic detection of occult fractures in the foot and ankle. *J Clin Ultrasound* 1999;**27**:421–5.

20. Senall JA, Failla JM, Bouffard JA, Van Holsbeeck M: Ultrasound for the early diagnosis of clinically suspected scaphoid fracture. *J Hand Surg* 2004;**29**(3):400–5.

21. Grassi E, Farina A, Filippucci E, Cervinin C: Sonographically guided procedures in rheumatology. *Semin Arthritis Rheum* 2001;**30**(5):347–53.

22. Smith SW: Emergency physician-performed ultrasonography-guided hip arthrocentesis. *Acad Emerg Med* 1999;**6**(1):84–6.

23. Mayekawa DS, Ralls PW, Kerr RM, et al.: Sonographically guided arthrocentesis of the hip. *J Ultrasound Med* 1989;**8**:665–7.

24. Miralles M, Gonzales G, Pulpeiro JR, et al.: Sonography of the painful hip in children: 500 consecutive cases. *AJR Am J Roentgenol* 1989;**152**(3):579–82.

25. Shavit I: Sonography of the hip-joint by the emergency physician: its role in the evaluation of children presenting with acute limp. *Pediatr Emerg Care* 2006;**22**(8):570–3.

26. Bialik V: Sonography in the diagnosis of painful hips. *Int Orthop* 1991;**15**(2):155–9.

27. Foldes K, Gaal M, Balint P, et al.: Ultrasonography after hip arthroplasty. *Skeletal Radiol* 1992;**21**(5):297–9.

28. Harcke HT, Grissom LE: Pediatric hip sonography: diagnosis and differential diagnosis. *Radiol Clin North Am* 1999;**37**(4):787–96.

29. Wu TS, Roque PJ, Green J, et al.: Bedside ultrasound evaluation of tendon injuries. *Am J of Emerg Med* 2012 Oct;**30**(8):1617–21.

30. Secko J, Diaz M, Paladino L: Ultrasound diagnosis of quadriceps tendon tear in an uncooperative patient. *J Emerg Trauma Shock* 2011 Oct-Dec;**4**(4):521–2.

31. Adhikari S, Marx J, Crum T: Point-of-care ultrasound diagnosis of acute Achilles tendon rupture in the ED. *Am J of Emerg Med* 2012;**30**:634.e3–e4.

32. Bomann JS, Tham E, McFadden P, et al.: Bedside ultrasound of a painful finger: Kanavel's fifth sign? *Acad Emerg Med* 2009 Oct;**16**(10):1034–5.

Chapter 26

Soft Tissue Ultrasound

Seric S. Cusick and Katrina Dean

The use of ultrasound in the evaluation of soft tissue structures has many potential applications. When used judiciously, soft tissue ultrasound may improve the clinician's diagnostic accuracy, result in more appropriate treatment, and improve patient comfort during diagnostic and therapeutic procedures. This modality serves as an extension to the clinician's physical exam and allows real-time visualization during procedures without the use of ionizing radiation. The role for ultrasound in disease states involving the soft tissues continues to expand with the increased utilization of bedside ultrasound in emergency medicine. This chapter focuses on three indications well documented in the literature: soft tissue infections, foreign bodies, and peritonsillar abscesses.

Skin and soft tissue infections

Indications

The patient presenting with signs or symptoms consistent with a soft tissue infection requires accurate diagnosis to facilitate appropriate management. Clinicians across disciplines are evaluating an increasing number of soft tissue infections, particularly those associated with community-acquired methicillin-resistant *Staphylococcus aureus* (1–4). Traditionally, the findings on physical examination of fluctuance or protuberant swelling were sought as indicators of a cutaneous abscess. In equivocal cases, needle aspirates could be employed to identify areas containing purulent collections. However, the use of ultrasound provides a noninvasive tool to distinguish between cellulitis and abscess. In certain clinical scenarios, the information obtained during a bedside ultrasound may also identify alternative diagnoses such as deep venous thrombosis, lymphadenitis, superficial phlebitis, hematoma, or even a strangulated hernia.

Diagnostic capabilities

The use of emergency ultrasound in the evaluation of soft tissue infections has been well reported in the literature (5–17). A prospective analysis of the comparative accuracy of clinical impression versus bedside ultrasound in the determination of abscess or cellulitis demonstrated that ultrasound is superior when compared with incision and drainage as the gold standard (6). Of the 100 patients enrolled in this study, there were 18 disagreements between clinician impression and ultrasound findings; in 17 of these cases, ultrasound was

accurate. A second study in 2007 suggested that the use of bedside soft tissue ultrasound may hold a profound impact on management. In those patients believed to be unlikely to have a fluid collection requiring drainage, ultrasound changed management in 48%. When clinicians believed a patient would require a drainage procedure, emergency ultrasound changed management in 73% of this patient group (7). The relative accuracy and potential for profound impact on patient care nearly mandates the use of bedside ultrasound in the patient with an undifferentiated soft tissue infection.

In addition to a well-documented role in the differentiation of cellulitis and abscess, there have been several reports of the use of bedside ultrasound in the management of complicated soft tissue infections. Recently, ultrasound in the diagnosis of necrotizing fasciitis has been described (8). In this single center study of 62 patients with suspected necrotizing fasciitis, the findings of diffuse subcutaneous thickening and at least 4 mm of fluid accumulating along the deep fascial layer had good sensitivity and specificity when compared with histologic diagnosis. In fact, a case report from 2014 describes a woman who presented with clinically suspected necrotizing fasciitis (9). This patient had an ultrasound that showed thickened deep fascia, fluid tracking, and fluid pockets measuring 6 mm in depth, consistent with necrotizing fasciitis. She then had a CT and MRI, which was read as cellulitis. This caused surgical treatment to be delayed, and the patient suffered septic shock and multisystem organ failure before being taken to the OR and found to have necrotizing fasciitis. Other authors have reported the utility of bedside ultrasound in the management of perirectal abscesses (16), complicated breast abscesses (10), and abscesses of the head and neck (5–17).

Although ultrasound may prove of great utility in the management of these soft tissue infections, certain clinical situations will require the use of further imaging studies. Plain radiography may be used to assess for underlying skeletal pathology, gas within the tissues, or retained foreign bodies. Similarly, cross-sectional imaging with CT or MRI may be warranted due to the location, severity, or extent of the suspected infection or even as a result of findings on bedside ultrasound (7).

The use of ultrasound in the management of these patients may be extended to afford procedural guidance. Incision and drainage of a cutaneous abscess can be performed using static or dynamic guidance and may prove of particular utility in difficult cases. Direct visualization of the needle or scalpel entering a fluid collection may result in increased patient comfort and permit avoidance of important surrounding structures. Reevaluation postprocedure may identify persistent fluid collections, particularly in those of a loculated nature.

Imaging considerations

When evaluating a soft tissue infection with ultrasound, consideration of several key principles will increase the potential for successful image acquisition. Prior to attempting the study, effective analgesia should be ensured. In the majority of cases, the use of a high-frequency linear probe (7 to 13 MHz) will allow for improved resolution of superficial structures. In the exceptional case of a particularly deep collection, a curved or phased array probe of lower frequency (3 to 5 MHz) may allow better visualization and a wider field of view. Regardless of the probe used, the sonologist should attempt to follow the convention of directing the indicator to the patient's right in transverse images and toward the head in longitudinal images. Because of the reliance on differences in echogenicity for accurate image interpretation, the ultrasound should be performed in a dim room, affording the use of minimal total gain. Appropriate use of image depth will improve visualization of the structures of interest, maximize frame rate, and allow accurate assessment of tissue involvement and the intended depth of any procedure to follow. Color, power, or spectral Doppler may be employed to verify the location of associated vascular structures. In particularly painful or superficial infections – such as the hand – the use of a commercially available standoff pad or water bath may be used to improve patient tolerance and enhance image quality by minimizing the effect of the near-field acoustic dead space (18). Alternatively, a latex glove filled with water or a 250-cc bag of intravenous fluids may be used.

During image acquisition, one should first evaluate the surrounding (or contralateral) normal tissue to appreciate the normal tissue planes and associated anatomical structures. The affected area is then evaluated in orthogonal planes, observing changes in echogenicity of the subcutaneous tissues, the presence of edema, and the location and size of any fluid collections. Cellulitis is characterized by an increased thickness of the subcutaneous layer that is relatively hyperechoic compared to normal tissue. As the infection – and associated swelling – increases, hyperechoic fat globules are outlined in hypoechoic edema, yielding the appearance described as *cobblestoning*. Abscesses are typically identified as spherical and anechoic to hypoechoic, often containing echogenic debris. However, atypical fluid collections may be near isoechoic and have complex loculations and septations. Gentle pressure over these complicated collections often allows the appreciation of free-flowing purulent material with real-time B-mode imaging.

Imaging pitfalls and limitations

Common pitfalls in scanning soft tissue infections include improper probe selection, poor use of depth and gain, failure

to recognize associated structures, and inadequate patient analgesia. Maximizing ultrasound system controls and appropriate patient preparation and positioning may alleviate many of these obstacles.

Although the role for bedside ultrasound in the management of soft tissue infections offers many advantages, it is not without limitations. Certain anatomical locations and patient conditions may not be amenable to sonographic evaluation, despite the measures mentioned previously and genuine attempts at analgesia. Furthermore, the optimal management of patients with small, poorly defined, subcutaneous fluid collections detected on ultrasound has yet to be defined. In the case of necrotizing fasciitis, the previously referenced report (8) describes encouraging results for the use of ultrasound in the assessment of this critical condition. However, further studies are being done to establish ultrasound as a primary diagnostic tool for necrotizing fasciitis and implementing a protocol (19).

Soft tissue foreign bodies

Indications

Soft tissue foreign bodies represent a troubling entity for emergency physicians. They often pose remarkable clinical challenges – in identification and removal – and represent a significant component of malpractice claims against emergency physicians (20–22). The traditional approach to these patients has often included a combination of plain radiography and local wound exploration at the bedside. However, wound exploration has potential disadvantages, including patient discomfort, damage to nearby structures, and increased possibility of infection. Difficult cases may require the use of cross-sectional imaging, surgical consultation, or fluoroscopy. Application of bedside ultrasound may facilitate efficient diagnosis and appropriate management of these patients.

Diagnostic capabilities

In evaluating the use of ultrasound in the detection of foreign bodies, one must consider the other imaging modalities available. Plain radiography has excellent sensitivity for metallic, glass, and mineral-based foreign bodies but variable – and generally poor – sensitivity for wooden, plastic, and organic materials. CT and MRI may be used with an additional set of positive and negative attributes. Both of these cross-sectional imaging modalities afford precise localization of foreign bodies in relation to adjacent anatomical structures and may be of particular use in deeply embedded objects. Their primary limitations include time, cost, and ionizing radiation (CT). In addition, the reported sensitivity of CT in the detection of foreign bodies – particularly those of radiolucent nature – is low, between 0% and 70% (23–26). Peterson and colleagues found that the best modality for detecting retained wooden foreign bodies is ultrasound, although it is frequently underused (27).

The use of ultrasound affords many benefits in the assessment, localization, and removal of soft tissue foreign bodies and has been reported across several disciplines (28–32). Although radiography holds excellent sensitivities for radiopaque foreign bodies, ultrasound has become the diagnostic modality of choice for radiolucent foreign bodies. In both tissue models and clinical investigations, ultrasound appears accurate. A study from the radiology literature described ultrasound to have sensitivities of 95.4% and specificities of 89.2% in the evaluation of 48 patients with negative radiographs and clinical suspicion of a foreign body (33). In two series evaluating ultrasound in the detection of wooden foreign bodies of the hand and foot, the sensitivity was 95% to 100%, and particles as small as 2 mm were visualized with ultrasound (29, 30). Within the emergency medicine literature, case reports describe its application in ED patients and utility at the bedside (34, 35), and studies of tissue models report variable test characteristics (21, 34, 36–38). The absence of clinical findings and an associated inflammatory reaction may be partly responsible for the low sensitivities demonstrated in these tissue models (35, 39). Despite its promised utility, further prospective evaluation of emergency physician-performed ultrasound for foreign body detection is needed to characterize the accuracy of this modality.

In addition to its role in the detection of foreign bodies, the use of bedside ultrasound may facilitate precise localization during removal, allowing concomitant identification and avoidance of associated structures. Several techniques have been described to facilitate localization and removal, including static (29, 31) and dynamic (28, 29, 31, 40) ultrasound guidance and ultrasound-guided needle localization (31, 32, 40–42).

Imaging considerations

As described previously, most soft tissue ultrasound is best performed with a high-frequency (7 to 13 MHz) linear probe. However, the use of an intracavitary probe with a standoff pad has been described (34), and deeper foreign bodies may require the use of a lower-frequency probe for adequate tissue penetration. Because of the superficial nature of many foreign bodies, the use of a water bath or standoff pad may be required to avoid the probe's dead space and ideally place the structures of interest near the focal zone.

Once the appropriate probe and scanning conditions are obtained, success is maximized by slow, orderly image acquisition. For many sonologists, soft tissue ultrasound affords the opportunity to insonate anatomical regions not routinely evaluated. As such, comparison with the contralateral side provides an understanding of the sonographic appearance of normal anatomical structures. For removal, identification of associated structures is critical to avoid iatrogenic injury during the procedure. Typically, the skin and subcutaneous tissue will appear relatively hyperechoic, with underlying muscle taking on a hypoechoic, organized, striated appearance. Tendons may appear of intermediate echogenicity and

demonstrate a linear organization, whereas fascial planes are brightly reflective linear echoes. Vascular structures may be identified as anechoic structures with characteristic Doppler signals, as described elsewhere in this text.

The appearance of soft tissue foreign bodies has been well described (27, 33, 36, 39). The majority of these objects will be hyperechoic and associated with artifacts cast into the far field. Metallic objects are hyperechoic and may cause reverberation (evenly spaced hyperechoic lines) or comet tail (tightly spaced or continuous reverberations) artifacts into the far field. Wood and mineral-based foreign bodies (rock, gravel) are often brightly reflective with dense posterior shadowing. Plastic and rubber are similarly hyperechoic with variable posterior shadowing, although plastic may, on occasion, cause reverberation. Glass has the widest range of sonographic appearances with variable echogenicities and the possibility of both shadowing and reverberation-based far-field artifacts. As the local tissue reaction develops, the foreign body will develop a characteristic hypoechoic halo (43) indicative of the surrounding inflammation and edema.

Ultrasound-guided removal of foreign bodies allows estimation of the object's depth and proximity to anatomical structures. Static – or indirect – guidance permits identification of larger, superficial structures using visual landmarks or a surgical skin marker to recall the location during the procedure to follow. Dynamic – or direct – guidance affords real-time visualization of the procedure. The clinician may begin by visualizing a needle that is directed toward the object during infiltration of local anesthetic. Often the anesthetic improves visualization of the hyperechoic foreign body by outlining it with anechoic fluid. Removal of the object may then occur using the appropriate instruments under direct ultrasound guidance. Alternatively, a finder needle may be placed under direct visualization. Teisen et al. (42) described the use of two needles placed on either side of the object at a 90-degree angle to each other. The foreign body is then retrieved by dissection guided by these needles without concomitant dynamic ultrasound guidance. A probe sheath should be used for the procedures with dynamic guidance, and the sonologist should ensure the probe indicator is directed to the left to avoid misinterpretation of the images and facilitate the procedure.

Imaging pitfalls and limitations

The detection of foreign bodies may prove difficult for the novice sonologist. The combination of irregularly shaped, superficial anatomical regions; wide probe footprints; and unfamiliar sonographic images creates a technical challenge. As described previously, the use of standoff pads or a water bath may remove some of these impediments and improve the sensitivity of the examination. In addition, misinterpretation of air, calcifications, and scar tissue may decrease the specificity. The use of the contralateral side as an example of normal anatomy is encouraged and may assist in the interpretation of otherwise unfamiliar images.

361

Peritonsillar abscess

Indications

The differentiation between peritonsillar cellulitis and abscess can be difficult based solely on clinical findings. Historical features of sore throat, odynophagia, and hot-potato voice – combined with the exam findings of trismus, swelling, erythema, and unilateral bulging of the soft palate – are suggestive but nonspecific. Historically, blind needle aspiration has been employed routinely as a diagnostic intervention, despite poor reported test characteristics. Ultrasound may be used at the bedside to facilitate both the accurate diagnosis and management of these patients.

Diagnostic capabilities

As mentioned previously, the diagnosis of peritonsillar abscess has often been established clinically or invasively via needle aspiration. Unfortunately, this practice may subject those with peritonsillitis to an unnecessary procedure with its inherent risks and is associated with a 10% to 24% false-negative rate (44–47). Recently, CT has become the diagnostic gold standard with sensitivities near 100% (48–49). Ultrasound provides the clinician with a noninvasive bedside tool that is cost-effective and does not subject the patient to ionizing radiation but holds sensitivities of 89% to 100% (49–53). A prospective analysis comparing ultrasound and CT scan with clinical outcome demonstrated a sensitivity and specificity of 89% and 100%, respectively, for intraoral ultrasound compared with 100% and 75%, respectively, for CT (49). Subsequently, Lyon and Blaivas (51) reported a retrospective review of 43 emergency ultrasounds for suspected peritonsillar abscess with 35 true positives, one false positive, and zero false negatives when compared with clinical outcome.

In addition to using ultrasound as a diagnostic modality, the clinician may perform needle aspiration of the abscess under direct ultrasound guidance. The use of ultrasound to assist in drainage was first suggested in the otolaryngology literature (54) and has since been well described by emergency physicians (50, 51). This establishes bedside ultrasound as the sole tool available to facilitate this procedure.

Imaging considerations

As with many soft tissue ultrasounds, appropriate patient preparation will improve both procedural tolerance and image acquisition. In the case of suspected peritonsillar abscess, the use of systemic and topical agents may reduce pain and trismus, and provide local anesthesia. An intracavitary transducer (4 to 8 MHz) may be used, covered in a commercially available sheath or nonlubricated condom, after sufficient ultrasound gel is placed on the probe's footprint to ensure efficient conduction of the sound. The peritonsillar region and soft palate are then insonated in both sagittal and transverse planes. The presence and extent of a fluid collection is established, as is the location of nearby anatomical structures. The internal carotid artery should be identified posterolateral to the tonsils, and its proximity may be verified using Doppler. Although abscesses have a variable appearance, the majority will demonstrate hypoechoic centers that are often heterogeneous in appearance (45, 50, 53). According to O'Brien and Summers (53), up to 30% of abscesses may be isoechoic when compared with surrounding tissues, but the finding of posterior acoustic enhancement is consistent across abscesses of varied appearances. Using these features and the contralateral side as a comparison, the sonologist is able to readily identify and localize abscesses and critical associated structures.

Aspiration may occur under dynamic ultrasound guidance, allowing identification of the maximal fluid collection and visualization of needle entry into this space. The use of a biopsy guide may aid in precise needle placement (54) but is not without its disadvantages; this equipment is an additional expense and may prove cumbersome when working intraorally.

Imaging pitfalls and limitations

The primary limitation in the sonographic evaluation of suspected peritonsillar abscess is patient tolerance. In a disease that is characterized by focal pain and swelling, with associated trismus, the clinician must ensure patient comfort prior to attempting image acquisition. The sonologist should remember to effectively lubricate the probe prior to sheath placement, minimize the depth settings, and use Doppler as needed to maximize image quality. Thorough interrogation of the peritonsillar area and soft palate, recognition of posterior acoustic enhancement in isoechoic abscesses, and comparison to the unaffected side will afford the greatest possible sensitivity and specificity.

Clinical images

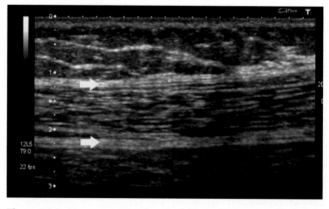

Figure 26.1. Upper extremity ultrasound demonstrating normal subcutaneous tissue (*above upper arrow*), which identifies the most superficial fascial plane. The normal-appearing striated appearance (*between arrows*) of muscle in longitudinal section is visualized.

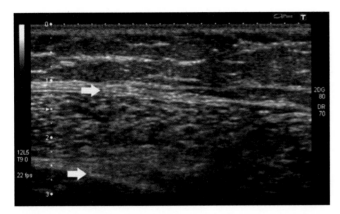

Figure 26.2. Oblique view through the same anatomical region as in Figure 26.1, demonstrating normal subcutaneous tissue, fascial planes (*arrows*), and striated appearance of muscle.

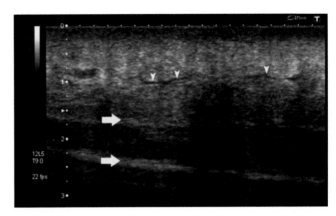

Figure 26.3. This image is from the contralateral upper extremity of the same patient imaged in Figures 26.1 and 26.2. Note the relative hyperechoic appearance of the subcutaneous tissue above the most superficial fascial plane (*upper arrow*) and the subtle areas of anechoic edema (*arrowhead*) tracking within this tissue.

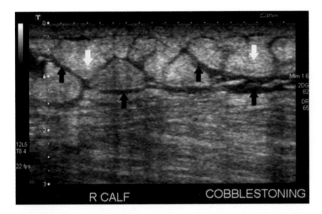

Figure 26.4. Image from lower extremity demonstrating hyperechoic subcutaneous tissue with anechoic edema (*black arrows*) tracking among the hyperechoic fat globules (*white arrows*), yielding the characteristic cobblestoning appearance of cellulitis.

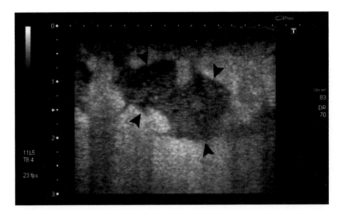

Figure 26.5. Soft tissue ultrasound demonstrating typical appearance of a subcutaneous abscess (*outlined by arrowheads*) – well-circumscribed, simple, hypo- or anechoic collection with or without echogenic debris.

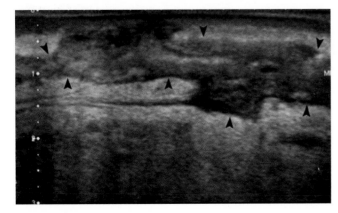

Figure 26.6. Atypical-appearing abscess (*outlined by arrowheads*) that is near isoechoic in select regions and has a complex, loculated shape. Applying gentle pressure with the probe allows visualization of free-flowing purulent material.

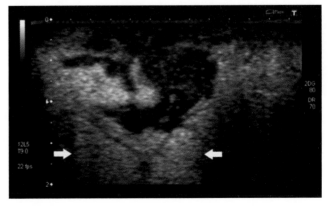

Figure 26.7. Complex cutaneous abscess that is hypoechoic and demonstrates posterior acoustic enhancement (*between arrows*).

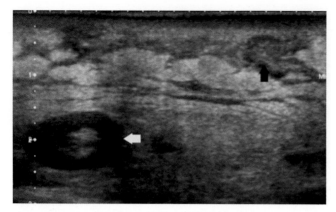

Figure 26.8. Soft tissue ultrasound of the thigh revealing a large, loculated abscess (*black arrow*). This image presents a good example of the characteristic appearance of an enlarged lymph node in far field (*white arrow*), an ovoid structure greater than 1 cm with a hyperechoic center, and surrounding hypoechoic rim.

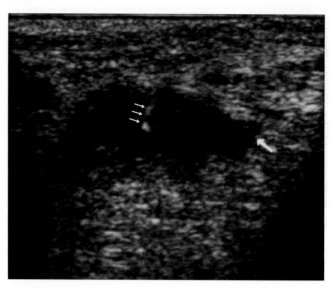

Figure 26.9. Ultrasound-guided drainage of a cutaneous abscess. The precise location of the maximal fluid collection was identified by ultrasound, and a needle (*white arrows*) was directed to the cavity during infiltration of anesthesia, facilitating incision and drainage.

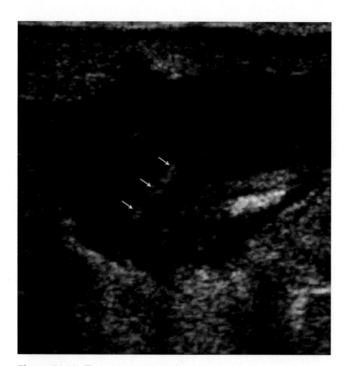

Figure 26.10. This patient presented with a breast abscess deep to the areola. A plastic surgeon directed an 18-gauge needle (*arrows*) into the abscess cavity – using the ultrasound guidance provided by the emergency physician – after puncturing the skin medial to the areola. The cavity was then incised by guiding a scalpel along this path.

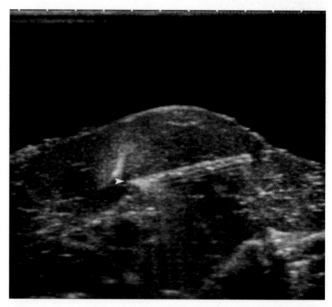

Figure 26.11. Soft tissue ultrasound of metallic foreign body (needle) imaged in a water bath. Note the hyperechoic nature of the foreign body (*arrowhead*) and the reverberation artifacts into the far field.

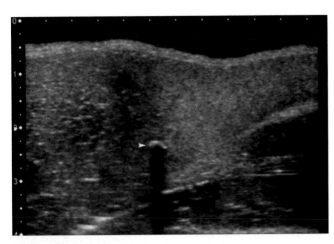

Figure 26.12. Wooden foreign body (toothpick, *denoted by arrowhead*) with characteristic hyperechoic nature and dense posterior acoustic shadowing. These images were obtained in a water bath.

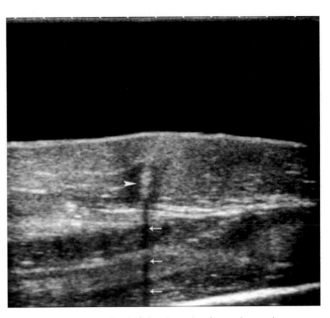

Figure 26.13. A large shard of glass (*arrowhead*), seen here to be hyperechoic with posterior acoustic shadowing (*arrows*), as imaged using a 250-cc bag of saline for a standoff pad. The sonographic appearance of glass foreign bodies varies widely, as do the artifacts that may arise in the far field.

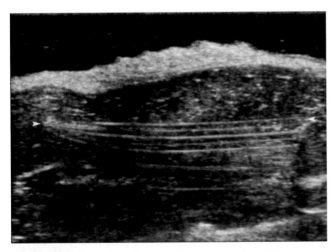

Figure 26.14. This image was obtained in a water bath and demonstrates a plastic foreign body (between *arrowheads*) that appears hyperechoic with reverberation artifacts.

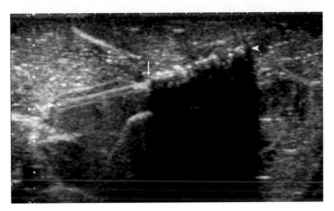

Figure 26.15. Soft tissue ultrasound identifies a foreign body of mixed composition. The large plastic piece (*right arrowhead*) produces dense posterior acoustic shadowing, likely due to the air contained within the foreign body. To the left of the arrow, the thin metallic foreign body is seen (*extending to the left arrowhead*) yielding subtle reverberation artifacts.

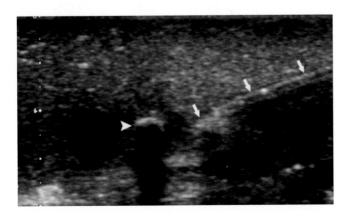

Figure 26.16. Ultrasound-guided removal of a foreign body. A wooden foreign body (*arrowhead*) is identified on ultrasound, and a needle (*arrows*) is directed under dynamic guidance for infiltration of local anesthesia and precise localization.

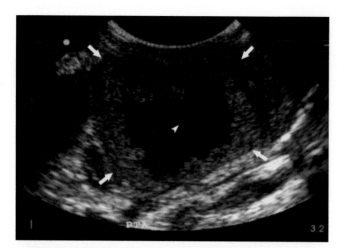

Figure 26.17. Image of a left peritonsillar abscess using a sheathed intracavitary probe. The extent of the inflammatory response is visualized (*arrows*), and the precise location of the maximal fluid collection is identified (*arrowhead*).

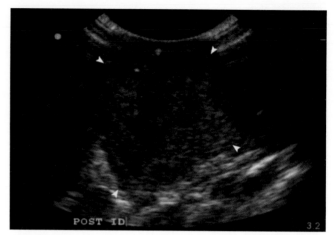

Figure 26.18. This is the same anatomical location in the patient imaged in Figure 26.17, immediately following incision and drainage. The extent of the soft tissue infection is still well visualized (*arrowheads*), but the anechoic fluid collection is absent.

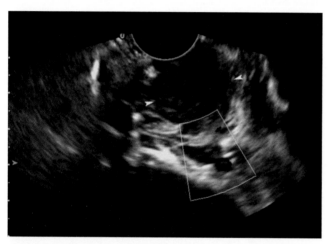

Figure 26.19. Color Doppler demonstrates the posterolateral position and proximity of the internal carotid artery to this left peritonsillar abscess (*arrowheads*).

References

1. Hasty MB, Klasner A, Kness S, et al.: Cutaneous community-associated methicillin-resistant Staphylococcus aureus among all skin and soft-tissue infections in two geographically distant pediatric emergency departments. *Acad Emerg Med* 2007;**14**(1):35–40.

2. Frazee BW, Lynn J, Charlebois ED, et al.: High prevalence of methicillin-resistant Staphylococcus aureus in emergency department skin and soft tissue infections. *Ann Emerg Med* 2005;**45**(3):311–20.

3. Moran GJ, Krishnadasan A, Gorwitz RJ, et al.: Methicillin-resistant S. aureus infections among patients in the emergency department. *N Engl J Med* 2006;**355**(7):666–74.

4. Jarvis WR, Jarvis AA, Chinn RY: National prevalence of methicillin-resistant Staphylococcus aureus in inpatients at United States health care facilities. *Am J Infect Control* 2012;**40**:194–200.

5. Yusa H, Yoshida H, Ueno E, et al.: Ultrasound-guided surgical drainage of face and neck abscesses. *Int J Oral Maxillofac Surg* 2002;**31**(3):327–9.

6. Squire BT, Fox JC, Anderson C: ABSCESS: applied bedside sonography for convenient evaluation of superficial soft tissue infections. *Acad Emerg Med* 2005;**12**(7):601–6.

7. Tayal VS, Hasan N, Norton HJ, Tomaszewski CA: The effect of soft-tissue ultrasound on the management of cellulitis in the emergency department. *Acad Emerg Med* 2006;**13**(4):384–8.

8. Yen ZS, Wang HP, Ma HM, et al.: Ultrasonographic screening of clinically-suspected necrotizing fasciitis. *Acad Emerg Med* 2002;**9**(12):1448–51.

9. Kehri, T: Point of care ultrasound diagnosis of necrotizing fasciitis missed by computed tomography and magnetic resonance imaging. *J Emerg Med* 2014;**47**(2):172–5.

10. Blaivas M: Ultrasound-guided breast abscess aspiration in a difficult case. *Acad Emerg Med* 2001;**8**(4):398–401.

11. Bureau NJ, Ali SS, Chhem RK, Cardinal E: Ultrasound of musculoskeletal infections. *Semin Musculoskelet Radiol* 1998;**2**(3):299–306.

12. Cardinal E, Bureau NJ, Aubin B, Chhem RK: Role of ultrasound in musculoskeletal infections. *Radiol Clin North Am* 2001;**39**(2):191–201.

13. Cardinal E, Chhem RK, Beauregard CG: Ultrasound-guided interventional procedures in the musculoskeletal system. *Radiol Clin North Am* 1998;**36**(3):597–604.

14. Chao HC, Lin SJ, Huang YC, Lin TY: Sonographic evaluation of cellulitis in children. *J Ultrasound Med* 2000;**19**(11):743–9.

15. Craig JG: Infection: ultrasound-guided procedures. *Radiol Clin North Am* 1999;**37**(4):669–78.

16. Chandwani D, Shih R, Cochrane D: Bedside emergency ultrasonography in the evaluation of a perirectal abscess. *Am J Emerg Med* 2004;**22**(4):315.

17. Gaspari RJ: Bedside ultrasound of the soft tissue of the face: a case of early Ludwig's angina. *J Emerg Med* 2006;**31**(3):287–91.

18. Blaivas M, Lyon M, Brannam L, et al.: Water bath evaluation technique for emergency ultrasound of painful superficial structures. *Am J Emerg Med* 2004;**22**(7):589–93.

19. Castleberg, E, Jenson N, Dinh VA: Diagnosis of necrotizing fasciitis with bedside ultrasound: the STAFF exam. *West J Emerg Med* 2014;**15**(1):111–3.

20. Anderson MA, Newmeyer WL III, Kilgore ES Jr: Diagnosis and treatment of retained foreign bodies in the hand. *Am J Surg* 1982;**144**(1):63–7.

21. Schlager D: Ultrasound detection of foreign bodies and procedure guidance. *Emerg Med Clin North Am* 1997;**15**(4):895–912.

22. Karcz A, Holbrook J, Auerbach BS, et al.: Preventability of malpractice claims in emergency medicine: a closed claims study. *Ann Emerg Med* 1990;**19**(8):865–73.

23. Bodne D, Quinn SF, Cochran CF: Imaging foreign glass and wooden bodies of the extremities with CT and MR. *J Comput Assist Tomogr* 1988;**12**(4):608–11.

24. Ginsburg MJ, Ellis GL, Flom LL: Detection of soft-tissue foreign bodies by plain radiography, xerography, computed tomography, and ultrasonography. *Ann Emerg Med* 1990;**19**(6):701–3.

25. Mizel MS, Steinmetz ND, Trepman E: Detection of wooden foreign bodies in muscle tissue: experimental comparison of computed tomography, magnetic resonance imaging, and ultrasonography. *Foot Ankle Int* 1994;**15**(8):437–43.

26. Oikarinen KS, Nieminen TM, Makarainen H, Pyhtinen J: Visibility of foreign bodies in soft tissue in plain radiographs, computed tomography, magnetic resonance imaging, and ultrasound: an in vitro study. *Int J Oral Maxillofac Surg* 1993;**22**(2):119–24.

27. Peterson JJ, Bancroft LW, Kransdorf MJ: Wooden foreign bodies: imaging appearance. *AJR Am J Roentgenol* 2002;**178**(3):557–62.

28. Bradley M, Kadzombe E, Simms P, Eyes B: Percutaneous ultrasound guided extraction of non-palpable soft tissue foreign bodies. *Arch Emerg Med* 1992;**9**(2):181–4.

29. Crawford R, Matheson AB: Clinical value of ultrasonography in the detection and removal of radiolucent foreign bodies. *Injury* 1989;**20**(6):341–3.

30. Rockett MS, Gentile SC, Gudas CJ, et al.: The use of ultrasonography for the detection of retained wooden foreign bodies in the foot. *J Foot Ankle Surg* 1995;**34**(5):478–84; discussion 510–11.

31. Shiels WE II, Babcock DS, Wilson JL, Burch RA: Localization and guided removal of soft-tissue foreign bodies with sonography. *AJR Am J Roentgenol* 1990;**155**(6):1277–81.

32. Yiengpruksawan A, Mariadason J, Ganepola GA, Freeman HP: Localization and retrieval of bullets under ultrasound guidance. *Arch Surg* 1987;**122**(9):1082–4.

33. Gilbert FJ, Campbell RS, Bayliss AP: The role of ultrasound in the detection of non-radiopaque foreign bodies. *Clin Radiol* 1990;**41**(2):109–12.

34. Dean AJ, Gronczewski CA, Costantino TG: Technique for emergency medicine bedside ultrasound identification of a radiolucent foreign body. *J Emerg* 2003;**24**(3):303–8.

35. Graham DD Jr: Ultrasound in the emergency department: detection of wooden foreign bodies in the soft tissues. *J Emerg Med* 2002;**22**(1):75–9.

36. Hill R, Conron R, Greissinger P, Heller M: Ultrasound for the detection of foreign bodies in human tissue. *Ann Emerg Med* 1997;**29**(3):353–6.

37. Manthey DE, Storrow AB, Milbourn JM, Wagner BJ: Ultrasound versus radiography in the detection of soft-tissue foreign bodies. *Ann Emerg Med* 1996;**28**(1):7–9.

38. Schlager D, Sanders AB, Wiggins D, Boren W: Ultrasound for the detection of foreign bodies. *Ann Emerg Med* 1991;**20**(2):189–91.

39. Jacobson JA, Powell A, Craig JG, et al.: Wooden foreign bodies in soft tissue: detection at US. *Radiology* 1998;**206**(1):45–8.

40. Blankstein A, Cohen I, Heiman Z, et al.: Localization, detection and guided removal of soft tissue in the hands using sonography. *Arch Orthop Trauma Surg* 2000;**120**(9):514–17.

41. Jones R: Ultrasound-guided procedures. *Crit Decisions Emerg Med* 2004;**18**:11–17.

42. Teisen HG, Torfing KF, Skjodt T: Ultrasound pinpointing of foreign bodies: an in vitro study. *Ultraschall Med* 1988;**9**(3):135–7.

43. Davae KC, Sofka CM, DiCarlo E, Adler RS: Value of power Doppler imaging and the hypoechoic halo in the sonographic detection of foreign bodies: correlation with histopathologic findings. *J Ultrasound Med* 2003;**22**(12):1309–13; quiz 1314–16.

44. Buckley AR, Moss EH, Blokmanis A: Diagnosis of peritonsillar abscess: value of intraoral sonography. *AJR Am J Roentgenol* 1994;**162**(4):961–4.

45. Kew J, Ahuja A, Loftus WK, et al.: Peritonsillar abscess appearance on intra-oral ultrasonography. *Clin Radiol* 1998;**53**(2):143–6.

46. Snow DG, Campbell JB, Morgan DW: The management of peritonsillar sepsis by needle aspiration. *Clin Otolaryngol Allied Sci* 1991;**16**(3):245–7.

47. Spires JR, Owens JJ, Woodson GE, Miller RH: Treatment of peritonsillar abscess: a prospective study of aspiration vs incision and drainage. *Arch Otolaryngol Head Neck Surg* 1987;**113**(9):984–6.

48. Friedman NR, Mitchell RB, Pereira KD, et al.: Peritonsillar abscess in early childhood: presentation and management. *Arch Otolaryngol Head Neck Surg* 1997;**123**(6):630–2.

49. Scott PM, Loftus WK, Kew J, et al.: Diagnosis of peritonsillar infections: a prospective study of ultrasound, computerized tomography and clinical diagnosis. *J Laryngol Otol* 1999;**113**(3):229–32.

50. Blaivas M, Theodoro D, Duggal S: Ultrasound-guided drainage of peritonsillar abscess by the emergency physician. *Am J Emerg Med* 2003;**21**(2):155–8.

51. Lyon M, Blaivas M: Intraoral ultrasound in the diagnosis and treatment of suspected peritonsillar abscess in the emergency department. *Acad Emerg Med* 2005;**12**(1):85–8.

52. Miziara ID, Koishi HU, Zonato AI, et al.: The use of ultrasound evaluation in the diagnosis of peritonsillar abscess. *Rev Laryngol Otol Rhinol (Bord)* 2001;**122**(3):201–3.

53. O'Brien VV, Summers RL: Intraoral sonography of peritonsillar abscesses: feasibility and sonographic appearance. *Ann Emerg Med* 1999;**34**:S26.

54. Haeggstrom A, Gustafsson O, Engquist S, Engstrom CF: Intra-oral ultrasonography in the diagnosis of peritonsillar abscess. *Otolaryngol Head Neck Surg* 1993;**108**(3):243–7.

367

Ultrasound in Resuscitation

Anthony J. Weekes and Resa E. Lewiss

Indications

Ultrasound in resuscitation is an important clinical diagnostic imaging tool for evaluating the emergent and unstable patient presenting to the emergency department or critical care unit. Ultrasound in resuscitation is not limited to one anatomic area or system. It integrates several well-established focused clinical ultrasound applications with the primary goal of understanding the patient's immediate hemodynamic physiology. Several combinations of various ultrasound application protocols have been proposed for hypotension, dyspnea, and shock states. Most of these protocols are similar with differences in sequence and emphasis of the individual applications. The focus of this chapter is to show how ultrasound in resuscitation offers an organized pathway to narrowing the differential diagnosis in the emergent undifferentiated adult patient. Management strategies described are mostly for conditions common in adult patients and may not fully apply to the pediatric patient or patients in the critical care unit. This chapter will discuss specific focused cardiac ultrasound applications and how the key cardiac ultrasound findings help with understanding shock physiology and peri-arrest resuscitation. This chapter will also discuss thoracic and peritoneal ultrasound applications and emergent ultrasound procedural guidance.

Concept

Several protocols have been published for using bedside ultrasound in undifferentiated dyspnea, hypotension, shock (1–8), and peri-arrest states (9–12). Most of the protocols are for nontraumatic medical resuscitation scenarios.

- All protocols include focused cardiac ultrasound.
- Although no traumatic conditions are suspected, the principles of the Focused Assessment of Sonography in Trauma (FAST) application may be used for free fluid detection.
- Thoracic ultrasound focuses on detecting pleural effusion, pneumothorax, and signs of pulmonary edema.
- Evaluate abdominal aorta evaluation for aortic aneurysm or aortic dissection (13, 14)
  - Thoracic aorta dissection is more critical than abdominal aortic dissection.
- Evaluate inferior vena cava and internal jugular vein evaluations

- Veins that are proximal to the right atrium provide indirect clues to volume status and cardiac outflow obstruction.

One report, a randomized control trial, did show improved emergency physicians' accuracy and narrowed differential diagnosis list when employing information from ultrasound protocol for patients with undifferentiated hypotension (5). A different study, a prospective trial of prehospital evaluations of patients undergoing cardiopulmonary resuscitation or in a shock showed that clinical management was influenced by ultrasound (mainly echo) protocol findings in 78% of the 204 subjects (15). Only a few of the above protocols have been researched for clinical efficacy or patient outcomes.

Ultrasound guidance, however, has been extensively researched and clearly improves safety and increases success for emergent procedures like central vascular catheter and transvenous pacer insertions, and pericardiocentesis.

Basic equipment includes an ultrasound machine with linear array and phased array broadband transducers. Also, 2D imaging is required. Doppler technology (color, pulsed wave, and continuous wave) and M-mode can add to the diagnostic certainty of some evaluations.

Focused cardiac ultrasound

Focused cardiac evaluation begins with the four-chamber view. Typically, the subcostal four-chamber view is the most readily obtained and most feasible in time-sensitive trauma and peri-arrest resuscitations. Other common windows include the parasternal long axis and the apical four-chamber views. The parasternal short axis views are particularly important in assessing the right ventricle (RV) free wall motion, RV size, and interventricular septal wall motion.

The main priorities of focused cardiac ultrasound are:

- Detection of pericardial effusion
- Assessment of global left ventricle contractility and size
- Detection of RV enlargement
- Assessment of volume status

  Other important features:

- Aortic root assessment
  - Enlargement >4.0 cm suggests proximal aortic aneurysm
  - Intimal flap detects dissection
- Descending aorta assessment
  - Enlargement

Pericardial effusion

The pericardial sac is fibrous and appears thin and echogenic with ultrasound. The sac surrounds most of the heart but tapers near the left atrioventricular region near the descending aorta. The normal amount of pericardial fluid is not usually visible with ultrasound. A pericardial effusion, however, shows up as a thin layer of echolucent fluid within the pericardial space, and larger accumulations fill the space surrounding the heart. Larger pericardial effusions lead to wider echolucent areas but do not extend posterior to the descending aorta when viewed in the parasternal windows. Patients with recent cardiac surgeries or previous histories of pericardial effusion and drainage may develop loculated effusions. Several views may be required to detect loculated pericardial effusions. Pericardial effusions may appear simply echolucent but can be heterogenous or echogenic if there are septation, debris, purulence or clotted blood within them.

When a pericardial effusion is discovered, the next step is to evaluate for signs of tamponade. The clinical significance of pericardial fluid accumulation depends on whether the intrapericardial pressure compromises cardiac function. The pressure within the pericardial space increases with rapid accumulations of fluid or when large volumes develop over time.

- Rapid pericardial accumulations may develop within seconds to minutes due to proximal aortic dissection rupture or penetrating cardiac injuries.
- Moderate to large fluid accumulations may develop over days to weeks due to subacute or chronic conditions such as cancer, infection, renal disease, or autoimmune disease.

Tamponade is detected in the unstable patient when the pericardial effusion decreases cardiac filling and output (16–18). Compared to the left, the right heart chambers are thinner walled and have less afterload resistance. Increased pericardial pressure from effusion accumulation can exceed that within the right atrium and ventricle, causing inward bowing of the right atrial wall or collapse of the RV free wall. When tachycardia makes it difficult to observe RV wall motion, options include:

- Frame-by-frame evaluation of RV wall motion on cine loop
- Use of a combination of different windows to view RV free wall (parasternal long and short, subcostal, and apical views)
- M-mode tracing of RV and LV in subcostal or parasternal view to detect if there is inward RV motion (abnormal) during LV diastole

Inadequate filling and emptying of the right heart ultimately affects LV output. Unlike the hypovolemic shock state, tamponade is an obstructive shock state. Inferior vena cava is plethoric (enlarged and with minimal or absent respiratory size).

Special conditions include:

- Tamponade physiology develops in the absence of pericardial effusion and in the presence of large pleural effusions.
- Tamponade physiology may be delayed in the presence of RV enlargement and RV hypertrophy (chronic pulmonary hypertension may feature pericardial effusion, RV dilation, RV hypertrophy, and IVC plethora without RV or RA wall collapse).

Overall left ventricle contractility

Quantitative measurements are not required or feasible during the resuscitation ultrasound of the unstable patient. Qualitative estimation of left ventricle contractility and the percentage change in diastolic to systolic chamber dimensions gives accurate and clinically useful information. The overall chamber size and wall thickness provide important information on overall cardiac function. The primary focus of echocardiography in resuscitation is usually limited to 2D assessments of overall systolic function. Basic focused cardiac ultrasound is not focused on diastolic function, regional wall motion, or valve interrogation.

The main categories of LV contractility are:

- Normal
- Hyperdynamic
- Moderately depressed
- Severely depressed

The physician must interpret the LV contractility within the clinical context of the patient and not simply according to normal range of values. For example, moderately depressed (and not hyperdynamic) cardiac contractility in a patient on inotropic medications suggests an underlying or preexisting cardiac dysfunction.

Multiple studies have shown that emergency medicine and critical care physicians' visual estimation of overall LV systolic function are as accurate as cardiologists' estimations (19–21).

Criteria for evaluating LV systolic function include:

- LV wall systolic thickening
- Movement of the wall of the LV along the minor axis (inward motion)
- Movement of the mitral annulus along the major axis of the LV (motion toward the apex)
- Approximation of the anterior mitral leaflet to septal wall

Normal LV systolic function involves:

- Approximately 50% LV wall thickening with systole
- Approximately 50% LV diameter decrease from diastole to systole
- Close approximation of the mitral valve anterior leaflet to septal wall less than 6 mm

Hyperdynamic LV systolic function involves relatively small LV chamber size with almost full emptying at end systole (inner walls touching). Hyperdynamic LV typically includes tachycardia, usually due to compensation to improve on suboptimal cardiac output. Hyperdynamic LV is found in patients with impaired filling states, including intravascular hypovolemia, and obstructive phenomena such as pericardial effusion provoking tamponade, resulting from impaired RV filling and emptying. Hyperdynamic LV is also found in vasodilated states of distributive shock (early stages of sepsis syndrome). Hyperdynamic LV function is shown in LV hypertrophy, severe mitral regurgitation, and patients receiving high doses of inotropic medications.

Severely depressed LV systolic function involves minimal (less than 30%) change in chamber size or dimensions between diastole and systole. LV wall thickening and mitral annular movements are minimal, and anterior mitral leaflet motion is not close to the septal wall. There are minimal movements of the mitral annulus along the long axis of the LV. Additionally, the LV is usually thin in patients with chronic dilated cardiac dysfunction.

Severe LV systolic dysfunction may be acute, chronic, or acute on chronic in the emergent patient. The presence of severely depressed LVF, however, must make one consider cardiogenic shock. Myocardial dysfunction can have several underlying causes, including sepsis, non-ischemic cardiomyopathy, toxidromes, and severe electrolyte disturbances.

Right ventricle assessment

Right ventricle assessment focuses on RV enlargement, RV free wall motion, and RV systolic function. The normal RV is about 60% the diameter of the normal LV. The normal RV apex occupies only a third of the overall cardiac apex, and its free wall is thin walled. RV systolic function is partly concentric contractions but mostly longitudinal toward the apex. The normal RA and RV fill easily from the venous return via the superior and inferior vena cava, and RV ejects blood into the typically lower resistance pulmonary vascular bed. Acute or chronic afterload increases to RV outflow will first lead to RV enlargement.

Enlargement of the RV is best appreciated and verified using multiple echo windows:

- RV apex shape becomes blunt rather than sharp
- RV apex extends toward the level of LV apex
- RV basal diameter approaches or exceeds basal diameter of LV (ratio greater than or equal to 1) on A4 view
  - Parasternal long view RV anterior-posterior width exceeds that of normal aortic outflow or left atrium
  - Parasternal short view
    - Normal RV has semilunar shape
    - Enlarged RV has diameter increase and altered shape
    - Septum may flatten during part or all of cardiac cycle
    - Septum may curve into LV

Diminished RV fee wall motion or systolic function can be detected with decreased apical movement of the tricuspid annulus decreased inward movement of the RV free wall during systole.

Significant RV enlargement can alter LV shape:

- D-shape septum in the parasternal short-axis view
- Diminished LV volume

If you find RV size enlargement, then you should look to see if the interventricular septum is flattened or bowing toward the left ventricle. This suggests increased RV pressure. The most common cause of RV enlargement is LV dysfunction and dilation. The other important cause is acute versus chronic pulmonary outflow obstruction. Chronic RV outflow obstruction is usually associated with RV hypertrophy (free wall width greater than 5 mm) with signs of RA enlargement. An important cause of acutely elevated RV enlargement includes, but is not limited to, significant pulmonary embolism. Most other causes of chronic and acute RV enlargement are associated with IVC plethora.

Hemodynamic profiles can suddenly change because of cardiopulmonary decompensation, disease progression. or therapeutic interventions. Sonography allows an assessment of preload, fluid status, right and left heart function, as well as pericardial and thoracic obstructions to cardiac output. The use of sonography allows for noninvasive and repeatable real-time hemodynamic monitoring. Recent sepsis goal-directed therapeutic guidelines emphasize the role of early central venous pressure (CVP) measurements and fluid resuscitation.

Inferior vena cava

Sonographic assessments of the inferior vena cava (IVC) can sometimes help determine fluid status. IVC assessment complements the above-mentioned cardiac assessments. IVC assessment consists of longitudinal and short-axis subcostal views of the proximal inferior vena cava focused on the IVC size (diameter) and its size variation during spontaneous or mechanically assisted breathing.

IVC size and its respiratory variability are influenced by:

- Increased intravascular volume status
- Elevated right-sided pressure
  - Cardiomyopathy
  - Valve dysfunction
  - Acute pulmonary embolism with right heart strain
  - Pulmonary hypertension
  - Acute respiratory distress syndrome
  - Pericardial effusion with tamponade
  - Right ventricle dysfunction
  - Mechanical ventilation with positive end expiratory pressure
  - Chronic obstructive pulmonary disease and asthma

Inferior vena cava assessment should be secondary to the assessments of the pericardium, ventricle contractility, and chamber size. The accuracy of IVC assessments of volume status is somewhat debatable. A normal range of IVC dimensions has not been clearly defined. Some reports on asymptomatic subjects have shown a wide range of IVC diameters and respiratory variability (22, 23). Larger IVC diameters with reduced respiratory variability are usually strongly influenced by elevated right-sided pressures. However, the small IVC with high collapsibility will gradually increase its size and gradually reduce its respiratory collapsibility during volume resuscitation.

The combined heart and IVC assessments can be used to categorize the patient's condition into physiologic categories of hypotension or shock. Physicians using ultrasound in resuscitation should be aware of important limitations of this approach: First, patients may have coexistent conditions that can prevent the simple assignment into one category of shock or symptomatic hypotension. Second, the findings described here are for classic and usually severe shock states; patients may have varying degrees of physiologic derangements.

Volume status determination can be challenging in the critically ill patient. Fluid challenges can increase the cardiac output and improve hemodynamic physiology. Patients with such a response are described as being "volume responsive." In contrast, volume unresponsive patients have no improvements in hemodynamic state or their clinical condition may worsen due to volume overload. Effectiveness of fluid loading can be assessed by monitoring increases in cardiac output and left ventricular filling. Passive leg-raising maneuvers can safely test for fluid-loading response without the risks of exogenous fluid challenge. The main value of goal-directed echocardiography in the ED is to quickly screen for patients with a low tolerance for fluid loading and determine if specific interventions – such as inotropic or fibrinolytic medications, thoracostomy, thoracentesis, or pericardiocentesis – are emergently indicated.

Clues to poor tolerance of fluid loading include:

- Severe RV enlargement
- Severe LV systolic dysfunction
- IVC plethora in the absence of tamponade

Focused cardiac ultrasound in categorizing shock states

Hypovolemic

This group of patients is likely to require aggressive fluid loading. Severe hypovolemia presents with hyperdynamic LV that is empty (low LV systolic and diastolic dimensions) and signs of low preload (small and highly collapsible IVC or IJ).

Obstructive

This group of patients is likely to benefit from diagnosis-specific therapy, and fluid loading may not be effective. The main causes of obstruction shock physiology are acute cor pulmonale (acute right-sided heart strain) and tamponade. Tamponade is mainly caused by pericardial disease (effusions being the most common) and rarely by constrictive pericarditis (thick pericardium). Less common causes include large pleural effusion and tension pneumothorax.

Cardiogenic

Poor systolic function is present usually with dilated LV. Most cases of ischemic or non-ischemic cardiomyopathy have dilated LV with thin walls. Dilated cardiomyopathies associated with RV dilation and dysfunction have a worse prognosis and an intolerance of fluid loading. Inotropic support and afterload reduction may be necessary. Valvular dysfunction may be present.

Distributive

Distributive shock is most commonly caused by sepsis and less commonly caused by anaphylaxis. Sepsis is a complex pathophysiologic state. Three classic physiologic conditions can occur within the clinical spectrum of sepsis:

- Hypovolemia
- LV myocardial insufficiency and RV myocardial insufficiency (alone or with LV dysfunction)
- Vasodilation
  - Vasodilation may be a critical issue if hypotension persists despite volume loading and normal or hyperdynamic LV function.
  - Vasopressor medication may be indicated.

These three conditions may coexist to varying degrees, making sepsis challenging to manage.

Special notes

You can *falsely diagnose* hypovolemia with ultrasound by:

- Compression of the IVC: Firm probe pressure may be used to displace bowel gas and allow a viewing of the abdominal aorta. If that same pressure is applied to look at the adjacent IVC, the IVC will be hard to find or narrowed due to your hand pressure. Use light pressure, and use the presence of the liver – an excellent acoustic window – to view the proximal IVC.
- Scanning off-plane of IVC: Scanning off-axis can give a falsely narrowed IVC and aortic "diameter." Either use the short axis or sweep to achieve the maximal anteroposterior dimensions of the long axis of the IVC or aorta.
- Scanning out-of-plane of heart: Scanning off-axis (obliquely) can give falsely low dimensions to the heart chambers. Attempt to open up (maximize) the chambers as much as possible. Use different cardiac windows to compare chamber sizes.
- Not keeping the clinical picture in mind: Poor cardiac filling does not necessarily mean low circulating volumes. Restrictive (diastolic myocardial dysfunction with intact systolic function) and constrictive cardiomyopathies (pericardial stiffening) should be considered.

Limits to evaluation of pulmonary embolism

Echocardiography is not sensitive enough to definitively diagnose pulmonary embolism (24–26). Definite signs of pulmonary embolism can be detected by transesophageal echocardiography or CT angiography of the thorax. Transthoracic echocardiography may detect thrombus in transit within the IVC and the right atrium or ventricle, or within the pulmonary outflow tract (27–29). This is a rare

Table 27.1: Ultrasound Findings and Shock Categories

Ultrasound Assessments	SHOCK CATEGORY			
Criterion assessed	Cardiogenic	Hypovolemic	Obstructive	Distributive/ Vasodilatory
Pericardial effusion	Absent	Absent	Present? Evaluate RA and RV for collapse (tamponade)	Absent
Overall LVF	Severely depressed	Normal to hyperdynamic	Normal to hyperdynamic	Hyperdynamic; moderate to severely depressed (sepsis myocardial dysfunction)
LV chamber size	Dilated	Small	Normal to small	Normal to dilated
Overall RV size	± Dilated but RV:LV ratio less than 0.7	Normal to small	Tamponade: decreased RV during diastole; Suspected RV strain; Enlarged RV: evaluate for coexistent LV dilation dysfunction	Normal; can be increased (if sepsis-induced myocardial dysfunction)
Relative RV size	Normal (less than LV)	Normal or reduced	Tamponade: normal to decreased; Strain: increased; RV: LV diameter> 0.9	Normal or reduced
IVC features	Plethora	Small with increased respiratory variation	Plethora	Normal size and inspiratory collapse, unless hypovolemia or myocardial impairment predominate
Abdominal aorta diameter assessment	Normal	Dilated dissection flap: assess aortic root, aortic arch, and descending thoracic aorta	Normal: Pericardial effusion present? Abdominal aorta may be abnormal if aneurysm dissection extends	Normal
Peritoneal free fluid assessment	Negative but may be positive if severe right-sided heart failure	Positive (consider cirrhosis, delayed traumatic bleed, ruptured ectopic pregnancy, AAA, ovarian cancer, etc.)	Negative	± Free fluid (suspect bacterial peritonitis or bowel injury purulence)
Pleural evaluation	+ Pleural sliding + Comet tails + Pleural effusion	+ Pleural sliding + Suspect hemothorax	Pneumothorax: NO pleural sliding and no B lines; large pleural effusions	+ Pleural sliding + Suspect pneumonia or infectious pleural effusion
DVT evaluation	Normal compressibility	Normal	No compressibility of CFV, PV, or IJ	Normal

RV = right ventricle; DVT = deep vein thrombosis; LV= left ventricle; LVF = left ventricle systolic function; RA = right atrium
CFV = common femoral vein; PV= popliteal vein; IJ = internal jugular vein, AAA= abdominal aortic aneurysm

finding. By itself, thrombus in transit does not serve as an indication for thrombolytic therapy. The important clinical finding of hypotension, respiratory failure, or RV failure signs (with resultant compromise of LV function) are the usual clinical indicators for thrombolytic intervention or surgical embolectomy. Echocardiography has low sensitivity and specificity for the detection of pulmonary embolism. The main and limited role of echocardiography in suspected or confirmed pulmonary embolism is to detect signs of acute right heart strain that are associated with acute and chronic morbidity and mortality (24, 30). Normal RV echocardiography indicates a better prognosis. McConnell's sign is a cardiac ultrasound finding that is very specific for a significant pulmonary embolism. McConnell's sign refers to the combination of a hypodynamic RV free wall with a hyperdynamic RV apex (also called apical sparing) (26, 31).

In summary, a submassive or massive pulmonary embolism is unlikely to be the cause of the patient's instability if the focused cardiac ultrasound reveals no RV enlargement.

Cardiac arrest

The main focus in peri-arrest resuscitation ultrasound is the cardiac evaluation. Ultrasound evaluations are very time sensitive and must be performed quickly. The explicit goal of focused echo in pulseless electrical activity and asystole resuscitation is to avoid any interruption to ongoing advanced life support. The resuscitation team leader must provide clear instructions to hold compressions, and then an assigned provider immediately performs the echo. Focused echo is performed during the brief 5-second pulse-check (while chest compressions are stopped) (9). A rapid bedside review and report of the echo is done. Serial cardiac evaluations monitor the response to chest compressions, volume expansion, medications, and procedure interventions. After a return of circulation, further noncardiac elements of ultrasound in resuscitation or other diagnostic imaging and testing can occur in the peri-resuscitation stage.

The search during peri-arrest echo is for detection of extreme or severe cases of the various categories of shock. The severity of the condition should explain the cause of the patient's peri-arrest state.

- Ventricular standstill
  - No organized cardiac movements
  - Other finding may include swirling echogenicity of coagulating blood, especially in the right heart chambers (Rouleaux formation)
  - Associated with poor outcome and death (32–34)
  - Repeat during next pulse check to see if cardiac standstill persists
- Severe myocardial insufficiency or myocardial stunning
  - Can be provoked by coronary artery disease
  - Reversible (if caused by toxicologic, electrolyte disturbances, etc.)

- Severe hypovolemia
  - Empty heart
  - Hyperdynamic heart (may be due to inotropic medications used)
  - Small, fully collapsing IVC
  - Consider hidden source of rapid hemorrhage
  - Look for fluid in hemithorax or free peritoneal fluid from ruptured abdominal aortic aneurysm (AAA) or ectopic pregnancy
- Tamponade
  - Consider aortic dissection if pericardial effusion increases in size during the resuscitation
  - Has an echogenic appearance to suggest clotting blood
- Massive pulmonary embolism
  - Obvious RV enlargement significantly greater than LV
  - Septal shift into LV
  - May be the result of a chronic disease, for example, pulmonary hypertension or acute RV infarction (LV function usually preserved except for inferior myocardial infarction)
  - Consider fibrinolytics for massive pulmonary embolism if no contraindications
- Tension pneumothorax
  - Absence of pleural sliding and absence of B lines (35, 36)
  - Absence of sliding extending lateral on the hemithorax suggests large pneumothorax (35)

Focused cardiac ultrasound may detect fine ventricular fibrillation that either did not show up clearly on the cardiac monitor or looked like asystole.

Focused lung ultrasound

Thoracic disease etiologies sought during resuscitation

Pneumothorax, pulmonary edema, and pleural effusion are some of the conditions within the thorax that can compromise cardiac output or provoke dyspnea. These conditions are identified by bedside lung ultrasound. Artifacts within the lung traditionally thought of as nuisances are now being analyzed to help determine whether pulmonary parenchyma is fluid filled.

Pneumothorax is deflation of the lung with separation of the pleural surfaces. Pleural sliding is noted on ultrasound just beneath the ribs when the lungs are inflated and the pleural surfaces are together. The combination of pleural sliding and the presence of B lines accurately proves the lung is inflated and no pneumothorax exists at the site of scanning. Thoracic ultrasound evaluation of the anterior chest for pleural sliding is more sensitive than supine plain chest x-ray in detecting pneumothorax (99% sensitive and 99% specific).

Pleural fluid accumulates in the posterior thorax of a supine patient, just cephalad to the diaphragm, and is accurately detected using mid-frequency ultrasound transducers. Pulmonary alveolar edema (wet lung) is shown on lung ultrasound as many prominent B lines projecting from the pleural line within the intercostal spaces.

Aorta assessment

Abdominal aorta evaluation

Aneurysm

Bedside ultrasound evaluation is accurate in determining the presence or absence of an abdominal aortic aneurysm. Most aortic wall dilations have a fusiform shape. The normal abdominal aorta is less than 3 cm and tapers distally. Most aortic aneurysms are fusiform. This fusiform shape is best appreciated on the long-axis view. The aorta diameter enlargement is also appreciated by comparing short-axis views of the proximal middle and distal abdominal aorta. Thrombosis adherent to the aortic wall can cause false underestimations of the actual aortic lumen. The outer wall–to–outer wall diameter measurement must be sought. A saccular aneurysm is a dilated outpouching of a segment of the aorta wall. The saccular aneurysm can be missed if its segment was out of plane in either long- or short-axis ultrasound views. Sweeping left to right on the long-axis imaging view and head to toe in each short-axis view can improve detection of a saccular aneurysm. Thrombosis within the saccular aneurysm can make it challenging to detect.

The majority of abdominal aortic bleeding enters the retroperitoneum. Retroperitoneal hematomas are not easily identified with ultrasound. In contrast, when an abdominal aortic aneurysm bleeds into the peritoneum, bleeding is not contained; it is rapid, and it can quickly cause hemorrhagic shock.

Most of the times, bedside ultrasound will not be able to tell if the wall of the AAA is intact or if there is a leak or rupture of the aortic wall. The mere detection of AAA by ultrasound will cause the physician to consider the possibility that an AAA leak or rupture is the cause of hypotension or shock. Computed axial tomography or MRI can determine the extent of the aneurysm and if and where bleeding has occurred. The presence of echo features of hypovolemia or free fluid within the peritoneal space with presence of AAA increases the likelihood of AAA rupture. An echolucent area immediately outside the aneurysm may suggest periaortic fluid accumulations.

Dissection

Aortic dissection is another acute aortic disaster that usually leads to acute severe symptoms. The term "dissection" refers to the separation of the inner wall from the outer wall as blood enters into, and widens, the middle layer of the aorta wall.

The aortic diameter may be normal in a patient with aortic dissection. The main finding in aortic dissection is the intimal flap. The intimal flap is an echogenic loose flap within the aorta. The intimal flap movement is sometimes not parallel to the rest of the aortic wall movements. The intimal flap detection may require both short- and long-axis views of the aorta to be fully appreciated. Color Doppler can distinguish the true lumen of the aorta from the false lumen (middle layer of the aorta wall).

The presence of an abdominal aortic dissection requires an evaluation for a proximal thoracic aortic dissection. Dissections that involve the aortic root and the ascending thoracic aorta usually require urgent cardiothoracic surgery. Transthoracic echocardiography can view different and limited segments of the thoracic aorta. Transesophageal echocardiography provides superior imaging details and a more extensive view of the thoracic aorta.

Different transthoracic echocardiography can evaluate different segments of the thoracic aorta. Parasternal long- and short-axis windows can evaluate:

- Aortic root dilation
- Aortic root intimal flap
- Aortic regurgitation (using color flow Doppler)
- Pericardial effusion
- Descending aorta intimal flap

Right parasternal and modified left parasternal long-axis views (one to two intercostal levels cephalad from the usual position) can evaluate the aortic root and the proximal ascending aorta. Suprasternal and modified apical two-chamber views can also detect intimal flaps at the aortic arch and descending thoracic aorta segments, respectively.

Principles of FAST: Look for fluid accumulations within the thoracic and peritoneal cavities. Free fluid within the peritoneum will create positive findings in the retrovesicular, perisplenic, or hepatorenal windows in the supine patient. Modified flank views (cephalad to the diaphragm) can detect unloculated fluid accumulations in each hemithorax. As in the trauma setting, the free fluid detection does not specifically identify the source of fluid leakage or bleeding; it simply detects the presence of free fluid within the abdomen. In the nontrauma setting, free fluid can be blood from a ruptured AAA, the corpus luteum, or an ectopic pregnancy, or it can be other fluid such as ascites from liver disease, congestive heart failure, or ovarian cancer.

Procedural guidance

Ultrasound aids in resuscitation procedures such as vascular access, transvenous pacer placement (37), pericardiocentesis and endotracheal tube placement, paracentesis, and thoracentesis. This section discusses CVC placement, pericardiocentesis, and endotracheal placement in further detail.

Central venous catheter placement

Central venous access can be challenging in some patients, especially during resuscitation when anatomical landmarks are unreliable. Ultrasound-guided vascular access is superior to anatomical landmark–guided central venous access in terms of safety, time to successful cannulation, and the reduction of complications and unsuccessful attempts. Indirect ultrasound guidance can warn the physician that a particular site or approach is not optimal due to thrombus, vessel caliber, or a precarious anatomical relationship.

Needle and guidewire insertion

Ultrasound guidance allows accurate identification and differentiation of adjacent common femoral artery and vein for femoral CVC placement and the carotid artery and internal jugular vein for IJ CVC placement (38). This leads to increased success and reduced number of needle insertion attempts (39–42). Ultrasound may assist in identifying a thrombus within a vein if the vein is noncompressible by transducer pressure. (For more information on deep vein thrombosis using ultrasound, see Chapter 16.) To identify the ideal site for needle entry, compare the left and right veins for size, and compare vein overlap to the artery. Choose the site with the least overlap with the artery. Ultrasound may guide adjustment of the needle-penetration angle to reduce the risk of posterior artery puncture.

Central venous catheter tip placement

Central venous catheters inserted via the IJ and subclavian approach may have aberrant positioning of the distal CVC tip. Inadvertent CVC insertion into the femoral artery during resuscitation may not be realized immediately and can have severe consequences to the patient.

During the procedure

- Subclavian or IJ approach:
  - View the distal guidewire near or within the right atrium and ventricle prior to passing the catheter over the guidewire and securing it in place (43).
- Femoral approach:
  - Look for the guidewire within the inferior vena cava.

After the procedure

- Venous CVC placement can be verified by saline flush of the CVC port and visualization of turbulence entering the right atrium into the right ventricle with echocardiography (44–46).
- The saline flush echo test is accurate in distinguishing femoral arterial catheterization versus femoral venous catheterization (47).
- Delayed or absent turbulence within the heart should provoke suspicion of CVC tip misplacement.
- Other ultrasound approaches to detect an aberrant CVC tip location include:

- Ultrasound evaluation of the subclavian and IJ veins for a direct view of an aberrant catheter
- Vascular turbulence within the IJ or subclavian vein after saline flush of the CVC port (48)

Iatrogenic pneumothorax can be a complication of IJ and subclavian CVC placement. Pleural sliding on each hemithorax of the supine is an accurate way of ruling out pneumothorax.

Pericardiocentesis

Pericardiocentesis is indicated in clinical deterioration when pericardial effusion and tamponade physiology is likely (49–51). It is less indicated when the pericardial effusion is suspected to be blood as in penetrating trauma or type A dissection. In that case, pericardial window or cardiothoracic surgery intervention is preferred.

Procedure

- Obtain the echo window that shows the deepest pericardial effusion.
- Direct the pericardiocentesis needle toward the highest-yield region of the effusion.
- The needle insertion site can be apical, subcostal, or parasternal.
- Ultrasound guidance can occur near the site of needle insertion or away from the sterile prepped area.

Needle tip positioning can be confirmed with echocardiography:

- Direct visualization
- Agitated saline turbulence within pericardial space
- Guidewire viewing within the pericardial space

After the procedure, repeat echo to monitor for:

- Decrease in pericardial effusion size
- Re-expansion of right ventricle and RA
- LV filling and hemodynamic status of patient

Confirmation of endotracheal tube placement

Inadvertent esophageal intubation can occur in challenging prehospital or emergency department airway cases. Anterior neck scanning will identify and distinguish an endotracheal tube within the trachea from a trachea without an endotracheal tube. The esophagus is located posterolateral to the trachea. An empty esophagus can be distinguished from an esophagus that is tunneled by an endotracheal tube. Bilateral pleural sliding in a mechanically ventilated patient suggests proper endotracheal intubation (52).

Imaging pitfalls and limitations

There are often space limitations during a code (e.g., ventilators, code carts, and multiple persons at the bedside are all competing for space).

Some possible solutions include:

Assigned role as ultrasound physician

Dedicated ultrasound machine(s) assigned to the resuscitation areas

Machine readiness

- Basic probes: linear probes and cardiac or abdominal probes
- Transesophageal probe – an option if further training and expertise are accessible
- Portable but high-quality machine selection
- Battery packs for ultrasound machine
- Retractable power cords

Emergency medicine resuscitation sonography moves from one anatomical region to another. Switching to and from cardiac and abdominal probe settings and orientation can lead to confusion; however, especially with apical cardiac viewing, where RV and LV size and morphology and function comparisons are crucial, it is important to know which side is left or right. We recommend using the probe marker pointed to the patient's right when doing the apical echo using the abdominal probe setting. The bigger, thicker ventricle on the monitor is not always the LV. Using the abdominal setting, rotate the probe marker to the 4 o'clock and 7 o'clock positions for the left parasternal long- and short-axis windows, respectively.

Technical limitations to imaging in the emergent patient may include:

- Patients may demonstrate intolerance or inability to hold their breath or exhale as instructed.
- The Valsalva maneuver, used to optimize CVC placement, is limited to awake and cooperative patients.
- Some patients may not be able to lie flat or turn to the left lateral decubitus (cervical immobilization, rib injuries, thoracic procedures).
- Likely comorbid or preexisting conditions, including abdominal tenderness, bowel gas, hyperinflated lungs, and obesity, can make scans technically difficult.
- Focused cardiac ultrasound must be quickly performed during the brief pulse checks in cardiac arrest. Saved video images can be reviewed while the resuscitation continues.

Transesophageal echocardiography (TEE) holds the advantage over transthoracic echocardiography (TTE) by providing better close-up images of the heart and can even be performed during chest compressions. TEE bypasses pulmonary interference and provides a better resolution viewing of the ascending and arching thoracic aorta, although the left main bronchus does limit its view of parts of the aortic arch. It also provides excellent images of major pulmonary arteries.

Clinical interpretation

Despite multiple studies that attempt to neatly categorize patients into etiologies of shock, it is ultrasound's ability to rule in conditions with certainty that becomes most helpful. Hypovolemia is often present in sepsis. Myocardial impairment can be found in one-third of sepsis cases. Hyperdynamic responses may be blunted by medications (aortic valve nodal blocking agents).

Positive ultrasound findings must be carefully interpreted within the clinical context. Positive ultrasound findings may not be the cause of the patient's condition. For example, a small pericardial effusion discovered after penetrating left-sided chest trauma may prompt an urgent call to a trauma surgeon, while a moderate-sized pericardial effusion may have little bearing on the management of a patient complaining of palpitations.

Solutions

- Allow information from the various goal-directed applications to complement each other.
- Use IVC size and respiratory variation, cardiac chamber size, systolic and diastolic function, and pericardial appearance as a package.
- Findings of hypovolemia should prompt a search for major vessel rupture – abdominal aortic aneurysm, free fluid in abdomen or thorax, and even sepsis sources when applicable.

Other clinical indications

We presented two clinical applications for ultrasound in resuscitation. Other emergent clinical applications for ultrasound in resuscitation may include dyspnea and chest pain. These conditions can benefit from focused cardiac and lung ultrasound, but their limitations must be recognized. Comprehensive echocardiography will evaluate for diastolic dysfunction and valvular dysfunction (both especially important for congestive heart failure assessment) and regional (segmental) ventricle wall motion abnormalities. Specialized echocardiography will evaluate for congenital heart abnormalities in pediatric and adult patients. In addition, comprehensive echocardiography will perform quantitative assessments of myocardial function using several different ultrasound technologies. In some situations, the dyspnea evaluation may include a DVT evaluation. Goal-directed DVT assessment is usually for lower extremities and is usually limited to compression of veins to the proximal thigh and the popliteal fossa. Comprehensive extremity venous assessments include long- and short-axis 2D views, direct compression and augmentation maneuvers, and spectral and color Doppler modalities.

Clinical images

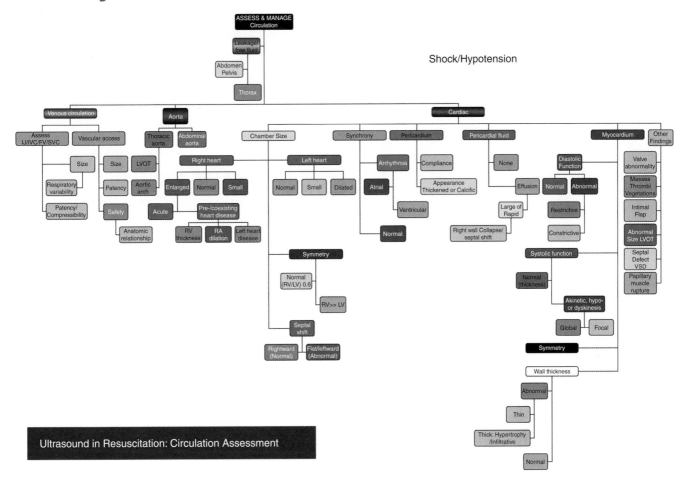

Shock/Hypotension

Ultrasound in Resuscitation: Circulation Assessment

Figure 27.1. Shock/hypotension algorithm.

Cardiac ultrasound	Clinical Diagnosis
Well filled hyperdynamic heart	Distributive shock-Sepsis, anaphylaxis
Well filled hypodynamic heart	Cardiogenic shock: sepsis, metabolic/ischemic, toxidrome
Barely filled hyperdynamic heart	Hypovolemia-hemorrhage, dehydration

Figure 27.2. Diagnosis corresponding to findings on cardiac ultrasound.

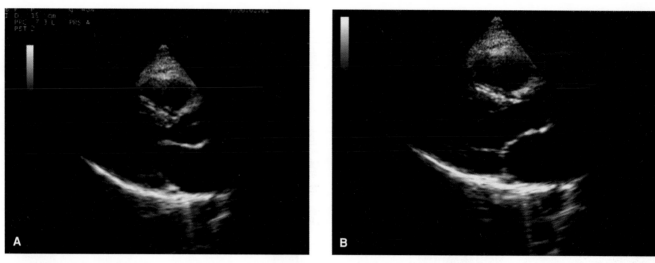

Figure 27.3A and B. (A) Normal heart (parasternal long-axis view [PLA]). The mitral valve (MV) leaflets are open, consistent with early LV diastole. Note the septal wall contour (bowing into the RV), as well as the size of the RV relative to the LV and the sinotubular appearance of the left ventricular outflow tract (LVOT). (B) Normal heart (PLA systolic phase). The ventricular myocardium thickens, and the endocardial surfaces move toward the center of the chamber. Note the appearance of a normal RV chamber and the septal wall, and how the septum varies with the appearance in diastole.

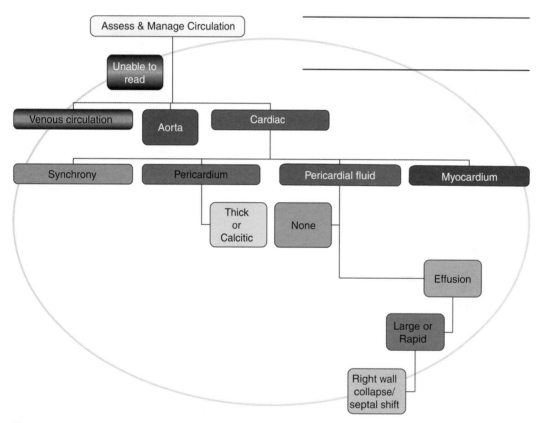

Figure 27.4. Hypotensive algorithm.

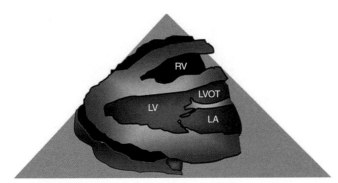

Figure 27.5. Schematic of heart in PLA shows positioning of descending aorta and pericardial (black) and left pleural (gray) effusions.

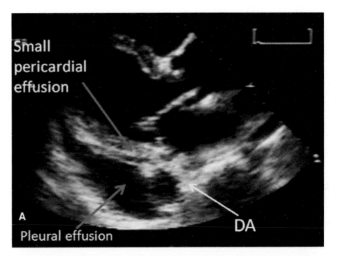

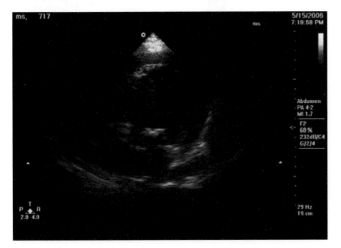

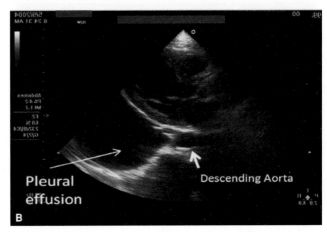

Figure 27.7. Pericardial effusion (apical four-chamber view [A4]). On dynamic imaging, the heart was empty with weakened myocardial contraction globally. This patient with a history of warfarin use presented with chest pain radiating to the back and hypovolemia. Examination of the abdomen and aortic arch could not confirm a reason for this patient's signs and symptoms.

Figure 27.6A and B. Pleural effusion versus pericardial effusion. Distinguish fluid in the pericardial space that tucks above and is limited by the descending aorta (Dao) versus fluid in the pleural space that extends beyond the Dao.

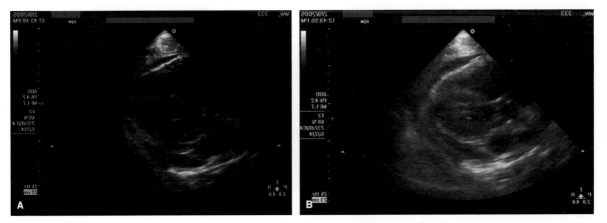

Figure 27.8A and B. (A) Pericardial effusion (PLA). The LV is barely filled, while the RV remains enlarged. Dynamic imaging showed poor cardiac output. Same patient on warfarin presenting with chest pain and hypovolemia. (B) Pericardial effusion (PLA systolic phase). The thick-walled LV is almost completely empty. The RV remains dilated. There is a pericardial effusion. Same patient on warfarin presenting with chest pain and hypotension.

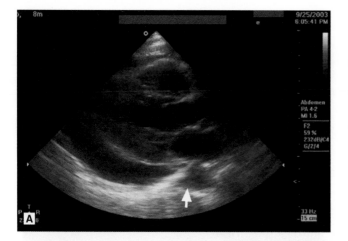

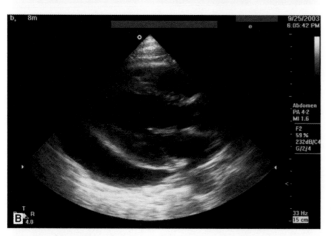

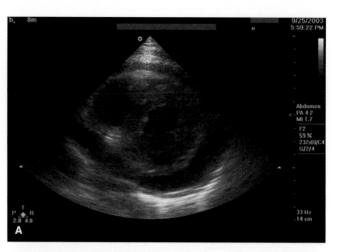

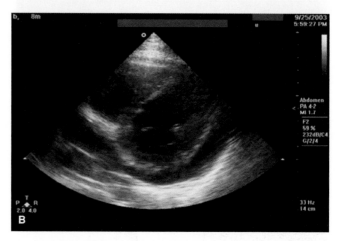

Figure 27.9A and B. (A) Pericardial effusion (PLA). Fluid extends around the heart but narrows at the Dao (*short arrow*) seen near the atrioventricular sulcus. (B) Pericardial effusion (PLA diastolic phase). RV and LV are dilated, and the myocardial walls are relatively thinner than during systole (see Fig. 27.9A). The heart was swinging within the pericardial sac. There were no signs of electrical alternans or low-voltage QRS complexes on the ECG.

Figure 27.10A and B. (A) Pericardial effusion (parasternal short-axis view [PSA] systolic phase). (B) Pericardial effusion (PSA diastolic phase). The RV assumes the expected semilunar appearance. There is no tamponade physiology evident. The intraventricular septal myocardium is curved toward the RV – this is normal when compared to Figure 27.9 (same heart).

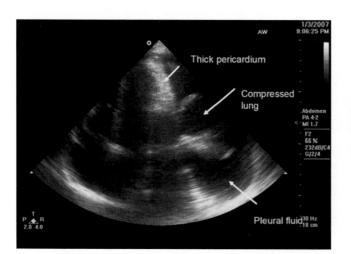

Figure 27.11. Pericardial calcification (A4). Note a thick calcified pericardium. Moderate to large left-sided pleural effusion with the left lung compressed by the fluid. Note the absence of pericardial fluid: a nondilated RV. The patient presented in cardiopulmonary arrest with distended neck veins and decreased breath sounds. The heart is barely able to fill – not because of hypovolemia – but because of diastolic dysfunction caused by the constricting thick calcified pericardium.

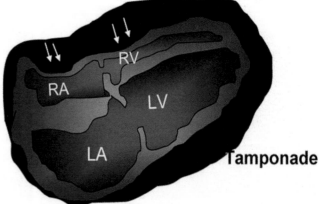

Figure 27.12. Schematic diagram demonstrating diastolic collapse of the right ventricle.

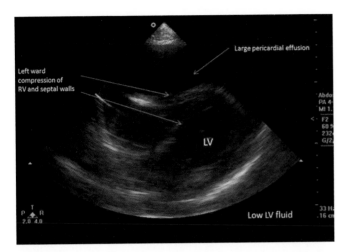

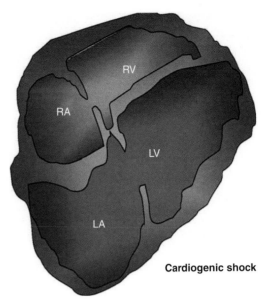

Figure 27.13. Pericardial effusion and tamponade in a patient with lung cancer on chemotherapy. He was vomiting frequently for 1 week and presented with weakness and hypotension. ECG showed low voltages. The LV size showed aggressive movements but barely any filling. His IVC was fairly flat, showing the severity of the hypovolemia (despite the tamponade), as well as how the GI losses and poor fluid intake hastened the development of tamponade. The size of the effusion shows it had slowly accumulated.

Figure 27.15. Schematic diagram illustrating a dilated heart in cardiogenic shock.

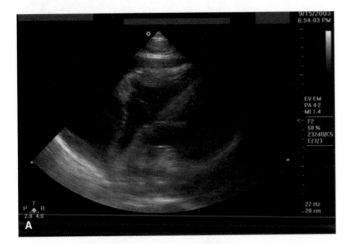

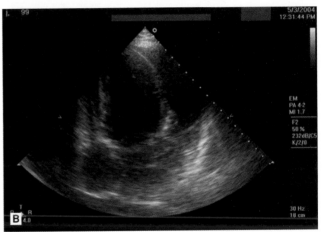

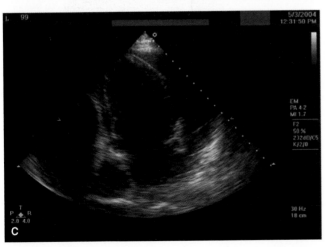

Figure 27.14A–C. (A) Pericardial effusion and tamponade (subxiphoid [subcostal] [SX]). Note low RV volume and a flattened thin-walled RA. (B) Pericardial effusion with tamponade (A4 diastolic phase). This patient had shortness of breath and a cough for several weeks despite outpatient antibiotics. Chest x-ray showed an enlarged heart with mild pulmonary congestion. On examination, the patient was hypotense without hypoxia. No jugular venous distension but rales throughout the lungs. The specialist drained more than 3 L of fluid. (C) Pericardial effusion and tamponade (A4 systolic phase). LV ejection fraction was poor.

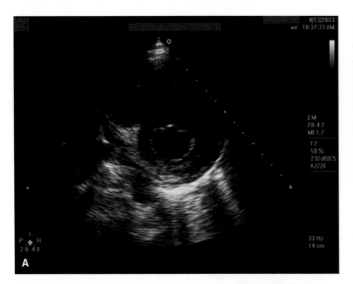
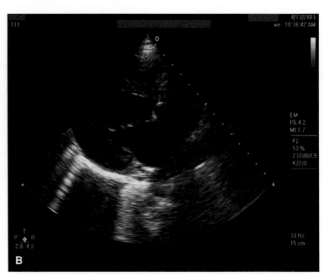

Figure 27.16A and B. Cardiomyopathy on parasternal long axis (PSLA). Movements are estimated at left ventricular ejection fraction (LVEF) of 40% – moderately depressed. (Normal to hyperdynamic LVEF: 55%–75%; moderately depressed LVEF: 30%–55%; depressed LVEF: <30%.)

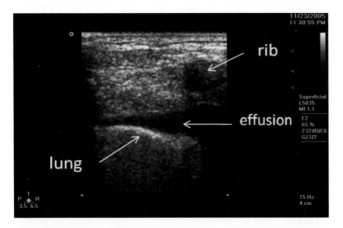

Figure 27.17. Pleural effusion. Loss of normal lung sliding of the parietal pleura over visceral pleura.

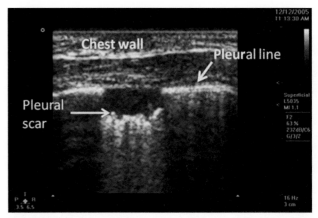

Figure 27.18. Pleural scar. Comet tail artifact is maintained in the area without scar.

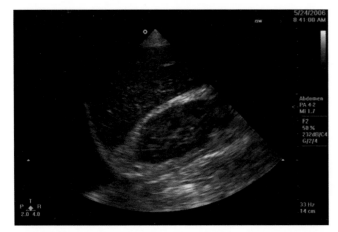

Figure 27.19. Pleural effusion. Normal hepatorenal space without appreciable fluid in either Morison's pouch or at the inferior pole of the kidney.

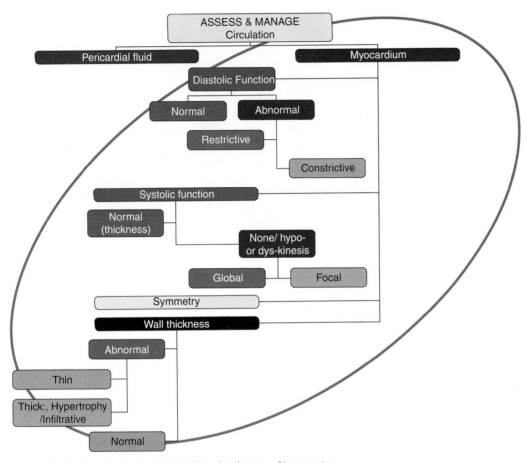

Figure 27.20. Algorithm for assessing cardiac-related causes of hypotension.

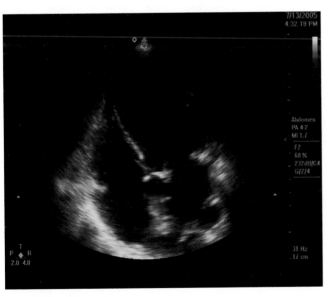

Figure 27.21. Myocardial infarction (A4). The apical and septal segments seen in this apical window showed thin and akinetic segments of the septal and apical walls of the LV. The region is also curved with a rightward bulge. The findings were consistent with an old myocardial infarction with subsequent ventricular aneurysm formation. There was thrombus in the LV. The RV is normal size and contour, with the usual tapering toward the apex of the heart. This patient had a complaint of dizziness and shortness of breath and was found to be hypotensive and hypoxic with bilateral rales. The ECG showed 4-mm elevations of the ST segments in the precordial leads.

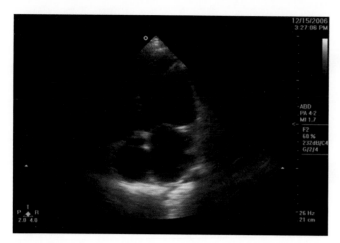

Figure 27.22. Dilated cardiomyopathy (A4). No RV strain pattern (RV is smaller than the LV), and the heart showed very poor systolic LV function. No pericardial effusion. The chamber sizes are neither dilated nor thickened or empty. Patient presented with dyspnea and hypotension.

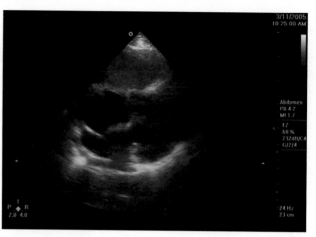

Figure 27.23. Pneumonia (SX). Markedly enlarged RA, normal RV size, and a low LV size and function. This patient was intubated soon after arrival in the ED for severe respiratory distress and worsening hypoxia. Chest CT ruled out significant PE. The hyperinflation of the lungs was consistent with chronic obstructive pulmonary disease.

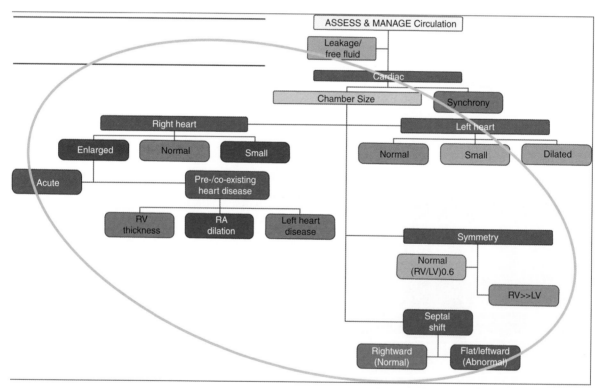

Figure 27.24. Algorithm for assessing cardiac chamber sizes.

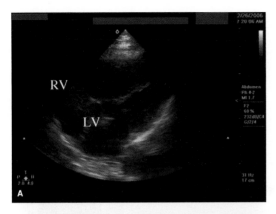

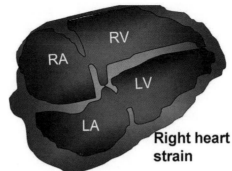

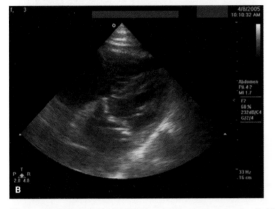

Figure 27.25A and B. (A) RV dilation. Ventricular septal wall shift is seen with bowing of the midsection of the septal wall into the LV. 1) Dyskinesis of a previously infarcted septal wall, 2) septal wall infarction in the setting of preexisting RV strain, or 3) an acute severe RV infarction. Preexisting or chronic RV strain would usually lead to RV hypertrophy and septal wall leftward shift. The normal RV:LV ratio of the heart is less than 0.6. The RV in this scan is larger than the LV (RV:LV diameter ratio >1.0) in diastole. Sonographic findings in RV strain:RV dilation, a leftward septal shift, the absence of RV hypertrophy, good LV contractions, large IVC diameter, and poor respiratory variation (IVC plethora). (B) RV strain (SX). Thick LV with an enlarged RA and widened RV. Stuttering contractions of the LV caused inadequate cardiac output. Patient presented with atrial fibrillation. With adequate anticoagulation already present, ventricular rate control leads to an improvement in clinical condition. Look for LV disease/dysfunction even if you see RV strain.

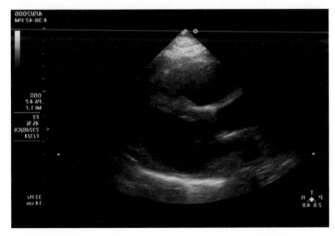

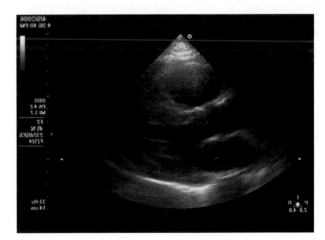

Figure 27.26. PE. RV dilation (PLA) during diastole. The overall left atrium (LA) and LV size and appearance are normal. The right-sided intraventricular pressure on the intraventricular septal wall is not sufficiently increased to overcome the left-sided pressures. The septal wall is not deviated toward the LV. The RV is thin.

Figure 27.27. RV dilation (PLA systolic phase). Compare the RV size to that of the LV (measured at the level where the mitral leaflets touch). The RV is dilated and larger than the LV.

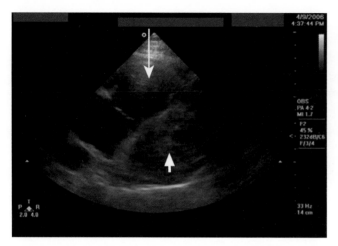

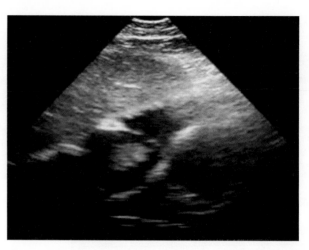

Figure 27.28. PE with significant RV dilation (*long arrow*) (PSA) view. The LV is markedly compressed (*short arrow*) due to the bulge of the septum into the LV. Note that the RV side of the septum is flatter than in Figure 27.27. The patient presented with severe dyspnea, hypoxia, tachycardia, and hypotension. Chest CT showed a large PE.

Figure 27.29. RA clot (SX). The mass may be a tumor, but in the setting of acute dyspnea, hypotension, and hypoxia, a clot in transit is more likely. This is an uncommon sonographic finding. Note there is no RV dilation.

Image courtesy of Chris Moore, Yale University, New Haven, CT.

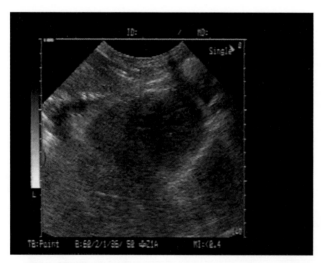

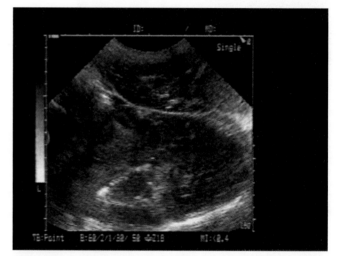

Figure 27.30. Hypovolemia (SX). Heart chambers are difficult to distinguish because the endocardial surfaces are very close together. The heart became hyperdynamic, but poor filling volumes led to a very low cardiac output. This patient presented with severe GI bleeding compounded by warfarin toxicity.

Figure 27.31. Ventricular standstill (SX). Clotted blood has a swirling, smoky appearance. Intraventricular blood has the same echogenicity as the ventricular myocardium. The swirling motion may be due to the presence of valve despite ventricular standstill. Ventricular standstill is associated with 100% in-hospital mortality. On a still image, the clotting blood may appear similar to the myocardium.

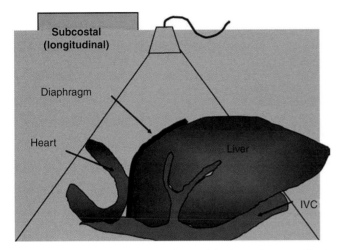

Figure 27.32. Diagram illustrating relation of diaphragm, heart, and liver in the subcostal four-chamber view.

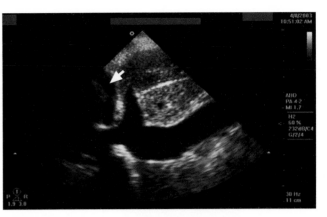

Figure 27.33. IVC plethora (SX longitudinal view). Minimal respiratory variation in IVC diameter. Note the pericardial effusion (*short arrow*) between the RA and the diaphragm, as well as the dilated hepatic veins branching off of the proximal IVC. No collapse of IVC during inspiration or on sniff test means elevated CVP. This may be found in cases of pure tamponade, massive PE, RV infarction, and congestive heart failure.

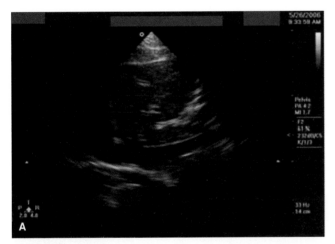

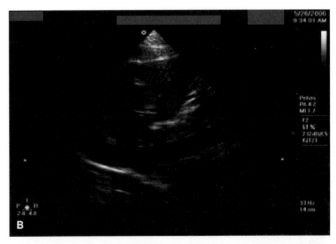

Figure 27.34A and B. (A) IVC (SX longitudinal view inspiratory phase). Note the respiratory variation in diameter. The normal caval index is usually about 40% or 0.4. Too much probe pressure can falsely narrow or even completely flatten the IVC. (B) IVC (SX longitudinal view expiratory phase). Compare the diameter during routine inspiration. IVC less than 1.5 cm with >50% inspiratory collapse has a CVP 0 to 5 mmHg. IVC diameter between 1.5 and 2.5 cm with >50% respiratory variation has a CVP of 5 to 10 mmHg. Larger IVC sizes of 1.5 to 2.5 cm with <50% respiratory variation tend to have a CVP of 10 to 15 mmHg. IVC plethora: Diameter <2.5 cm and very little respiratory variation corresponds to CVP of 15 to 20 mmHg.

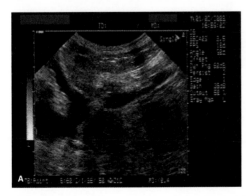

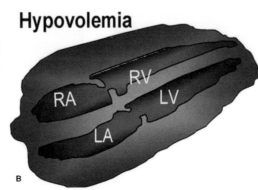

Figure 27.35A and B. Hypovolemia (SX longitudinal view). Make measurements about 2 to 3 cm away from the IVC/diaphragm juncture. The proximal IVC was a maximum of 0.5 cm, with complete collapse on the patient's inspiratory efforts. The caval index is nearly 1, suggestive of low right atrial pressures or CVPs.

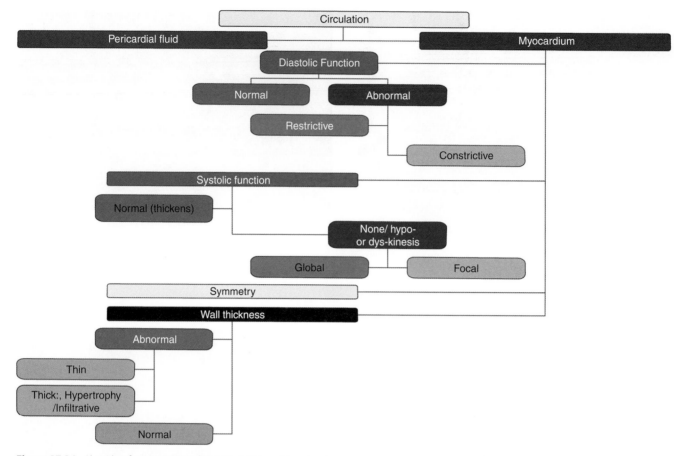

Figure 27.36. Algorithm for assessing cardiac-related causes of hypotension.

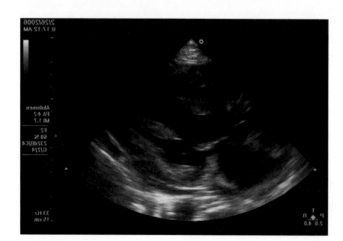

Figure 27.37. LV hypertrophy (PLA diastolic phase). Septal and posterior walls are each more than 2 cm thick.

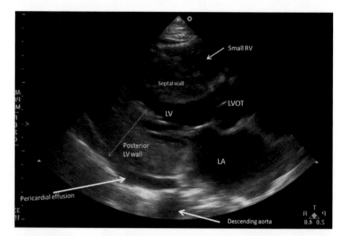

Figure 27.38. Compared to the previous image, this heart has a more pronounced cardiomyopathy with thicker walls and more pronounced septal hypertrophy – hence, LV outflow tract obstruction. Note the small LV. The small pericardial effusion is clinically insignificant. There are multiple types of cardiomyopathies that may present with chest pain, palpitations, arrhythmias, syncope, and dyspnea. Diffuse LV hypertrophy, isolated subaortic septal wall thickening, and dilated thin walls are just a few examples of cardiomyopathy. This patient is preload dependent, and chest pain arrhythmia treatment may involve more fluid, beta-blocker use, cardiac catheterization, cardioversion, or avoidance of nitrates. It depends on the clinical scenario and the dynamics witnessed on real-time 2D scanning.

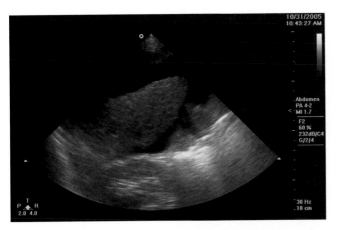

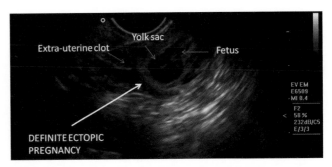

Figure 27.40. Ectopic pregnancy. Transvaginal coronal view of the right adnexa confirms a fetal pole with yolk sac outside the uterus.

Figure 27.39. Abdominal free fluid. In this view of the right upper quadrant of the abdomen, note that free fluid surrounds most of the contracted liver, the lobulated appearance of bowel loops, and the fluid between the inferior pole of the kidney. This image can belong to several patients, including the blunt abdominal trauma victim, a female of childbearing age with abdominal pain and near syncope, and the elderly male with abdominal pain radiating to the back. The contracted liver suggests to the clinician that there may be preexisting portal hypertension and ascites. The free fluid may not be due to internal hemorrhage.

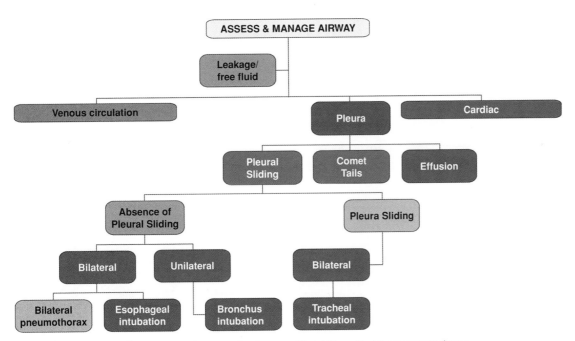

Figure 27.41. Algorithm for assessing pulmonary-related causes of instability as it relates to pneumothorax.

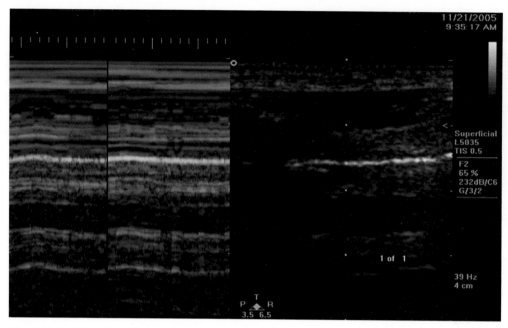

Figure 27.42. Normal lung M-mode characteristic seashore sign. Real time shows characteristic lung sliding and comet tail artifact. A lines are present.

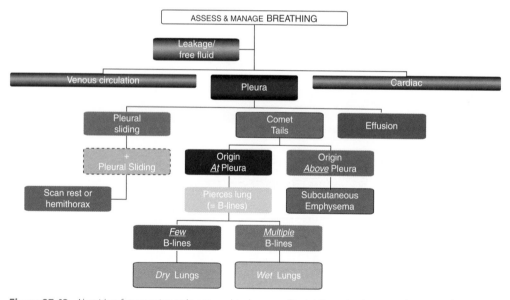

Figure 27.43. Algorithm for assessing pulmonary-related causes of instability as it relates to pulmonary edema.

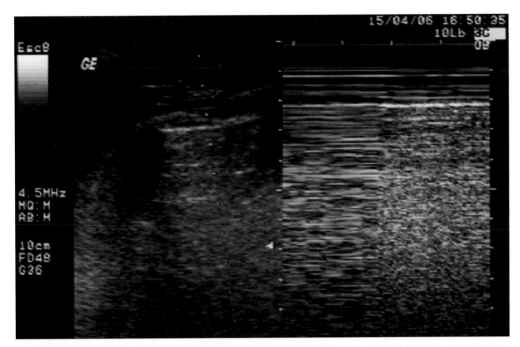

Figure 27.44. Lung point sign is shown on this M-mode tracing as a transition between the granular wavy pattern of sliding pleural surfaces (seashore sign) and smoother linear lines of the separated pleural surfaces seen in pneumothorax, mainstem intubation, pleurodesis, and other disorders.

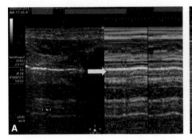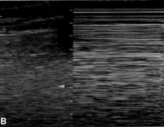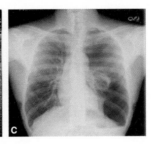

Figure 27.45A–C. (A) Seashore sign on M-mode at the pleural line of the right anterior chest scan. (B) No pleural sliding is evident at the left anterior chest M-mode scan. (C) A very large left-sided pneumothorax was seen on the chest x-ray. There will be no lung point sign on ultrasound.

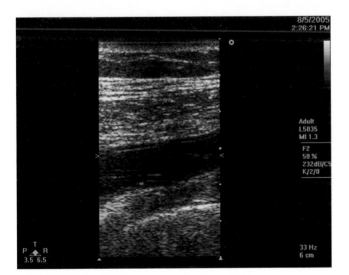

Figure 27.46. Fluid is seen above the pleural line but within the anterior chest wall. The pleural line slides. This was a patient with complications after coronary artery bypass graft.

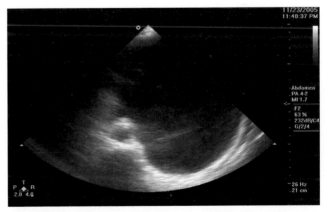

Figure 27.47. Massive pleural effusion. The probe placed on the anterior chest wall displayed an unusually good acoustic window. The heart was discovered on the right parasternal window. Note that the depth of the pleural effusion was 20 cm when measured in the anteroposterior plane. The vertebral body is shown in the posterior midline. Lungs and heart were displaced to the right hemithorax. The patient was being scanned for several reasons: the low voltages on ECGs, absent breath sounds on the left lung fields, hypoxia, and borderline hypotension.

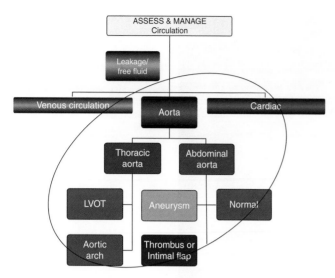

Figure 27.48. Algorithm for assessing aortic-related causes of instability.

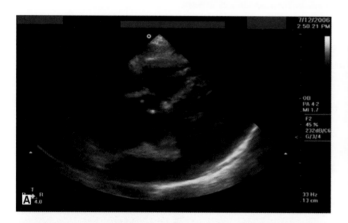

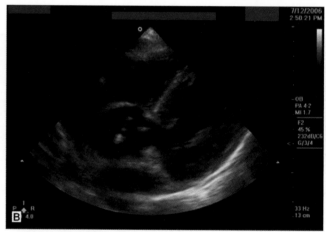

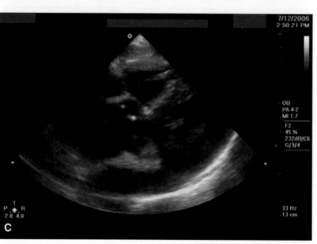

Figure 27.49A–C. (A) Thoracic aortic dissection (TAD). Mobile intimal flap is distal to the AV opening in the sinotubular region of the LVOT. The separated aortic layers are seen in cross section, and the loosened intimal layer appears as a thin echogenic line. The separation of the medial layer from the intimal layer created the false lumen (anechoic region). The false lumen widens and flattens, and its movements are distinguished from the regular opening and closing of the AV leaflets. A small pericardial effusion is seen between the RA and liver. The patient presented in shock with sudden chest pain migrating to the abdomen and left leg, which was pulseless. (B) TAD. Anterograde dissection from the thoracic to the abdominal aorta, with the left iliac artery then occluding the left femoral artery. The pericardial effusion suggests the release of blood as it tears through the adventitial layer in retrograde TAD.

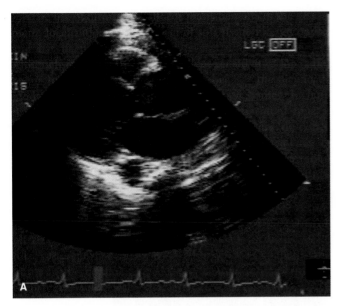
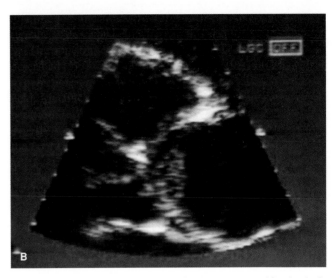

Figure 27.50A and B. (A) TAD (PLA). Mobile intimal flap at the proximal LVOT. The intimal tear site and loosened intimal surface become a raised flap that looks a sheet of tissue. (B) LVOT close-up shows an aortic intimal flap raised "en face" toward the viewer. The flap is immediately distal to the AV leaflets.

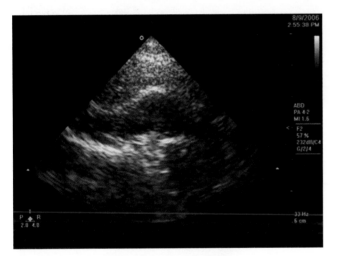
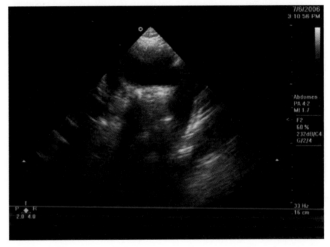

Figure 27.51. Normal thoracic aortic arch (longitudinal view). The echogenic apex of the arch is the echolucent curved band. Sections of the ascending aorta (AAO) and Dao are similar in diameter. (See abnormalities of aortic arch in Figs. 27.52 and 27.53.)

Figure 27.52. TAA. The aorta dilates as it ascends, including the top of the arch. The thoracic aorta tapers to normal as it descends from the arch. The patient presented with chest pain but had a normal ECG. Chest CT of her thorax confirmed the aneurysm extending from the LVOT to the aorta arch.

393

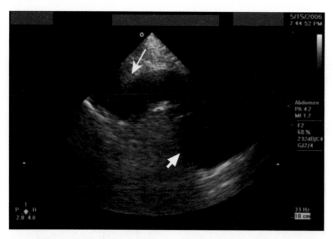

Figure 27.53. Distal TAA (suprasternal view). Normal AAO and arch (*long arrow*). The Dao shows a sudden dilation (*short arrow*). This patient walked into the ED triage area and collapsed after saying he was having chest and back pain. His complaints were likely due to a ruptured TAA.

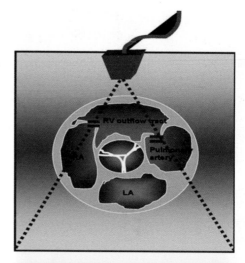

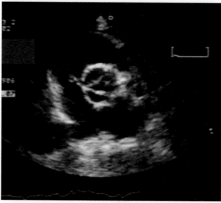

Figure 27.54. Schematic diagram with probe placed in the suprasternal notch. Normal AV and normal LVOT (PSA).

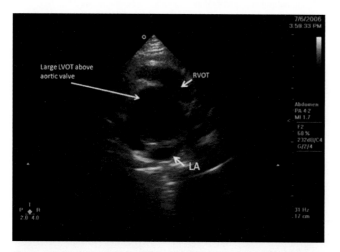

Figure 27.55. TAA (PLA). Note dilated LVOT (>4 cm diameter). The right ventricular outflow tract and LA are located anterior and posterior, respectively, to the centrally located LVOT and the AV. The patient presented with sudden onset of back pain, mild chest pain, and deteriorating mental status.

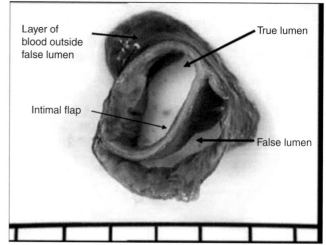

Figure 27.57. Aorta in cross section showing the intimal flap between the true and false lumina.

Image courtesy of Leslie Davidson, Consultant Histopathologist, The General Infirmary, Leeds, England.

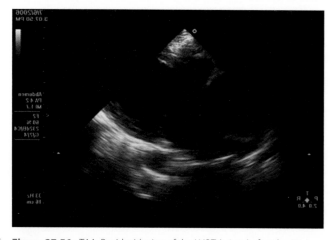

Figure 27.56. TAA. Rapid widening of the LVOT (>6 cm) after the AV. A normal LVOT on transthoracic cardiac scanning does not rule out a TAD or TAA.

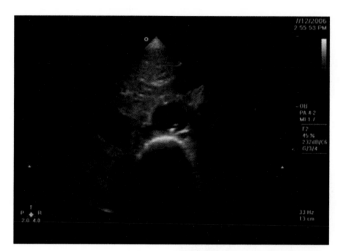

Figure 27.58. Abdominal aortic dissection (transverse view). The intimal flap's movement is different from the aortic pulsations. The aorta is not dilated at this level. This patient presented in shock after the sudden onset of chest pain that migrated down to her abdomen, then to her left leg. Although the patient's pulseless and painful leg was a major concern, the presence of a pericardial effusion and an intimal flap in the proximal ascending thoracic aorta prompted emergent surgical intervention.

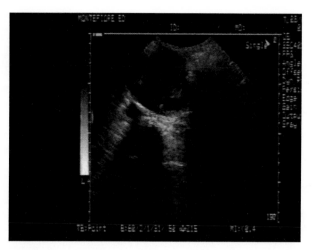

Figure 27.59. Abdominal aortic aneurysm (AAA) with thrombus (transverse view). Two channels (at 5-o'clock and 7-o'clock positions) are noted within the large thrombus and occupy most of the aorta. The aorta is >5 cm in diameter. The IVC is situated between the aorta and the prominent vertebral body shadow.

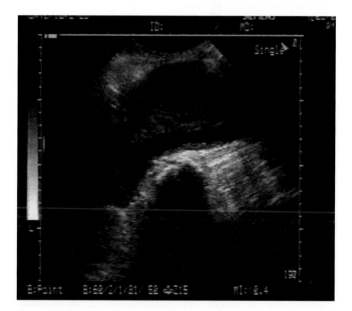

Figure 27.60. AAA with thrombus (longitudinal view). Seventy-five percent of the true aortic lumen is filled with thrombus. The remaining lumen may be mistaken for the entire aorta.

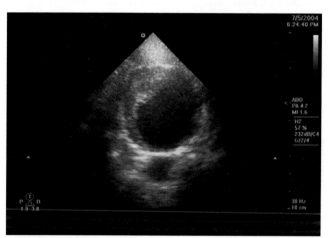

Figure 27.61. AAA with thrombus (transverse view). A thrombus is attached to the inner anterior and lateral walls. The patient presented with the abrupt onset of abdominal pain, diaphoresis, and near syncope. The cardiac ultrasound revealed a partially empty heart, normal cardiac contractions, and no fluid in the pericardial, pleural, and peritoneal spaces.

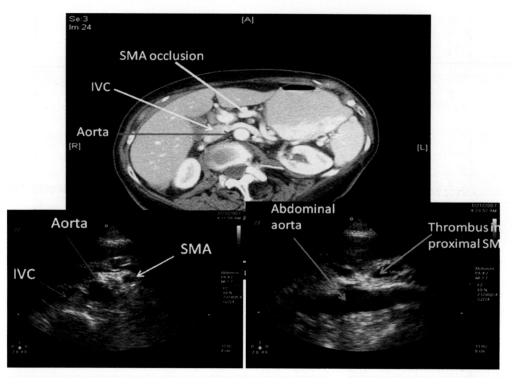

Figure 27.62. Superior mesenteric artery (SMA) thrombus seen on long view of aorta and SMA. An IVC thrombus is also seen on the transverse view. The patient's severe abdominal pain – with no abdominal tenderness – was due to mesenteric ischemia. She had no leg swelling, pain, chest pain, or dyspnea before going to the operating room. Due to a misunderstanding, she had stopped taking her warfarin for her atrial fibrillation.

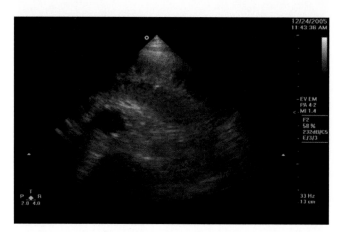

Figure 27.63. Bowel obstruction. Dilated loops of bowel with prominent haustral markings. The patient presented with hypotension, abdominal pain, and lethargy. The abdomen was distended, tense, and diffusely tender.

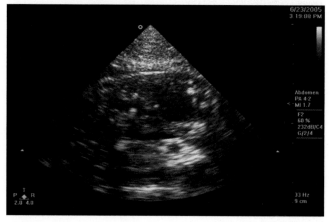

Figure 27.64. Pancreatitis. Markedly enlarged and heterogeneous pancreas: with visible internal calcifications and small cysts.

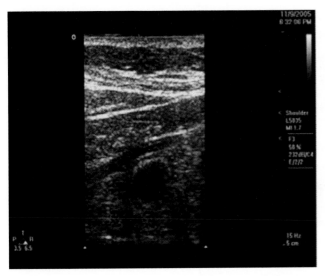
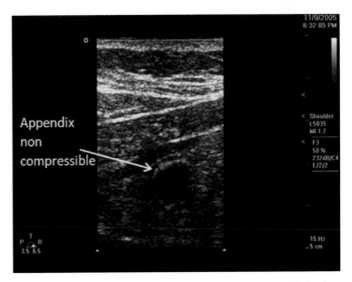

Figure 27.65. Appendicitis. Connects with cecum and distal blind loop. Features: Lack of peristalsis (compare to adjacent bowel), edematous wall thicker than 3 mm, diameter >6 mm, noncompressible, and may have a fecalith with shadowing.

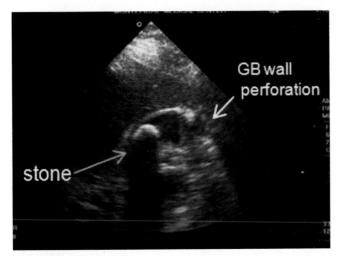

Figure 27.66. Acute cholecystitis. Thickened gallbladder wall with air and a stone. The patient presented with hypotension and laboratory white blood cell count of 38,000.

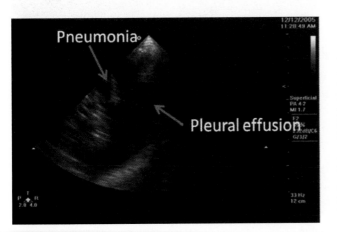
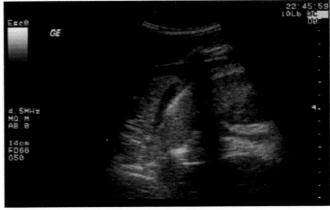

Figure 27.67. Pneumonia with effusion. The lingual lung tissue is visualized as a wedge-shaped structure that is surrounded by a small hypoechoic effusion. Courtesy of Fernando Silva, Porto Alegre, Brazil.

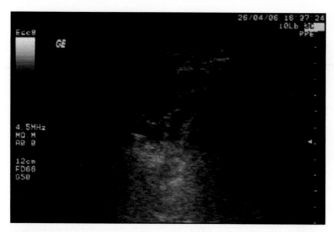

Figure 27.68. Pneumonia. A heterogeneous collection of internal echoes within the lung parenchyma is a pattern typical for pneumonia on 2D mode.

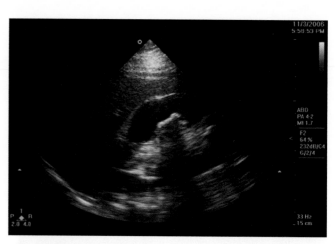

Figure 27.69. Renal calculus with hydronephrosis. Unilateral enlarged kidney and large stone with prominent shadowing consistent with a staghorn calculus and urinary tract-provoked sepsis. This patient had a high fever, uroseptic shock, and extreme lethargy.

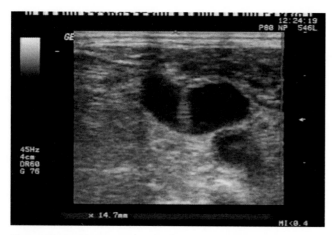

Figure 27.70. Central access (transverse view, right internal jugular). Note tenting of the venous vascular wall and ring-down artifact from the entering needle. The thicker-walled and noncompressible carotid artery (CA) is medial and deeper.

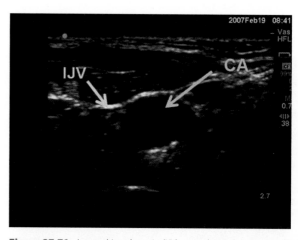

Figure 27.71. Internal jugular vein (IJV) cannulation/access is unlikely to be successful in this patient with a flat IJV, even with Valsalva maneuver and Trendelenburg position. The IJV is imperceptible and inaccessible. Attempts at this site will lead to the puncture of the carotid artery.

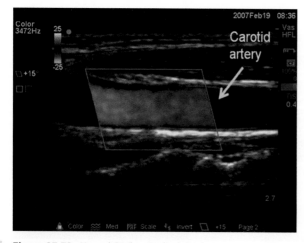

Figure 27.72. Normal CA (longitudinal view).

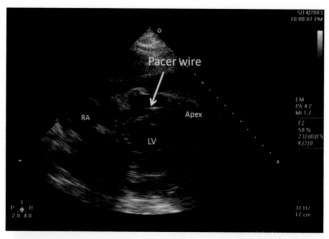

Figure 27.73. Transvenous pacer wire insertion is confirmed as an echogenic line entering the RV and touching the apex of the RV endocardium.

References

1. Atkinson PR, McAuley DJ, Kendall RJ, et al.: Abdominal and cardiac evaluation with sonography in shock (ACES): an approach by emergency physicians for the use of ultrasound in patients with undifferentiated hypotension. *Emerg Med J* 2009;**26**:87–91.

2. Bahner DP: Trinity: a hypotensive ultrasound protocol. *J Diagn Med Sonography* 2002;**18**:193–8.

3. Carr BG, Dean AJ, Everett WW, et al.: Intensivist bedside ultrasound (INBU) for volume assessment in the intensive care unit: a pilot study. *J Trauma* 2007;**63**:495–500; discussion 500–2.

4. Gunst M, Ghaemmaghami V, Sperry J, et al.: Accuracy of cardiac function and volume status estimates using the bedside echocardiographic assessment in trauma/critical care. *J Trauma* 2008;**65**:509–16.

5. Jones AE, Tayal VS, Sullivan DM, Kline JA: Randomized, controlled trial of immediate versus delayed goal-directed ultrasound to identify the cause of nontraumatic hypotension in emergency department patients. *Crit Care Med* 2004;**32**:1703–8.

6. Perera P, Mailhot T, Riley D, Mandavia D: The RUSH exam: rapid ultrasound in shock in the evaluation of the critically ill. *Emerg Med Clin North Am* 2010;**28**:29–56, vii.

7. Pershad J, Myers S, Plouman C, et al.: Bedside limited echocardiography by the emergency physician is accurate during evaluation of the critically ill patient. *Pediatrics* 2004;**114**:e667–71.

8. Rose JS, Bair AE, Mandavia D, Kinser DJ: The UHP ultrasound protocol: a novel ultrasound approach to the empiric evaluation of the undifferentiated hypotensive patient. *Am J Emerg Med* 2001;**19**:299–302.

9. Breitkreutz R, Walcher F, Seeger FH: Focused echocardiographic evaluation in resuscitation management: concept of an advanced life support-conformed algorithm. *Crit Care Med* 2007;**35**:S150–61.

10. Hernandez C, Shuler K, Hannan H, et al.: C.A.U.S.E.: cardiac arrest ultra-sound exam–a better approach to managing patients in primary non-arrhythmogenic cardiac arrest. *Resuscitation* 2008;**76**:198–206.

11. Lanctôt J-F, Valois M, Beaulieu Y: EGLS: Echo-guided life support. *Crit Ultrasound J* 2011;**3**:123–9.

12. Robson R: Echocardiography during CPR: more studies needed. *Resuscitation* 2010; **81**:1453–4.

13. Blaivas M, Sierzenski PR: Dissection of the proximal thoracic aorta: a new ultrasonographic sign in the subxiphoid view. *Am J Emerg Med* 2002;**20**:344–8.

14. Tayal VS, Graf CD, Gibbs MA: Prospective study of accuracy and outcome of emergency ultrasound for abdominal aortic aneurysm over two years. *Acad Emerg Med* 2003;**10**:867–71.

15. Breitkreutz R, Price S, Steiger HV, et al.: Focused echocardiographic evaluation in life support and peri-resuscitation of emergency patients: a prospective trial. *Resuscitation* 2010;**81**:1527–33.

16. Blaivas M: Incidence of pericardial effusion in patients presenting to the emergency department with unexplained dyspnea. *Acad Emerg Med* 2001;**8**:1143–6.

17. Tayal VS, Beatty MA, Marx JA, et al.: FAST (focused assessment with sonography in trauma) accurate for cardiac and intraperitoneal injury in penetrating anterior chest trauma. *J Ultrasound Med* 2004;**23**:467–72.

18. Tayal VS, Kline JA: Emergency echocardiography to detect pericardial effusion in patients in PEA and near-PEA states. *Resuscitation* 2003;**59**:315–8.

19. Moore CL, Rose GA, Tayal VS, et al.: Determination of left ventricular function by emergency physician echocardiography of hypotensive patients. *Acad Emerg Med* 2002;**9**:186–93.

20. Randazzo MR, Snoey ER, Levitt MA, Binder K: Accuracy of emergency physician assessment of left ventricular ejection fraction and central venous pressure using echocardiography. *Acad Emerg Med* 2003;**10**:973–7.

21. Weekes AJ, Tassone HM, Babcock A, et al.: Comparison of serial qualitative and quantitative assessments of caval index and left ventricular systolic function during early fluid resuscitation of hypotensive emergency department patients. *Acad Emerg Med* 2011;**18**:912–21.

22. Moreno FL, Hagan AD, Holmen JR, et al.: Evaluation of size and dynamics of the inferior vena cava as an index of right-sided cardiac function. *Am J Cardiol* 1984;**53**:579–85.

23. Weekes AJ, Lewis MR, Kahler ZP, et al.: The effect of weight-based volume loading on the inferior vena cava in fasting subjects: a prospective randomized double-blinded trial. *Acad Emerg Med* 2012;**19**:901–7.

24. Jaff MR, McMurtry MS, Archer SL, et al.: Management of massive and submassive pulmonary embolism, iliofemoral deep vein thrombosis, and chronic thromboembolic pulmonary hypertension: a scientific statement from the American Heart Association. *Circulation* 2011;**123**:1788–830.

25. Jackson RE, Rudoni RR, Hauser AM, et al.: Prospective evaluation of two-dimensional transthoracic echocardiography in emergency department patients with suspected pulmonary embolism. *Acad Emerg Med* 2000;**7**:994–8.

26. Dresden S, Mitchell P, Rahimi L, et al.: Right ventricular dilatation on bedside echocardiography performed by emergency physicians aids in the diagnosis of pulmonary embolism. *Ann Emerg Med* 2014;**63**:16–24.

27. Brodmann M, Stark G, Pabst E, et al.: Pulmonary embolism and intracardiac thrombi – individual therapeutic procedures. *Vasc Med* 2000;**5**:27–31.

28. Fisman DN, Malcolm ID, Ward ME: Echocardiographic detection of pulmonary embolism in transit: implications for institution of thrombolytic therapy. *Can J Cardiol* 1997;**13**:685–7.

29. Madan A, Schwartz C: Echocardiographic visualization of acute pulmonary embolus and thrombolysis in the ED. *Am J Emerg Med* 2004;**22**:294–300.

30. Kline JA, Steuerwald MT, Marchick MR, et al.: Prospective evaluation of right ventricular function and functional status 6 months after acute submassive pulmonary embolism: frequency of persistent or subsequent elevation in estimated pulmonary artery pressure. *Chest* 2009;**136**:1202–10.

31. Unluer EE, Senturk GO, Karagoz A, et al.: Red flag in bedside echocardiography for acute pulmonary embolism: remembering McConnell's sign. *Am J Emerg Med* 2013;**31**:719–21.

32. Blaivas M, Fox JC: Outcome in cardiac arrest patients found to have cardiac standstill on the bedside emergency department echocardiogram. *Acad Emerg Med* 2001;**8**:616–21.

33. Salen P, Melniker L, Chooljian C, et al.: Does the presence or absence of sonographically identified cardiac activity predict resuscitation outcomes of cardiac arrest patients? *Am J Emerg Med* 2005;**23**:459–62.

34. Salen P, O'Connor R, Sierzenski P, et al.: Can cardiac sonography and capnography be used independently and in combination to predict resuscitation outcomes? *Acad Emerg Med* 2001;**8**:610–5.

35. Blaivas M, Lyon M, Duggal S: A prospective comparison of supine chest radiography and bedside ultrasound for the diagnosis of traumatic pneumothorax. *Acad Emerg Med* 2005;**12**:844–9.

36. Lichtenstein DA, Menu Y: A bedside ultrasound sign ruling out pneumothorax in the critically ill. Lung sliding. *Chest* 1995;**108**: 1345–8.

37. Aguilera PA, Durham BA, Riley DA: Emergency transvenous cardiac pacing placement using ultrasound guidance. *Ann Emerg Med* 2000;**36**:224–7.

38. Troianos CA, Hartman GS, Glas KE, et al.: Guidelines for performing ultrasound guided vascular cannulation: recommendations of the American Society of Echocardiography and the Society of Cardiovascular Anesthesiologists. *J Am Soc Echocardiogr* 2011;**24**:1291–318.

39. Denys BG, Uretsky BF, Reddy PS: Ultrasound-assisted cannulation of the internal jugular vein. A prospective comparison to the external landmark-guided technique. *Circulation* 1993;**87**:1557–62.

40. Hind D, Calvert N, McWilliams R, et al.: Ultrasonic locating devices for central venous cannulation: meta-analysis. *BMJ* 2003;**327**:361.

41. Randolph AG, Cook DJ, Gonzales CA, Pribble CG: Ultrasound guidance for placement of central venous catheters: a meta-analysis of the literature. *Crit Care Med* 1996;**24**:2053–8.

42. Milling TJ Jr, Rose J, Briggs WM, et al.: Randomized, controlled clinical trial of point-of-care limited ultrasonography assistance of central venous cannulation: the Third Sonography Outcomes Assessment Program (SOAP-3) Trial. *Crit Care Med* 2005;**33**: 1764–9.

43. Bedel J, Vallee F, Mari A, et al.: Guidewire localization by transthoracic echocardiography during central venous catheter insertion: a periprocedural method to evaluate catheter placement. *Intensive Care Med* 2013;**39**:1932–7.

44. Vezzani A, Brusasco C, Palermo S, et al.: Ultrasound localization of central vein catheter and detection of postprocedural pneumothorax: an alternative to chest radiography. *Crit Care Med* 2010;**38**:533–8.

45. Weekes AJ, Johnson DA, Keller SM, et al.: Central vascular catheter placement evaluation using saline flush and bedside echocardiography. *Acad Emerg Med* 2014;**21**:65–72.

46. Cortellaro F, Mellace L, Paglia S, et al.: Contrast enhanced ultrasound vs chest x-ray to determine correct central venous catheter position. *Am J Emerg Med* 2014;**32**:78–81.

47. Horowitz R, Gossett JG, Bailitz J, et al.: The FLUSH study – flush the line and ultrasound the heart: ultrasonographic confirmation of central femoral venous line placement. *Ann Emerg Med* 2014;**63**(6):678–83.

48. Rath GP, Bithal PK, Toshniwal GR, et al.: Saline flush test for bedside detection of misplaced subclavian vein catheter into ipsilateral internal jugular vein. *Brit J Anaesthesia* 2009;**102**:499–502.

49. Drummond JB, Seward JB, Tsang TS, et al.: Outpatient two-dimensional echocardiography-guided pericardiocentesis. *J Am Soc Echocardiogr* 1998;**11**:433–5.

50. Maggiolini S, Bozzano A, Russo P, et al.: Echocardiography-guided pericardiocentesis with probe-mounted needle: report of 53 cases. *J Am Soc Echocardiogr* 2001;**14**:821–4.

51. Price S, Via G, Sloth E, et al.: Echocardiography practice, training and accreditation in the intensive care: document for the World Interactive Network Focused on Critical Ultrasound (WINFOCUS). *Cardiovascular Ultrasound* 2008;**6**:49.

52. Weaver B, Lyon M, Blaivas M: Confirmation of endotracheal tube placement after intubation using the ultrasound sliding lung sign. *Acad Emerg Med* 2006;**13**:239–44.

Chapter

28

CT in the ED: Special Considerations

Tarina Kang and Melissa Joseph

The annual per-capita radiation exposure due to diagnostic imaging increased six-fold from 0.5 to 3.0 millisieverts (mS) from the 1980s to mid-2000s, carrying with it not only the risk of cancer but also the risks of intravenous (IV) contrast in patients susceptible to radiographic contrast-induced neprothpathy (RCIN) (1). Emergency physicians routinely obtain CT scans to evaluate many types of patients in daily practice, such as those who present with abdominal pain, neurological symptoms, or chest pain. This chapter focuses on some of the special populations commonly seen in everyday practice. We start by reviewing the renal effects of radiological contrast media and pretreatment options in the patient with underlying renal insufficiency. We then review the systematic approach to the patient who has a history of a contrast reaction. Finally, we review guidelines regarding diagnostic image ordering and acquisition in pregnant and pediatric patients.

Radiographic contrast-induced nephropathy

RCIN is a significant complication in at-risk patients who receive IV contrast. It is the third most common cause of hospital-acquired renal failure, after surgery and hypotension (2), and is associated with prolonged hospitalizations, worsened renal function at discharge, and increased mortality. One study found that patients with RCIN were 2.7 times more likely to die before the 28-day follow-up (3–6).

Because serial creatinine clearance measurements (glomerular filtration rates) are not practical or cost-effective in an acute care setting, isolated serum creatinine levels are used to measure renal function for most ED patients receiving CT scans. In general, the literature defines RCIN as an increase in total serum creatinine by 25%, or 0.5 mg/dL within 48 hours after an IV contrast load (7–9). Typically, the creatinine in RCIN peaks within 3 to 5 days, then returns to baseline approximately by day 10 after administration (10).

Epidemiology and risk factors

Several studies have described patients at risk for RCIN. Most of these studies have been conducted on patients who underwent cardiac catheterization, not on patients who typically present to the ED. Contrast administered intra-arterially, as

Table 28.1: List of risk factors that predispose patients to RCIN (8, 9, 15)

- Renal insufficiency
- Longstanding diabetes mellitus
- Hypovolemia or anemia
- Age older than 55 years
- Proteinuria
- Multiple myeloma
- Patients taking metformin or nephrotoxic drugs
- Liver disease
- Heart failure

in cardiac catheterizations, is more nephrotoxic than intravenous administration performed for the average CT evaluation (11). These differences make it difficult to generalize risk for ED patients. In a study by Mitchell and colleagues in 2010, of 633 consecutive ED patients receiving contrast CT, the overall risk of RCIN was 11% (12).

Underlying renal insufficiency and longstanding diabetes are the most important risk factors for development of RCIN. Other risk factors, such as advanced age and hypovolemia, are shown in Table 28.1 (13, 14). Patients are at increased risk if they have more than one risk factor or receive large doses or multiple injections of contrast within 72 hours (8, 9, 11, 15). In patients with no risk factors, the risk of RCIN is less than 1% (13, 14).

Special considerations with IV contrast

Pregnant and breastfeeding women

Special considerations should be made for pregnant or lactating women who require IV contrast media. There is a theoretical risk of fetal and neonatal thyroid depression due to contrast crossing the placenta, and some suggest checking neonatal thyroid function within the first week if iodinated contrast was given during the pregnancy (16, 17). Although it is always important to consider clinical necessity when ordering imaging studies with contrast in pregnant patients, there is no contraindication to use contrast media in all trimesters of pregnancy (17–19). Contrast dye can also be excreted in breast milk. Some centers instruct pregnant women to discard breast milk for 12 to 24 hours after receiving IV contrast, but this precaution is not mandated by the American College of Gynecology (ACOG) (19, 20).

Patients with multiple myeloma

Patients with multiple myeloma and underlying renal insufficiency may be particularly predisposed to RCIN (18, 21). The literature lists several specific factors that predispose patients with multiple myeloma to the development of RCIN, including levels of beta-2 microglobulin, dehydration, hypercalcemia, infection, and Bence-Jones proteinuria (21, 22). The overall incidence of RCIN in multiple myeloma patients with a normal creatinine is 5% to 15% (22). The risk of RCIN may be decreased if the patient has been intravenously hydrated prior to the injection of contrast media, with close follow-up and repeat renal-function tests.

Patients with diabetes mellitus on metformin

Non-insulin-dependent diabetics who are taking metformin have historically been considered at high risk for developing RCIN after receiving contrast media. Metformin is a biguanide that is primarily excreted by the kidneys. Metformin also promotes conversion of glucose to lactate in the small intestine and inhibits lactate use in gluconeogenesis (23, 24). Patients on metformin can infrequently develop lactic acidosis from the resultant excess amount of lactate, which can result in renal insufficiency (20). The current recommendations of the American College of Radiology (ACR) are to suspend metformin for 48 hours following a contrast study if the patient has one or more comorbidities that affect lactate production or clearance (Table 28.2). In patients with normal creatinine and no comorbidities, metformin does not need to be held. In patients with known renal dysfunction, metformin

Table 28.2: Risk factors for development of lactic acidosis in patients taking metformin (18)

Liver dysfunction
Alcohol abuse
Cardiac failure
Muscle ischemia (including cardiac)
Sepsis or severe infection

should be held indefinitely until follow-up studies of renal function deem it safe to be reinstated (18).

Contrast dye

Specific properties of contrast media can increase the risk of developing RCIN. First-generation contrast media with high ionicity and osmolality (>1,500 mOsm/kg), large-volume injections, and repeated doses of contrast were all associated with a higher incidence of RCIN (11, 25). More recently, nonionic, low-osmolar solutions have replaced early generation contrast media (Table 28.3) (11, 14).

Prevention of contrast-induced nephropathy

Identification of high-risk patients, judicious use of contrast in CT studies, discontinuation of any nephrotoxic medications, adequate prehydration, use of low or iso-osmolar contrast, and avoidance of repeated doses of IV contrast are the most important steps clinicians can take to prevent contrast-induced renal insufficiency.

When the use of contrast media is needed, several prophylactic methods have been used to prevent the development of RCIN, including hydration therapy, dialysis, N-acetyl cysteine, diuretics, endothelin antagonists, adenosine, calcium channel blockers, prostaglandin E1, and ascorbic acid (26, 27).

Hydration therapy

Prehydration with IV fluids has been shown to be the most effective intervention to prevent the development of contrast-induced nephropathy in high-risk patients requiring contrast CT scans, although a widely accepted protocol has not been specified (26, 28). Oral hydration alone is likely inadequate (29). The literature does not support superior efficacy in hydration therapy between isotonic normal saline and sodium bicarbonate; however, half-normal saline has been shown to be not as effective as normal saline in the prevention

Table 28.3: Ionicity and osmolality of different contrasts

	Name	Type	Iodine Content	Osmolality	
Ionic	Diatrizoate (Hypaque 50)	Ionic monomer	300	1550	High
	Metrizoate (Isopaque Coronar 370)	Ionic	370	2100	Osmolar
	Ioxaglate (Hexabrix)	Ionic dimmer	320	580	Low osmolar
Nonionic	Iopamidol (Isovue 370)	Nonionic monomer	370	796	
	Iohexol (Omnipaque 350)	Nonionic	350	884	
	Optiray Iopromide	Nonionic	350	741	
	Iodixanol (Visipaque 320)	Nonionic dimmer	320	290	Iso-osmolar

Courtesy of the Beth Israel Deaconess Medical Center, Department of Radiology, Boston.

of RCIN (28, 30–35). While longer duration of hydration both before and after contrast administration decreases the likelihood for development of RCIN, prolonged hydration regimens are not practical in the ED (32, 33). There is some literature that shows a protective benefit of IV prehydration in a shorter time period as well, such as the sodium bicarbonate regimen listed in the next paragraph (32, 33).

The European Society of Urogenital Radiology (ESUR) suggests the following protocols for high-risk patients: normal saline 1.0–1.5 ml/kg/h for at least 6 hours before and after injection of contrast medium, or isotonic sodium bicarbonate (154 mEq/L in dextrose 5% water): 3 ml/kg/h for 1 hour before contrast medium and 1 ml/kg/h for 6 hours after contrast medium (36).

N-acetylcysteine

The protective effects of N-acetylcysteine (NAC) has been studied for its ability to reduce the production of oxygen-free radicals that cause nephrotoxicity (37). The efficacy of NAC in preventing contrast-induced nephropathy, however, is not clear (38, 39). The use of oral NAC may be justified due to the favorable side effect profile and low cost. The current recommendation by the RCA is to initiate oral NAC 12 hours prior to outpatient contrast studies. This regimen, however, is not practical in the ED setting (18).

Hemodialysis and renal replacement therapies

Studies have also looked at prophylactic hemodialysis (HD) and hemofiltration in non–end stage renal disease (ESRD) patients to help prevent RCIN (40). Such therapies, however, even when performed immediately after injection of a contrast load, have not been shown to decrease incidence of RCIN and are not currently recommended (41). Hemodialysis may be beneficial in patients with stage 4 or 5 CKD; however, it is not supported well in the literature (41). It has been proposed that the lack of benefit for RRT or HD may be due to the toxicity of renal replacement therapy (RRT) itself with release of inflammatory mediators, or secondary to the fact that the damage with IV contrast may be very early, possibly within minutes of contrast administration (28). Renal replacement therapy begun prior to contrast administration may be helpful, if only because it allows for aggressive hydration in patients at risk for fluid overload, but this requires further study (28). In patients already on dialysis, there is no need for urgent dialysis post-contrast unless the patient received a significant amount of volume or is at significant risk for heart disease (18).

Allergic-type and anaphylactoid reactions to contrast

Many patients will report an allergic reaction to contrast media. These adverse reactions vary from minor skin reactions to severe, anaphylactoid reactions with bronchospasm and angioedema (42). Previously, these reactions were considered "allergic-type" reactions and not a true allergy, because contrast molecules were thought to be too small to act as true antigens to stimulate an IgE response (20). There is recent literature, however, that documents positive skin tests that confirm immediate allergic hypersensitivity (anaphylaxis) to contrast media in some patients (43, 44).

Although a previous reaction to contrast is the most important risk factor for a subsequent reaction, with up to a five-fold increased likelihood of a repeat reaction (18), patients who are atopic (i.e., have asthma, food allergies) or have a history of allergic-type reactions are at three times higher risk for IV contrast reactions in general (18, 20). If a patient with active asthma develops bronchospasm following IV contrast media, this typically resolves quickly with beta-agonist.

There is a common perception that patients allergic to shellfish should not receive IV contrast, because shellfish are rich in iodine. Iodine is an essential element, making it extremely difficult to have an allergic reaction to it (20). Patients with shellfish allergies are allergic to the muscular proteins found in shellfish, such as parvalbumin (in scaly fish) and tropomyosin (in crustaceans). The ACR recommends that providers focus on patients with severe prior allergic reactions from any cause, not necessarily about seafood or shellfish, prior to injection of contrast media (18). Additionally, sensitivity to Betadine and other externally used iodine-based solutions do not place patients at higher risk for IV contrast dye reactions (18).

Use of nonionic or low-osmolality agents may reduce the risk of allergic-type reactions by approximately 80% (18, 45). In high-risk patients, such as those with a previous allergy to IV contrast, a history of severe allergic reaction in the past, or a history of asthma, premedication with steroids or antihistamines may be beneficial (18, 36). Suggested regimens are described in Table 28.4. Note that, in the ED setting, steroids

Table 28.4: ACR-recommended pretreatment protocols (18)

1. Emergency premedication (in order of decreasing preference)

  a. Methylprednisolone sodium succinate 40 mg or hydrocortisone sodium succinate 200 mg IV every 4 hours until contrast study, plus diphenhydramine 50 mg IV 1 hour prior to contrast injection.

  b. Dexamethasone sodium sulfate 7.5 mg or betamethasone 6 mg IV every 4 hours prior to contrast study in patients with known allergy to the above medications, NSAIDs, or aspirin, especially if asthmatic, in addition to diphenhydramine 50 mg IV 1 hour prior to contrast.

  c. Omit steroids entirely and give diphenhydramine 50 mg IV.

  **Steroids have not been shown effective when administered less than 4 to 6 hours prior to contrast.

2. Elective premedication (both are accepted)

  a. Prednisone 50 mg PO at 13 hours, 7 hours, and 1 hour prior to contrast, plus diphenhydramine 50 mg IV/IM/PO 1 hour prior to contrast.

  b. Methylprednisolone 32 mg PO 12 and 2 hours prior to contrast +/- diphenhydramine as above

Table 28.5: Measures of radiation

Measure	Unit	SI Unit
Exposure	Roentgen (R)	Coulomb
Dose	Rad	Gy
Effective dose	Rem	Sv

Table 28.6: Fetal radiation exposure of common diagnostic tests

Study	Fetal Exposure
Chest x-ray	0.02–0.07 mrad
Abdominal x-ray (single view)	100 mrad
Lumbar spine x-ray (single view)	50–150 mrad
Hip x-ray (single view)	200 mrad
Extremity x-ray	0.05 mrad
CT of the head/chest	<1 rad
CT of the abdomen/lumbar spine	3.5 rad
CT of the pelvis	250 mrad

may not be feasible, as they must be given 4 to 6 hours prior to contrast.

Even though the overall incidence of allergic-type reactions to IV contrast media is low (approximately 0.2% to 3% with low-osmolality contrast agents), they can be severe and potentially life threatening, so it is important to be prepared to treat the patient with beta-agonists, steroids, and antihistamine medications if such reactions develop (46).

Radiation and CT scanning

Radiation dose

X-rays are a form of electromagnetic radiation with sufficient energy to ionize matter. In contrast to nonionizing radiation, ionizing radiation can displace orbital electrons and results in electrically charged ions in matter. Ionizing radiation dose is commonly measured in rads (radiation-absorbed dose), which is defined as the energy absorbed per kilogram of tissue. Other measures of radiation dose include the effective dose (rem), which takes into account the biological effect of the radiation and the sensitivity of the organ exposed. In the Systeme International d'Unites (SI) classification system, 1 gray (Gy) = 100 rads, and 1 sievert (Sv) = 100 rem (Table 28.5) (19).

Risk in pregnant patients

The primary risk of ionizing radiation is direct damage to DNA. A fetus with rapidly dividing and differentiating cells is more sensitive to radiation effects, and large doses of radiation can potentially lead to miscarriage, birth defects, severe mental retardation, intrauterine growth retardation, or childhood cancers (47). ACOG has issued a committee bulletin statement that summarizes general guidelines regarding diagnostic imaging during pregnancy. In summary, fetal exposure to less than 5 rads has not been associated with an increase in fetal anomalies or pregnancy loss (19, 47). Current diagnostic imaging studies are well below this threshold, with radiation exposure of a CT abdomen averaging 3.5 rads (48). Other common radiation exposures are listed in Table 28.6. The American College of Radiology concluded that no single diagnostic x-ray procedure results in radiation exposure to a degree that would threaten the well-being of the developing pre-embryo, embryo, or fetus (19, 48). Thus, exposure to a single x-ray during pregnancy is not an indication for therapeutic abortion.

Development of childhood cancer after radiation exposure as a fetus is a risk. Goldberg-Stein and colleagues estimated a 1.5- to 2-fold increase in childhood leukemia in a fetus who was exposed to a single CT abdomen or pelvis (48). The use of radioactive isotopes of iodine are contraindicated in pregnancy, and the use of fluoroscopy should be limited (19).

In general, ultrasound and MRI are preferable to CT when feasible (49). An important exception to these recommendations occurs when the patient was involved in a severe trauma. CT should not be delayed due to radiation concerns alone, as the risks of delayed-diagnosis of trauma far outweigh the risks of radiation to the developing fetus (49, 50).

Risk in pediatric patients

CT should be used judiciously in the pediatric population. Not only are tissues and organs continuing to develop, making them more prone to deleterious effects of ionizing radiation, but children have a longer life expectancy in which to develop malignancies (51).

The risk of solid cancers from a CT scan is estimated to be as high as 1 in 760 for an abdominal and pelvic CT scan (51). The risk of developing leukemia from noncontrast head CT scans is estimated to be 1.9 cases per 10,000 CT scans, depending on age (51). Overall, the excess relative risk of cancer from the ionizing radiation from CT scans is approximately 1% to 10% (52). Risks are higher with younger age, female sex, and radiation to the abdomen and pelvis (51, 52).

ALARA, or as low as reasonably achievable, was developed in 1980 in an effort to decrease ionizing radiation exposure in the pediatric population (51, 53). Several other practice guidelines have been developed in the past 20 years, most notably by the Pediatric Emergency Care Applied Research Network (PECARN). Several publications by PECARN describe considerations for use of CT in children and offer decision rules such as one for the identification of children at low risk for intracranial hemorrhage and, thus, in whom CT may be avoided (54–56). Lastly, the safety and use of low-dose CT scans in selected pediatric populations is currently being studied and may offer additional, safer imaging alternatives (57).

Conclusion

Special considerations should be made when determining whether contrast media should be given to patients with renal insufficiency, diabetes, or allergic-type or anaphylactic reactions to contrast. Additionally, pregnant and pediatric patients should be given special consideration in determining whether alternative radiographic modalities such as MRI or ultrasound should be performed prior to a CT scan to save the patient from exposure to ionizing radiation.

References

1. Crownover BK, Bepko JL: Appropriate and safe use of diagnostic imaging. *Am Fam Physician* 2013;**87**(7):494–501.

2. Tublin ME, Murphy ME, Tessler FN: Current concepts in contrast media-induced nephropathy. *AJR Am J Roentgenol* 1998;**171**(4):933–9.

3. Pannu N, Wiebe N, Tonelli M: Alberta Kidney Disease Network. Prophylaxis strategies for contrast-induced nephropathy. *JAMA* 2006;**295**(23):2765–79.

4. Gruberg L, Mehran R, Dangas G, et al.: Acute renal failure requiring dialysis after percutaneous coronary interventions. *Catheter Cardiovasc Interv Off J Soc Card Angiogr Interv* 2001;**52**(4):409–16.

5. McCullough PA, Wolyn R, Rocher LL, et al.: Acute renal failure after coronary intervention: incidence, risk factors, and relationship to mortality. *Am J Med* 1997;**103**(5):368–75.

6. Hoste EAJ, Doom S, De Waele J, et al.: Epidemiology of contrast-associated acute kidney injury in ICU patients: a retrospective cohort analysis. *Intensive Care Med* 2011;**37**(12):1921–31.

7. Morcos SK, Thomsen HS, Webb JA: Contrast-media-induced nephrotoxicity: a consensus report. Contrast Media Safety Committee, European Society of Urogenital Radiology (ESUR). *Eur Radiol* 1999;**9**(8):1602–13.

8. Jakobsen JA, Lundby B, Kristoffersen DT, et al.: Evaluation of renal function with delayed CT after injection of nonionic monomeric and dimeric contrast media in healthy volunteers. *Radiology* 1992;**182**(2):419–24.

9. Cochran ST, Wong WS, Roe DJ: Predicting angiography-induced acute renal function impairment: clinical risk model. *AJR Am J Roentgenol* 1983;**141**(5):1027–33.

10. De Freitas do Carmo LP, Macedo E: Contrast-induced nephropathy: attributable incidence and potential harm. *Crit Care Lond Engl* 2012;**16**(3):127.

11. Gleeson TG, Bulugahapitiya S: Contrast-induced nephropathy. *AJR Am J Roentgenol* 2004;**183**(6):1673–89.

12. Mitchell AM, Jones AE, Tumlin JA, Kline JA: Incidence of contrast-induced nephropathy after contrast-enhanced computed tomography in the outpatient setting. *Clin J Am Soc Nephrol* 2010;**5**(1):4–9.

13. Parfrey PS, Griffiths SM, Barrett BJ, et al.: Contrast material-induced renal failure in patients with diabetes mellitus, renal insufficiency, or both. A prospective controlled study. *N Engl J Med* 1989;**320**(3):143–9.

14. Rudnick MR, Goldfarb S, Wexler L, et al.: Nephrotoxicity of ionic and nonionic contrast media in 1196 patients: a randomized trial. The Iohexol Cooperative Study. *Kidney Int* 1995;**47**(1):254–61.

15. Traub SJ, Kellum JA, Tang A, et al.: Risk factors for radiocontrast nephropathy after emergency department contrast-enhanced computerized tomography. *Acad Emerg Med* 2013;**20**(1):40–5.

16. Atwell TD, Lteif AN, Brown DL, et al.: Neonatal thyroid function after administration of IV iodinated contrast agent to 21 pregnant patients. *AJR Am J Roentgenol* 2008;**191**(1):268–71.

17. Webb JAW, Thomsen HS, Morcos SK: Members of Contrast Media Safety Committee of European Society of Urogenital Radiology (ESUR). The use of iodinated and gadolinium contrast media during pregnancy and lactation. *Eur Radiol* 2005;**15**(6):1234–40.

18. American College of Radiology: Manual on contrast media, version 10. 2015. Available at: www.acr.org/~/media/37D8442 8BF1D4E1B9A3A2918DA9E27A3.pdf

19. ACOG Committee on Obstetric Practice: ACOG Committee Opinion. Number 299, September 2004 (replaces No. 158, September 1995). Guidelines for diagnostic imaging during pregnancy. *Obstet Gynecol* 2004;**104**(3):647–51.

20. Bettmann MA: Frequently asked questions: iodinated contrast agents. *Radiogr Rev Publ Radiol Soc N Am Inc* 2004;**24** Suppl 1:S3–10.

21. McCarthy CS, Becker JA: Multiple myeloma and contrast media. *Radiology* 1992;**183**(2):519–21.

22. Pahade JK, LeBedis CA, Raptopoulos VD, et al.: Incidence of contrast-induced nephropathy in patients with multiple myeloma undergoing contrast-enhanced CT. *AJR Am J Roentgenol* 2011;**196**(5):1094–101.

23. Bailey CJ, Wilcock C, Day C: Effect of metformin on glucose metabolism in the splanchnic bed. *Br J Pharmacol* 1992;**105**(4):1009–13.

24. Sirtori CR, Pasik C: Re-evaluation of a biguanide, metformin: mechanism of action and tolerability. *Pharmacol Res Off J Ital Pharmacol Soc* 1994;**30**(3):187–228.

25. Barrett BJ, Carlisle EJ: Metaanalysis of the relative nephrotoxicity of high- and low-osmolality iodinated contrast media. *Radiology* 1993;**188**(1):171–8.

26. Briguori C, Airoldi F, D'Andrea D, et al.: Renal insufficiency following contrast media administration trial (REMEDIAL): a randomized comparison of 3 preventive strategies. *Circulation* 2007;**115**(10):1211–7.

27. Ludwig U, Riedel MK, Backes M, et al.: MESNA (sodium 2-mercaptoethanesulfonate) for prevention of contrast medium-induced nephrotoxicity – controlled trial. *Clin Nephrol* 2011;**75**(4):302–8.

28. Ellis JH, Cohan RH: Prevention of contrast-induced nephropathy: an overview. *Radiol Clin North Am* 2009;**47**(5):801–11.

29. Trivedi HS, Moore H, Nasr S, et al.: A randomized prospective trial to assess the role of saline hydration on the development of contrast nephrotoxicity. *Nephron Clin Pract* 2003;**93**(1):C29–34.

30. From AM, Bartholmai BJ, Williams AW, et al.: Sodium bicarbonate is associated with an increased incidence of contrast nephropathy: a retrospective cohort study of 7977 patients at Mayo Clinic. *Clin J Am Soc Nephrol* 2008;**3**(1):10–8.

31. Gomes VO, Lasevitch R, Lima VC, et al.: Hydration with sodium bicarbonate does not prevent contrast nephropathy: a multicenter clinical trial. *Arq Bras Cardiol* 2012;**99**(6):1129–34.

32. Merten GJ, Burgess WP, Gray LV, et al.: Prevention of contrast-induced nephropathy with sodium bicarbonate: a randomized controlled trial. *JAMA* 2004;**291**(19):2328–34.

33. Adolph E, Holdt-Lehmann B, Chatterjee T, et al.: Renal insufficiency following radiocontrast exposure trial (REINFORCE): a randomized comparison of sodium bicarbonate versus sodium chloride hydration for the prevention of contrast-induced nephropathy. *Coron Artery Dis* 2008;**19**(6):413–9.

34. Mueller C, Buerkle G, Buettner HJ, et al.: Prevention of contrast media-associated nephropathy: randomized comparison of 2 hydration regimens in 1620 patients undergoing coronary angioplasty. *Arch Intern Med* 2002;**162**(3):329–36.

35. Weisbord SD, Palevsky PM: Prevention of contrast-induced nephropathy with volume expansion. *Clin J Am Soc Nephrol* 2008;**3**(1):273–80.

36. Stacul F, van der Molen AJ, Reimer P, et al.: Contrast induced nephropathy: updated ESUR Contrast Media Safety Committee guidelines. *Eur Radiol* 2011;**21**(12):2527–41.

37. Tepel M, van der Giet M, Schwarzfeld C, et al.: Prevention of radiographic-contrast-agent-induced reductions in renal function by acetylcysteine. *N Engl J Med* 2000;**343**(3):180–4.

38. Bagshaw SM, Ghali WA: Acetylcysteine for prevention of contrast-induced nephropathy after intravascular angiography: a systematic review and meta-analysis. *BMC Med* 2004;**2**:38.

39. Traub SJ, Mitchell AM, Jones AE, et al.: N-acetylcysteine plus intravenous fluids versus intravenous fluids alone to prevent contrast-induced nephropathy in emergency computed tomography. *Ann Emerg Med* 2013;**62**(5):511–520.e25.

40. Cruz DN, Perazella MA, Ronco C: The role of extracorporeal blood purification therapies in the prevention of radiocontrast-induced nephropathy. *Int J Artif Organs* 2008;**31**(6):515–24.

41. Cruz DN, Goh CY, Marenzi G, et al.: Renal replacement therapies for prevention of radiocontrast-induced nephropathy: a systematic review. *Am J Med* 2012;**125**(1):66–78.e3.

42. Morcos SK, Thomsen HS, Webb JA: Contrast Media Safety Committee of the European Society of Urogenital Radiology. Prevention of generalized reactions to contrast media: a consensus report and guidelines. *Eur Radiol* 2001;**11**(9):1720–8.

43. Dewachter P, Laroche D, Mouton-Faivre C, et al.: Immediate reactions following iodinated contrast media injection: a study of 38 cases. *Eur J Radiol* 2011;**77**(3):495–501.

44. Brockow K: Immediate and delayed reactions to radiocontrast media: is there an allergic mechanism? *Immunol Allergy Clin North Am* 2009;**29**(3):453–68.

45. Caro JJ, Trindade E, McGregor M: The risks of death and of severe nonfatal reactions with high- vs low-osmolality contrast media: a meta-analysis. *AJR Am J Roentgenol* 1991;**156**(4):825–32.

46. Katayama H, Yamaguchi K, Kozuka T, et al.: Adverse reactions to ionic and nonionic contrast media. A report from the Japanese Committee on the Safety of Contrast Media. *Radiology* 1990;**175**(3):621–8.

47. Nguyen CP, Goodman LH: Fetal risk in diagnostic radiology. *Semin Ultrasound CT MR* 2012;**33**(1):4–10.

48. Goldberg-Stein SA, Liu B, Hahn PF, Lee SI: Radiation dose management: part 2, estimating fetal radiation risk from CT during pregnancy. *AJR Am J Roentgenol* 2012;**198**(4):W352–6.

49. Masselli G, Derchi L, McHugo J, et al.: Acute abdominal and pelvic pain in pregnancy: ESUR recommendations. *Eur Radiol* 2013;**23**(12):3485–500.

50. Sadro C, Bernstein MP, Kanal KM: Imaging of trauma: part 2, abdominal trauma and pregnancy–a radiologist's guide to doing what is best for the mother and baby. *AJR Am J Roentgenol* 2012;**199**(6):1207–19.

51. Miglioretti DL, Johnson E, Williams A, et al.: The use of computed tomography in pediatrics and the associated radiation exposure and estimated cancer risk. *JAMA Pediatr* 2013;**167**(8):700–7.

52. Journy N, Ancelet S, Rehel J-L, et al.: Predicted cancer risks induced by computed tomography examinations during childhood, by a quantitative risk assessment approach. *Radiat Environ Biophys* 2014;**53**(1):39–54.

53. Winkler NT: ALARA concept – now a requirement. *Radiol Technol* 1980;**51**(4):525.

54. Lyttle MD, Crowe L, Oakley E, et al.: Comparing CATCH, CHALICE and PECARN clinical decision rules for paediatric head injuries. *Emerg Med J* 2012;**29**(10):785–94.

55. Kuppermann N, Holmes JF, Dayan PS, et al.: Identification of children at very low risk of clinically-important brain injuries after head trauma: a prospective cohort study. *Lancet* 2009;**374**(9696):1160–70.

56. Garcia M, Taylor G, Babcock L, et al.: Computed tomography with intravenous contrast alone: the role of intra-abdominal fat on the ability to visualize the normal appendix in children. *Acad Emerg Med* 2013;**20**(8):795–800.

57. Morton RP, Reynolds RM, Ramakrishna R, et al.: Low-dose head computed tomography in children: a single institutional experience in pediatric radiation risk reduction: clinical article. *J Neurosurg Pediatr* 2013;**12**(4):406–10.

Chapter 29

CT of the Spine

Michael E. R. Habicht and Samantha Costantini

CT of the spine is becoming one of the most common studies in the modern ED. Typically, CT is more sensitive than plain film for many pathologies, less expensive and faster than MRI, and usually available at all hours of the day. With multislice helical scanners in many EDs, it is possible to get a complete scan with multiple protocols in less than 15 minutes door to door. This has obvious advantages over taking multiple plain films of the head, neck, chest, spine, and abdomen. Although the fixed cost of a CT scan is more expensive, a single trip to CT may save time, decreasing nursing and technologists' costs over multiple plain films with multiple trips to radiology (1). More importantly, CT yields a faster and more accurate diagnosis, leading to increased patient safety and satisfaction.

Clinical indications

Trauma is one of the most common presentations to the ED that indicates the use of spinal CT to rule out, confirm, or further evaluate injury. There are very well-established protocols that should be followed before resorting to the use of imaging to evaluate injury in the trauma patient. The National Emergency X-Radiography Utilization Study was conducted to evaluate the need for radiographic images in trauma patients with suspected mechanisms of spinal injury (2). This large multicenter study used clinical protocol to evaluate the likelihood of a C-spine injury that would mandate further studies with C-spine plain films. The study group discovered that, if the patient met certain criteria, no further radiological study was indicated. Another study with similar goals, but altered clinical criteria, is the Canadian C-spine Rule (3). Both are fairly simple to follow and give the clinician guidelines to direct the next step in imaging (see Chapter 5, Tables 5.2 and 5.3).

Traditionally, if patients do not meet these criteria, plain film of the cervical spine is indicated with three views: odontoid (open-mouth), lateral, and anteroposterior. However, new recommendations specifically for the C-spine are moving to CT first. The Eastern Association for the Surgery of Trauma (EAST) has officially recommended CT over plain films as the initial evaluation of the cervical spine, citing several studies that found plain films inferior to CT, even missing many significant injuries (4–7). Several studies have shown that CT is more sensitive than plain film in detecting clinically significant fractures and suggest that CT should replace plain film as the standard of care. Plain films are only 70% sensitive in some studies compared with greater than 99% for CT, with plain films missing some unstable fractures leading to poor outcomes (1, 8–11). In particular, CT is more sensitive than plain film at visualizing bony intrusion into the spinal canal, small retropulsed fragments, and ligamentous and disc injury, and it is better at providing information for possible procedures or surgical intervention. A few studies even suggest that, with appropriate reconstructions in modern helical scanners, it is possible to view the chest, abdomen, thoracic, and lumbar spine in one pass, reducing costs and radiation exposure by eliminating multiple plain films and repeated CT scans (12).

Along with trauma, CT is a valuable tool in assessing other spinal pathologies. Back pain is a common presentation to the ED, and CT is indicated in only a few of these cases. Nearly 95% of lower back pain is musculoskeletal and commonly resolves with physical therapy, rest, and anti-inflammatory medication. Nonspecific low back pain is not an indication for imagining, and routine x-rays or advanced imaging is not associated with improved outcomes or satisfaction (13).

However, the remaining 5% deserve a workup that includes CT of the spine (14). These include cauda equina syndrome, spinal stenosis, perispinal infection or abscess, radiculopathies, and cancer metastasis. An absolute indication for imaging of the spine is a history that includes a combination of back pain with a history of cancer, even if distant (14). Relative indications include a history of back pain with osteoporosis or injection drug use. Any patient who presents to the ED with sudden onset neurological deficits not related to stroke deserves a workup that includes imaging of the spine.

CT is also indicated whenever detailed imaging of the spine is required but MRI is contraindicated. This is commonly due to known ferromagnetic material or sensitive electronics such as steel implants or pacemakers. Lead is not magnetic, so a gunshot wound is not a contraindication to MRI; however, an unknown foreign body consistent with metal is a relative contraindication to MRI. One option in such cases is a CT myelogram. This is becoming a rare study due to the capabilities of modern MRI. By injecting contrast into the subdural space prior to CT, it becomes possible to visualize the outline of the spinal cord, nerve roots, and cauda equina. The process of CT myelogram is similar to a lumbar puncture with similar risks and is only useful in the lower spine because it is best to avoid allowing contrast to enter the cranial space, and the availability of safe injection sites is limited.

Table 29.1: Sensitivity and specificity of certain imaging modalities

Technique	Sensitivity	Specificity
Plain radiography		
Cancer	0.6	0.95–0.995
Infection	0.82	0.57
Ankylosing spondylitis	0.26–0.45	1
Computed tomography		
Herniated disc	0.62–0.9	0.7–0.87
Stenosis	0.9	0.8–0.96
Magnetic resonance imaging		
Cancer	0.83–0.93	0.90–0.97
Infection	0.96	0.92
Ankylosing spondylitis	0.56	1
Herniated disc	0.6–1.0	0.43–0.97
Stenosis	0.9	0.72–1.0
Radionuclide		
Cancer		
Planar imaging	0.74–0.98	0.64–0.81
SPECT	0.87–0.93	0.91–0.93
Infection	0.90	0.78
Ankylosing spondylitis	0.26	1.0

Diagnostic capabilities

The best use of CT is visualization of bony lesions. The high contrast of bone to the surrounding soft tissue and the computer-generated coronal, sagittal, and even 3D reformatting allows for extremely detailed views of what would otherwise be obscured on plain films. Less dense tissue lesions are more subtle on CT, but a well-trained radiologist should be able to visualize disc herniation, stenosis of the spinal cord, bony erosion from infection, or cancer with approximately equal sensitivity as MRI (14). Ligamentous injury, cord injury, infections such as discitis or paraspinous infections, and muscle strains or sprains are best visualized with MRI. If a patient clearly demonstrates focal neurological impairment such as loss of reflex, sensation, or motor deficits, MRI with CT is indicated as the initial evaluation to visualize the extent of soft tissue and spinal cord involvement along with any bony lesions (14, 15). Table 29.1 shows the estimated sensitivity and specificity of a variety of imaging modalities in the lumbar region (14).

Imaging pitfalls and limitations

In today's litigious environment, clinicians image patients to confirm a suspicion of what they already believe to be a clinically insignificant finding. It is important to keep in mind that CT is not a harmless study. The risk of future cancers is often ignored in favor of confirming clinical observations. There is significant radiation exposure with one complete image of the spine, and the risk of radiation-related thyroid cancer is not insignificant (2, 16). If the patient is stable and can wait for another study such as MRI, lower

radiation plain films, or clinical reevaluation, this may save the patient radiation exposure and reduce hospital and patient expenses.

Time is critical in trauma victims, and it is often tempting to rush a patient to the scanner when the operating room or continued resuscitation is required. Transport to a remote scanner where the patient can only be viewed from several yards away behind protective glass is contraindicated in a patient with unstable vitals and is associated with a poor outcome if the patient should suddenly decompensate. CT scans also require the patient to remain motionless for long periods, which may be impossible for an altered trauma victim. This leads to aggressive sedation, which carries risks that could be avoided with other imaging modalities such as bedside plain films. Appropriate clinical judgment is required prior to sending the patient to the scanner (16).

CT is exactly as its name implies – a mathematical approximation of the multiple densities seen as the x-ray beam rotates around the patient. If the data entered into the equation have large gaps, the approximation becomes less accurate and can miss fractures. Most institutions have specific criteria on how to capture spine images, which should include a maximum slice thickness of 2 to 3 mm for the spine. Images captured at 5 mm slices can miss up to 75% of fractures (4). This is important when doubling the use of a chest or abdominal CT for thoracic and lumbar spine images. Frequently, chest and abdominal views have protocol for larger slice thickness, and only modern helical scanners can reformat these data appropriately for viewing the lumbar and thoracic spine (12).

It is easy to dismiss symptoms when the event history is not traumatic or typical for a spinal column injury. However, even a minor trauma, light lifting, or an occult event can cause severe spinal pathology in select patients. Presentations that combine back pain and a history of cancer are an absolute indication for imaging of the spine. It is simple for a patient to fail to mention a distant history of a "cured" cancer or a chronic condition such as osteoporosis, and it is the clinician's duty to complete a detailed history in every case to determine if imaging is indicated. Conversely, a false sense of security can come from a negative CT image of the spine in the face of clinical symptoms. Back pain can be the initial presentation in abdominal aortic aneurysms, pyelonephritis, renal stones, and pancreatitis, but these pathologies may be missed with selective spinal imaging. Pathologies that involve the cord alone, such as spinal shock or multiple sclerosis, often have a negative CT but are easily visualized on MRI. Guillain–Barré syndrome may have negative imaging on both CT and MRI and requires a thorough history and clinical suspicion (14, 15).

The pediatric population presents a wide array of pitfalls for the clinician when evaluating the spine. The pediatric population on the whole has a different pattern of spinal injuries than adults and frequently requires a different imaging workup. Dislocations and ligamentous injury are more common in the pediatric population; they can be occult on CT and require MRI more frequently. They also present with multiple levels of injury, and complete imaging of the spine is indicated if injury is found at any level of the spine (17).

Because the NEXUS criteria were developed primarily with adults, any attempt to translate this to the pediatric population should be done with caution. One recent study suggests that use of the NEXUS criteria for the pediatric population is appropriate and 100% sensitive, provided that the patient is capable of answering questions appropriately. This excludes any patient younger than 2 years (18).

Spinal cord injury without radiological abnormality (SCIWORA) is an entity that is more common in the pediatric population and, as its name implies, involves injury to the spinal cord without evidence on plain film or CT. Typically, it presents 24 to 48 hours after a trauma with a wide range of neurological dysfunctions. It is believed to be related to the variable stretch between the spinal cord and its surrounding structures. SCIWORA can be treated with steroids but is only seen on MRI and, therefore, requires suspicion by the clinician (19).

Conclusion

CT images of the spine have become ubiquitous in the ED, and justly so. CT is arguably the fastest, most cost-effective method of imaging the spine and provides the most accurate information for diagnosis, with the exception of some soft tissue or spinal cord lesions. This is especially true for trauma patients who require multiple studies in a short period of time. However, when a clinician has access to a large, powerful imaging hammer, each pathology begins to look a lot like a nail. Correct clinical judgment is required prior to sending a patient to the scanner to avoid excess costs, radiation exposure, or adverse outcomes from delayed transport to the operating room or resuscitation.

Recent changes from the Eastern Association for the Surgery of Trauma rate plain films as inferior to CT of the cervical spine. Evidence suggests that CT of the cervical spine should be the study of choice for suspected spinal column injury that cannot be cleared clinically (4–11).

Clinical images

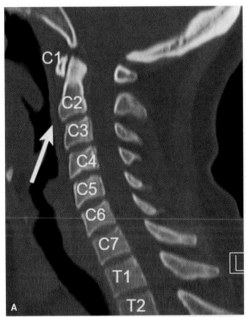

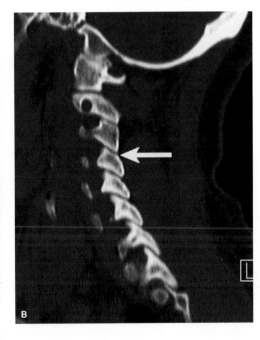

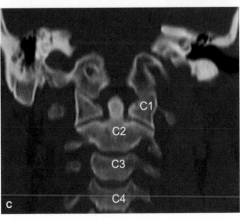

Figure 29.1. A: Normal sagittal view of the C-spine in a 36-year-old female. The arrow is pointing toward the normal prevertebral soft tissue thickness. A simple mnemonic to remember is 6 at 2 and 22 at 6; that is, 6 mm of soft tissue at the level of C2 and 22 mm of soft tissue at C6 is normal. B: Normal alignment of the facet joints (*arrow*) on the right side in this sagittal view. C: Normal view of the basilar condyles, C1/2–dens relationships. A significant portion of all spine injuries occurs at this C1/2 level or at the C6/7 level, depending on the type of injury and age of the patient.

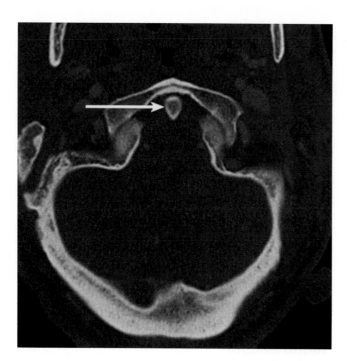

Figure 29.2. Normal axial view of the skull, C1–dens relationship, with the arrow pointing to the dens or odontoid process of C2.

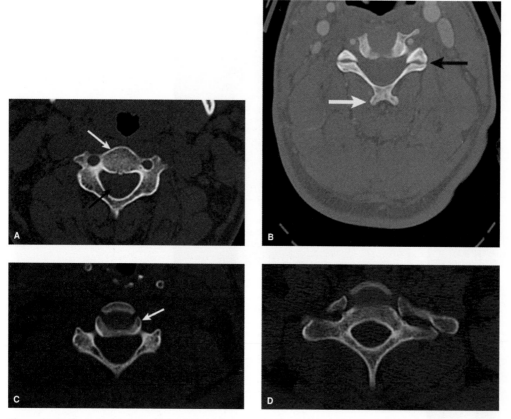

Figure 29.3. Normal axial views of C3. A: Thin but intact cortical layer of the body of C3 (*white arrow*) and spinal canal (*black arrow*). B: The biped spinous process (*white arrow*) is constant from C2 to C6. C1 has no spinous process, and C7 has the largest, usually single-tipped, spinous process. The normal facet joint in axial view (*black arrow*). C: Normal axial view of the superior portion of C6 (*white arrow*) and a small part of the inferior body of C5 (*black arrow*). The less dense material between them is the disk space. D: Normal axial view of T1. Note the ribs laterally. This indicates a complete study from the base of the skull to the T1–C7 interface.

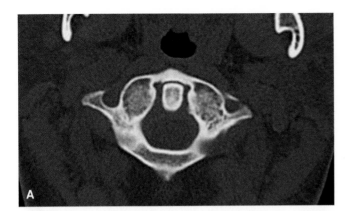

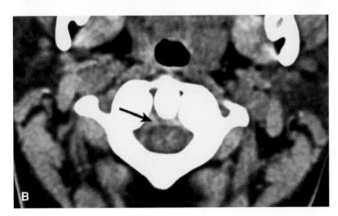

Figure 29.4. A: Normal axial soft tissue view of the dens–C1 interface using the bone-view setting, which changes the computer contrast. Unlike MRI, the CT scanner makes only one scan with axial slices, and then the computer generates every image of the region from that initial scan (B). It is important to note that the important transverse ligament (*arrow*), like all ligaments, is not ideally visualized with CT either in the soft tissue view or the bone view. B: Normal axial soft tissue view of the dens–C1 interface. Note that the prevertebral area and other soft tissues are well visualized, whereas the bone lacks details and is completely white.

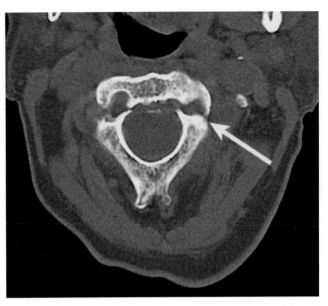

Figure 29.5. "Hangman's fracture." This is a classic fracture of the bilateral pedicles or posterior arch of C2 common with hanging injuries. It is also seen in hyperextension and compression injuries associated with trauma, such as an unrestrained passenger hitting his or her head on a windshield, which involves extending the head back and compressing it at the same time. This is a highly unstable injury. The fracture (*arrow*) involves the transverse foramen where the vertebral arteries course. An angiogram is indicated in this patient.

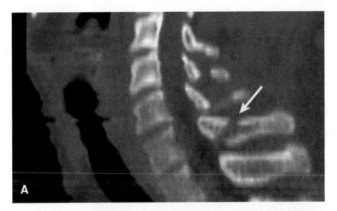

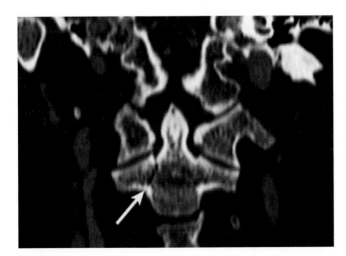

Figure 29.6. A 30-year-old female trauma victim with a type 2 dens fracture. This type of injury is unstable and associated with a fracture extending into the body of C2. Type 2 fractures are avulsions of the tip of the dens, and type 2 are transverse fractures at the base of the dens. This fracture was treated with external fixation with a halo. Type 1 fractures are often stable, and type 2 or 3 fractures also require halo traction or internal fixation.

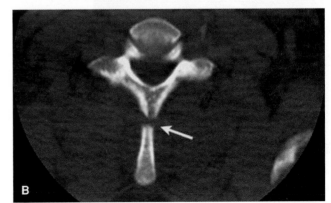

Figure 29.7. A and B: A 20-year-old male who suffered an abrupt flexion of the neck in a fall where he hit his occiput, causing this "clay shoveler's fracture." This injury occurs when the spinous process is avulsed by the powerful supraspinous ligament. This injury commonly occurs at the C7 level. The fracture (*arrow*) is visible in both axial and sagittal views. It is necessary to confirm that the fracture only involves the spinous process with CT because the patient will likely have tenderness in the area; however, it is considered a stable fracture.

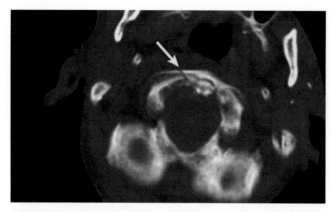

Figure 29.8. Nondisplaced fracture through the right anterior ring of C1, also known as a Jefferson's fracture. Classically, this fracture involves bilateral anterior or bilateral posterior arches of C1; however, here we see only the anterior right arch (*arrow*). This type of injury is associated with axial loading on the cranium that one might see in a diving accident or in a blow to the top of the head.

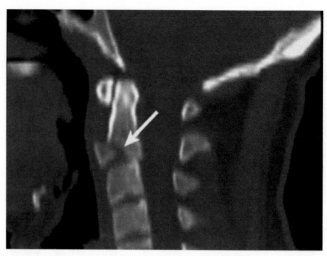

Figure 29.9. A 32-year-old male who was thrown from his motorcycle and sustained a C2 teardrop fracture (*arrow*). This type of injury is associated with extreme extension injuries where the anterior ligament remains in place and avulses the anterior inferior corner of the body of the vertebrae. MRI is indicated to view the extent of the ligamentous injury.

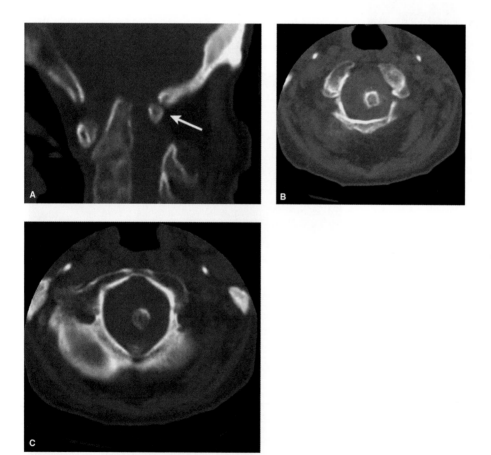

Figure 29.10. A: A 69-year-old male with history of rheumatoid arthritis status post minor fall with C1/2 subluxation, where the displaced arch of C1 (*arrow*), which moved anterior and superior, can be visualized. B: The normal location of the dens is just posterior to the anterior arch of C1, but here it has moved 6 mm posteriorly. C: The dens can be seen entering the foramen magnum, indicating the severity of this injury. Movement of the dens without a fracture indicates injury to the transverse ligament, but the only evidence seen on this CT is the displaced C1/2. This type of ligamentous injury is more common in rheumatoid patients and in Down syndrome and is associated with shearing-type forces. An MRI is clearly indicated in this patient to visualize ligaments and cord damage.

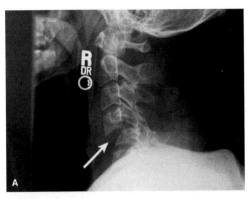
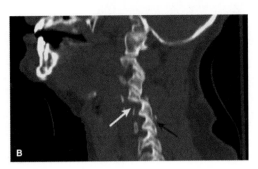

Figure 29.11. A 36-year-old trauma patient. A: An incomplete x-ray that lacks a good view of the C7–T1 interface, but the pathology at the C4/5 with a subluxation of C4/5 level indicates immediate CT. B: The C4 facet is now completely anterior to the C5 facet. This type of injury is a bilateral facet joint dislocation or "locked" facets. The dislocation (*white arrow*) compared with the normal arrangement and 45-degree plane of the C5/6 facet (*black arrow*) can be seen.

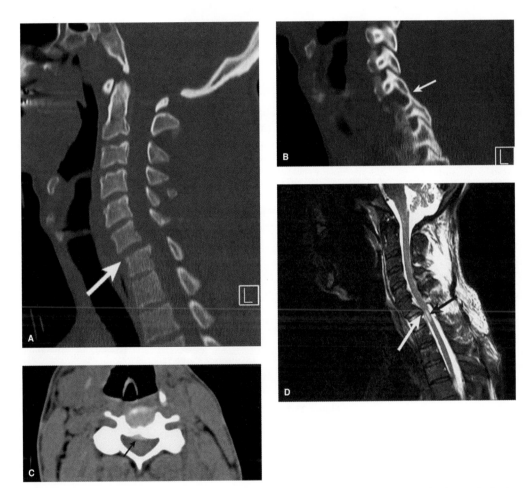

Figure 29.12. A 40-year-old male who fell while intoxicated and riding a skateboard. A: A sagittal reformat clearly shows edema of prevertebral soft tissues anterior to C5/6/7 and a 4 mm anterolisthesis of C6 on C7 (*white arrow*). B: Pathology with C6 "perched" on top of C7 at the left facet joint (*arrow*). C: A small disc protrusion at C4/5 just hinting at the severity of the injury (*black arrow*). D: MRI of the same region shows the enhanced view of the soft tissue with protrusion into the spinal canal (*white arrow*) and edema within the cord (*black arrow*) at the C6/7. There is also impressive edema/hemorrhage of the extensor spinous musculature. Traction was applied for a long period before the joint was able to settle back into the correct anatomical location.

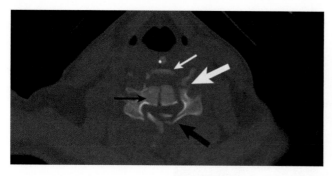

Figure 29.13. Multiple pathologies can be seen here. The inferior portion of C4 (*thin white arrow*) is 12 mm anterior to C5; it has subluxed more than 50% of the width of the vertebral body. Subluxation of 25% or greater of one vertebral body on another is associated with unilateral facet dislocation. Greater than 50% is associated with bilateral dislocation, as seen here. C4 also has a left pedicle fracture (*thick white arrow*), C5 has a burst-type fracture of the body (*thin black arrow*), and both posterior arches have multiple fractures (*thick black arrow*). Each pathology is associated with different forces on the body that are possible in an extremely violent traumatic event. A burst-type fracture is associated with a force oriented in the axial plain, such as landing on top of the head in a fall or the blow of a blunt object. Facet dislocations are associated with extreme flexion combined with a shearing force. This constellation of injuries is highly unstable, and the patient became quadriplegic from the shoulders down.

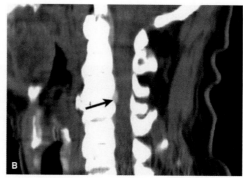

Figure 29.14. A 52-year-old male trauma patient. No acute bony abnormalities were seen on (A), but when visualized with the soft tissue view on (B), a C3/4 disc protrusion becomes obvious as it enters the spinal canal, possibly causing acute compromise of the cord at that level.

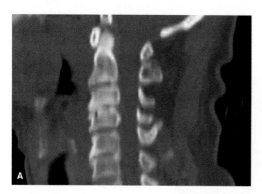

Figure 29.15. A 34-year-old male who landed on his head after a 12-ft fall. A good CT of the spine will cover the region just superior to the occipital condyle down to the C7–T1 interface. In this film, a skull base fracture was discovered on C-spine imaging.

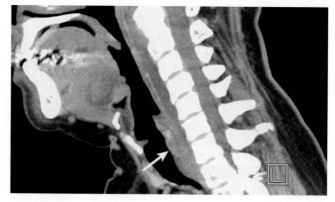

Figure 29.16. A 57-year-old female with obvious neck swelling received a CT for suspicion of a neck abscess. CT revealed prevertebral soft tissue swelling, but no focal collection of fluid can be seen.

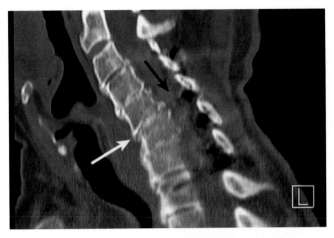

Figure 29.17. A 66-year-old female complaining of neck pain. She was found to have degenerative disease, subluxation, and a mild kyphosis at C5/6, which together form cervical spinal canal stenosis (*black arrow*). Note the almost total collapse of the intervertebral discs and osteophytes (*white arrow*).

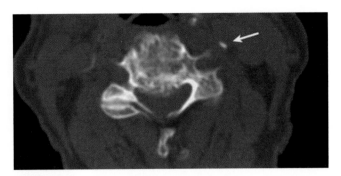

Figure 29.18. An 80-year-old male with a history of neck pain. Seen here are C5 degenerative changes with bony protrusions into the spinal canal, likely causing his pain. These bony changes are similar appearing to osteomyelitis, except the soft tissue is notably not swollen in this image. Note the intramuscular calcifications seen with normal aging (*white arrow*).

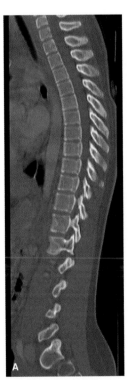
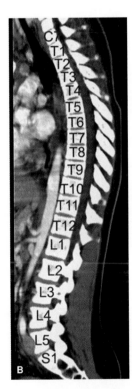

Figure 29.19. A and B: Normal curve of the thoracic and lumbar spine is seen in this bone and soft tissue view. This image of a young patient shows none of the chronic changes of aging and has the normal lordosis curve of the lumbar region, kyphosis of the thoracic, and lordosis of the cervical spine. The patient was not straight on the table, leading to midline imaging of the upper spine and slightly lateral images of the lower spine.

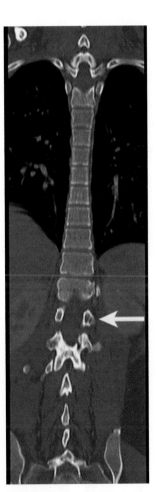

Figure 29.20. Normal coronal view. The normal curves of the spine bring different parts of the spine into view with each cut in this reformatted image. All bodies of the thoracic spine are in view, whereas only the pedicles of L1 (*arrow*) and the spinous processes of L4 and L5 are visualized. Note the motion artifact in the right hemidiaphragm, as the patient continued to breathe during this scan.

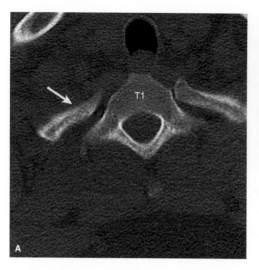

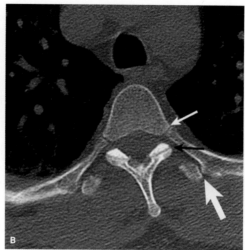

Figure 29.21. A: Normal T1 vertebra showing the first pair of ribs meeting the vertebral body (*arrow*). B: Normal T5 vertebra showing a multitude of joints: the rib joining the body of T5 (*thin white arrow*), the T5/6 facet (*thin black arrow*), and the rib joining the transverse process (*thick white arrow*). The thoracic spine is a very complex structure with 12 joints on every vertebral body, except for T1 and T12, where there is no superior or inferior rib joints.

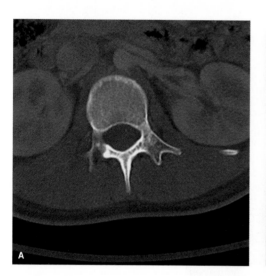

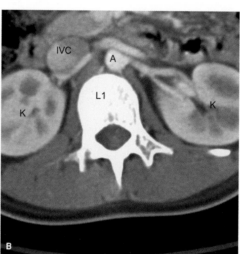

Figure 29.22. A and B: These two images are taken from an abdominal CT and zoomed into the spine region, providing an excellent view of the lumbar spine. They are normal axial views in both soft tissue and bony views of L1. Note how well the anatomy of the region is highlighted in the soft tissue view, which should never be ignored, even in a dedicated spine view.

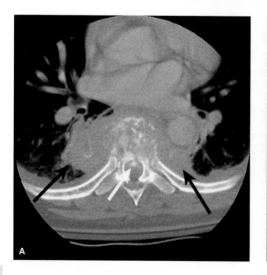

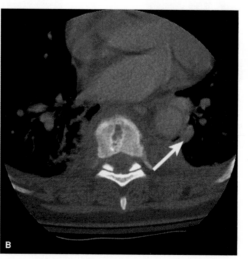

Figure 29.23. A 48-year-old female complaining of decreased rectal tone, urinary retention, and inability to ambulate after a minor fall. A: A bony view of C6 showing that the body of C6 has lost density, and there is soft tissue swelling bilaterally (*black arrows*). Destruction of the bone cortex has led to intrusion of the spinal canal (*white arrow*). B: Spondylodiskitis at T6/7. Note the lower-density disk with a central black lesion and an enlarged lymph node (*arrow*). This is a case of Pott disease or tuberculosis of the spine.

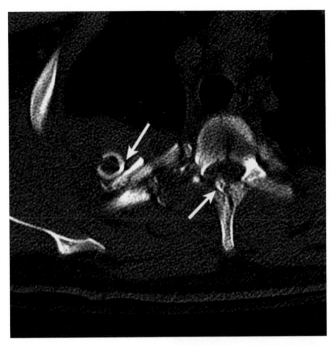

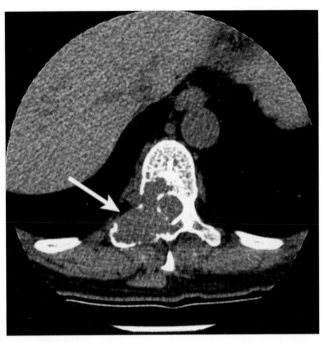

Figure 29.24. A 14-year-old male gunshot victim with paraplegia from the level of the nipples down. He has multiple T2 fractures that include bony protrusion into the spinal canal (*black arrow*). Note the bright dot and semicircle-like structure (*white arrow*). This is a chest tube draining a medium-density substance or hemothorax.

Figure 29.26. A 44-year-old female with history of uterine leiomyosarcoma with obvious metastasis to the spine involving the right posterior T10 vertebral body, with multiple cortical destructions and complete loss of symmetry. Again, history of a primary tumor with spinal lesions is metastatic disease until proven otherwise.

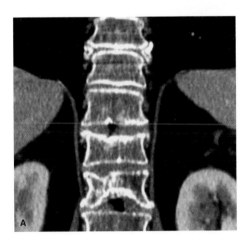

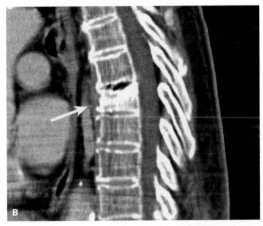

Figure 29.25. A 67-year-old female with history of pancreatic cancer with lytic lesions of the thoracic spine. A: A coronal view clearly showing black lesions in the intervertebral disks indicating air, which can be a normal sign of aging called "vacuum phenomenon." B: A significant loss of height of the T7 vertebral body with prevertebral swelling or mass (*arrow*). Although these could be normal signs of aging, the patient is young for such severe degeneration, and with her history of cancer, this is metastatic disease until proven otherwise.

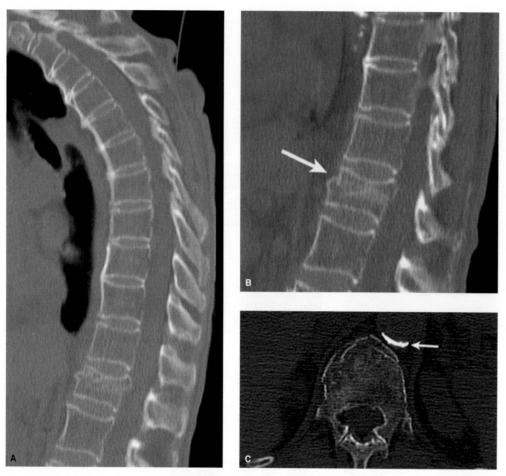

Figure 29.27. A: An 87-year-old female with severe kyphosis. B: An acute collapse of the T12 vertebral body (*white arrow*). C: This appears to be a burst-type fracture with no intrusion into the canal. The small crescent-shaped fleck (*arrow*) is not bone but the descending aorta with calcifications. This type of injury is common in osteoporosis or metastatic disease of the spine, and it frequently occurs at T12 or lower because these structures support the most weight. Frequently, these injuries occur with very minor trauma or when the patient tries to lift a heavy object.

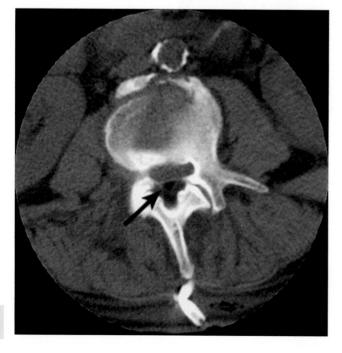

Figure 29.28. A 56-year-old male with a history of lower extremity numbness. Bilateral ligamentum flavum hypertrophy at L3 (*tip of arrow*) can be seen causing stenosis and cauda equina syndrome. Also shown is a compression fracture of the L4 vertebral body of indeterminate age.

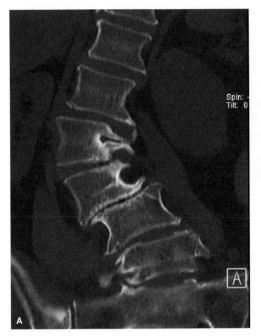
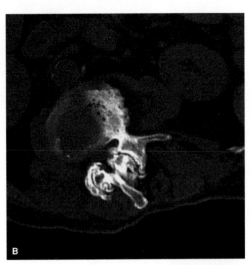

Figure 29.29. Patient with severe dextroscoliosis of the lumbar spine in coronal view obvious in (A). This pathology would be obvious clinically, but the osteophytes caused by uneven pressures on the left aspect of the spine are also causing spinal canal stenosis and cauda equina syndrome, seen in the axial view in (B).

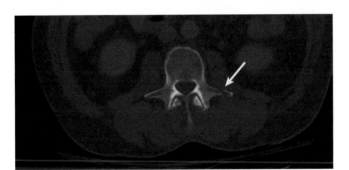

Figure 29.30. A 50-year-old trauma victim who had a blunt abdominal injury and a positive focused assessment by sonography for trauma scan and immediately went to the operating room. After a splenectomy, she had an abdominal CT, which was sufficient to visualize the spine. This patient had a fracture of several spinous processes and the 12th rib on the left side, a common cause of splenic laceration. There is evidence to show that chest and abdominal CT are just as sensitive as dedicated spine images at detecting bony pathology, and they have the advantage of capturing the required images in one pass, which is faster and exposes the patient to less radiation than multiple dedicated films.

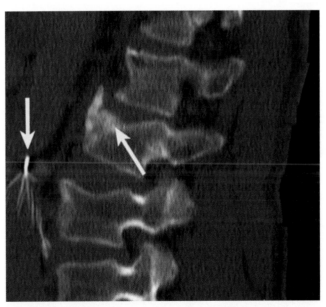

Figure 29.31. A wedge-type fracture of the anterior body of L1 (*white arrow*). These fractures are caused by severe flexion-compression injuries and are considered unstable injuries. Note the IVC filter in place (*black arrow*).

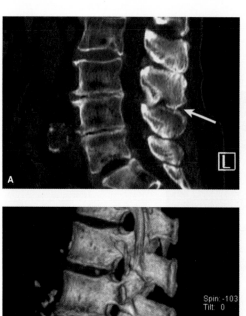

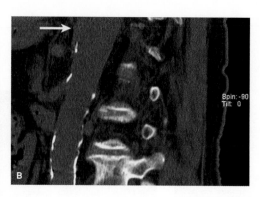

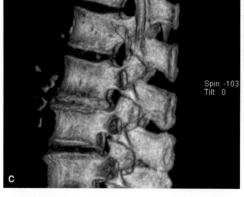

Figure 29.32. A 72-year-old female with back pain. Severe degenerative changes with narrow disc spaces and multiple osteophytes can be seen. Osteoarthritis between the spinous processes of L2 through L5 is compatible with Baastrup disease, or "kissing spines" (A, *arrow*). This is a rare cause of back pain; however, this patient may have another more common reason for back pain, which is her expanding aorta (B, *arrow*). Incidental findings such as the dilated aorta on a dedicated lumbar scan should not be ignored, especially in a case of back pain. C: 3D reformatting of the spine to analyze the patient's extensive arthritis for surgery. This type of computer-generated image is very useful in planning complex orthopedic surgeries but has little value in the ED. This patient needs a complete image of her aorta prior to any surgery.

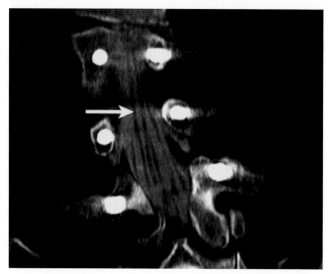

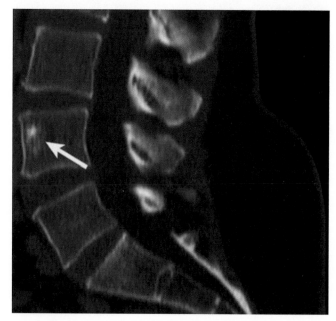

Figure 29.33. CT myelogram in an 87-year-old female with back pain and neurological deficits. Myelograms are not frequently used in the ED, but they are extremely useful for imaging the spinal cord in patients with contraindications to MRI, such as the screws seen in this patient's lumbar spine, electronics, or magnetic material. By injecting dye into the subdural space in the desired region, it is possible to outline the spinal cord with contrast. Note the clearly outlined cauda equina (*arrow*).

Figure 29.34. Enostosis, otherwise known as a bone island, is usually a benign dense region of bone frequently found in the thoracic and lumbar spine (*arrow tip*). Enostosis can also represent metastatic disease and can be differentiated using a bone scan or clinical correlation with primary tumor findings. If, on subsequent films, the dense lesion is noted to be enlarging, a biopsy may be warranted.

References

1. Antevil JL, Sise MJ, Sack DI, et al.: Spiral computed tomography for the initial evaluation of spine trauma: a new standard of care? *J Trauma-Injury Infect Crit Care* 2006;**61**(2):382–7.

2. Hoffman JR, Mower WR, Wolfson AB, et al.: Validity of a set of clinical criteria to rule out injury to the cervical spine in patients with blunt trauma. National Emergency X-Radiography Utilization Study Group. *N Engl J Med* 2000;**343**(2):94–9.

3. Stiell IG, Wells GA, Vandemheen KL, et al.: The Canadian C-spine Rule for radiography in alert and stable trauma patients. *JAMA* 2001;**286**:1841–8.

4. Harris JH Jr, Harris WH: *The radiology of emergency medicine*, 4th ed. Philadelphia: Lippincott Williams & Wilkins, 2000: 307–8.

5. Barrett T, Mower W, Zucker M, Hoffman J: Injuries missed by limited computed tomographic imaging of patients with cervical spine injuries. *Ann Emerg Med* 2006;**47**(2):129–33.

6. Griffen MM, Frykberg ER, Kerwin AJ, et al.: Radiographic clearance of blunt cervical spine injury: plain radiograph or computed tomography scan? *J Trauma* 2003;**55**:222–7.

7. Diaz JJ, Gillman C, Morris JA Jr, et al.: Are five-view plain films of the cervical spine unreliable? A prospective evaluation in blunt trauma patients with altered mental status. *J Trauma* 2003;**55**: 658–64.

8. Brown CVR, Antevil JL, Sise MJ, Sack DI: Spiral computed tomography for the diagnosis of cervical, thoracic, and lumbar spine fractures: its time has come. *J Trauma-Injury Infect Crit Care* 2005;**58**(5):890–6.

9. Brohi K, Healy M, Fotheringham T, et al.: Helical computed tomographic scanning for the evaluation of the cervical spine in the unconscious, intubated trauma patient. *J Trauma-Injury Infect Crit Care* 2005;**58**(5):897–901.

10. Gale SC, Gracias VH, Reilly PM, Schwab CW: The inefficiency of plain radiography to evaluate the cervical spine after blunt trauma. *J Trauma-Injury Infect Crit Care* 2005;**59**(5):1121–5.

11. Holmes JF, Akkinepalli R: Computed tomography versus plain radiography to screen for cervical spine injury: a meta-analysis. *J Trauma-Injury Infect Crit Care* 2005;**58**(5):902–5.

12. Sheridan R, Peralta R, Rhea J, et al.: Reformatted visceral protocol helical computed tomographic scanning allows conventional radiographs of the thoracic and lumbar spine to be eliminated in the evaluation of blunt trauma patients. *J Trauma-Injury Infect Crit Care* 2003;**55**(4):665–9.

13. Chou R, Qaseem A, Snow V, et al.: Diagnosis and treatment of low back pain: a joint clinical practice guideline from the American College of Physicians and the American Pain Society. *Ann Intern Med* 2007 Oct;**147**(7):478–91.

14. Jarvik JG, Deyo RA: Diagnostic evaluation of low back pain with emphasis on imaging MPH. *Ann Intern Med* 2002;**137**: 586–97.

15. Agency for Healthcare Research and Quality: American College of Radiology appropriateness criteria. 2016. Available at: https://www.guideline.gov/content.aspx?id=37931

16. Berne JD, Velmahos GC, El-Tawil Q, et al.: Value of complete cervical helical computed tomographic scanning in identifying cervical spine injury in the unevaluable blunt trauma patient with multiple injuries: a prospective study. *J Trauma-Injury Infect Crit Care* 1999;**47**(5):896.

17. Martin BW, Dykes E, Lecky FE: Patterns and risks in spinal trauma. *Arch Dis Child* 2004;**89**:860–5.

18. Viccellio P, Simon H, Pressman BD, et al.: NEXUS Group: A prospective multicenter study of cervical spine injury in children. *Pediatrics* 2001;**108**(2):e20.

19. Veena K, Sheffali G, Mahesh K, Ajay G: SCIWORA – spinal cord injury without radiological abnormality. *Ind J Pediatr* 2006;**73**(9);829–31.

Chapter 30

CT Imaging of the Head

Marlowe Majoewsky and Stuart Swadron

Indications

Head CT is one of the most common imaging studies ordered from the emergency department. It is indicated in the evaluation of patients with head injury as well as in a variety of nontraumatic presentations.

In most U.S. centers, the clinical threshold for obtaining a head CT in the traumatized patient is very low. Although three clinical decision rules have been developed to identify low-risk patients for whom imaging is unnecessary, none is in widespread use. The criteria identified by the Canadian Head CT Investigators (1), the National X-Ray Utilization investigators (2), and the New Orleans group (3) are listed in Table 30.1. Utilization of head CT in the pediatric population is of particular concern given the risks of radiation exposure in this demographic. Children are more radiosensitive than adults and have more years of life available to develop cancer. It is estimated that the lifetime risk of mortality from malignancy due to a single pediatric head CT ranges from 1:2000 in infants to 1:5000 in older children (4). Multiple clinical prediction rules have been proposed for head CT in children, but these have been limited by a lack of validation and heterogeneous variables (5). The recommendations of the PECARN study are summarized in Table 30.2 (6).

Head CT is also used in the evaluation of the patient who presents with headache, altered mental status, suspected stroke, or other acute neurological abnormalities. As in patients with head injury, head CT is used rather liberally in emergency departments in the United States. Although some guidelines for its use exist, they are generally the product of consensus panels rather than randomized controlled trials. In patients with altered mental status or acute neurological abnormalities, there is little controversy about the need for emergent head CT scanning. In patients with headache, it is generally recommended that emergent CT be limited to patients with certain high-risk features to their presentation (7). Table 30.3 contains the most recent recommendations of the American College of Emergency Physicians on the indications for emergent CT in the setting of acute headache.

Head CT may be obtained emergently in other circumstances. For example, a head CT may be obtained prior to the administration of fibrinolytic medications in a patient with a history of malignancy to look for metastatic disease that may make such therapy dangerous. In the evaluation of an immune-compromised patient with a fever, head CT may be of value to determine the safety of a subsequent lumbar puncture. In this patient population, space-occupying lesions are more common and may represent a contraindication.

Diagnostic capabilities

Current CT scanners are very sensitive for the detection of acute hemorrhage and bony injury, the two principal pathologies sought in evaluation of patients with head injury. CT continues to be superior to more expensive technologies, such as MR, in the acute setting due to its sensitivity, speed, and accessibility (8, 9). It should be noted that CT is much less sensitive than MR in the detection of subacute hemorrhage (e.g., ≥6 hours after injury), axonal shear injury, and lesions of the posterior fossa. However, these limitations should not diminish its dominant role in the decision-making process for acute head injury.

In the patient with head injury, head CT will identify skull fractures although fractures through the thinnest areas of the base of the skull may be missed in the axial cuts. Extracranial lesions such as hematomas and soft tissue edema are also apparent. Acute hemorrhage appears hyperdense (white) on CT. The head CT is very sensitive for all intracranial collections of blood: extraaxial (epidural and subdural), subarachnoid, intraparenchymal, and intraventricular. Although the CT is relatively insensitive for the early signs of axonal injury and cellular injury, the mass effect that results from such injury is clearly seen so that clinical decision making can be facilitated. Pneumocephalus is also readily identified and represents a violation of the dura mater, typically by a skull fracture.

In patients with altered mental status and other neurological abnormalities, head CT is extremely valuable in detecting pathology that requires emergent intervention. Although CT is not sensitive enough to identify or characterize all space-occupying lesions, those of relevance in the emergency department will be readily identified because of their size or the mass effect of surrounding edema. At times, it may not be clear whether a mass is infectious (e.g., abscess), vascular (e.g., arteriovenous malformation), or neoplastic (e.g., metastatic disease), and further investigation must be done to delineate the lesion. Regardless of pathology, it is the resultant mass effect on brain architecture that is most important for the initial management in the ED. Acute hemorrhagic stroke is readily identified on head CT. Subarachnoid hemorrhage from spontaneous rupture of a cerebral aneurysm or arteriovenous malformation is also usually identified. However, in patients with new, sudden-onset headache, a small but persistent number of false-negative

Table 30.1: National Criteria for Obtaining Head CT in Patients with Head Injuries

	Patients with minor head injury can be identified at two levels of risk:
	1) **Patients with any one of the following five findings are at substantial risk for requiring neurosurgical intervention. Head CT is mandatory in these cases.** • GCS score <15 at 2 h after injury • Suspected open or depressed skull fractures • Any sign of basal skull fracture (hemotympanum, cerebrospinal fluid, otorrhea/rhinorrhea, Battle's sign) • Vomiting > two episodes • Age > 65 years
Canadian Head CT Investigators (1)	2) **Patients with either of the following two characteristics could have clinically important lesions identified with CT but are not at risk for requiring neurological intervention. Management with CT versus close observation depends on local resources.** • Amnesia before impact >30 min • Dangerous mechanism (pedestrian struck by motor vehicle, occupant ejected from motor vehicle, fall from height >3 feet or five stairs)
National X-ray Utilization Investigators (2)	**Patients with blunt head trauma who do not meet any of the following eight criteria are unlikely to have significant injuries revealed by CT scanning and do not require imaging.** • Evidence of significant skull fracture • Scalp hematoma • Neurologic deficit • Altered level of alertness • Abnormal behavior • Coagulopathy • Persistent vomiting • Age 65 years or more
New Orleans Group (3)	**Patients with minor head injury should undergo CT in the presence of one or more of the following seven clinical findings:** • Headache • Vomiting • Age over 60 years • Drug or alcohol intoxication • Deficits in short-term memory • Physical evidence of trauma above the clavicles • Seizure

studies support the recommendation for a lumbar puncture following CT to rule out hemorrhage (10–13).

In the first several hours after an ischemic stroke (and in transient ischemic attack), head CT lacks the sensitivity to detect abnormalities in the majority of patients. Nonetheless, the initial CT is critical to rule out the presence of hemorrhage, masses, and other pathologies. CT may also identify signs of edema that point to a stroke that is older than the clinical presentation suggests and for which fibrinolytic therapy may have a higher likelihood of resulting in catastrophic hemorrhage. Augmentations of standard CT protocols (e.g., perfusion CT with contrast) and MR hold greater promise for use in stratifying stroke patients into various interventions.

Imaging pitfalls and limitations

The vast majority of head CTs performed in the ED are done without contrast. Intravenous contrast confounds the detection of acute hemorrhage. If contrast will be administered, CT without contrast should be performed first. Contrast administration may enhance the ability to detect subacute blood collections and to better characterize space-occupying lesions, but because of the superiority of MR in these situations, it may be limited to settings where MR is unavailable. In both head injury and nontraumatic indications for CT, acute pathologies are not static – the CT appearance of an acute cerebral contusion or acute ischemic stroke will evolve with time, and repeat imaging is often necessary in the initial stages of management.

Artifact is an important consideration in the interpretation of head CTs. There is always some degree of linear streak artifact in the areas of brain that are surrounded or bordered by thick, irregular bone. These areas include the posterior fossa and the caudal tips of the frontal and temporal lobes. This can result in either the masking or the mistaken identification of hemorrhage in these areas. Other structures that may be difficult to distinguish from blood include thickened

Table 30.2: Recommendations for Obtaining Head CT in Children with Blunt Head Trauma

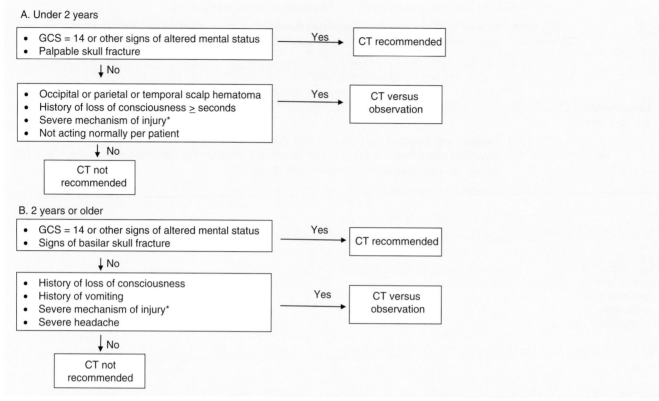

A. Under 2 years

- GCS = 14 or other signs of altered mental status
- Palpable skull fracture

→ Yes → CT recommended

↓ No

- Occipital or parietal or temporal scalp hematoma
- History of loss of consciousness ≥ seconds
- Severe mechanism of injury*
- Not acting normally per patient

→ Yes → CT versus observation

↓ No

CT not recommended

B. 2 years or older

- GCS = 14 or other signs of altered mental status
- Signs of basilar skull fracture

→ Yes → CT recommended

↓ No

- History of loss of consciousness
- History of vomiting
- Severe mechanism of injury*
- Severe headache

→ Yes → CT versus observation

↓ No

CT not recommended

* Severe mechanism of injury is defined as motor vehicle crash with patient ejection, death of another passenger, rollover, pedestrian or bicyclist with a helmet struck by motorized vehicle, falls of more than 3 ft (under 2 years) or 5 feet (2 years or older), or head struck by a high-impact object.

Table 30.3: ACEP Clinical Policy for Obtaining Head CT in Patients with Headache

Which patients with headache require neuroimaging in the ED?

Patient Management Recommendations.

Level A recommendations. None specified.

Level B recommendations.

1. Patients presenting to the ED with headache and new abnormal findings in a neurologic examination (e.g., focal deficit, altered mental status, altered cognitive function) should undergo emergent* noncontrast head CT.

2. Patients presenting with new, sudden-onset, severe headache should undergo an emergent* head CT.

3. HIV-positive patients with a new type of headache should be considered for an emergent* neuroimaging.

Level C recommendations. Patients who are older than 50 years and presenting with new type of headache but with a normal neurologic examination should be considered for an urgent** neuroimaging study.

*Emergent studies are those essential for a timely decision regarding potentially life-threatening or severely disabling entities. **Urgent studies are those that are arranged prior to discharge from the emergency department (scan appointment is included in the disposition) or performed prior to disposition when follow-up cannot be assured.

From:

American College of Emergency Physicians (ACEP). Clinical policy: critical issues in the evaluation and management of patients presenting to the emergency department with acute headache. Ann Emerg Med 2002 Jan;39(1):108–22.

areas of the falx cerebri, tentorium cerebelli, and dural venous sinuses, all of which appear hyperdense on CT.

Attention to all available windows is important. Windows are used to bring out certain details on the scan: bone, parenchyma, or blood. Fractures may be missed in a trauma patient if the bone windows are not inspected. It may be more difficult to detect a subdural hematoma if the blood windows are not inspected.

Clinical images

Basic principles and normal anatomy

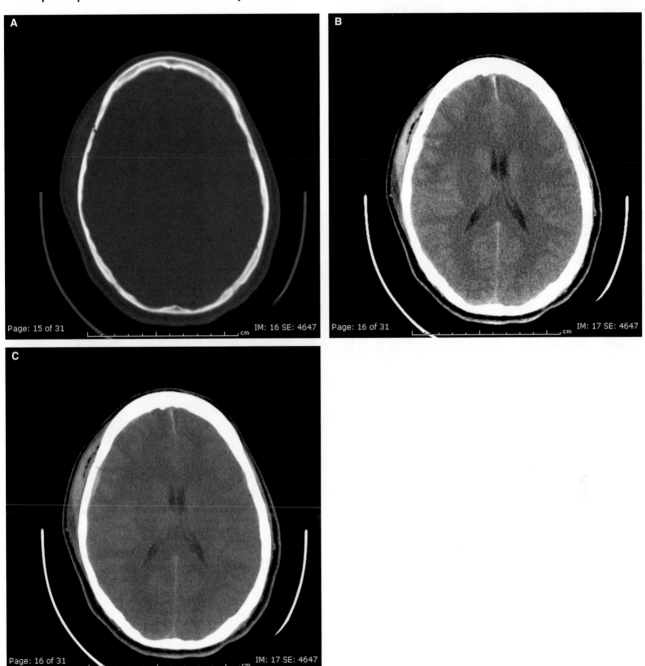

Figure 30.1. *Windows.* The three window settings commonly used for head CT. The *bone window* (left) is helpful to identify fractures, sinus pathology, and intracranial air (pneumocephalus). With the parenchymal or *brain window* (middle), gray matter can be differentiated from the white matter. Early signs of stroke and other processes that result in edema are best seen on the parenchymal window. The subdural or *blood window* is most sensitive for detecting subdural and other intracranial hemorrhage. In this example, a small fracture is seen in the right parietal area on the bone window. This corresponds to an area of soft tissue edema and subcutaneous emphysema (visible on all three windows), and to a small underlying epidural hematoma, distinguishable only on the blood window.

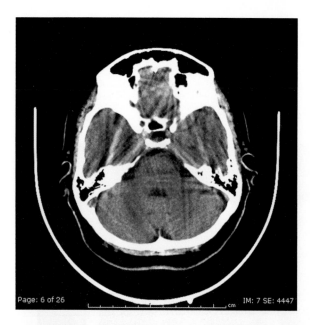

Figure 30.2. *Beam-hardening artifact.* The linear streaks in the brain parenchyma are seen in areas where thick bone surrounds much less dense brain tissue. This artifact is commonly seen at the base of the brain and in the posterior fossa, leading many clinicians to look less carefully in these areas.

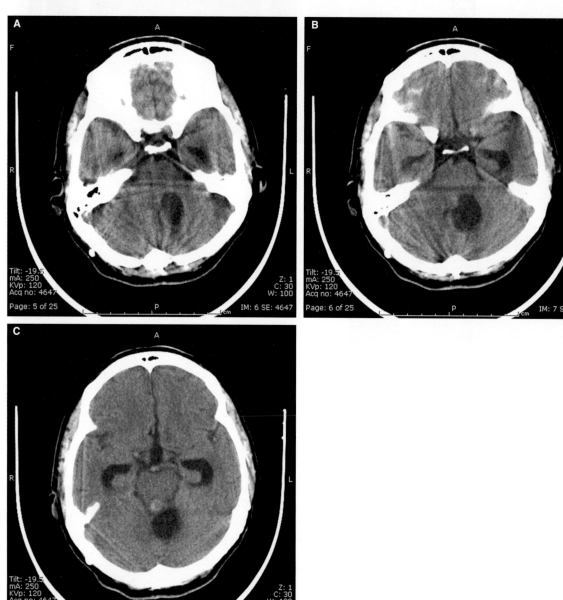

Figure 30.3. *Volume-averaging artifact.* When CT cuts are widely spaced, volume-averaging artifact may cause the appearance of blood. This typically occurs at the base of the brain. In this example, artifact is seen at the base of the frontal lobes, superior to the orbits. A cyst in the fourth ventricle is also present, resulting in non-communicating hydrocephalus and dilation of the temporal horns of the lateral ventricles.

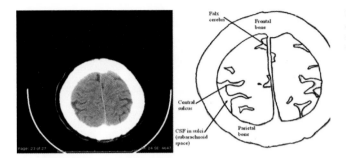

Figure 30.4. *Normal anatomy*. The following sequence demonstrates normal anatomical structures. The first image demonstrates bony anatomy at the level of the frontal sinus (bone window). The remainder of the images (parenchymal window) reveal normal structures in a caudal to rostral progression of cuts.

Trauma

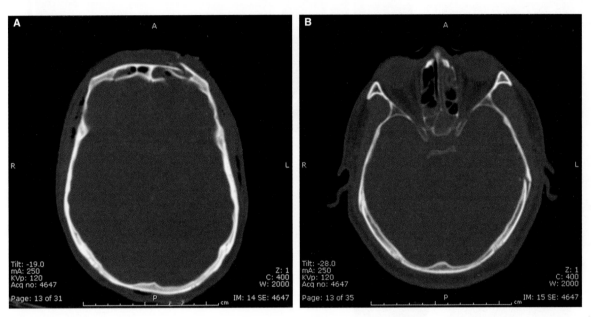

Figure 30.5. *Fractures*. Fractures of the skull can be classified as *linear, depressed, basal*, or *diastatic*. In the first example (A), a fracture through both the outer and inner walls of the left frontal sinus can be seen. In the second example (B), there is a fracture of the left temporal bone. The opacities in the sinuses represent blood from facial fractures, which are not seen in this particular cut.

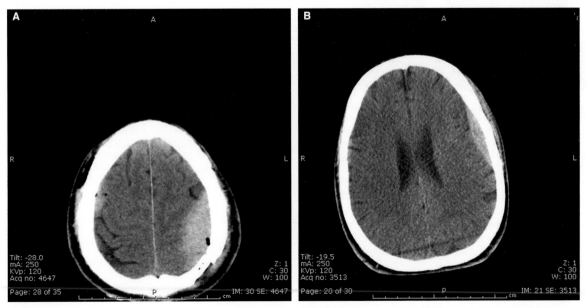

Figure 30.6. *Epidural hematoma*. Epidural hematomas can be seen anywhere along the convexities of the skull, with or without an associated skull fracture. In the first example, an epidural hematoma is seen along with pneumocephalus. This implies the presence of a fracture, which may be apparent only on bone window.

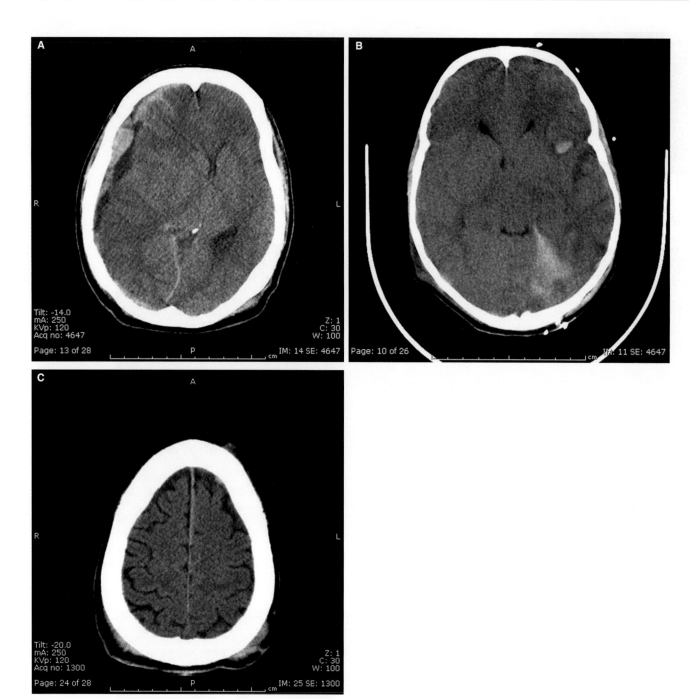

Figure 30.7. *Subdural hematoma.* Subdural hematomas may be seen around the cerebral convexities, adjacent to the tentorium and the falx (intercerebral). They are crescent shaped, not lens shaped like epidural hematomas. Subdural hematomas do not cross the midline but rather invaginate inward alongside the falx cerebri and the tentorium cerebelli. They are also associated with a much greater degree of underlying brain edema. In the first example (A), a chronic (black) and acute (white) component to the right-sided subdural is seen. The underlying edema has resulted in significant edema shift of the midline. In the second example (B), acute subdural blood has layered along the tentorium cerebelli. In the third example (C), subdural blood is found between the two hemispheres. An intercerebral subdural can often be differentiated from calcification of the falx by the mass effect (narrowing of the sulci) on the affected side.

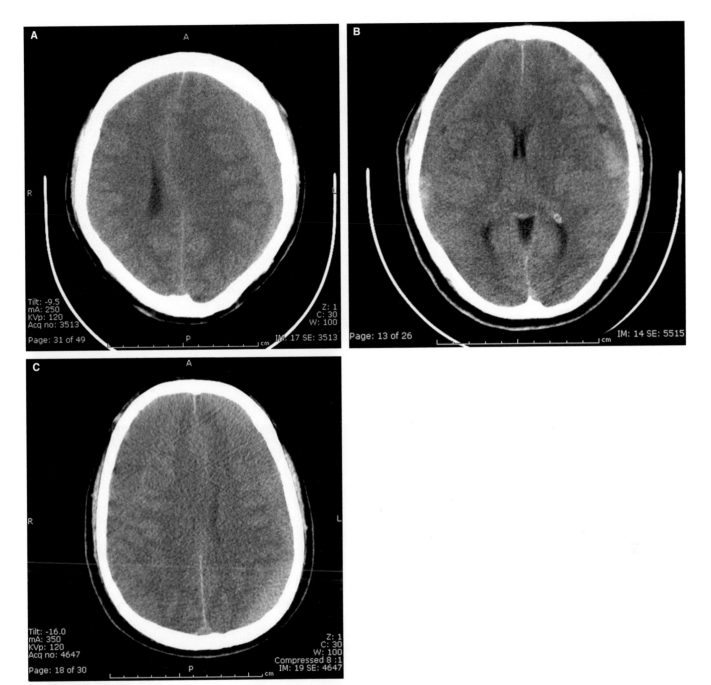

Figure 30.8. *Isodense subdural hematoma.* Subdural hematomas may be difficult to see when they are subacute, typically a week or more old, as they transition from an acute hyperdense (white) to a chronic hypodense (black) density. In the first example (A), below, a large isodense subdural hematoma is seen on the left side. It has resulted in significant mass effect and a shift of the midline. In the second example (B), bilateral subacute subdural hemorrhages are seen, with an acute component to the left-sided subdural. When bilateral hematomas are present, there is a balancing effect, and a midline shift may not be seen. The third example (C) demonstrates bilateral isodense subdural hematomas.

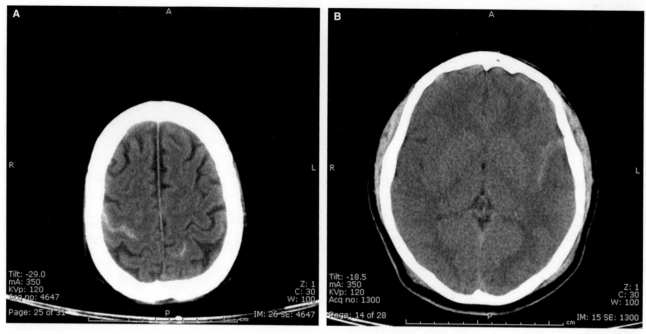

Figure 30.9. *Traumatic subarachnoid hemorrhage.* Blood is seen invaginating between the cerebral convolutions in both of these examples of traumatic subarachnoid hemorrhage. On the right, blood is seen in the left Sylvian fissure.

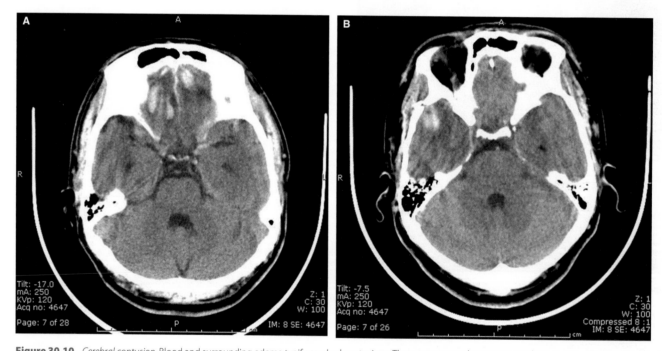

Figure 30.10. *Cerebral contusion.* Blood and surrounding edema typify cerebral contusions. These may expand over time, resulting in mass effect and herniation. Contusions at the base of the brain are more easily missed because of the dense adjacent bone. Here are examples of frontal (A) and temporal (B) cerebral contusions.

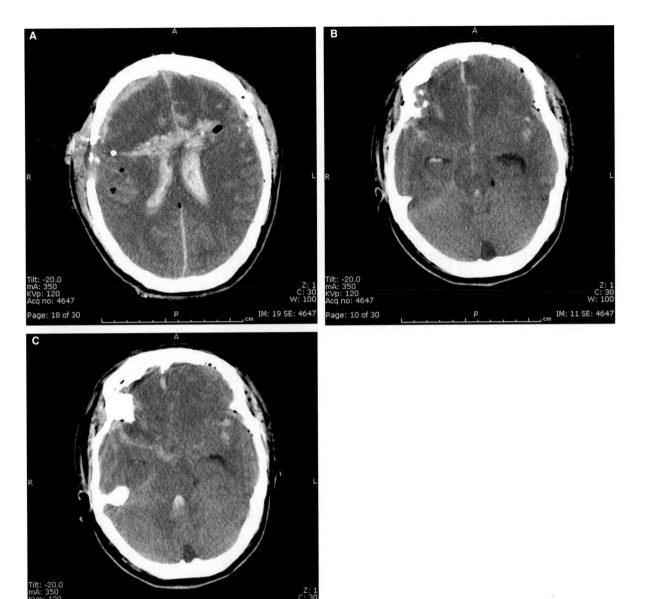

Figure 30.11. *Gunshot wound to the head*. This sequence of cuts from the same patient demonstrates changes typical in a gunshot wound that crosses the midline of the brain. In the first image (A), the trajectory of the missile can be seen, as well as hemorrhage throughout the lateral ventricles. In the lower cuts (B and C), subarachnoid blood and intraventricular blood is seen along with their devastating effects, hydrocephalus (indicated by the dilation of the temporal horns of the lateral ventricles) and transtentorial herniation (indicated by the loss and asymmetry of the basal cisternae around the brainstem).

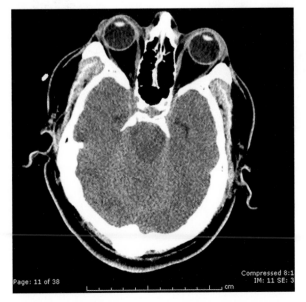

Figure 30.12. *Diffuse axonal injury*. Initial CT and MR scans are often normal in patients with diffuse axonal injury. Only about 10% will show characteristic punctate hemorrhagic lesions. These are most often located in the corpus callosum, the gray-white matter junction of the cerebrum, and the pontine-mesencephalic junction. The sequelae of diffuse axonal injury such as edema may be seen. In the image below, diffuse edema, loss of the gray-white matter junction and herniation is seen in a patient who presented with a GCS of 3 after a high-velocity motor vehicle accident.

Non-trauma

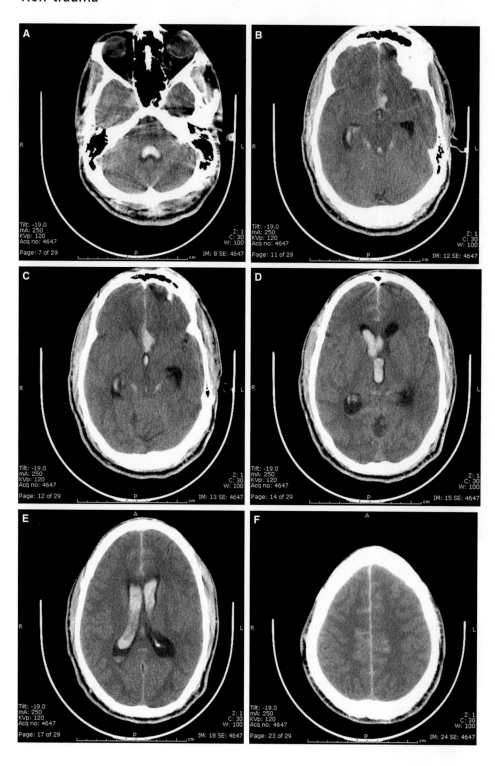

Figure 30.13. *Subarachnoid hemorrhage secondary to aneurysmal rupture complicated by intraventricular involvement and non-communicating hydrocephalus.* In contrast to traumatic subarachnoid hemorrhage, which is often isolated to the cerebral convexities, subarachnoid hemorrhage from a ruptured aneurysm is usually found in the basal cisternae. Cerebral aneurysms are found on the vessels of the Circle of Willis, which lies in the suprasellar cistern. This sequence of six cuts from a patient with a ruptured aneurysm demonstrates some of the typical findings. The first cut (A) demonstrates blood filling the fourth ventricle. Moving rostrally (B), blood in the cerebral aqueduct and temporal horn of the right lateral ventricle can be seen. The obstruction of the ventricular system by clotted blood at the level of the cerebral aqueduct has resulted in hydrocephalus evidenced by the dilated temporal horns. Blood is also seen in the cisternae surrounding the brainstem and in the fissures that surround them (anterior interhemispheric and Sylvian). The greatest density is seen at the level of the anterior communicating artery, a common site for aneurysms, and the likely cause in this case. In the third cut (C), blood can be seen in the third ventricle. In the subsequent cuts (D–F), blood can be seen extending into both lateral ventricles, and on the highest cut (F), blood can be seen to replace the cerebrospinal fluid in the sulci.

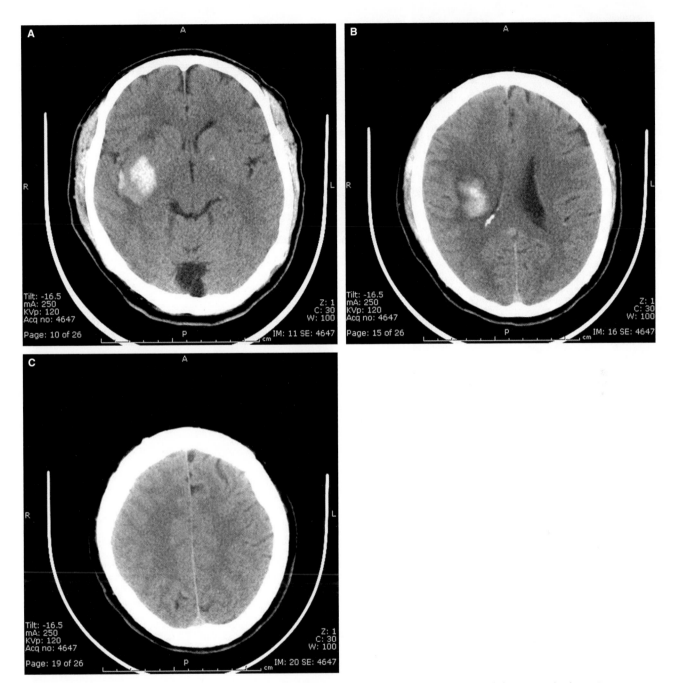

Figure 30.14. *Hypertensive hemorrhage.* Spontaneous hemorrhage secondary to longstanding hypertension and chronic vascular disease is seen most commonly in the basal ganglia (*upper panel*), thalamus (*lower left*), pons (*lower middle*), and cerebellum (*lower right*). In the upper panel, the mass effect of the hemorrhage and surrounding edema is evident in the loss of CSF-filled sulci on the right side. In the last image (*lower right*), the cerebellar hemorrhage has extended into the fourth ventricle.

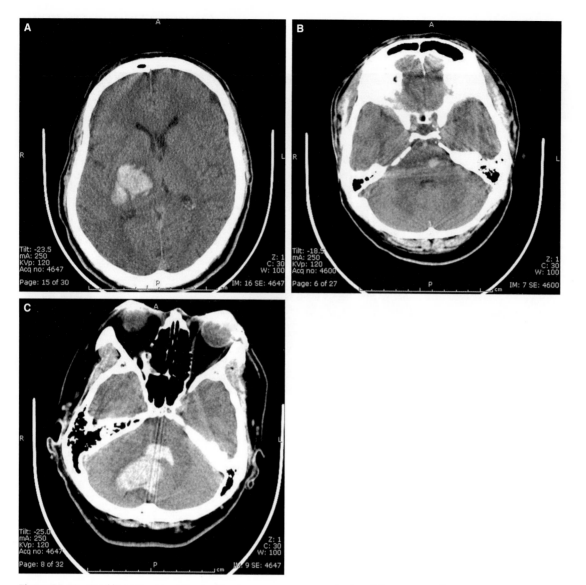

Figure 30.15. *Uncal herniation.* Herniation results when compensatory mechanisms fail to accommodate an expanding space-occupying lesion. Radiographic signs of herniation may precede clinical signs and may provide a small window of opportunity for clinical intervention. This would be unlikely in the case depicted here. In this patient, a massive hypertensive hemorrhage in the basal ganglia has dissected into the ventricular system. The mass effect of the hemorrhage and surrounding edema has resulted in uncal herniation, demonstrated by the loss of space around the brainstem. Also seen are hemorrhages in the midbrain, possibly representing Duret hemorrhages (caused by a tearing of the vessels that supply the brainstem as the brain moves caudally through the foramen magnum and suggesting an irreversible process). Also seen is a dilatation of the temporal horn of right lateral ventricle, a form of hydrocephalus resulting from the herniation.

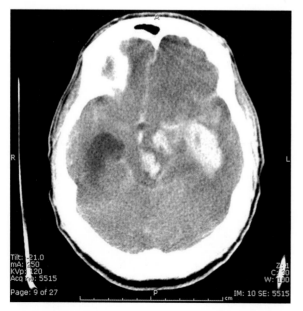

Figure 30.16. *Ischemic stroke.* Noncontrast CT is not sensitive for the detection of ischemic stroke in the first minutes and hours. The earliest changes are related to edema and include an obscuration of the gray-white matter junction and a loss of sulci in the affected area. With time, the affected area becomes hypodense. Old infarcts appear as a loss of parenchymal volume ("ex-vacuo" changes).

In the upper panels, CT changes in a patient both an acute stroke and old stroke are shown. In the lower cut (*upper right*), significant volume loss in the right occipital region suggests an old stroke. In the higher cut, obscuration of the gray-white matter junction and a loss of sulci in the left occipital region when compared with other areas suggest an acute ischemic stroke.

A second patient is depicted in the second panel. In this patient, in addition to the early signs of edema, the area of infarction is hypodense – this implies an older, subacute ischemic stroke, usually more than a few hours old to days old. Very little mass effect is evident.

The third panel demonstrates a cerebellar infarct. CT is less sensitive than MRI for detection of infarction in the posterior fossa. Limitations of CT include bony artifact in this region.

The lower panel shows an older-appearing infarct in the territory of the middle cerebral artery with relatively little edema. The time of maximal mass effect from an ischemic stroke is typically 2 to 4 days following the initial insult.

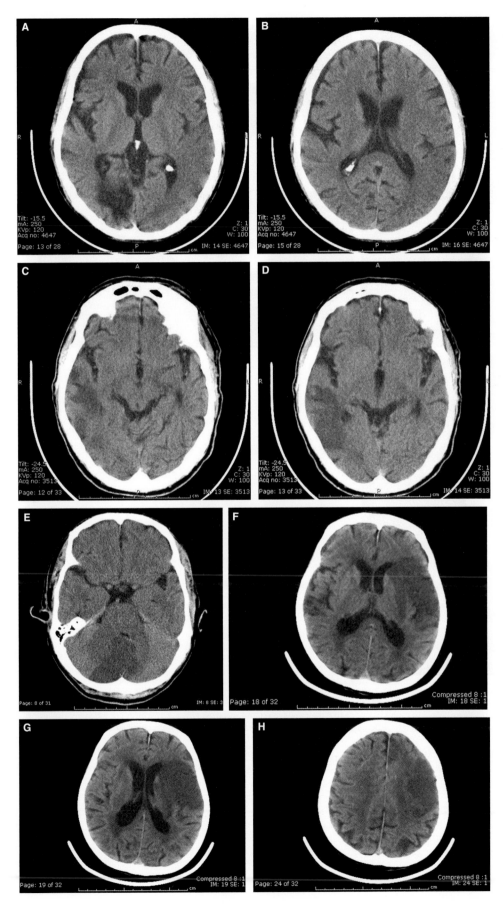

Figure 30.17. *Hydrocephalus with a non-functioning shunt.* This panel shows a patient with an intraventricular shunt in the lateral ventricles. The marked dilation of the lateral and third ventricles suggests that it is not functioning well, although comparison with previous CT studies may be helpful to confirm this.

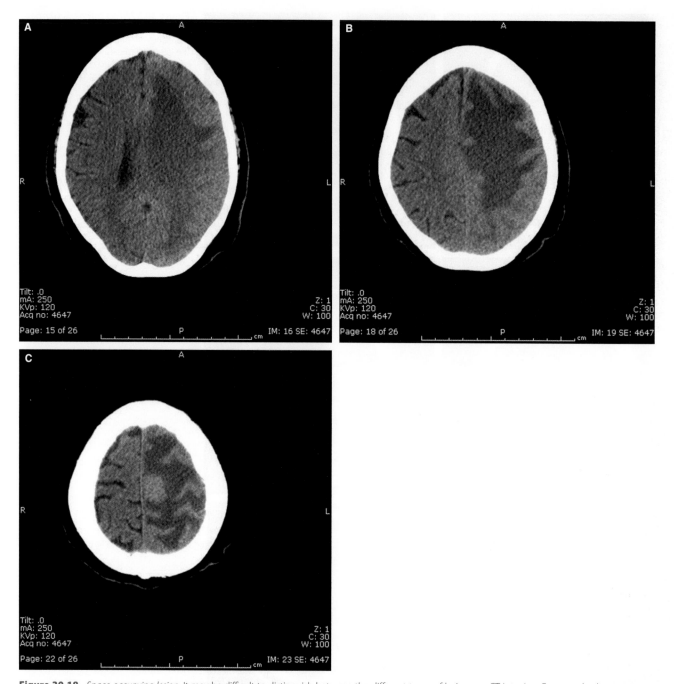

Figure 30.18. *Space-occupying lesion.* It may be difficult to distinguish between the different types of lesions on CT imaging. Fortunately, the most emergent priorities are often unrelated to the nature of the lesion itself and more related to its mass effect. Tumors, both primary and metastatic; vascular malformations; and infectious lesions, such as toxoplasmosis and abscesses, are all examples of lesions that may result in edema and mass effect. In this example, a hyperdense lesion is seen adjacent to the falx (C). The surrounding hypodensity represents edema and can be seen on several cuts below the lesion itself (A and B).

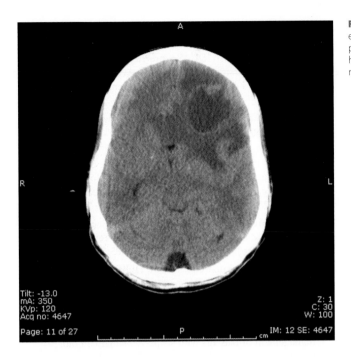

Figure 30.19. *Ring-enhancing lesion.* The differential diagnosis of ring-enhancing lesions includes abscess (bacterial, fungal, and parasitic), metastases, primary brain tumor such as glioblastoma, multiple sclerosis, infarction, resolving hematomas, and necrosis secondary to radiation therapy. This image shows likely metastases in a patient with a history of lung cancer.

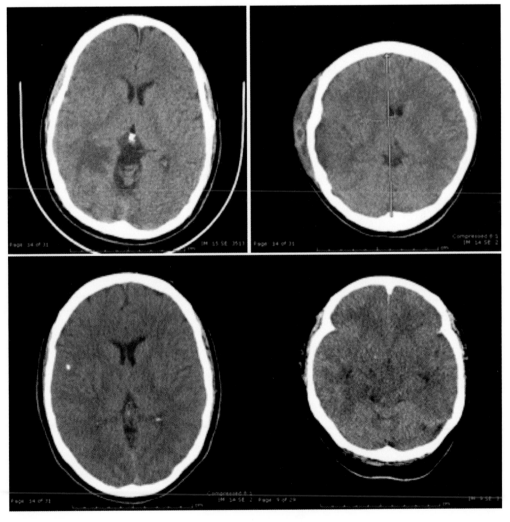

Figure 30.20. *Infection.* Findings on head CT in intracranial infection may be subtle. In the upper left image, diffuse cerebral edema and effacement of the basilar cisterns consistent with herniation are seen in a patient with encephalitis. In the upper right image, a crescent-shaped hypodensity and midline shift indicate a subdural empyema in a patient who presented with a severe facial infection following wisdom tooth extraction.

In the lower left image, a hypodense lesion and surrounding edema are seen in a patient who was found to have a brain abscess. In the lower right image, calcified lesions indicate inactive neurocysticercosis. Active lesions are cystic and may be found in the meninges, parenchyma, and ventricles.

References

1. Stiell IG, Wells GA, Vandemheen K, et al.: The Canadian CT Head Rule for patients with minor head injury. *Lancet* 2001;**357** (9266):1391–6.

2. Mower WR, Hoffman JR, Herbert M, et al.: Developing a decision instrument to guide computed tomographic imaging of blunt head injury patients. *J Trauma* 2005;**59**(4):954–9.

3. Haydel MJ, Preston CA, Mills TJ, et al.: Indications for computed tomography in patients with minor head injury. *N Engl J Med* 2000;**343**(2):100–5.

4. Brenner DJ, Hall EJ: Computed tomography—an increasing source of radiation exposure. *N Engl J Med* 2007 Nov;**357**(22): 2277–84.

5. Maguire JL, Boutis K, Uleryk EM, et al.: Should a head-injured child receive a head CT scan? A systematic review of clinical prediction rules. *Pediatrics* 2009 Jul;**124**(1):e145–54.

6. Kuppermann N, Holmes JF, Dayan PS, et al.: Identification of children at very low risk of clinically-important brain injuries after head trauma: a prospective cohort study. *Lancet* 2009 Oct;**374**(9696):1160–70.

7. American College of Emergency Physicians: Clinical policy: critical issues in the evaluation and management of patients presenting to the emergency department with acute headache. *Ann Emerg Med* 2002;**39**:108–22.

8. Mohamed M, Heasly DC, Yagmurlu B, Yousem DM: Fluid-attenuated inversion recovery MR imaging and subarachnoid hemorrhage: not a panacea. *Am J Neuroradiol* 2004;**25**:545–50.

9. Go JL, Zee CS: Unique CT imaging advantages. Hemorrhage and calcification. *Neuroimaging Clin N Am* 1998;**8**:541–58.

10. Heasley DC, Mohamed MA, Yousem DM: Clearing of red blood cells in lumbar puncture does not rule out ruptured aneurysm in patients with suspected subarachnoid hemorrhage but negative head CT findings. *Am J Neuroradiol* 2005;**26**:820–4.

11. O'Neill J, McLaggan S, Gibson R: Acute headache and subarachnoid haemorrhage: a retrospective review of CT and lumbar puncture findings. *Scott Med J* 2005;**50**:151–3.

12. Morgenstern LB, Luna-Gonzales H, Huber JC Jr, et al.: Worst headache and subarachnoid hemorrhage: prospective, modern computed tomography and spinal fluid analysis. *Ann Emerg Med* 1998;**32**(3 Pt 1):297–304.

13. Foot C, Staib A: How valuable is a lumbar puncture in the management of patients with suspected subarachnoid haemorrhage? *Emerg Med (Fremante)* 2001;**13**:326–32.

Chapter 31

CT Imaging of the Face

Monica Kathleen Wattana and Tareg Bey

CT has surpassed plain film radiography as the method of choice for rapid and efficient facial fracture identification in the multitrauma patient and the patient with isolated injuries to the face. One key reason is that plain film radiography facial views, such as the Waters' view, require repositioning to overcome the problem of overlapping structures obscuring fracture assessment. This is problematic because trauma patients often arrive with a rigid cervical collar in place. CT bypasses this problem and allows for simultaneous evaluation of facial trauma during emergent assessment for intracranial and cervical spine injury. CT images depict all areas of the facial skeleton without the need for repositioning, allow for accurate identification of exact bones involved in a facial fracture, and provide detail into the degree of fracture displacement and the extent of soft tissue involvement. In addition, 3D images constructed from CT images are useful to direct presurgical planning. The qualities listed here make CT the preferred diagnostic tool in suspected fractures involving the thin bones of the orbit and midface. CT is also preferred for multitrauma patients exhibiting clinical signs of orbital involvement and when soft tissue swelling prevents adequate clinical assessment (1–4).

In the multitrauma patient, a head CT is routinely performed to screen for intracranial injury. In these patients, determining the necessity for a simultaneous facial CT can be difficult because a complete physical exam is often complicated by restrictions such as a cervical-spine collar, intubation, and intoxication (5, 6). Therefore, other indicators such as the presence of soft tissue deformities can serve to screen and determine whether a trauma patient requires both an immediate head and a face CT scan. Holmgren and colleagues established an acronym that stands for lip laceration, intraoral laceration, periorbital contusion, subconjunctival hemorrhage, and nasal laceration (LIPS-N) (5). These soft tissue injuries are highly suggestive of an underlying facial fracture.

A recent study also evaluated the ability of head CT to diagnose nonnasal bone midfacial fractures as compared with that of facial CT. The sensitivity and specificity of head CT were 90% (95% CI = 79%–96%) and 95% (95% CI = 84%–99%), respectively; the positive and negative predictive values were 96% (95% CI = 86%–99%) and 89% (95% CI = 76%–95%), respectively. The rate of accuracy was 92% (7).

This chapter focuses on fractures involving the midface and mandible. A brief overview of the methods for obtaining CT images of the face and the facial buttress system of analysis

is provided, and the four main categories of midfacial fractures are presented in separate sections: 1) orbital blowout, 2) zygoma, 3) maxilla, and 4) mandible. Each section consists of general guidelines for the indications and pertinent findings for each type of facial fracture. At the end of the chapter, facial CT images are included to demonstrate the important pathological findings.

Methods for obtaining facial CT images

The technique consists of obtaining noncontrast axial slices 5 mm apart originating from the hard palate to the posterior fossa, followed by contiguous 100-mm axial slices from the hard palate to the skull vertex. The coronal plane is 90 degrees, and the axial plane is 0 degrees from the orbitomeatal line (8). Optimal visualization occurs when a structure is perpendicular to the imaging plane; structures parallel to the imaging plane are not well visualized. The coronal plane detects horizontally directed fractures and long vertical segments. Images in both planes should be viewed in soft-tissue and bony-window settings. The lung-window setting can also be used to distinguish orbital emphysema from fat and some wooden foreign bodies from air (8).

After the patient is stabilized, a more detailed CT exam can be performed to look specifically for facial trauma, or a facial CT can be ordered simultaneously. Facial images are obtained in the axial and coronal planes from the skull base to the clavicles in sequential 2- to 3-mm slices. A small field of view of 5 × 5 mm is used for face evaluation, as opposed to the 10 × 10 mm used in brain scanning, to allow for appreciation of the small facial bones in finer detail; however, the slices are still large enough to permit adequate visualization of the mandibular condyles.

A computed tomographic scan (1- to 2-mm axial slices) from the menton to the vertex with or without 3D reconstruction is the criterion standard for evaluation of facial fractures (9).

Structures such as the orbit, pterygoid plates, nasal septum, and mandibular rami are viewed well in the coronal plane. Optimal coronal imaging requires the patient to hyperextend the neck; if this is not possible, images of the coronal plane can be obtained by reformatting axial images. Images in the axial plane are useful in evaluating the zygomatic arch, posterior walls of the maxillary and frontal sinuses, and degree of posterior displacement in Le Fort fractures and the zygomaticomaxillary complex (ZMC) fractures (4, 8).

Analysis of CT facial anatomy

Gentry and colleagues developed the facial buttress system of facial analysis by observing normal facial anatomy on cadavers using CT (10). Interconnected bony buttresses are oriented in the horizontal, sagittal, and coronal planes to allow for sequential comprehensive evaluation of the face. Three horizontal, two coronal, and five sagittally oriented struts are typically described. Vertical reinforcement consists of the nasomaxillary, zygomaticomaxillary, and pterygomaxillary pillars. Horizontal reinforcement consists of the mandibulosymphyseal arch, palatoalveolar complex, and infraorbital and supraorbital buttresses. The buttress system provides for methodological examination of the face, but description of a facial fracture is still based on identifying the actual anatomical structures involved (2, 4, 10).

Orbital blowout fractures

Indications

In-depth scrutiny of orbital structures must be performed for a patient with suspected facial trauma. The orbit is involved in most types of facial fractures, with the exception of isolated nasal, mandibular, zygomatic arch, maxillary fractures, and the Le Fort I fracture (8). The orbital blowout type of fracture is discussed in more detail within this section. Orbital blowout describes fracture of the orbital floor with bone fragments displaced away from the orbit (11). A key diagnostic distinction with regard to blowout fractures is the integrity of the infraorbital rim. By definition, the orbital rim is intact with blowout fractures (12).

This type of fracture represents 3% of all craniofacial traumas (13). There are two types of blowout fracture: inferior blowout and medial blowout. The inferior blowout consists of fracture involving the middle horizontal strut and is the third most common isolated type of midfacial fracture (3). The isolated medial blowout fracture involves trauma to the parasagittal strut of the orbit (8). In mechanical engineering, a strut describes a structural component that is designed to resist longitudinal compressions.

Table 31.1 describes the three classically proposed mechanisms to cause orbital blowout: hydraulic, globe-to-wall theory, and buckle mechanism (14). All three of these mechanisms have been shown to cause orbital blowout fractures, and some are mutually exclusive (11, 14).

Emergent assessment of visual acuity and extraocular motility must be performed in these patients. The key clinical findings of an orbital blowout fracture include enophthalmos, decreased ocular movement during upward gaze, diplopia, and hypoesthesia or anesthesia in the distribution of the infraorbital nerve. These findings may not be apparent on physical examination due to periorbital swelling or unconsciousness. For the inferior blowout fracture, 10% to 20% are accompanied by entrapment of inferior rectus muscle (8). Pure medial blowout fractures usually do not cause entrapment because a minimal amount of bone is displaced (15).

Table 31.1: Three theories proposed to explain the mechanical mechanism of a blowout fracture

• Hydraulic theory	Increased orbital soft tissue pressure results in fracture of the thin-walled orbital floor and/or medial wall.
• Globe-to-wall contact theory	An external force delivered to the globe pushes it backwards into the orbit. The globe strikes and fractures the orbital walls.
• Bone conduction theory, or "buckle theory"	A force is delivered to the orbital rim and causes "buckling" of the rim, which then causes a fracture to the orbital walls.

Modified from He D, Blomquist PH, Ellis E III: Association between ocular injuries and internal orbital fractures. *J Oral Maxillofac Surg* 2007;65:713–20.

Diagnostic capabilities

CT is the first-line imaging modality in orbital trauma assessment to assess for both bone fracture and soft tissue injury. The orbits are best viewed in the coronal plane because this orientation provides detailed information about the patency of the medial wall and orbital floor, and visualization of the superior and inferior rectus muscles, optic nerves, paranasal sinuses, and cribriform plate (3, 16, 17). Entrapment is seen with small, narrow fractures, where the muscle can be immobilized in the fracture and is seen on CT scan as an abrupt kink in the muscle (12). If a foreign body is suspected, CT also allows for localization within the globe and orbit (16, 18). The findings indicative of an inferior orbital blowout fracture on CT include displaced bony fragments and a soft tissue mass displaced into the adjacent sinus (8, 17). For medial blowout fracture, herniation of orbital contents toward the ethmoid sinus can be seen as well as swelling and deviation of the medial rectus muscle (19). Lee and colleagues found that CT played a major role in determining the cause of decreased vision seen in patients with blowout fractures that can be attributed to globe rupture, retrobulbar hemorrhage, optic nerve edema and impingement, and intraorbital emphysema (16).

Imaging pitfalls and limitations

One major limitation is that axial images may need to be reformatted into the coronal orientation because a direct coronal scan is sometimes unobtainable in young children and in patients with head injury or limited neck mobility (16). Another limitation is that MRI is superior to CT in characterization of orbital soft tissue injuries, despite its lower sensitivity in bone disruption detection (16). Advantages of multiplanar imaging, ability to differentiate edema from hemorrhage, and greater soft tissue visualization make MRI superior to CT in characterization of orbital soft tissue injuries (16). MRI is especially useful in evaluating the presence of an intraocular hematoma because it is able to detect choroidal retinal and posterior hyaloid detachments (7). The third limitation is that, although CT is the main modality of choice to identify and localize foreign bodies within the globe, studies have shown that certain materials such as metal are easier to identify. Myllylä and colleagues found that wood is sometimes mistaken for gas bubbles on CT (18).

Figures 31.1 to 31.6 at the end of this chapter are CT images of trauma to the orbit.

Zygoma

Indications

The zygoma is the second most common fractured midfacial bone after the nasal bones and represents 13% of all craniofacial fractures (13). The body of the zygoma is usually spared in facial trauma. Most fractures involving the zygoma occur within areas of articulation with other facial bones. Fractures of the zygoma are grouped into two categories: isolated arch fractures and zygomaticomaxillary complex (ZMC) fractures. Zingg and colleagues provided a classification scheme for zygomatic fractures (20). The ZMC fracture is the most common type of zygomatic fracture, accounting for 40% of all midfacial fractures. ZMC fractures are the result of a direct blow to the malar eminence (21). The principal lines of fracture involve the orbital, zygomatic, and maxillary processes of the zygoma (1, 8). Displaced ZMC fractures are associated with fracture of the pterygoid process of the sphenoid bone. Clinically, suspicion for a fracture involving multiple articulations of the zygoma should be suspected in a patient who had direct force to the malar eminence. The fracture may present with edema and ecchymosis involving the cheek and lower eyelid, with flattening of the malar eminence (1, 4, 8). A fracture to the zygoma may also be felt during palpation of the infraorbital margin and intraorally in the buccal mucosa (1, 4, 8). Fractures limited to the zygomatic arch account for 10% of all midfacial fractures (13). Zygomatic arch fractures are usually due to impact from a horizontal force applied to the side of the face. Palpation reveals flatness localized to the lateral area of the cheek, and patients are unable to open their mouths due to impingement of the zygomatic arch fragment on the coronoid process of the mandible or the temporalis muscle (1, 8).

Diagnostic capabilities

Although fractures of the zygoma are adequately visualized on plain film, CT still offers the advantage of demonstrating the degree of fracture segment displacement (3). ZMC fractures are graded based on magnitude of displacement and degree of rotation of the disconnected fragment. The simple ZMC fracture is minimally displaced, whereas the complex ZMC fracture is severely comminuted or displaced (8). CT reveals the fracture lines and identifies the degree of rotation and displacement of fractured segments (8). This is especially important for treatment because repair of the ZMC fracture requires evaluation of the fractured segment in relation to the cranial base posteriorly and the midface anteriorly. ZMC and zygomatic arch fractures are best appreciated in the coronal orientation. The axial orientation does not allow for adequate visualization of the zygomatic arch (8).

Imaging pitfalls and limitations

A ZMC fracture may be accompanied by fracture of the ipsilateral greater sphenoid wing and may raise earliest consideration of a clinically silent epidural hematoma due to close relation with the middle meningeal artery. Therefore, CT imaging of the head and face must be obtained in both the coronal and axial orientations (3, 4, 8). Figures 31.7 to 31.11 at the end of this chapter are CT images of trauma to the zygoma.

Maxilla

Fractures to the maxilla occur unilaterally or bilaterally. Isolated unilateral fractures are uncommon (4). Isolated fractures occur as an isolated injury to the anterior wall of the maxillary sinus or to one side of the maxillary alveolar ridge. Bilateral fractures involving the maxilla are more severe and fall either into the Le Fort categorization or under "smash fracture" (20, 22). The Le Fort fractures may be found in isolation but are more commonly associated with other fractures such as orbital blowout, ZMC, and mandibular fractures (20, 22). The Le Fort injuries share common clinical and radiographic features (20, 23). The facial skeleton is severely disrupted, resulting in bilateral soft tissue swelling clinically. All types of Le Fort fractures result in instability and dissociation of a portion of the midface from the cranium due to involvement of the pterygoid processes. The posterior wall of the maxillary sinuses, formed by the pterygoid plates, is also fractured in each of the three Le Fort fractures. All Le Fort fractures also result in malocclusion of the maxilla and mandible (20, 23).

Indications

Le Fort I is a bilateral transmaxillary fracture that results in dislocation of the tooth-baring portion of the maxilla from the rest of the face. The physical findings associated with a Le Fort I fracture include facial edema and mobility of the hard palate. The palate is dislocated in a posterior or lateral direction, causing malocclusion and a floating palate. Grasping and pushing in and out on the incisors assesses the mobility of the hard palate (4, 8, 22).

Le Fort II is a pyramidal-shaped fracture that creates a separation of the maxilla and nasal skeleton from the remainder of the midface. The fracture extends posteriorly to the pterygoid plates at the base of the skull. On physical exam, a patient with a Le Fort II injury will have marked facial edema, with an abnormally increased distance between the medial canthi of the eye, bilateral subconjunctival

441

hemorrhages, and mobility of the maxilla. Epistaxis or cerebrospinal fluid rhinorrhea may also be present (3, 4, 8).

Le Fort III represents the most severe form of the Le Fort fractures, resulting in complete disassociation of the facial skeleton and zygoma from the cranium. Clinical evaluation of the patient is difficult due to the large extent of damage to the midfacial skeleton and overlying soft tissue (3, 4, 8).

Please refer to Figure 31.24, which is a schematic diagram that illustrates the three Le Fort classifications.

Diagnostic capabilities

Le Fort I

Coronal CT will show a fracture line of the zygomaticoalveolar arch and the piriform sinus (1). Coronal CT is the best orientation because horizontal fractures involving the sagittal buttresses can be observed (8). Dental root fractures are also appreciated on coronal CT (8).

Le Fort II

On CT, fracture lines along the nasal bones, inferomedial orbital rims, and posterolateral maxillary walls are appreciated on both axial and coronal CT images (8).

Le Fort III

Images obtained in both the coronal and axial orientations adequately visualize the fractured segments (4, 8).

Imaging pitfalls and limitations

Le Fort I

Axial CT may not adequately detect fracture unless the bones are comminuted or displaced (8). Axial sectioning is able to detect fractures of the maxillary wall and hard palate in this type of fracture.

Le Fort II and III

The proximity to the infraorbital foramen causes the Le Fort II fractures to have the highest incidence of infraorbital nerve damage. The Le Fort II fracture is also commonly associated with a ZMC fracture on the side of facial impaction, with the shared fractures being those of the anterolateral wall of the maxilla and inferior orbital rim and floor. Due to the extent of fracture, hyperextension of the neck may not be possible, resulting in reconstruction of coronal images from images taken in the axial orientation. Le Fort II and III fractures involve the base of the skull and have the potential for more severe neurosurgical complications. These fractures also have the potential of more severe ophthalmic trauma due to involvement of the orbit (1, 4, 8).

Le Fort III

CT images must be scrutinized for potential optic canal, cribriform plate, and ethmoid roof involvement.

Concomitant head CT should also be ordered to rule out injury to the brain (1, 4, 8).

Mandible

Indications

The anatomy of the mandible consists of a U-shaped body and two rami. The U shape of the mandible results in fractures that are bilateral, occurring at the site of impact and at a contralateral site due to dissipation of the impact force.

However, a recent study showed unifocal mandible fractures occur with greater frequency than anticipated by most radiologists. Of all 102 eligible patients, 43 fractures were unifocal (42%; 95% CI, 33%–52%) and 59 were multifocal (58%). The angle was the most frequently involved site, and many of these fractures involved the sockets of the posterior molars (Fig. 31.22. The body was the next most frequent site (24). Panoramic x-ray views and plain films provide adequate visualization of isolated mandibular injuries.

The incidence of unifocal fractures in a recent study was concordant with the existing plain film, panoramic tomography, and mixed-technique literature, despite the assumed higher sensitivity of CT that might be expected to yield a lower incidence of unifocal fractures (24).

The use of CT to identify isolated mandibular fractures has been increasing (1). Traditionally, however, CT is used only if the patient is undergoing evaluation for intracranial or other types of facial trauma because this type of fracture is well visualized on plain film radiography (21).

Diagnostic capabilities

Nondisplaced symphyseal fractures are better viewed using CT because the problem of overlapping spine lucency on plain film is not an issue when using CT. Restricted mouth opening also inhibits adequate visualization on plain film posteroanterior view. CT is helpful in this situation and also allows for reconstruction along the alveolar ridge to enable acquisition of images similar to those seen in panoramic radiographs (1).

On plain film, condylar fractures are the easiest to overlook. In a comparison of CT and panoramic radiographs conducted in 37 children between 2 and 15 years of age, CT provided consistently greater accuracy (90% vs. 73%) and sensitivity (87% vs. 77%) than panoramic photographs. Condylar fractures may be intracapsular or extracapsular. CT is able to precisely identify a condylar fracture and its degree of dislocation (1).

Imaging pitfalls and limitations

In rare occasions, a force directed to the symphysis can posteriorly displace the condyles into the external auditory canal or through the mandibular fossa into the middle cranial fossa superiorly (1). These types of fractures are best detected with CT, and head CT imaging should also be obtained.

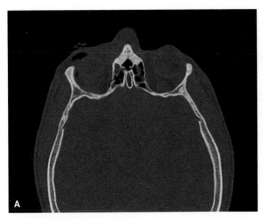 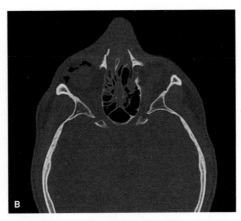

Figure 31.1. A and B: These two images taken from a series depict a multiple comminuted and minimally displaced fracture that involves the roof, floor, and medial wall of the right orbit. Soft tissue swelling with air and deformity of the periorbital and supraorbital regions of the right is also present in both pictures. Additionally, in B, a comminuted fracture of the nasal bones causes mild displacement of the nasal septum.

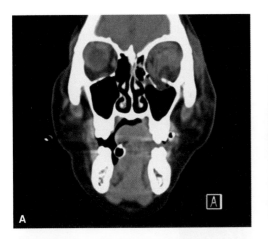 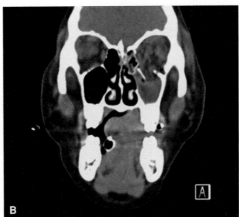

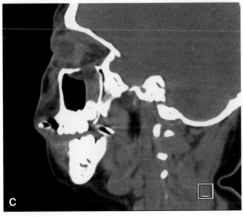

Figure 31.2. A and B: Images that depict approximately 1 cm herniation of orbital contents through a large defect in the inferior wall of the left orbit. The contents that are herniated include the inferior rectus and, to a lesser extent, the medial rectus muscle. C: A sagittal view that shows formation of an extensive retrobulbar hematoma and orbital contents within the left maxillary sinus.

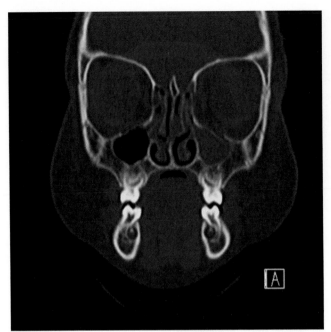

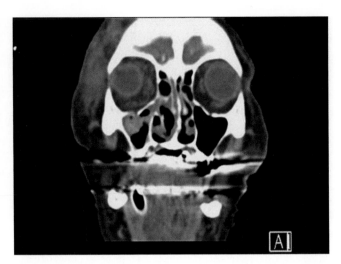

Figure 31.4. This image shows a displaced fracture within the right orbital floor. Blood is also present within the right maxillary sinus.

Figure 31.3. Left orbital blowout fracture through the inferior wall. Herniation of fat through the defect has occurred.

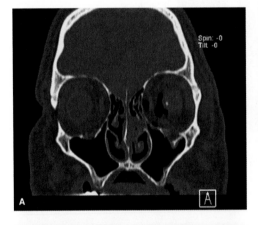

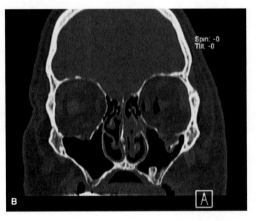

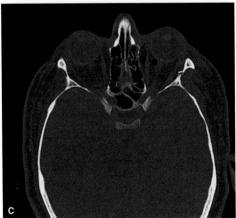

Figure 31.5. These images are from a series depicting bilateral orbital blowout. A and B: Coronal images that show a comminuted fracture of the left lateral orbital wall with mild medial displacement and a fracture of the left orbital floor. Intraorbital fat without extraocular muscle herniation has occurred through the defect as well as displacement of the fracture fragment. Left intraconal and extraconal air is also seen without deformity of the left globe. Injury is also accompanied by soft tissue swelling within the left periorbital region. The right globe also shows fracture with herniation of intraorbital fat through the defect. C: An image taken within the same series that shows left intraconal and extraconal air and fracture of the left lateral orbital wall depicted in the axial view.

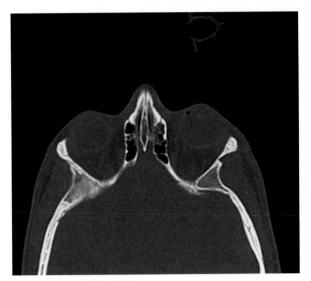

Figure 31.6. This image shows a 1 mm radiopaque foreign body next to air under the medial left eyelid. The orbit is intact.

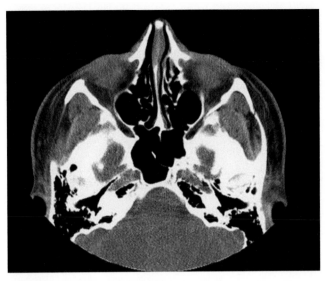

Figure 31.7. Fracture of the left temporozygomatic suture.

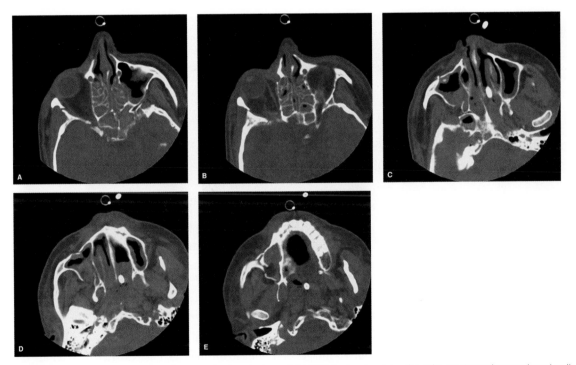

Figure 31.8. A–E: These images are from a series that depicts a right ZMC fracture involving the right anterior and posterolateral wall of the right zygoma.

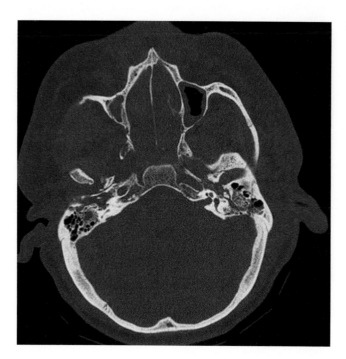

Figure 31.9. This image depicts fracture of the left zygomatic arch.

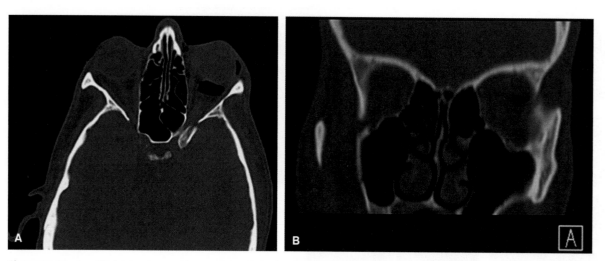

Figure 31.10. A and B: Axial and coronal images, respectively, that depict multiple fractures to the left zygomatic arch and fracture to the temporal processes with accompanied displacement. The fracture to the anterior portion of the arch is nondisplaced, whereas the fracture to the temporal process is displaced approximately by 5 mm.

Internal derangement or ligamentous or capsular injury to the temporomandibular joints may occur, but without a malalignment of the mandibular condyle within the condylar fossa, CT would be insensitive to this. MR imaging could potentially reveal injuries such as these (24).

Figures 31.12 to 31.19 at the end of this chapter are CT images of trauma to the maxilla. Figures 31.20 to 31.21 are CT images corresponding to smash fractures. Figures 31.22 to 31.23 are CT images of trauma to the mandible.

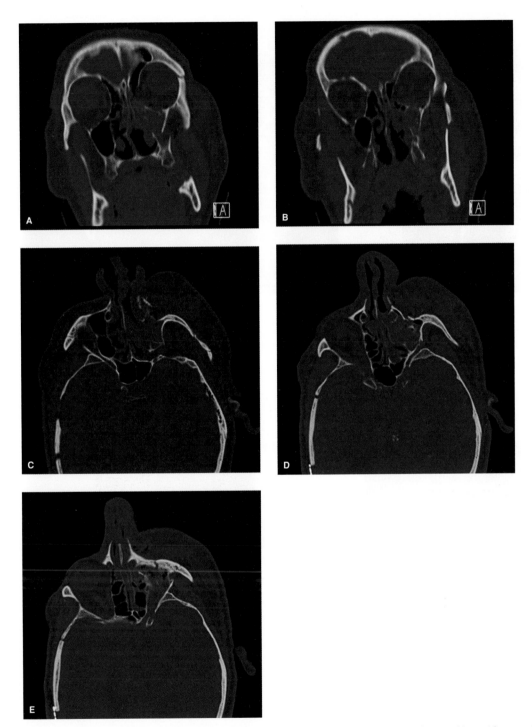

Figure 31.11. These images depict a left ZMC fracture and fracture of the left zygomatic arch. There is additional fracture of the inferior orbital rim and diastasis and angulation at the frontozygomatic suture. Figure A is a coronal section that shows fracture of the left ZMC as well as comminuted fractures through the medial, lateral, and anterior walls of the left maxillary sinus. Figure B is a coronal section that shows fracture has also occurred to the inferior orbital rim. Figures C, D, and E are images in the axial plane that depict fracture to the left ZMC and left zygomatic arch. Diastasis and angulation at the frontozygomatic suture is also seen in images C, D, and E.

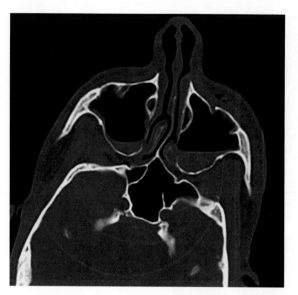

Figure 31.12. Axial depiction of a minimally displaced fracture of the left maxillary sinus anterior wall with associated soft tissue swelling and subcutaneous emphysema. The patient also has sinus mucosal disease, which is seen by bilateral air fluid levels within the maxillary sinus and minimal mucosal thickening.

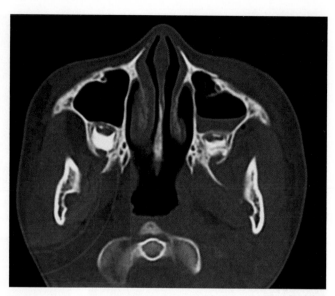

Figure 31.13. This axial image shows fracture to the anterior wall of the left maxillary sinus. There is also mild right maxillary sinus mucosal thickening, which indicates a nontraumatic chronic inflammatory process.

Figure 31.14. Axial image that depicts fracture of the lateral wall of the right maxillary sinus.

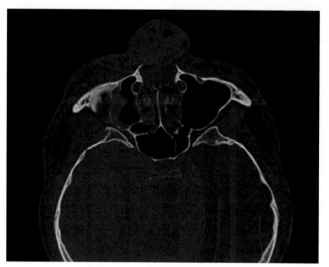

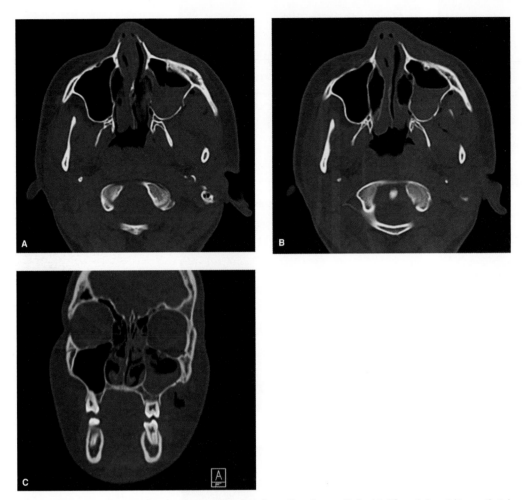

Figure 31.15. Part of a series that depicts fracture to the left maxillary sinus and left orbital floor. A: An axial image that shows fracture to the lateral wall of the left maxillary sinus as well as bilateral fracture of the nasal bones. B: An axial image that better depicts fracture of both the lateral and medial wall of the left maxillary sinus. C: A coronal image that shows fracture of the medial and lateral wall of the left maxillary sinus. This image also shows that there is a minimally displaced fracture of the left orbital floor with a small amount of fat protruding through the defect.

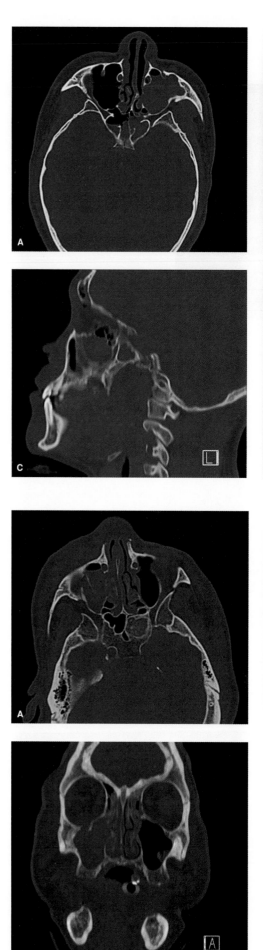

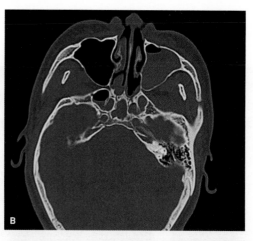

Figure 31.16. These images depict an obliquely oriented fracture through the anterior wall of the left maxillary sinus. The inferior component of this fracture involves the lateral wall of the maxillary antrum and the superior component involves the inferior orbital rim. Figures A and B are axial images, whereas C and D are sagittal images reconstructed from the axial plane.

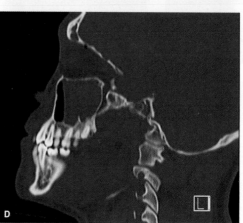

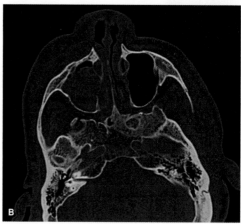

Figure 31.17. This series depicts fracture to the right maxillary sinus and right orbital blowout fracture. A and B: Axial images that depict a fracture of the medial wall of the right maxillary sinus. The right maxillary sinus is filled with hemorrhage. C: A reformatted coronal image that shows right orbital blowout fracture with the defect occurring in the orbital floor. The fracture fragment of the floor of the right orbit is associated with a small hematoma that protrudes superiorly into the inferior portion of the right orbit that is next to the right inferior rectus muscle. There is no evidence of extraocular muscle entrapment through the defect, and the orbital globe is still intact. The right orbital blowout fracture is accompanied by significant soft tissue swelling around the right periorbital region with mild proptosis.

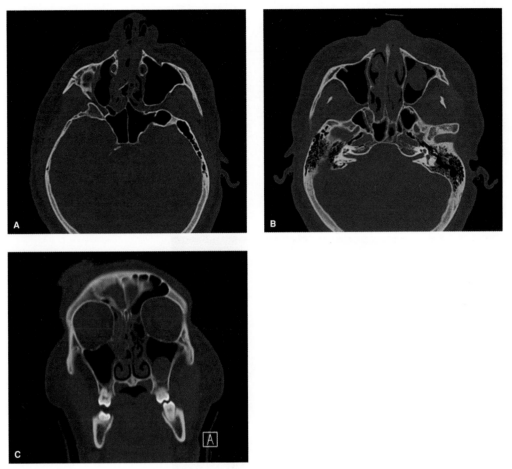

Figure 31.18. Figure A is an axial image depicting fracture of the nasal process of the right maxillary bone. Figure B is an axial image, and C is a coronal image of a retention cyst consistent with mucosal sinus disease that is present within the left maxillary antrum, which should not be confused with hemorrhage or a hematoma.

Figure 31.19. This image shows a comminuted fracture of the anterior wall and lateral wall of the right maxillary sinus. There is also a minimally displaced fracture of the zygomatic process of the right maxilla.

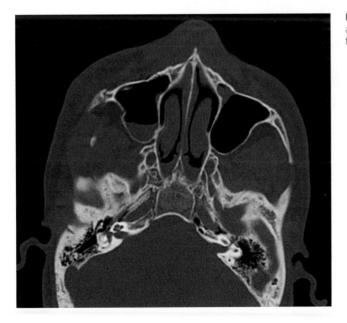

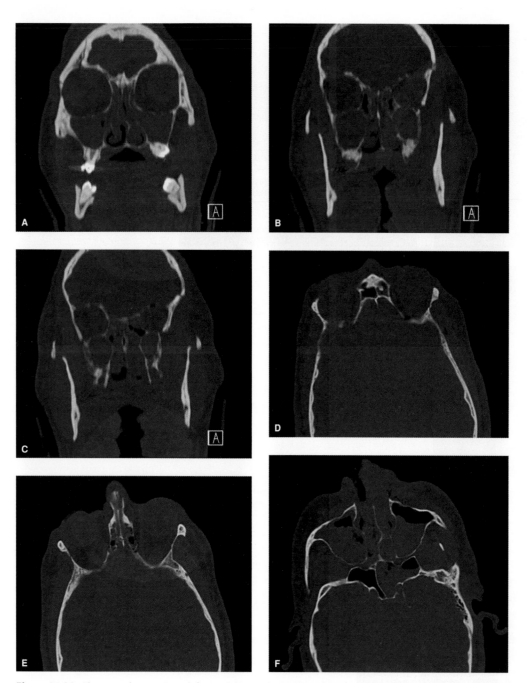

Figure 31.20. This series depicts a "smash fracture" that involves multiple facial fractures. The fractures sustained by this patient include: 1. fracture of right lateral orbital wall; 2. fracture of right inferior orbital rim; 3. fracture of left nasal bone and nasal process of left maxilla; 4. fracture of lateral wall of left orbit; 5. fracture of medial walls of maxillary sinuses bilaterally; 6. diastasis of left frontozygomatic suture with 2 mm depression of zygoma into anterior cranial fossa; 7. fracture of the right frontal bone with extension to the superior rim of right orbit.

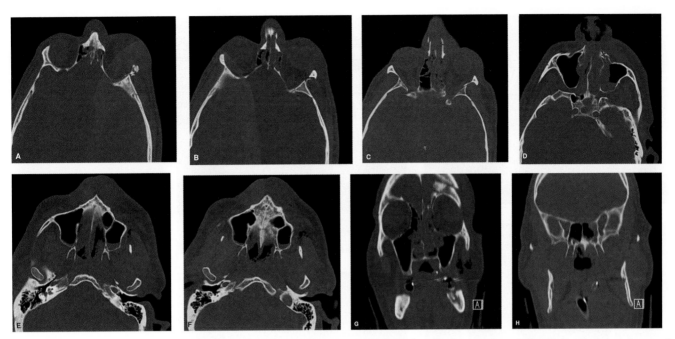

Figure 31.21. Smash fracture series depicting multiple facial fractures in the coronal and axial plane. The fractures shown in these images include: 1. fracture of the lateral orbital rim, lateral orbital wall, inferior orbital rim, and probably orbital floor on the left; 2. left orbital emphysema without evidence of herniation of orbital contents; 3. multiple fracture of the left lamina papyracea with associated swelling of the left medial rectus muscle, suggesting an intramuscular hematoma; 4. comminuted fracture of the anterior maxillary wall, nasal process of the left maxillary bone, and fractures of the lateral and posterolateral walls of the left maxillary sinus with associated hemorrhage within the sinus; 5. bilateral nasal bone fractures and fracture of the nasal septum.

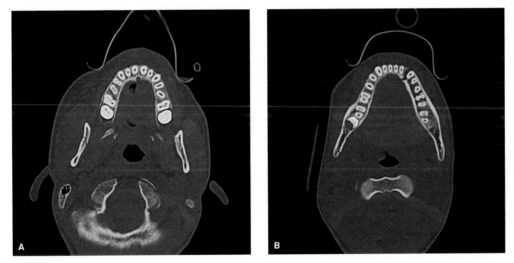

Figure 31.22. These axial images depict fracture to the mandible. Figure A shows fracture to the right mandibular ramus. Figure B shows fracture to the left parasymphyseal mandible.

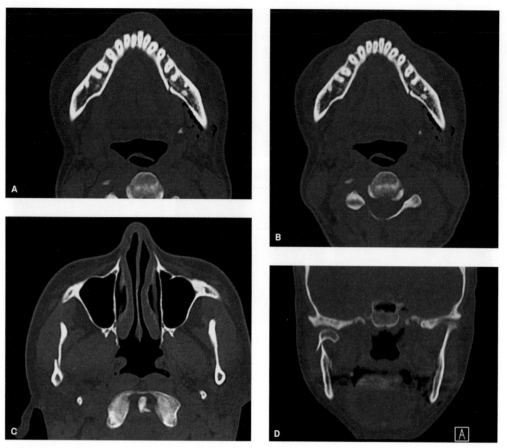

Figure 31.23. These axial and coronal images depict fracture of the right mandibular condyle and fracture of the left body of the mandible. Figures A and B are axial images that show fracture to the left body of the mandible that is minimally displaced. There is also extensive soft tissue air deep to the left mandibular angle within the region of the left submandibular gland. Figure C is an axial image, and Figure D is a coronal image that shows fracture of the right mandibular condyle has resulted in dislocation of the right temporomandibular joint anteriorly.

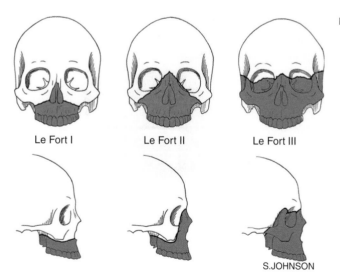

Figure 31.24. Schematic diagram illustrating the three Le Fort classifications.

References

1. Schuknecht B, Graetz K: Radiologic assessment of maxillofacial, mandibular, and skull base trauma. *Eur Radiol* 2005;**15**:560–8.

2. Kassel EE, Cooper PW, Rubernstein JD: Radiologic studies of facial trauma associated with a regional trauma centre. *J Can Assoc Radiol* 1983;**34**:178–88.

3. Russell J, Davidson M, Daly B, Corrigan AM: Computed tomography in the diagnosis of maxillofacial trauma. *Br J Oral Maxillofac Surg* 1990;**28**:287–91.

4. Salvolini U: Traumatic injuries: imaging of facial injuries. *Eur Radiol* 2002;**12**:1253–61.

5. Holmgren EP, Dierks EJ, Assael LA, et al.: Facial soft tissue injuries as an aid to ordering a combination head and facial computed tomography in trauma patients. *J Oral Maxillofac Surg* 2005;**63**:651–4.

6. Holmgren EP, Dierks EJ, Homer LD, Potter BE: Facial computed tomography use in trauma patients who require a head computed tomogram. *J Oral Maxillofac Surg* 2004;**62**: 913–8.

7. Marinaro J, Crandall CS, Doezema D: Computed tomography of the head as a screening examination for facial fractures. *Am J Emerg Med* 2007;**25**(6):616–9.

8. Laine FJ, Conway WF, Laskin DM: Radiology of maxillofacial trauma. *Curr Probl Diagn Radiol* 1993;**22**:145–88.

9. Ellstrom CL, Evans GR: Evidence-based medicine: zygoma fractures. *Plast Reconstr Surg* 2013 Dec;**132**(6):1649–57.

10. Gentry LR, Manor WF, Turski PA, Strother CM: High-resolution CT analysis of facial struts in trauma: 1. Normal anatomy. *AJR Am J Roentgenol* 1983;**140**:523–32.

11. Bullock JD, Warwar RE, Ballal DR, Ballal RD: Mechanisms of orbital floor fractures: a clinical, experimental, and theoretical study. *Trans Am Ophthalmol Soc* 1999;**97**:87–110.

12. Avery LL, Susarla SM, Novelline RA: Multidetector and three-dimensional CT evaluation of the patient with maxillofacial injury. *Radiol Clin North Am* 2011 Jan;**49**(1):183–203.

13. Hussain K, Wijetunge DB, Grubnic S, Jackson IT: A comprehensive analysis of craniofacial trauma. *J Trauma* 1994;**36**:34–47.

14. He D, Blomquist PH, Ellis E III: Association between ocular injuries and internal orbital fractures. *J Oral Maxillofac Surg* 2007;**65**:713–20.

15. Jank S, Schuchter B, Emshoff R, et al.: Clinical signs of orbital wall fractures as a function of anatomic location. *Oral Surg Oral Med Oral Pathol Oral Radiol Endod* 2003;**96**:149–53.

16. Lee HJ, Mohamed J, Frohman L, Baker S: CT of orbital trauma. *Emerg Radiol* 2004;**10**:168–72.

17. Ng P, Chu C, Young N, Soo M: Imaging of orbital floor fractures. *Australas Radiol* 1996;**40**:264–8.

18. Myllylä V, Pyhtinen J, Päivänsalo M, et al.: CT detection and location of intraorbital foreign bodies: experiments with wood and glass. *Rofo* 1987;**146**:639–43.

19. Tanaka T, Morimoto Y, Kito S, et al.: Evaluation of coronal CT findings of rare cases of isolated medial orbital wall blow-out fractures. *Dentomaxillofac Radiol* 2003;**32**:300–3.

20. Zingg M, Laedrach K, Chen J, et al.: Classification and treatment of zygomatic fractures: a review of 1,025 cases. *J Oral Maxillofac Surg* 1992;**50**:778–90.

21. Newman J: Medical imaging of facial and mandibular fractures. *Radiol Technol* 1998;**69**:417–35.

22. Bagheri SC, Holmgren E, Kademani D, et al.: Comparison of the severity of bilateral Le Fort injuries in isolated midface trauma. *J Oral Maxillofac Surg* 2005;**63**:1123–9.

23. Le Fort R: Etude experimentale sur les fractures de la machoire superieure. *Rev Chir Paris* 1901;**23**:208–27.

24. Escott EJ, Branstetter BF: Incidence and characterization of unifocal mandible fractures on CT. *AJNR Am J Neuroradiol* 2008 May;**29**(5):890–4.

Chapter 32

CT of the Chest

Jonathan Patane and Megan Boysen-Osborn

Indications

CT of the chest accounts for approximately 6% to 13% of CT scans ordered in the ED (1, 2). The most common indications for thoracic CT in the ED are the suspicion of pulmonary embolism (PE) or aortic dissection (AD) and the evaluation of trauma (3). CT angiography for the diagnosis of PE and AD are discussed in Chapter 34. Thus, the majority of this chapter will focus on trauma and other indications for CT chest.

Supine chest radiography is the accepted initial imaging modality in the evaluation of chest trauma (4–6). Chest radiographs are able to diagnose or suggest many traumatic injuries, including pneumothorax, hemothorax, diaphragmatic rupture, flail chest, pulmonary contusion, pneumopericardium, and pneumo- and hemomediastinum (7).

Computed tomography has superior sensitivity for detecting intrathoracic pathology after trauma (7–9). Many physicians include a chest CT with the initial imaging of trauma patients (7, 10–12). CT detects many injuries that may be missed on chest radiographs (13). Chest CT is extremely useful in the assessment of injuries to the aorta, chest wall, lung parenchyma, airway, pleura, and diaphragm (5).

While chest CT has a high sensitivity for detecting intrathoracic injuries, unnecessary chest CT may expose the patient to ionizing radiation, possible adverse reactions to contrast, and delays in patient care (6). A standardized protocol, such as the NEXUS chest decision instrument, may reduce the use of unnecessary thoracic CT in blunt trauma (4). The NEXUS chest decision instrument has a sensitivity of 98.8% in detecting chest injury (4).

Chest radiograph may be sufficient in the diagnosis of pneumonia. Many patients, especially immunocompromised patients, may undergo CT when there is high clinical suspicion for pneumonia in the absence of positive radiographic findings (14, 15). Pneumonia may also be discovered when CT is performed to rule out other causes of chest pain, such as pulmonary embolism (16). Chest CT may also characterize the extent of pleural effusions, empyemas, and infectious lung processes, such as tuberculosis.

Diagnostic capabilities

Helical multidetector CT (MDCT) facilitates the comprehensive acquisition of high-quality images at a rapid rate (17). The improved technology enables the expeditious assessment of critically ill patients and allows for more specialized examinations. Intravenous contrast enhancement is used in the setting of trauma, and CT angiography is employed for suspected aortic injuries. Oral contrast is sometimes indicated for the characterization of esophageal pathology.

CT is two to three times more sensitive than chest radiograph in detecting intrathoracic injuries following trauma (6). The clinical significance of this increased sensitivity is debated. Some studies indicate that patient management does not change significantly as a result of these findings (18, 19), whereas others demonstrate critical findings – such as pulmonary contusions, diaphragmatic rupture, myocardial rupture, hemothorax, pneumothorax, and aortic injuries – that are missed on radiograph (10, 13, 20). Furthermore, in patients with penetrating chest trauma, up to 12% may have delayed complications from injuries undetected on chest radiograph (21).

CT is very sensitive in detecting pleural effusions and empyema. Its sensitivity in diagnosing pneumonia, however, has been reported to be as low as 59% (22). No single CT finding is sufficient to diagnose pneumonia (22, 23).

Imaging pitfalls and limitations

Inherent in thoracic imaging is the necessity for breath holding during image acquisition; however, MDCT has minimized this limitation (17). The applications of CT continue to increase with its advancing technology. CT angiography has replaced ventilation-perfusion scans and catheter angiography for the diagnoses of pulmonary embolism and aortic dissection/transection, respectively (2). Many authors suggest CT chest should accompany CT abdomen and pelvis in the evaluation of trauma patients (10, 13), especially in patients with a rapid deceleration mechanism.

The radiation effective dose for CT chest is approximately 7 mSv (24), whereas the dose for lateral PA radiography is between 0.05 and 0.25 mSv (25). Although radiation doses less than 100 mSv may have no carcinogenic harm, many authors believe in a "linear, no threshold" theory for carcinogenic risk (2). Up to 2% of patients undergoing chest CT have undergone the same procedure at least three times in a 5-year period (2). Furthermore, when chest CT is performed in trauma patients, it typically accompanies several other studies, including CT head, cervical spine, and abdomen/pelvis. The radiation dose for these procedures is 2 mSv, 1.5 mSv, and 12 mSv, respectively (24, 26). Thus, when considering the potential carcinogenic risk, judicious use of CT should be practiced, especially in children and young adults.

Clinical images

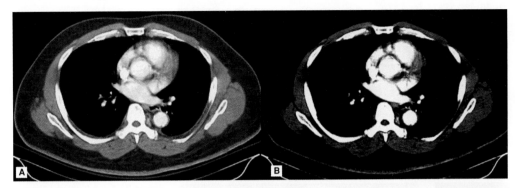

Figure 32.1. Window levels commonly employed in chest CT. A: Original window level. B: Mediastinal window. The mediastinal structures are apparent, but lung detail is poorly visualized. C: Lung window. The lung vasculature and parenchyma is better seen. D: Bone window. This window is commonly used to detect fractures and dislocations of the vertebrae, sternum, ribs, clavicles, and scapulae.

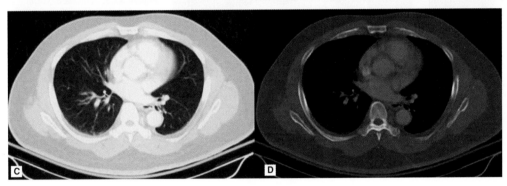

Lung parenchyma

Pulmonary contusions

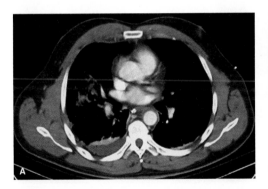
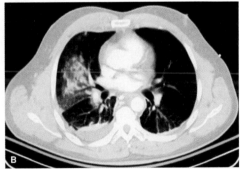

Figure 32.2. Right-sided pulmonary contusion and hemothorax on (A) original and (B) lung windows.

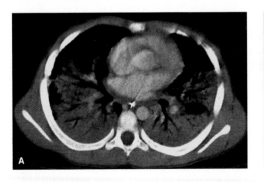
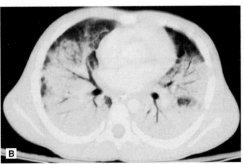

Figure 32.3. Extensive bilateral pulmonary contusions on (A) original and (B) lung windows.

457

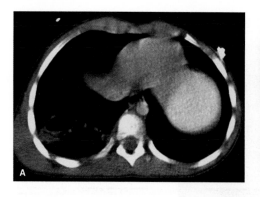
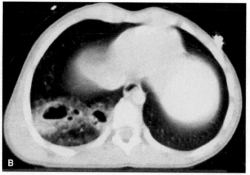

Figure 32.4. Lung laceration surrounded by contusion in original and lung windows.

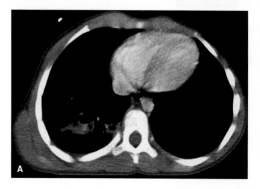
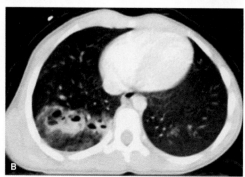

Figure 32.5. Multiple small lung lacerations creating a "Swiss cheese" appearance.

Pulmonary contusions occur when blood leaks into the alveolar and interstitial space as a result of injury to the walls of the alveoli and pulmonary vessels (27). On CT, pulmonary contusions can be unilateral or bilateral; patchy or diffuse (28); and usually peripheral, nonsegmental, and nonlobar in distribution (7). Their location generally correlates to the site of impact (29) and proximity to dense structures, such as the spine (7). They may appear similar to fat embolism; however, contusions become visible within 6 hours of the injury, whereas the appearance of fat embolisms usually takes at least 24 hours (29). In children, several air-space diseases can cause similar opacification, including aspiration, atelectasis, and infection. Subpleural sparing can usually (95%) distinguish contusions from these alternative diagnoses (30). CT is very useful in estimating the extent of contusion, which is important in predicting the degree of posttraumatic respiratory insufficiency (29). The sensitivity of CT in detecting pulmonary contusions is very high (6, 11, 13, 28, 29, 31), estimated to be 100% in one study (32).

Pulmonary lacerations

A laceration results from a ruptured alveolar wall, creating an empty space (29). They are typically ovoid radiolucencies, surrounded by a thin pseudomembrane and contused lung (28) (Fig. 32.4). Multiple small lacerations amidst pulmonary contusion create a "Swiss cheese" appearance (7) (Fig. 32.5). If hemorrhage occurs into the cavity, an air-fluid level may be present (28). If a clot forms in the laceration, it may create an air-meniscus sign (28). If the air space is filled completely with blood and is well circumscribed, it is called a "pulmonary hematoma"

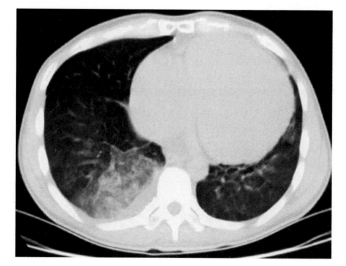

Figure 32.6. Area of right lower-lobe consolidation.

(29). CT is more sensitive than chest radiograph in detecting pulmonary lacerations (7, 28, 29). It is usually difficult to visualize lung lacerations on chest radiograph until the accompanying contusion resolves (28).

Pneumonia

Although CT is more sensitive than radiograph in detecting community-acquired pneumonia (33), CT is usually not indicated unless chest radiograph provides insufficient evidence of pneumonia in the presence of high clinical suspicion (15). The most common finding on CT is air-space consolidation

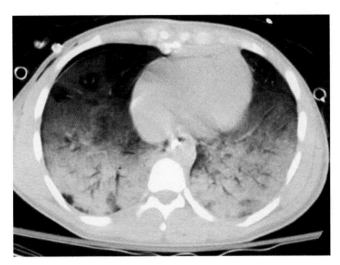

Figure 32.7. Extensive bilateral consolidation with right-sided pneumothorax.

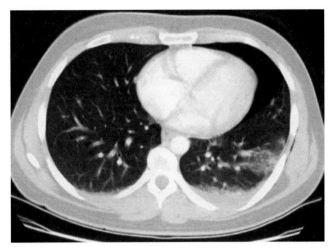

Figure 32.8. Left-sided pneumothorax.

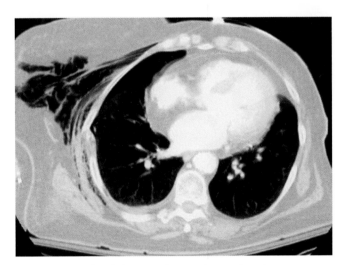

Figure 32.9. Right-sided pneumothorax with extensive subcutaneous emphysema.

(15) (Fig. 32.6). Other common findings include centrilobular nodules in viral and *Mycoplasma pneumoniae* pneumonias and ground-glass attenuation in *Pneumocystis carinii* (15). Ground-glass attenuation is otherwise rare (34).

Pleural space

Pneumothorax

Pneumothorax succeeds rib fractures as the second most common injury seen in chest trauma (31). CT is able to detect pneumothoraces missed by initial chest radiograph in 5% to 15% of trauma patients (6, 13). Most of these are small, but their detection is important. Many can progress to a tension pneumothorax, especially in patients undergoing general anesthesia or positive-pressure ventilation (27, 35).

Pleural air collects in the most nondependent part of the chest (5) (Fig. 32.8). In the upright patient, this is the apical or lateral hemithorax (28); in the supine patient, this is the anterior costophrenic sulcus (28). The pneumothorax is usually accompanied by a flattened ipsilateral diaphragm on CT. Pneumothorax may be accompanied by subcutaneous emphysema, especially in the case of chest wall injury (Fig. 32.9).

Tension pneumothorax and hydropneumothorax

The diagnosis of tension pneumothorax should be made clinically and not by CT. During this potentially life-threatening condition, air progressively accumulates in the pleural space as the result of a one-way valve mechanism, causing high intrathoracic pressures (27). The visualization of intrathoracic air accompanied by a shift of the mediastinum to the contralateral side (27, 28) helps make the diagnosis on CT (Figs. 32.10 and 32.11). CT and radiograph may also demonstrate a flattened or inverted ipsilateral diaphragm (27, 28).

Hemothorax and traumatic effusions

Posttraumatic effusions are usually hemothoraces (28). While arterial bleeds progress over time and may cause mediastinal shift, venous bleeds tend to self-terminate (27). Other etiologies of traumatic effusions include chylothorax, symptomatic serous pleural effusion, or, rarely, bilious effusions or urinothorax (27, 28). MDCT attenuation differentiates hemothorax (35–70 Hounsfield units [HU]) (21, 27) from serous effusions (<15 HU) (27). Chylothorax typically has low or negative fluid attenuation values (21). MDCT is not very useful in distinguishing among bilious, chylous, serous, and urinary effusions (27). Hemothoraces visible only on CT may not need to be evacuated (31).

Transudates, exudates, and empyemas

In the nontraumatic setting, pleural effusions are classified as transudates or exudates. Transudates are usually secondary to

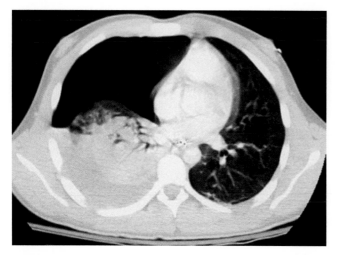

Figure 32.10. Right-sided tension hydropneumothorax.

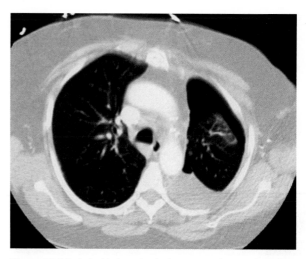

Figure 32.11. Left-sided tension hydropneumothorax.

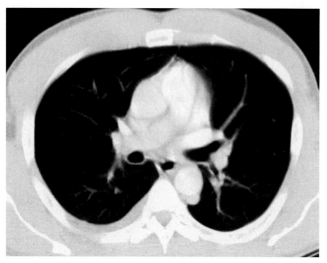

Figure 32.12. Small right-sided hemothorax.

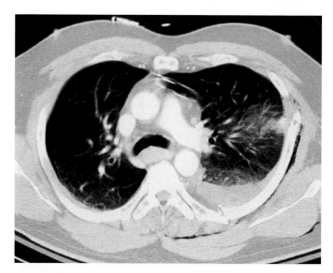

Figure 32.13. Large left-sided hemothorax with lung contusion, posterior rib fracture, and pneumothorax.

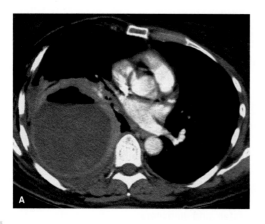

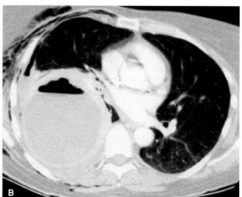

Figure 32.14. Original (A) and lung (B) windows. Large empyema with an air-fluid level.

congestive heart failure, and exudates are usually due to inflammatory or neoplastic processes (36). Although the criterion reference for distinguishing these entities is diagnostic thoracocentesis, several studies suggest that contrast-enhanced CT can help differentiate between them (36–38). Factors associated with exudates are parietal pleural thickening (≥2 mm), visceral pleural thickening, and extrapleural fat thickening (≥2 mm) (37); loculation of the effusion; or nodules in a pleural surface (36). These factors, however, are not very sensitive (36, 37). Factors associated with exudates of infectious origin are visceral pleural thickening, increased density in the extrapleural fat, and pulmonary consolidation (36). Likewise, these factors are somewhat specific (98%, 91%, and 90%, respectively) but not very sensitive (20%, 25%, and 48%, respectively) (36).

Empyemas are exudates associated with pulmonary infections; thoracocentesis demonstrates macroscopic pus, a positive culture, or positive Gram stain (36). On CT, they usually have a regularly shaped lumen and a smooth inner surface (39); an air-fluid level may be present (Fig. 32.14). As opposed to lung abscesses, empyemas have a sharply defined border separating them from lung parenchyma (39) (Fig. 32.15). Although not entirely specific, most empyemas demonstrated enhancement of the parietal pleura on contrast-enhanced CT (38).

Mediastinum

Pneumomediastinum

Pneumomediastinum can be either traumatic or spontaneous (40). Air can enter the mediastinum directly from esophageal or tracheal injuries, or it may track from ruptured alveoli through the pulmonary interstitium (the Macklin effect) (5). In addition, pneumomediastinum can be the result of neck or retroperitoneal injuries (5).

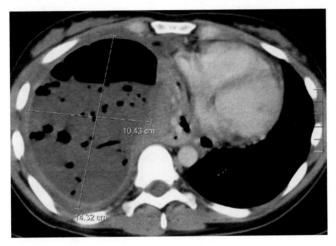

Figure 32.15. Large empyema.

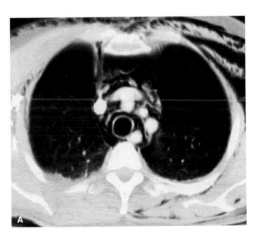

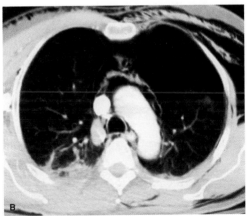

Figure 32.16. Air outlining the trachea (A) and vasculature (B).

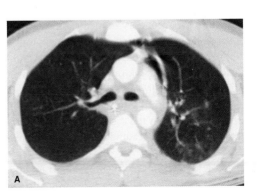

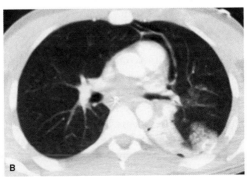

Figure 32.17. Air outlining the pericardium and parietal pleura.

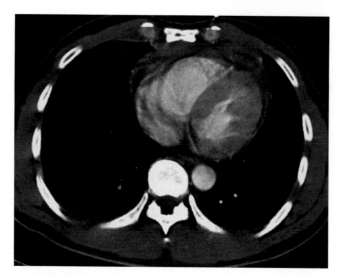

Figure 32.18. Pericardial effusion after trauma.

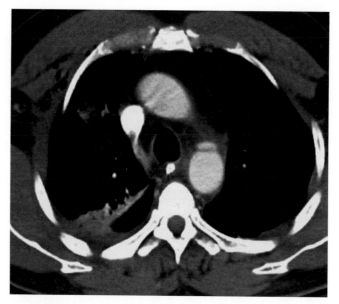

Figure 32.19. Pericardial effusion with sternal fracture.

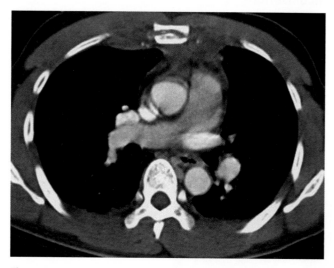

Figure 32.20. Incomplete aortic tear in a trauma patient.

Pericardial effusion

Echocardiography is the criterion reference for the diagnosis and evaluation of pericardial effusion. CT is useful when echocardiogram findings are nondiagnostic or difficult to interpret, or when a loculated or hemorrhagic effusion is present (41). In addition, pericardial effusion may be found incidentally on CT performed for trauma or chest pain.

Aortic tear

Traumatic rupture of the aorta (TRA) implies the complete transaction of the aortic wall. TRA is rarely visualized on CT because patients expire from exsanguination before reaching medical facilities. In incomplete aortic tears, the adventitia maintains the integrity of the aorta, while the intima and media may be compromised (35). In blunt injuries, the site of the injury is typically at the aortic isthmus. Survival of traumatic aortic injuries is usually less than 5% (35).

Tracheobronchial injuries

Tracheobronchial trauma can result from blunt, penetrating, or iatrogenic trauma, or from inhalation injuries (42). Bronchial fracture is more common than tracheal, and the right side is more commonly injured (29). Up to 10% of affected patients have no evidence of tracheobronchial injury on physical exam or chest radiograph (42). One small study demonstrated that, compared with chest radiograph, CT more sensitively diagnosed acute tracheobronchial tear and better identified the location of injury (43). Bronchoscopy is the preferred diagnostic modality. Signs of tracheal injury on CT include overdistension of the endotracheal cuff, lateral or posterior herniation of the endotracheal cuff, tracheal wall discontinuity, and displacement of the endotracheal tube (42–44). In cases of bronchial injury, CT may show discontinuity or enlargement of the bronchial wall, a "fallen lung" sign (collapse of the lung distal to the tear) (44), or an "air leak" (43). Accompanying signs include pneumothorax, pneumomediastinum with subcutaneous emphysema, fracture of the first three ribs (29), deep cervical emphysema, and a heightened hyoid bone above the level of the third cervical vertebrae (42).

Esophagus

Most esophageal ruptures are secondary to medical instrumentation (40). Other causes are Boerhaave syndrome, toxic ingestions and radiation, penetrating trauma, and, rarely, blunt chest trauma (41, 44, 45). Esophageal perforations usually present with pneumomediastinum and subcutaneous emphysema (40, 44). Pneumothorax, hydropneumothorax, or pleural effusion may also be apparent, especially in the case of esophagopleural fistula (40). Esophageal injury after trauma is usually associated with other injuries to the heart, great vessels, trachea, or spine (45). Although the role of CT in the diagnosis of traumatic esophageal perforations is not established, CT findings may

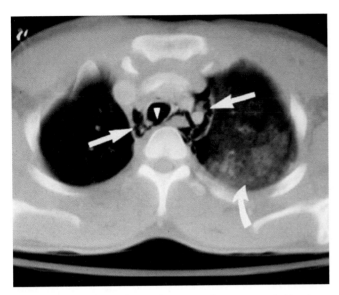

Figure 32.21. Defect in the membranous trachea accompanied by air tracking and mediastinal emphysema.

Image courtesy of Chen JD, Shanmuganathan K, Mirvis SE, et al.: Using CT to diagnose tracheal rupture. *AJR Am J Roentgenol* 2001;176(5):1273–80.

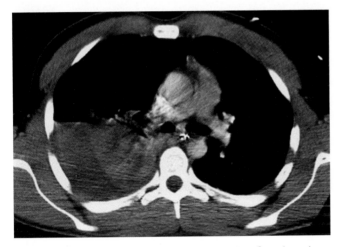

Figure 32.23. Air in posterior mediastinum, suggestive of esophageal perforation.

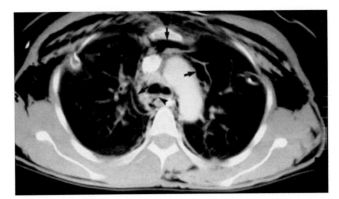

Figure 32.22. Air tracking and mediastinal emphysema.

Image courtesy of Chen JD, Shanmuganathan K, Mirvis SE, et al.: Using CT to diagnose tracheal rupture. *AJR Am J Roentgenol* 2001;176(5):1273–80.

include pneumomediastinum; subcutaneous emphysema; esophageal thickening at the area of perforation (44); extravasation of oral contrast material into the mediastinum (21); a wound track and proximal esophageal wall defect (21); or, as in Figure 32.23, air bubbles in the mediastinum proximal to the esophagus (28). Although CT can suggest esophageal lesions, patients with suspected injury should be evaluated by esophagography and possibly esophagoscopy (45).

Diaphragmatic rupture

Diaphragmatic rupture can occur following blunt or penetrating thoracoabdominal trauma (5, 21, 29, 31). Diaphragmatic injuries are usually left sided (90%) (31) (Figs. 32.24 and 32.25). Right-sided injuries are less common,

secondary to apparent protection by the liver (29) (Fig. 32.26). The most common locations for tears are at the junction of the diaphragmatic tendon and posterior leaves, as well as at the central tendon (31). Plain films may miss up to 37% of left-sided and 83% of right-sided injuries (46). The sensitivity of CT has improved with the advent of helical CT and now ranges from 71% to 100% (47). On CT, the most common finding is a discontinuity of the diaphragm (48) (Fig. 32.24), although this finding is not very specific (29). Other findings include diaphragmatic thickening, segmental nonrecognition of the diaphragm, herniation of intraabdominal contents, elevation of the diaphragm, and the combination of hemothorax and hemoperitoneum (49). Right-sided diaphragmatic injuries are more difficult to visualize (31). A line of decreased density within the liver parenchyma may indicate an injury to the right hemidiaphragm (7). Rupture or herniation of the liver into the chest cavity may also occur with these injuries (31).

Bone

Sternoclavicular dislocations and clavicular fractures

Anterior sternoclavicular dislocation (Fig. 32.27) is more common than posterior dislocation (27), although most anterior dislocations do not have major clinical significance (7). They are, however, evidence of high-energy trauma, and most are associated with other chest injuries, including pneumothorax, hemothorax, rib fractures, or pulmonary contusions (27). Posterior dislocations are less common and are more easily diagnosed on CT (7, 27). Posterior dislocations can be associated with injuries to the great vessels, brachial plexus, trachea, and esophagus (7). On CT, clavicular fractures and sternoclavicular dislocations can be associated with a retrosternal hematoma (5).

Rib fractures

Single rib fractures usually have little clinical significance. However, because fractures of the first through third ribs are indicative of high-velocity trauma, other intrathoracic

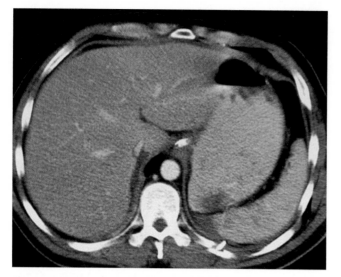

Figure 32.24. Rib punctures left hemidiaphragm.

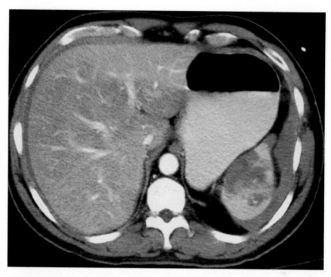

Figure 32.25. Interrupted diaphragm.

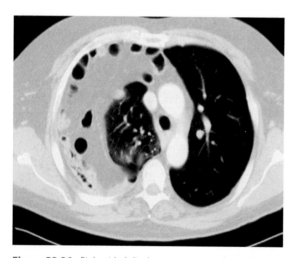

Figure 32.26. Right-sided diaphragm rupture with intrathoracic herniation of bowel.

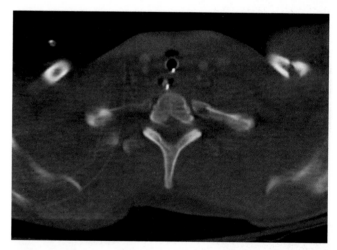

Figure 32.28. Left-sided clavicular fracture on bone window.

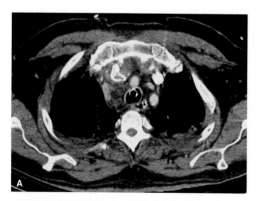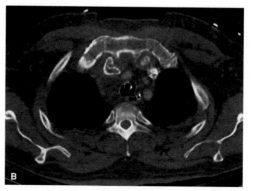

Figure 32.27. Right-sided posterior dislocation in original (A) and bone (B) windows.

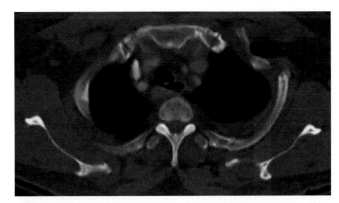

Figure 32.29. Posterior third and anterior second rib fractures.

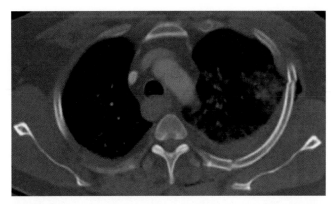

Figure 32.30. Lateral fourth and posterior fifth rib fractures on bone windows.

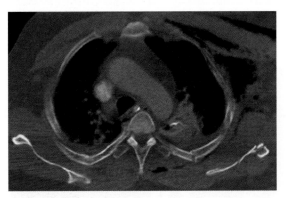

Figure 32.31. Left-sided scapular fracture with posterior rib fractures.

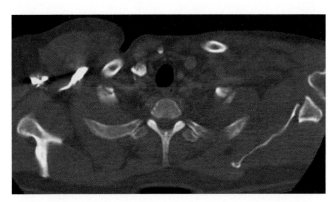

Figure 32.32. Left-sided scapular fracture.

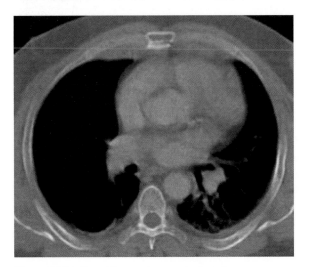

Figure 32.33. Sternal fracture in coronal orientation.

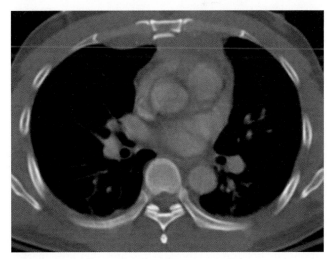

Figure 32.34. Sternal fracture in a similar orientation.

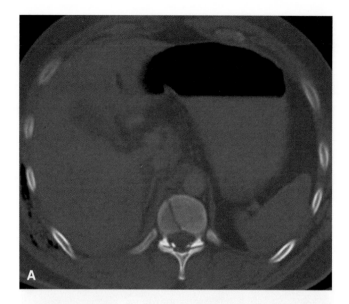

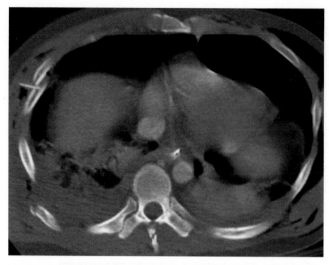

Figure 32.36. Fracture of the spinous process.

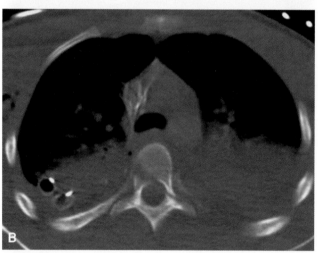

Figure 32.35. Vertebral body fractures.

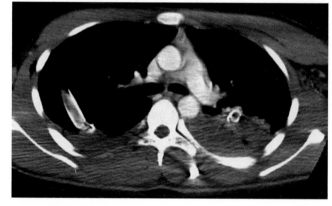

Figure 32.37. Bullet fragment in left posterior thorax with surrounding air.

injuries should be investigated (27). These injuries are some-times associated with brachial plexus injuries (50) or other neurovascular lesions (17, 27). Fractures of the eighth through eleventh ribs may be associated with upper abdominal visceral injury (27). Flail chest occurs when multiple rib fractures occur to three or more ribs. The paradoxical motion of the flail segment is associated with respiratory compromise.

Scapular fractures

Scapular fractures are frequently overlooked on the interpre-tation of chest radiographs (51). Like sternoclavicular dislo-cations and first through third rib fractures, they are a marker of significant impact (7) and are often associated with other injuries (51). The surgical management of these fractures depends on the particular center's orthopedic preference (35).

Sternal fractures

Sternal fractures usually occur in the coronal plane (7) (Figs. 32.33 and 32.34). Lateral chest radiographs have

a relatively high sensitivity in diagnosing sternal fractures (52). However, a frontal chest radiograph misses most sternal fractures, unless they are transversely displaced (7). Sternal fractures are usually detected on CT (5).

Vertebral fractures

The most common vertebral fractures are transverse process, compression, and burst fractures (53). Although dedicated spinal CT may be performed when there is high clinical suspi-cion, vertebral fractures can usually be identified on routine chest, abdominal, and pelvic CT (53). A series by Berry and colleagues demonstrated that routine CT identified 100% of patients with vertebral fractures compared with 73% on radio-graph (53).

Special images

Wound tracks

On CT, air, hemorrhage, and bone or bullet fragments can help identify the course of a bullet or knife (21).

Malpositioned chest tubes

Chest tube thoracostomy is often a necessary procedure after blunt trauma to evacuate hemothorax, monitor thoracic blood loss, and prevent tension pneumothoraces (54). Supine AP chest x-ray has been shown to detect as few as 45% of malpositioned chest tubes when compared with thoracic CT (54).

References

1. Sosna J, Slasky BS, Bar-Ziv J: Computed tomography in the emergency department. *Am J Emerg Med* 1997;**15**:244–7.

2. Broder J, Warshauer DM: Increasing utilization of computed tomography in the adult emergency department, 2000–2005. *Emerg Radiol* 2006;**13**:25–30.

3. Wilson T, Larsen B, Blecha M, et al.: Computed tomography of the chest: indications and utilization in the community hospital emergency department. *Chest* 2014;**145**:533A.

4. Rodriguez R, Anglin D, Langdorf MI, et al.: NEXUS Chest, validation of a decision instrument for selective chest imaging in blunt trauma. *JAMA Surgery* 2013;**148** (10):940–6.

5. Zinck SE, Primack SL: Radiographic and CT findings in blunt chest trauma. *J Thorac Imaging* 2000;**15**:87–96.

6. Traub M, Stevenson M, McEvoy S, et al.: The use of chest computed tomography versus chest x-ray in patients with major blunt trauma. *Injury Int J Care Injured* 2007;**38**:43–7.

7. Mirvis SE: Diagnostic imaging of acute thoracic injury. *Semin Ultrasound CT MRI* 2004;**25**:156–79.

8. Andruszkiewicz P, Sobczyk D: Ultrasound in critical care. *Anesthesiology Intensive Therapy* 2013;**45**(3):177–81.

9. Blaivas M, Lyon M, Duggal S: A prospective comparison of supine chest radiograph and bedside ultrasound for the diagnosis of traumatic pneumothorax. *Acad Emerg Med* 2005;**12**(9):844–9.

10. Trupka A, Waydhas C, Hallfeldt KK, et al.: Value of thoracic computed tomography in the first assessment of severely injured patients with blunt chest trauma: results of a prospective study. *J Trauma* 1997;**43**:405–11.

11. Brink M, Kool DR, Deunk J, et al.: Predictors of abnormal chest CT after blunt trauma: a critical appraisal of the literature. *Clin Radiol* 2009;**64**:272–83.

12. Scaglione M, Pinto A, Pedrosa I, et al.: Multidetector row computed tomography and blunt chest trauma. *Eur J Radiol* 2008;**65**:377–88.

13. Exadaktylos AK, Sclabas G, Schmid SW, et al.: Do we really need routine computed tomographic scanning in the primary evaluation of blunt chest trauma in patients with "normal" chest radiograph? *J Trauma* 2001;**51**:1173–6.

14. Washington L, Palacio D: Imaging of bacterial pulmonary infection in the immunocompetent patient. *Semin Roentgenol* 2007;**42**:122–45.

15. Reittner P, Ward S, Heyneman L, et al.: Pneumonia: high-resolution CT findings in 114 patients. *Eur Radiol* 2003;**13**:515–21.

16. Richman PB, Courtney DM, Friese J, et al.: Prevalence and significance of nonthromboembolic findings on chest computed tomography angiography performed to rule out pulmonary embolism: a multicenter study of 1,025 emergency department patients. *Acad Emerg Med* 2004;**11**:642–7.

17. Abbuhl SB: Principles of emergency department use of computed tomography. In: Tintanelli JE, Kelen GD, Stapczynski JS (eds), *Emergency medicine: a comprehensive study guide*. New York: McGraw-Hill, 2004:1878–83.

18. Holscher CM, Faulk LW, Moore EE, et al.: Chest computed tomography imaging for blunt pediatric trauma: not worth the radiation risk. *J Surg Res* 2013;**184**:352–7.

19. Kea B, Gamarallage R, Vairamuthu H, et al.: What is the clinical significance of chest CT when the chest x-ray result is normal in patients with blunt trauma? *Am J Emerg Med* 2013;**31**:1268–73.

20. Omert L, Yeaney WW, Protetch J: Efficacy of thoracic computerized tomography in blunt chest trauma. *Am Surg* 2001;**67**:660–4.

21. Shanmuganathan K, Matsumoto J: Imaging of penetrating chest trauma. *Radiol Clin North Am* 2006;**44**:225–38.

22. Winer-Muram HT, Steiner RM, Gurney JW, et al.: Ventilator-associated pneumonia in patients with adult respiratory distress syndrome: CT evaluation. *Radiology* 1998;**208**:193–9.

23. Lahde S, Jartti A, Broas M, et al.: HRCT findings in the lungs of primary care patients with lower respiratory tract infection. *Acta Radiol* 2002;**43**:159–63.

24. Smith-Bindman R, Lipson J, Marcus R, et al.: Radiation dose associated with common computed tomography examinations and the associated lifetime attributable risk of cancer. *Arch Intern Med* 2009;**269**:2078–86.

25. Sarma A, Heilbrun ME, Conner KE, et al.: Radiation and chest CT scan examinations. *Chest* 2012;**142**(3):750–60.

26. Mulkens TH, Marchal P, Daineffe S, et al.: Comparison of low-dose with standard-dose multidetector CT in cervical spine trauma. *AJNR* 2007;**28**:1444–50.

27. Miller LA: Chest wall, lung, and pleural space trauma. *Radiol Clin North Am* 2006;**44**:213–24.

28. Shanmuganathan K, Mirvis SE: Imaging diagnosis of nonaortic thoracic injury. *Radiol Clin North Am* 1999;**37**:533–51.

29. Kang E-Y, Muller NL: CT in blunt chest trauma: pulmonary, tracheobronchial and diaphragmatic injuries. *Semin Ultrasound CT MRI* 1996;**17**:114–18.

30. Donnelly LF, Klosterman LA: Subpleural sparing: a CT finding of lung contusion in children. *Radiology* 1997;**204**:385–7.

31. Tocino IM, Miller MH: Computed tomography in blunt chest trauma. *J Thorac Imaging* 1987;**2**:45–59.

32. Schild HH, Strunk H, Weber W, et al.: Pulmonary contusion: CT vs. plain radiographs. *J Comput Assist Tomogr* 1989;**13**:417–20.

33. Syrjala J, Braos M, Suramo I, et al.: High-resolution computed tomography for the diagnosis of community-acquired pneumonia. *Clin Infect Dis* 1998;**27**:358–63.

34. Tanaka N, Matsumoto T, Kuramitsu T, et al.: High-resolution CT findings in community-acquired pneumonia. *J Comput Assist Tomogr* 1996;**20**:600–8.

35. Chan O, Hiorns M: Chest trauma. *Eur Radiol* 1996;**23**:23–34.

36. Arenas-Jimenez J, Alonso-Charterina S, Sanchez-Paya J, et al.: Evaluation of CT findings for diagnosis of pleural effusions. *Eur Radiol* 2000;**10**:681–90.

37. Aquino SL, Web WR, Gushiken BJ: Pleural exudates and transudates: diagnosis with contrast-enhanced CT. *Radiology* 1994;**192**:803–8.

38. Waite RJ, Carbonneau RJ, Balikian JP, et al.: Parietal pleural changes in empyema: appearances at CT. *Radiology* 1990;**175**: 145–50.

39. Baber CE, Hedlund LW, Oddson TA, Putnam CE: Differentiating empyemas and peripheral pulmonary abscesses. *Radiology* 1980;**125**:755–8.

40. Tocino IM, Miller MH: Mediastinal trauma and other acute mediastinal conditions. *J Thorac Imaging* 1987;**2**:79–100.

41. Wang ZJ, Reddy GP, Gotway MB, et al.: CT and MR imaging of pericardial disease. *Radiographics* 2003;**23**:S167–80.

42. Stark P: Imaging of tracheobronchial injuries. *J Thorac Imaging* 1995;**10**:206–19.

43. Scaglione M, Romano S, Pinto A, et al.: Acute tracheobronchial injuries: impact of imaging on diagnosis and management implications. *Eur J Radiol* 2006;**59**:336–43.

44. Ketai L, Brandt M-M, Schermer C: Nonaortic mediastinal injuries from blunt chest trauma. *J Thorac Imaging* 2000;**15**: 120–7.

45. Euthrongchit J, Thoongsuwan N, Stern E: Nonvascular mediastinal trauma. *Radiol Clin North Am* 2006;**44**:251–8.

46. Gelman R, Mirvis SE, Gens D: Diaphragmatic rupture due to blunt trauma: sensitivity of plain chest radiographs. *AJR Am J Roentgenol* 1991;**156**:51–7.

47. Sliker CW: Imaging of diaphragm injuries. *Radiol Clin North Am* 2006;**44**:199–211.

48. Worthy SA, Jang EY, Hartman TE, et al.: Diaphragmatic rupture: CT findings in 11 patients. *Radiology* 1995;**194**:885–8.

49. Nchimi A: Helical CT of blunt diaphragmatic rupture. *AJR Am J Roentgenol* 2005;**184**:24–30.

50. Fermanis GG, Deane SA, Fitgerald PM: The significance of first and second rib fractures. *Aust N Z J Surg* 1985;**55**:383–6.

51. Collins J: Chest wall trauma. *J Thorac Imaging* 2000;**15**:112–9.

52. Huggett JM, Roszler MH: CT findings of sternal fracture. *Injury* 1998;**29**:623–6.

53. Berry GE, Adams S, Harris MB, et al.: Are plain radiographs of the spine necessary during evaluation after blunt trauma? Accuracy of screening torso computed tomography in thoracic/lumbar spine fracture diagnosis. *J Trauma* 2005;**59**:1410–13.

54. Ball C, Lord J, Laupland KB, et al.: Chest tube placement: How well trained are our residents? *Can J Surg* 2007;**50**(6):450–8.

Chapter 33

CT of the Abdomen and Pelvis

Nichole S. Meissner and Matthew O. Dolich

Indications

Since its inception, CT has greatly aided in the diagnosis of intraabdominal and pelvic pathology. The rapid diagnosis of underlying pathology in the "acute abdomen" is critical to help reduce the rates of morbidity and mortality from delayed diagnosis. Physical examination and laboratory findings are often nonspecific, so efficient diagnostic tools are essential. CT scanning has widely become the diagnostic test of choice for patients presenting with abdominal or pelvic pain and for the stable trauma patient to evaluate for intraabdominal injury; its use has increased dramatically in the two decades. Various studies show sensitivities of 69% to 95% and specificities of 95% to 100% for the diagnosis of bowel and mesenteric injuries with CT (1). The sensitivities for diagnosing solid organ injuries are even higher.

Because of the limitations of plain radiographs, CT scanning is also being increasingly used in cases of bowel obstruction to help delineate the location, severity, and underlying cause of the obstruction. For high-grade small bowel obstructions, CT has high sensitivity and specificity; it is less accurate for low-grade obstructions. In addition, CT with water-soluble contrast may be both therapeutic and diagnostic because the contrast material may favor intraluminal absorption of water and diminution of bowel wall edema, allowing resolution of mechanical small bowel obstruction. The ability to generate reconstructions in different planes on multidetector CT (MDCT) has enabled radiologists and clinicians to determine more easily whether a closed-loop obstruction is present. Findings suggestive of closed-loop intestinal obstruction include a C-shaped, U-shaped, or "coffee bean" appearance to the bowel, as well as a "whirlpool sign" of mesentery spiraling out from the point of strangulation. This information is vital, as closed-loop bowel obstructions generally mandate emergent surgical intervention.

Diagnostic capabilities

First-generation, single-slice CT scanners have been almost completely replaced with MDCT scanners. The faster acquisition of images has reduced motion artifact because the entire abdomen can be scanned on a single breath-hold. Thinner slices can be obtained, which increases resolution and gives better visualization of certain areas of interest within the abdomen and pelvis. The high resolution of today's MDCT scanners is an important feature for detection of malignancy, uncovering subtle foci of inflammation

or infection, and revealing traumatic injuries not seen with earlier generation scanners. This ability, in turn, allows more accurate triage and patient flow within hospitals, and it may help prevent unnecessary admissions from emergency departments. In the setting of abdominal trauma, high-resolution images from MDCT scanners facilitate determination of which patients require surgical intervention, angiographic embolization for hemorrhage control, and admission to the intensive care unit.

More information can be gathered from MDCT with the use of intravenous (IV) contrast in evaluating for certain diagnoses, such as intraabdominal abscesses or other inflammatory processes. Scanning without intravenous contrast generates the fastest, but most limited, images. Often, noncontrasted studies need to be later repeated with contrast, which not only delays diagnosis but also increases ionizing radiation exposure to the patient (see discussion on radiation in the "Imaging pitfalls and limitations" section). Outside of specific indications, we recommend the use of IV contrast to obtain the best-quality images possible, to help most effectively resolve the clinical question. Avoiding the use of IV contrast is appropriate in suspected or confirmed renal insufficiency or if trying to diagnose nephrolithiasis or ureterolithiasis. In the latter circumstance, renal excretion of the contrast material may opacify the collecting system and ureters, obscuring small stones from view. In almost all other cases, contrast is indicated. Oral contrast material facilitates delineation of pathology involving the stomach, small intestine, and colon. However, use of enteral contrast in the setting of blunt abdominal trauma has diminished over recent years as the added benefit is relatively small and the risk of aspiration is higher in this patient population. Water-soluble rectal contrast may be administered for cases of suspected colonic or rectal perforation from penetrating abdominal, flank, or back trauma. Caution is warranted in using oral contrast in suspected cases of bowel obstruction due to the increased risk of emesis and aspiration, and barium-containing contrast material should not be used when hollow viscus perforation is suspected. To obtain the highest quality images and to answer the clinical question efficiently, consultation with a radiologist should be considered if the type of contrast to be used is in question.

Conditions in the right upper quadrant that can be easily diagnosed by CT are pancreatitis, cholecystitis, ascending cholangitis, perforated hollow viscus, hepatic tumor or abscess, and, occasionally, acute appendicitis.

In cases of pancreatitis, a CT scan can help determine if there is sterile or infected necrosis, the latter being indicated by gas bubbles within a nonenhancing, necrotic pancreas. If the scan is performed with IV contrast, a "dark" unenhanced pancreas is visualized, indicating pancreatic necrosis of varying percentages. In acute pancreatitis, when the pancreas demonstrates normal enhancement with IV contrast, peripancreatic inflammation or fat stranding is usually noted. Depending on the severity of the pancreatitis, the inflammation can extend to the surrounding structures, such as the transverse colon, duodenum, or stomach, or inflammation can be seen tracking down either paracolic gutter or in the pararenal spaces. Due to the small size of the pancreas, a CT scan with pancreatic protocol is often useful in visualizing all portions of the organ. With MDCT, image thickness can be set as small as 2 mm with image acquisition as small as 0.5 mm (2). A discussion with the radiologist about a specific pancreatic CT protocol may be helpful in obtaining the highest quality images when pancreatitis or pancreatic necrosis are on the list of differential diagnoses.

The most sensitive findings in acute cholecystitis are gallbladder wall thickening greater than 3 mm and increased attenuation of the wall in the setting of a distended gallbladder. Other findings include increased attenuation of the surrounding liver from inflammation, subserosal edema, and pericholecystic fluid (3). Gallbladder calculi may be frequently detected on CT imaging, and both the intrahepatic and extrahepatic biliary tree may be assessed as well.

Because of the dual blood supply of the liver, multiphase contrast studies are best to study suspected liver lesions. A normal liver receives 75% of its blood flow from the portal vein and 25% from the hepatic artery. Most hepatic tumors receive their blood supply from the hepatic artery exclusively. How a liver lesion appears on CT depends on the vascularity of the lesion and delay in obtaining images after IV contrast administration (2). Metastatic tumors are the most common malignant liver lesion. The most common primary liver tumor is hepatocellular carcinoma. Focal nodular hyperplasia is not associated with symptoms and is generally noted to enhance on arterial phase CT. These lesions are rarely symptomatic, so if they are found on CT in a patient with abdominal pain, another source should be sought. Hemangiomas often cause chronic low-grade right upper quadrant abdominal pain, especially when they become very large. When small, hepatic hemangiomas are usually asymptomatic and are typically found incidentally.

While the vast majority of cases of acute appendicitis will present in the right lower quadrant, there are instances where the appendix is located in the right upper quadrant; these may cause clinical confusion if the provider is not aware of possible anatomical variations. If the appendix is quite long, it can track up along the right paracolic gutter and reach as high as the hepatic flexure. In this circumstance, inflammation isolated to the distal end of the appendix, or "tip appendicitis," will cause right upper quadrant pain. In cases of subclinical malrotation or cecal bascule, the cecum and therefore the appendix can be located in the right upper quadrant.

Right lower quadrant pathology readily imaged by CT includes appendicitis, mesenteric adenitis, ectopic pregnancy, hernia, diverticulitis, uretrolithiasis, ovarian pathology, and psoas abscess. Inflammation of small bowel lymph nodes from viral infection is common, especially in children, and is probably the most common cause of pain severe enough to lead to the diagnosis of "acute abdomen." In patients with right lower quadrant abdominal pain, a number of findings are indicative of acute appendicitis, including appendiceal dilation of greater than 1 cm in diameter, periappendiceal fat "stranding" or inflammation, and presence of an appendicolith. In more severe cases of appendicitis, the presence of a right lower quadrant phlegmon, fluid, extraluminal air bubbles, or an abscess all suggest the diagnosis of perforated appendicitis. Imaging in sagittal and coronal planes may help visualize the appendix in challenging cases.

Left upper quadrant pathologies include pancreatitis, splenic infarct or abscess, peptic ulcer disease, hiatal hernias, cecal volvulus, and gastric malignancy. Pancreatitis may present with a wide spectrum of severity, from mild, self-limited cases to life-threatening necrosis with septic shock. Abscesses of the spleen are very uncommon, with an incidence of 0.14% to 0.7% (4). Patients typically present with fever, left upper quadrant pain, and leukocytosis. Diagnosis is frequently delayed with most patients enduring symptoms for several days or weeks prior to diagnosis. The spleen may become infected by hematogenous infection, contiguous infection, hemoglobinopathy, immunosuppression, and trauma. Cases of cecal volvulus require urgent surgical evaluation because it is a closed-loop obstruction; delay in treatment could lead to gangrene and free perforation.

Disorders of the left lower quadrant include diverticulitis, ectopic pregnancy, ovarian pathology, hernia, psoas abscess, and nephrolithiasis. In cases of acute renal stones, 15% do not cause the classic sign of hematuria (4). In particular, CT is quite helpful in grading cases of acute diverticulitis. Uncomplicated colonic diverticulitis may be managed on either an inpatient or outpatient basis with antibiotics, while those with significant pericolonic or pelvic abscess on CT generally require drainage by interventional radiographic techniques. Uncontained perforated diverticulitis may be diagnosed by CT and typically requires early surgical intervention.

Diffuse abdominal pain can be caused by small bowel obstruction, abdominal aortic aneurysm, pancreatitis, aortic dissection, and urosepsis. Intussusception, a cause of abdominal pain and bowel obstruction in both children and adults, is revealed by a characteristic "target sign" on CT. In cases of aortic dissection, the onset of the dissection is often associated with severe chest or back pain, described as tearing that moves distally as the dissection propagates. Most abdominal aortic aneurysms are asymptomatic and are often found incidentally during workup of another ailment. In the few times where they are symptomatic, the most common symptom is new-onset low back and abdominal pain. The pain is the result of stretching retroperitoneal tissues and is associated with increased risk of rupture, so rapid evaluation and treatment are warranted.

Hernias of the abdominal wall and groin, when not evident clinically (such as in obese patients), may be well delineated by CT imaging (5). In this instance, no oral or intravenous contrast is necessary; however, it may be helpful to have the patient perform a Valsalva maneuver during image acquisition to accentuate the hernia.

CT is now the diagnostic modality of choice for patients with blunt abdominal trauma, particularly in the setting of concomitant head injury or alcohol intoxication in whom physical examination may be unreliable. Solid organ injury after blunt abdominal trauma can be graded according to standard radiologic scales, and stable patients with lower grade injuries may frequently be managed nonoperatively. In addition, contrast-enhanced CT may reveal a "blush" consistent with active extravasation of contrast; these patients typically require emergent intervention with angioembolization or surgery for hemorrhage control. Focal small bowel thickening, free fluid without solid organ injury, and mesenteric bleeding may signal intestinal injury and typically prompt further diagnostic studies or early surgical intervention. Free intraperitoneal air is a relatively rare occurrence in the early period after blunt trauma to the abdomen, and its absence should not falsely reassure the clinician. CT provides detailed imaging of the bony structures and soft tissues of the pelvis in trauma, and a large retroperitoneal hematoma with active extravasation may trigger an aggressive multidisciplinary approach including trauma surgeons, interventional radiologists, and orthopedic surgeons.

Imaging pitfalls and limitations

The administration of contrast in a patient with undiagnosed renal insufficiency may precipitate renal failure. Because of less developed fat planes in children and in very thin patients, CT scanning in these populations may be less accurate. CT scanning has a lower diagnostic yield in the morbidly obese patient because of increased scatter from the amount of fat present, although the limitations are far less than those encountered with ultrasonography. The limiting factor may ultimately be the technical specification of the scanner table because patients over a certain weight may interfere with movement of the table during the scan.

There is concern for ionizing radiation exposure in patients, especially the pediatric population, leading to increased risk for development of certain malignancies later in life (6). Radiation dose from CT scans varies widely based on the type of procedure, the size of the body part, the CT scanner itself, and how it is used. Ultimately it is difficult to estimate

cancer risks because cancer induction rates are approximated from historical data from occupational and wartime exposures. A single average CT scan nearly triples the patient's yearly radiation exposure (7); therefore, it is reasonable to anticipate a statistically significant increase in cancer induction. For this reason alone, it is important to emphasize again the judicious, but appropriate, use of this technology.

Clinical images

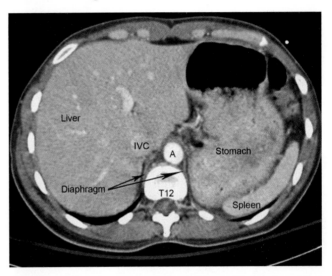

Figure 33.1. Normal anatomy at the level of the twelfth thoracic vertebral body (T12). A, aorta; IVC, inferior vena cava.

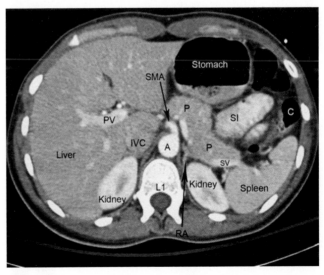

Figure 33.2. Normal anatomy at the level of the first lumbar vertebral body (L1). A, aorta; C, splenic flexure of colon; IVC, inferior vena cava; P, pancreas; PV, portal vein; RA, right adrenal gland; SMA, superior mesenteric artery; SI, small intestine; SV, splenic vein.

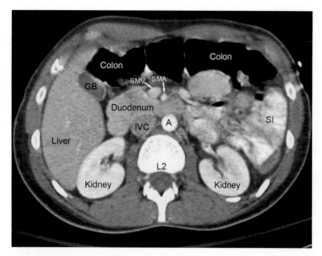

Figure 33.3. Normal anatomy at the level of the second lumbar vertebral body (L2). A, aorta; C, splenic flexure of colon; GB, gallbladder; IVC, inferior vena cava; SI, small intestine; SMA, superior mesenteric artery; SMV, superior mesenteric vein.

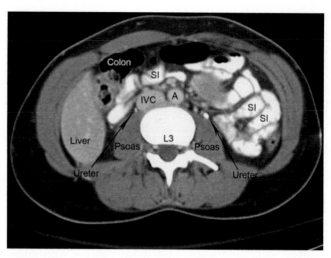

Figure 33.4. Normal anatomy at the level of the third lumbar vertebral body (L3). A, aorta; IVC, inferior vena cava; SI, small intestine.

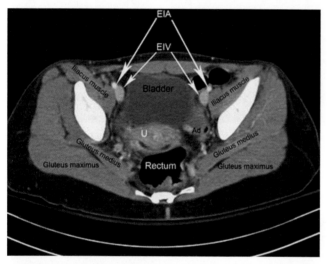

Figure 33.5. Normal pelvic anatomy. Ad, left adnexa; EIA, external iliac artery; EIV, external iliac vein; U, uterus.

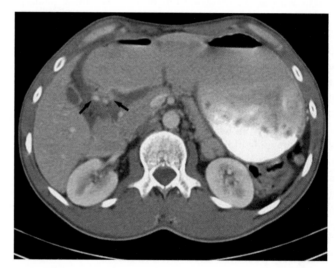

Figure 33.6. Gastric outlet obstruction. A dilated, contrast-filled stomach is noted in conjunction with a strictured pylorus secondary to peptic ulcer disease (*arrows*).

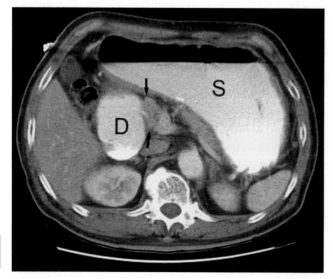

Figure 33.7. Duodenal obstruction secondary to neoplasm (*arrows*). Dilated, contrast-filled stomach (S) and proximal duodenum (D) are noted.

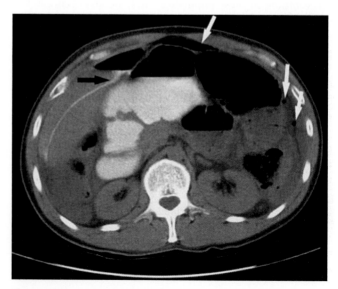

Figure 33.8. Duodenal perforation with free intraperitoneal air (*white arrows*) and extravasation of oral contrast material (*black arrow*).

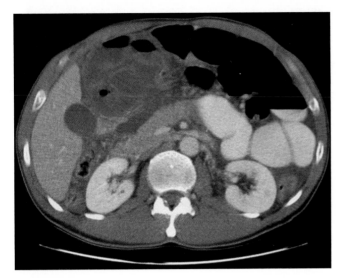

Figure 33.9. Small bowel obstruction. Multiple dilated loops of small bowel are filled with fluid and oral contrast material. The colon is collapsed.

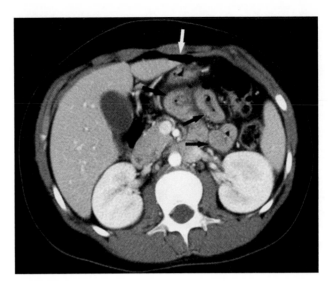

Figure 33.10. Jejunal perforation secondary to blunt abdominal trauma. Note thickened jejunal loops (*black arrows*) and free intraperitoneal air (*white arrow*).

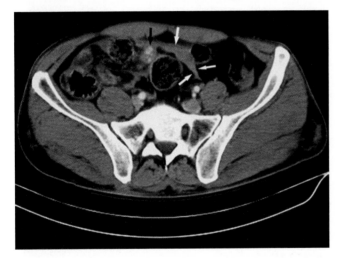

Figure 33.11. Mesenteric injury secondary to blunt abdominal trauma. Free fluid is present between bowel loops (*white arrows*), as well as active extravasation of contrast (*black arrow*).

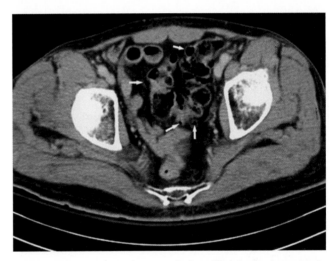

Figure 33.12. Diverticular disease. Multiple air-filled diverticula are noted throughout the sigmoid colon (*arrows*).

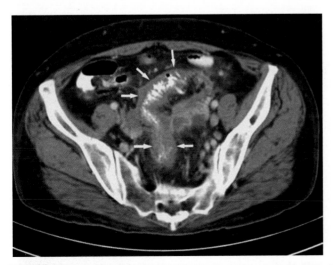

Figure 33.13. Acute diverticulitis. The sigmoid colon is markedly thickened (*arrows*).

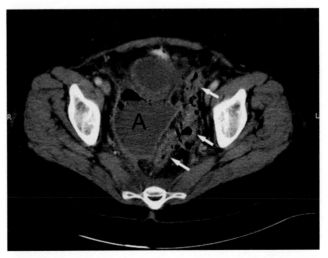

Figure 33.14. Perforated diverticulitis with pelvic abscess. Note the thickened sigmoid colon (*arrows*); adjacent is a large pelvic abscess (A) containing fluid and air.

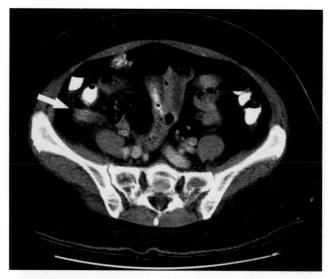

Figure 33.15. Acute appendicitis. Note the enlarged appendix (*white arrow*) and periappendiceal fat stranding.

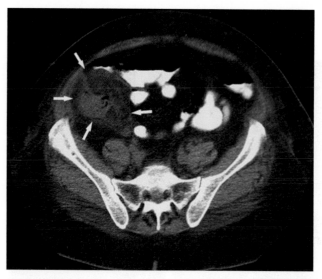

Figure 33.16. Perforated appendicitis. Note right lower quadrant phlegmon (*arrows*) containing fluid and bubbles of air.

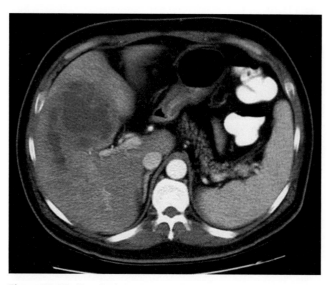

Figure 33.17. Hepatic abscess.

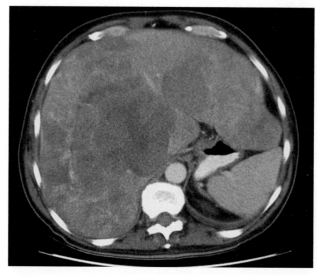

Figure 33.18. Liver neoplasm (metastatic adenocarcinoma).

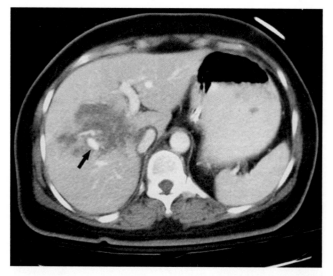

Figure 33.19. Liver laceration secondary to blunt abdominal trauma. Note active extravasation of contrast (*arrow*). The absence of intraperitoneal fluid prevented diagnosis by focused assessment with sonography in trauma.

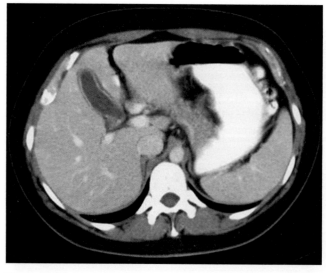

Figure 33.20. Acute cholecystitis. Note prominent gallbladder wall with pericholecystic fluid.

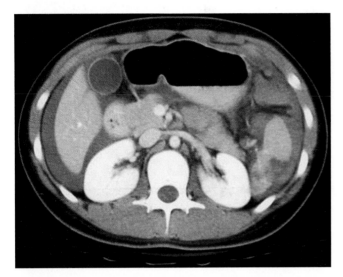

Figure 33.21. Splenic laceration with hemoperitoneum secondary to blunt abdominal trauma. Note free intraperitoneal blood surrounding both the spleen and liver.

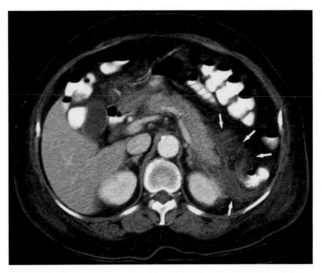

Figure 33.22. Acute pancreatitis. The pancreatic tail enhances with contrast; however, significant peripancreatic edema is present (*arrows*).

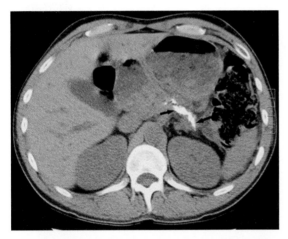

Figure 33.23. Chronic pancreatitis. Extensive calcification of the pancreatic tail is present (*arrows*).

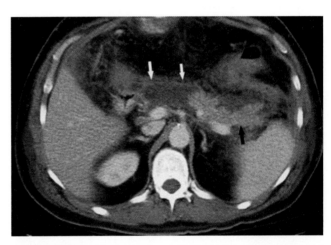

Figure 33.24. Necrotizing pancreatitis. The body of the pancreas is necrotic and does not enhance (*white arrows*). The pancreatic tail remains viable (*black arrow*).

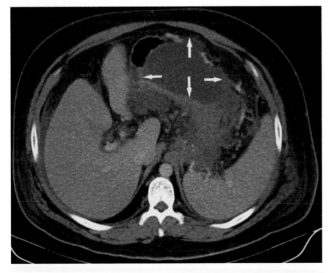

Figure 33.25. Pancreatic pseudocyst (*arrows*). Residual inflammation of the pancreatic tail is present.

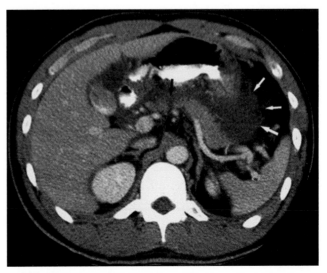

Figure 33.26. Pancreatic transection secondary to blunt abdominal trauma. The body of the pancreas is transected in the midline from compression against the spine (*black arrows*). Peripancreatic fluid is noted along the tail of the pancreas as well (*white arrows*).

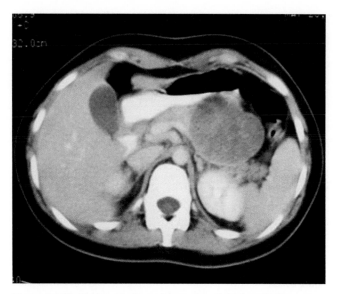

Figure 33.27. Benign neoplasm of the pancreatic body and tail.

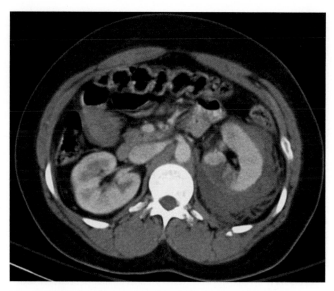

Figure 33.28. Renal injury secondary to blunt abdominal trauma. A moderate amount of perinephric hemorrhage is present.

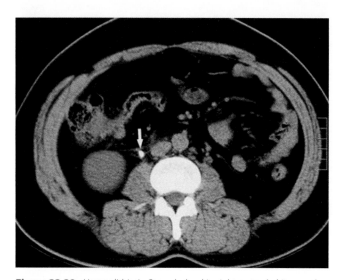

Figure 33.29. Ureterolithiasis. Stone lodged in right ureter (*white arrow*), easily visualized on noncontrast CT scan.

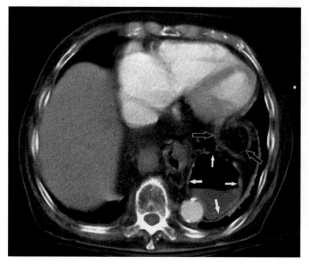

Figure 33.30. Chronic paraesophageal hiatal hernia. Portions of the stomach (*white arrows*) and left colon (*black arrows*) have herniated into the left thorax.

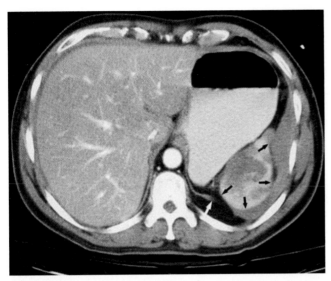

Figure 33.31. Rupture of the left hemidiaphragm secondary to blunt abdominal trauma (*white arrow*). A portion of the stomach has herniated into the left thorax (*black arrows*). A left pleural effusion is present.

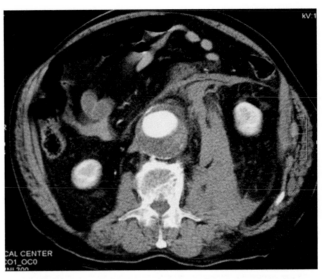

Figure 33.32. Infrarenal abdominal aortic aneurysm with contained retroperitoneal leak. Note extensive anterior displacement of the left kidney, as well as mural thrombus within the aortic lumen.

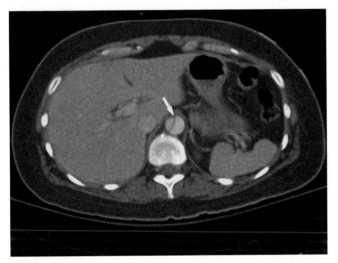

Figure 33.33. Aortic dissection. Note intimal flap separating the true and false lumens (*arrow*).

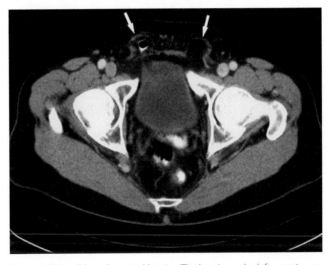

Figure 33.34. Bilateral inguinal hernias. The hernia on the left contains an air-filled bowel loop.

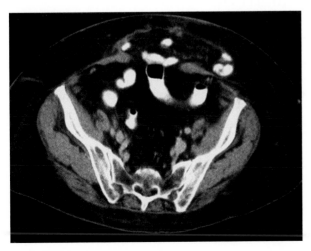

Figure 33.35. Ventral hernia containing multiple contrast-filled bowel loops.

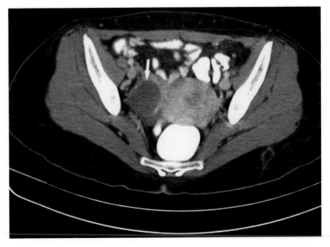

Figure 33.36. Right tuboovarian abscess. Note enhancing rim surrounding lower-density abscess cavity.

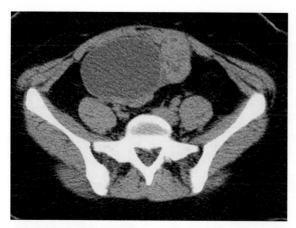

Figure 33.37. Ovarian cyst.

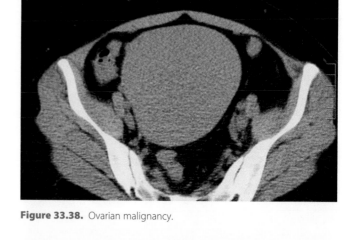

Figure 33.38. Ovarian malignancy.

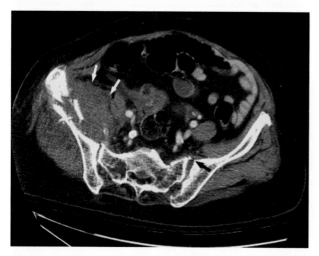

Figure 33.39. Pelvic fracture after motor vehicle collision. The right iliac wing has a comminuted fracture with adjacent retroperitoneal hematoma (*white arrows*). The left sacroiliac joint is widened as well (*black arrow*).

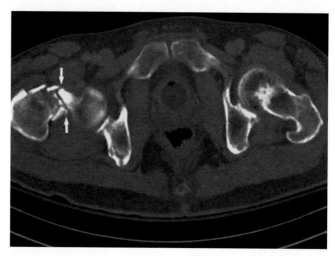

Figure 33.40. Comminuted fracture of the femoral neck (*arrows*).

References

1. Brofman N, Atri M, Hanson JM, et al.: Evaluation of mesenteric and bowel blunt trauma with multi-detector CT. *Radiographics* 2006;**26**:1119–31.

2. Gore RM: *Textbook of gastrointestinal radiology.* Philadelphia: Saunders Elsevier, 2008.

3. Leschka S, Alkhadi A, Wildermuth S, Marincek B: Multidetector computed tomography of acute abdomen. *Eur Radiol* 2005;**15**: 2435–47.

4. Kim K, Kim, Y, Kim S: Low-dose abdominal CT for evaluating suspected appendicitis. *New Engl J Med* 2012;**366**(17):1596–605.

5. Burkhardt JH, Arshanskiy Y, Munson JL, Scholz FJ: Diagnosis of inguinal hernias with axial CT: the lateral crescent sign and other key findings. *Radiographics* 2011;**31**(2):E1–E12.

6. Brenner D, Elliston C, Hall E, Berdon W: Estimated risks of radiation-induced fatal cancer from pediatric CT. *AJR Am J Roentgenol* 2001;**178**(2):289–96.

7. U.S. Food and Drug Administration: Radiation-Emitting Products: What are the radiation risks from CT? 2009. Available at: www.fda.gov/radiation-emittingproducts/radiationemitting productsandprocedures/medicalimaging/medicalx-rays /ucm115329.htm

CT Angiography of the Chest

Swaminatha V. Gurudevan and Reza Arsanjani

Indications

The most common clinical indication for a CT scan of the chest in the emergency department is to assist with the rapid diagnosis and treatment of a potentially life-threatening cause of chest pain. The three most common life-threatening conditions facing patients with chest pain in the ED are myocardial ischemia, pulmonary embolism, and aortic dissection. With the advent of multidetector row CT technology and improvements in the temporal and spatial resolution of modern CT scanners, all three entities can be diagnosed with excellent reliability.

Diagnostic capabilities

Coronary heart disease is the leading cause of death in the United States, responsible for about 817,000 deaths each year (1). Multidetector CT (MDCT) coronary angiography has emerged as a highly sensitive tool to diagnose both obstructive and nonobstructive coronary artery disease. Modern scanners that employ 16-slice and 64-slice multidetector row technology with cardiac gating enable rapid and continuous coverage of the heart with excellent visualization of both the lumen and vessel wall of the coronary arteries (2, 3). The sensitivity and specificity of 64-slice CT exceed 95% for the diagnosis of significant coronary artery disease (4). With adequate patient preparation, reliable images can be obtained with a rapid 8- to 10-second scan time.

Pulmonary embolism is a common disorder, with an estimated annual incidence of 25 to 70 per 100,000 (5).

Prompt diagnosis and institution of anticoagulant therapy is crucial to a favorable clinical outcome. Since its introduction in 1992, CT angiography of the pulmonary arteries has become the diagnostic test of choice for the evaluation of acute pulmonary embolism (6, 7). The improved spatial and temporal resolution of MDCT enables the clinician to obtain comprehensive visualization of the pulmonary arterial tree in 4 to 10 seconds. The sensitivity and specificity of CT for the detection of pulmonary embolism exceeds 90%, and a negative spiral CT is associated with a good prognosis when anticoagulation is withheld (8).

Aortic dissection is an uncommon disease, with a peak incidence of 3 to 5 cases per 1 million people per year. Approximately 2,000 new cases are reported each year in the United States (9). The mortality of untreated aortic dissection involving the ascending aorta (Stanford type A dissection) can approach 1% to 2% per hour after symptom onset (10, 11). This underscores the need for prompt diagnosis and treatment. MDCT enables rapid visualization of the entire aorta, localizing the site of intimal tear and the extent of anatomic involvement. The sensitivity and specificity of MDCT has been reported near 100% for the diagnosis of aortic dissection (12).

Imaging pitfalls and limitations

Multidetector CT coronary angiography requires significant technical expertise and attention to detail to yield diagnostic image quality. Patients should be capable of at least an 8- to 9-second breath-hold during image acquisition. As the study

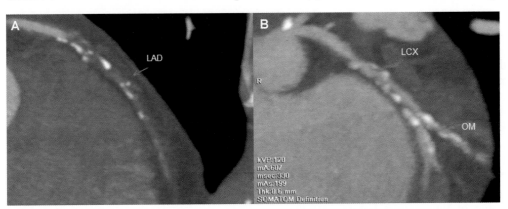

Figure 34.1. 2D oblique maximum intensity projection (MIP) of the (A) left anterior descending coronary artery (LAD) and (B) left circumflex (LCX) and obtuse marginal (OM) arteries from the MDCT study performed in a 58-year-old man with abnormal electrocardiogram. LAD appears sub-totally occluded with no contrast in distal segments of the artery. In addition, severe stenosis noted in LCX and OM. Diagnosis and interpretation of CT coronary angiography studies is typically done using 2D images.

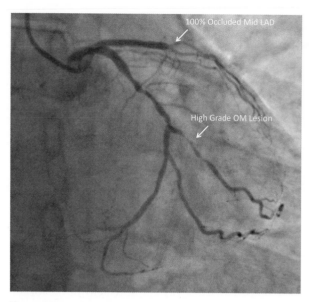

Figure 34.2. Invasive coronary angiography of the left anterior descending (LAD) and obtuse marginal (OM) arteries performed in the same 58-year-old man, confirming 100% occlusion of LAD and high-grade stenosis in the OM.

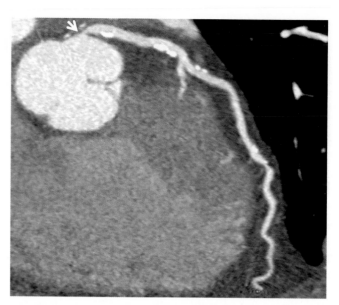

Figure 34.3. 2D oblique maximum intensity projection (MIP) of the left main and left anterior descending coronary arteries from MDCT study performed in a 64-year-old man with history of hypertension and hyperlipidemia referred for atypical chest pain. There is evidence of a large plaque in the ostium of the left main artery causing a severe degree of luminal obstruction, approximately 90% *(arrow)*.

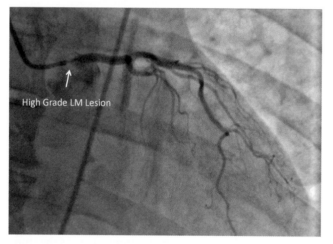

Figure 34.4. Invasive coronary angiography of the left coronary system performed in the same 64-year-old man, confirming high-grade left main stenosis.

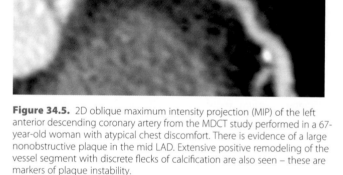

Figure 34.5. 2D oblique maximum intensity projection (MIP) of the left anterior descending coronary artery from the MDCT study performed in a 67-year-old woman with atypical chest discomfort. There is evidence of a large nonobstructive plaque in the mid LAD. Extensive positive remodeling of the vessel segment with discrete flecks of calcification are also seen – these are markers of plaque instability.

is ECG gated, patients should ideally have a slow, steady heart rate to avoid motion artifacts that can preclude effective visualization of the entire coronary arterial tree. Beta-blockers such as metoprolol are often given to patients prior to the initiation of the CT scan to achieve a heart rate less than 70 beats per minute. Significant coronary calcification can also limit the diagnostic accuracy of studies due to beam-hardening artifacts that can occur.

During CT pulmonary angiography, the major limitation to imaging is proper timing of the contrast bolus and scan acquisition to maximize visualization of the central and peripheral pulmonary arteries. The accuracy for diagnosis of subsegmental pulmonary emboli is also limited, but the clinical significance of these emboli have been debated. Spiral CT artifacts from the motion of the aorta can also masquerade as a dissection flap, making it essential to perform cardiac gating in aortic dissection studies.

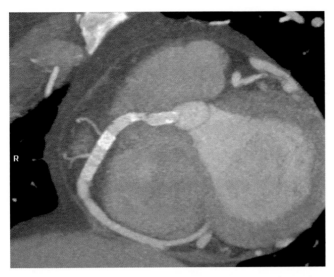

Figure 34.6. 2D oblique maximum intensity projection (MIP) of the right coronary artery (RCA) from the MDCT study performed in a 57-year-old man with prior history of percutaneous coronary intervention. There is evidence of a large stent in the mid RCA, which appears patent without significant in-stent restenosis.

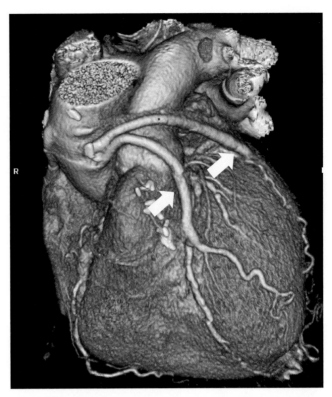

Figure 34.7. A 3D volume-rendered image of a 64-slice MDCT performed in a 73-year-old man with known coronary artery disease who underwent coronary artery bypass surgery 4 years earlier. The images show patent saphenous venous grafts to the diagonal and obtuse marginal branches (*arrows*).

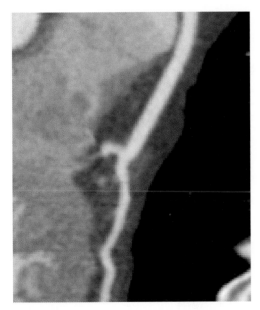

Figure 34.8. A curved-multiplanar image performed in the same 73-year-old man with known coronary artery bypass surgery demonstrating a patent saphenous venous graft to diagonal branch.

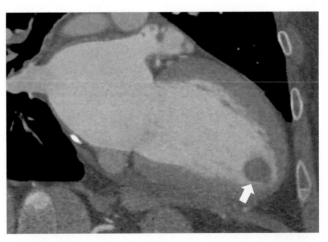

Figure 34.9. A 2D image of a 64-slice MDCT performed in a 48-year-old man who presented with shortness of breath and abnormal electrocardiogram. The patient was noted to have normal coronaries; however, evaluation of the left ventricle demonstrated a large thrombus *(arrow)*.

481

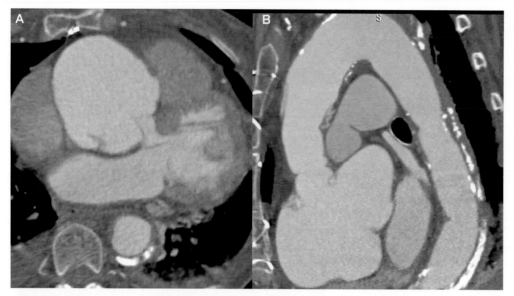

Figure 34.10. A 2D image of a 64-slice MDCT performed in an 71-year-old woman who presented with exertional chest discomfort. The axial (A) and sagittal oblique (B) projections demonstrate a massive fusiform aortic aneurysm involving the aortic root measuring 7.8 cm in diameter, which portends a high risk for subsequent fatal rupture.

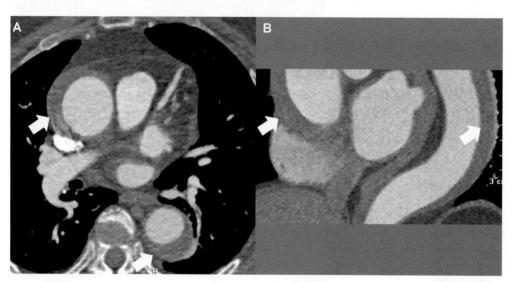

Figure 34.11. A 2D image of a 64-slice MDCT performed in 58-year-old man who presented with chest pain. The axial (A) and sagittal oblique (B) projections demonstrate significant intramural hematoma *(arrows)* involving the ascending and descending aorta, a variant form of classic aortic dissection and potentially fatal entity. Based on the involvement of both the ascending and descending aorta, this is classified as a Stanford type A aortic dissection.

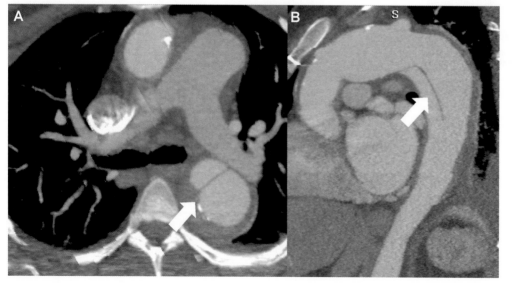

Figure 34.12. Axial (A) and sagittal oblique (B) projections of a thoracic and abdominal MDCT with contrast performed in a 61-year-old man with a history of hypertension who presented with severe back pain. A complex spiral dissection involving the descending aorta can be appreciated *(arrow)*. Based on the lack of ascending aorta involvement, this is classified as a Stanford type B aortic dissection.

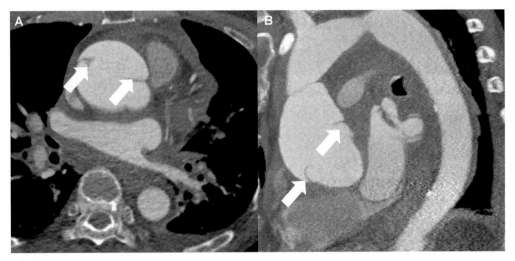

Figure 34.13. Axial (A) and sagittal oblique (B) projections of a thoracic and abdominal MDCT with contrast performed in a 66-year-old man with a history of hypertension who presented with severe chest pain. A complex spiral dissection involving the ascending aorta can be appreciated (*arrow*). Based on the ascending aorta involvement, this is classified as a Stanford type A aortic dissection.

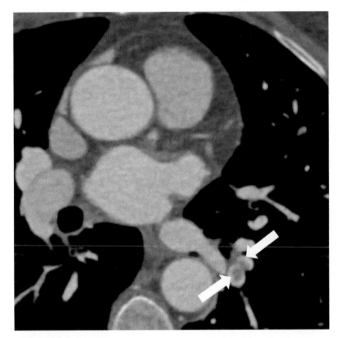

Figure 34.14. Axial maximum intensity projection of the thoracic MDCT performed in a 57-year-old woman with chest pain and dyspnea. The images show a filling defect in the right segmental pulmonary arteries (*arrows*), consistent with acute pulmonary embolism.

References

1. Rosamond W, Flegal K, Friday G, et al.: Heart disease and stroke statistics – 2007 update: a report from the American Heart Association Statistics Committee and Stroke Statistics Subcommittee. *Circulation* 2007;**115**:e69–171.

2. Achenbach S: Computed tomography coronary angiography. *J Am Coll Cardiol* 2006;**48**:1919–28.

3. Johnson TR, Nikolaou K, Wintersperger BJ, et al.: ECG-gated 64-MDCT angiography in the differential diagnosis of acute chest pain. *AJR Am J Roentgenol* 2007;**188**:76–82.

4. Raff GL, Gallagher MJ, O'Neill WW, Goldstein JA: Diagnostic accuracy of noninvasive coronary angiography using 64-slice spiral computed tomography. *J Am Coll Cardiol* 2005;**46**:552–7.

5. Schaefer-Prokop C, Prokop M: MDCT for the diagnosis of acute pulmonary embolism. *Eur Radiol* 2005;**15**(Suppl 4):D37–41.

6. Schoepf UJ: Diagnosing pulmonary embolism: time to rewrite the textbooks. *Int J Cardiovasc Imaging* 2005;**21**:155–63.

7. Schoepf UJ, Goldhaber SZ, Costello P: Spiral computed tomography for acute pulmonary embolism. *Circulation* 2004;**109**:2160–7.

8. Quiroz R, Kucher N, Zou KH, et al.: Clinical validity of a negative computed tomography scan in patients with suspected pulmonary embolism: a systematic review. *JAMA* 2005;**293**:2012–7.

9. Nienaber CA, Eagle KA: Aortic dissection: new frontiers in diagnosis and management. Part I: from etiology to diagnostic strategies. *Circulation* 2003;**108**:628–35.

10. Hagan PG, Nienaber CA, Isselbacher EM, et al.: The International Registry of Acute Aortic Dissection (IRAD): new insights into an old disease. *JAMA* 2000;**283**:897–903.

11. Hirst AE Jr, Johns VJ Jr, Kime SW Jr: Dissecting aneurysm of the aorta: a review of 505 cases. *Medicine (Baltimore)* 1958;**37**:217–79.

12. Hayter RG, Rhea JT, Small A, et al.: Suspected aortic dissection and other aortic disorders: multi-detector row CT in 373 cases in the emergency setting. *Radiology* 2006;**238**:841–52.

Chapter 35

CT Angiography of the Abdominal Vasculature

Kathleen Latouf, Steve Nanini, and Martha Villalba

Introduction

The development of multidetector computed tomography angiography (MDCTA), as opposed to single-row computed tomography angiography (CTA), is responsible for a drastic change in diagnostic imaging protocol of the abdomen. Coupled with a variety of 3D reformatting techniques, it has taken the place of catheter angiography in the assessment of both central and peripheral circulation. MDCTA has the capability to re-create 3D reconstructions of the vessels in question. Catheter angiography is now mostly reserved for interventional purposes or for dynamic imaging (1).

Renal and mesenteric artery pathologies – diagnoses that once required invasive techniques – can now be diagnosed within 3 minutes using MDCTA (2). The many benefits of MDCTA are expanding, but some of the common current indications include vascular mapping of invasive tumors, planning for hepatic resection, preoperative evaluation and planning of liver transplantation, diagnosing ischemic bowel disease and Crohn's disease, and visualizing the anatomy of collateral vessels in cirrhosis (3). Some of the other indications more specific to emergency medicine include the investigation for vascular injury following trauma; abdominal aortic aneurysm; and dissection, occlusion, and stenosis.

Normal anatomy

The abdominal aorta is the distal continuation of the thoracic aorta that enters the abdominal cavity by piercing the diaphragm at the aortic hiatus at T12. At L4, it bifurcates to the right and left common iliac arteries. The main branches of the abdominal aorta are the celiac trunk at the inferior endplate of T12, the superior mesenteric artery at the superior endplate of L1, the paired renal arteries at L1–L2 level, and the inferior mesenteric artery (IMA) at the level of L3-L4 (4).

The celiac artery branches from the anterior aspect of the aorta just below the aortic hiatus. It extends anteriorly for only 1 to 2 cm before dividing into the common hepatic, left gastric, and splenic artery. The splenic artery is distinctively tortuous, and it runs along the superior border of the pancreas toward the spleen. The left gastric artery passes retroperitoneal toward the esophageal hiatus, piercing through the lesser omentum. The common hepatic artery extends laterally to the right from the celiac trunk and bifurcates into the proper hepatic artery going to the liver and the gastroduodenal artery supplying the duodenum and pancreas (4).

The superior mesenteric artery (SMA) branches anteriorly from the abdominal aorta at the level of L1. It extends antero-inferiorly behind the neck of the pancreas and the splenic vein, crossing anterior to the left renal vein. It emerges anterior to the uncinated process of the pancreas and crosses anterior to the third part of the duodenum. Several branches to the left supply the jejunum and ileum, while those branching to the right supply the proximal and mid-colon (5).

The inferior mesenteric artery branches from the abdominal aorta at the level of L3–L4 approximately 8 cm below the SMA. It continues inferiorly to the left of the abdominal aorta. The left colic artery and two to four sigmoid arteries extend out to supply the hindgut. It continues and terminates as the superior rectal artery (5).

The renal arteries arise between L1 and L2. Both renal arteries divide near the hilum into five branches of segmental arteries that supply the segments of the kidney (6). Many common renal artery variations exist, including unilateral multiple (accessory) renal arteries (24%), bilateral multiple renal arteries (5%), and early division of the segmental arteries (8%) (7).

Patient preparation

When considering any form of CTA for a patient, several things should first be taken into consideration and discussed with the patient.

Kidney function should be evaluated before a CTA is performed. Contrast-induced nephropathy is often defined as an acute decline in renal function generating a rise of 0.5 mg/dL in serum creatinine or a >25% increase from baseline, occurring after the administration of contrast medium in the absence of an alternative cause (8). Acute reductions in renal function are of special concern in individuals with combined diabetes and preexisting renal insufficiency (9). Rarely, in the case of severe preexisting renal impairment, prophylactic dialysis may be required (8).

Adverse reactions to contrast media can occur in many forms. It is important to discuss the possibility of contrast allergy with the patient and to determine if the patient has a history of reactions to intravascular contrast media. If there is significant concern for a severe adverse reaction, skin testing is available to confirm an allergy (10).

Premedication is common practice, in which antihistamines and corticosteroids are given before the procedure (11). We recommend 50 mg of oral Prednisone at 13 hours, 7 hours, and 1 hour prior to the study, along with 50 mg of PO Benadryl and 20 mg of PO Pepcid 1 hour prior to the study. In emergent cases, we administer 125 mg of IV Solumedrol along with 50 mg of IV Benadryl. In the case of a previous life-threatening reaction, an MDCTA is not advised.

CTA technique

MDCTA is preferred over single-detector, incremental, or helical CTA in that it allows for the rapid, simultaneous acquisition of large volumetric datasets with submilimeter isotropic spatial resolution within a single breath-hold. This is especially true for the 16-slice or greater MDCTAs (12). The higher slice MDCT refers to the greater number of sections that are being obtained simultaneously. This in turn leads to greater visibility and higher spatial resolution (13).

Additionally, CTA has replaced digital subtraction angiography (DSA) because it is noninvasive and widely available (14). Unlike DSA, intra-arterial access is not required. Instead, a contrast agent is administered through a peripheral vein, and this contrast highlights blood flow throughout the body as a CT image is taken. Consequently, the risk of perforating an artery, infection, and nerve damage – as is seen in other more invasive techniques – is greatly lowered.

The scanning and data acquisition lasts approximately 5 minutes, and the processing of the images, with programs such as maximum intensity projection and shaded surface display, allows for the re-creation and mapping of the vasculature with great quality (3).

Indications

Trauma

Most large trauma centers do no routinely obtain CTA images of the abdomen. Due to its protected retroperitoneal location, the abdominal aorta is rarely injured with trauma, but when it happens, it mostly involves the infrarenal aorta, causing aortic injury and dissection.

On a CTA, an active bleed is seen as a high-attenuating region, and a pseudoaneurysm can be seen as a focal, rounded region equal in attenuation to the aorta (Figs. 35.1 to 35.3).

Abdominal aortic aneurysm

An abdominal aortic aneurysm (AAA) is the widening of an abdominal aorta to a diameter of 3 cm or greater (Fig. 35.4). An ectatic aorta is an abdominal aorta of 2.6 to 2.9 cm in diameter. It is recommended that individuals older than 65 years of age with an ectatic aorta be screened every four years (15). Operative intervention is recommended in AAA larger than 5.5 cm (15). For AAA, the larger the diameter, the greater the expansion rate and risk of rupture (16). Within an aneurysm, there is often a thrombus, which can rupture and become fatal if not resolved quickly (Figs. 35.5 and 35.6).

Evaluation of the abdominal aorta is one of the most common uses of an abdominal CTA. CTA is helpful in the diagnosis, characterization, and surgical preparation of an abdominal aortic aneurysm. For example, the exact location, existence of anomalous renal arteries, existence of stenosis in the vasculature, and extension of the aneurysm into the iliac arteries can be determined (17). Postoperatively, CTA is useful in examining stent placement and in evaluating for the presence of an endo-leak (Figs. 35.7 to 35.12).

Dissection

Aortic dissections are rarely limited to the abdominal aorta (<2%), with the ascending aorta being involved in 70% of cases (18). Aortic dissection is commonly associated with hypertension and preexisting aneurysmal degeneration of the abdominal aorta. Risk factors include connective tissue disorders (e.g., Marfan syndrome), deceleration trauma, or atherosclerosis. Isolated dissection of the abdominal aorta often presents with early nonspecific signs and symptoms. These include back pain, peripheral ischemia, distal embolization, and an easily detectable pulsatile mass (18). Symptomatic aortic dissections are at a greater risk of rupture, and complications and in-hospital mortality are common for such patients. Similar to atherosclerotic aneurysms, endovascular therapy is a viable treatment (19, 20).

The celiac artery and SMA can be involved in an aortic dissection (Figs. 35.13 and 35.14). For example, the flap can extend into the proximal portion of the vessel and decrease the blood flow. Although rare, a spontaneous dissection of the SMA can easily be detected by CTA. If not corrected surgically, it has a relatively high mortality rate (21).

Gastrointestinal bleeding

Nearly 300,000 patients present to the hospital in the United States each year for the management of gastrointestinal (GI) bleeding. Bleeding occurs more frequently in men and correlates with age. The clinical presentation varies significantly from asymptomatic to those requiring immediate intervention (22). Upper GI bleeds originate from branches of the celiac artery and present with hematemesis and melena; however, clinical presentation depends on the rate of the bleed. The causes for an upper GI bleed are extensive, but the most common include peptic ulcer disease (Figs. 35.15 and 35.16), gastritis, duodenitis, and esophageal varices. Lower GI bleeds originate from branches of the SMA and IMA. These also have many causes, but the most common are diverticulosis, arteriovenous malformations, neoplasms, anorectal abnormalities, and colitis (22). CTA is required for the definitive diagnosis of many of these pathologies.

Stenosis and occlusion: mesenteric ischemia

Mortality related to acute mesenteric arterial occlusion is high, and survival depends on revascularization time. An elderly individual with postprandial pain, food avoidance, or weight loss should prompt the consideration of intestinal ischemia. Underlying comorbidities include atherosclerosis, low cardiac output states, cardiac arrhythmias, severe cardiac valvular disease, recent myocardial infarction, and intraabdominal malignancy (23). CTA allows for imaging of all of the mesenteric arterial system and has shown to be as accurate as other techniques including angiography (24). Causes of acute mesenteric ischemia include embolic occlusion of the SMA (30%–50%), in situ SMA thrombosis in the setting of underlying atherosclerosis (15%–30%), non-occlusive (vasospastic) ischemia (20%–30%), superior mesenteric venous thrombosis (5%–10%), and spontaneous dissection (rare). If detected, this will likely need to be resolved surgically (25).

Stenosis and occlusion: median arcuate ligament syndrome (celiac artery compression syndrome)

Median arcuate ligament syndrome (MALS) presents with a clinical triad of postprandial abdominal pain, weight loss, an abdominal bruit in a middle-aged (40–60 years) female (26). Nausea and vomiting may also be present, and presumably all symptoms originate form foregut ischemia (27). It is thought that a fibrous band of the celiac plexus or of the diaphragmatic muscles compresses the celiac axis, especially during expiration, and causes ischemia.

CTA has improved the ability to obtain high-resolution images of the aorta and its branches, and it is useful for the diagnosis of MALS (28). With CTA, it is possible to clearly see the difference between a saccular aneurysm of the celiac trunk (Fig. 35.17) and the post-stenotic dilatation associated with a stenosis in MALS (Figs. 35.18 and 35.19).

Stenosis and occlusion: reno vascular hypertension, atherosclerosis, and fibromuscular dysplasia

In patients with suspected renovascular hypertension, it is the standard of care to assess all renal arteries for the presence of luminal stenosis (25). Recently, it was concluded that MDCTA studies have a sensitivity and specificity of 96% and 90%, respectively, to detect >50% renal artery stenosis (29). Thus, renal CTA provides a way to evaluate for renovascular hypertension (Figs. 35.20 and 35.21) (25). However, renal artery stenosis does not always cause hypertension, and, commonly, the diagnosis of renovascular hypertension is made only after the improvement that comes following surgical or interventional treatment.

In patients with fibromuscular dysplasia, there tends to be a web-like stenosis within the lumen of the artery. With improvements of CTA, however, it is suggested that CTA is the preferred imaging modality for diagnostic, screening, and procedure-guiding tasks in renal artery fibromuscular dysplasia. For detection, the sensitivity and specificity is 64% to 99% and 89% to 98%, respectively (30).

Inflammation: aortitis and arteriovenous malformation and fistula

Aortitis is a vasculitis of infectious or noninfectious origin of the vessel wall. It presents with nonspecific symptoms like pain, fever, weight loss, vascular insufficiency, and elevated acute phase reactant levels. Due to the ambiguity of these symptoms, imaging is often required to make the final diagnosis of aortitis. CTA can depict early changes in the vessel wall, such as thickening, thrombosis, stenosis, occlusion, vessel ectasia, aneurysms, and ulcers. Because the CTA uses iodinated contrast, it allows for the rapid exclusion of aortic pathologies that may clinically mimic acute aortitis. These include aortic dissection, intramural hematoma, and penetrating atherosclerotic ulcers (31).

Arteriovenous malformations (AVMs) are congenital communications between the arteries and veins with a vascular nidus that bypasses the capillary bed. Arteriovenous fistulas (AVFs) are a single direct communication between an artery and a vein (32). The majority of renal vascular abnormalities are AVFs, while AVMs are less common (>1%) (33). Congenital AVFs are high-flow shunts with enlarged compromised vessels, occasionally associated with venous aneurysms. Acquired AVFs are the most common and generally result from a penetrating trauma, percutaneous renal biopsy, surgery, malignancy, or inflammation. AVFs after percutaneous renal biopsy are reported to be as high as 18% (32). About 39% of AVFs are symptomatic, and the majority resolve spontaneously (32). If untreated, persistent AVFs will tend to have an increase in blood flow. Symptoms from both AVFs and AVMs vary from asymptomatic to hypertension with renal masses.

Primary aortoduodenal fistulas are a fatal cause of upper gastrointestinal hemorrhage. Although uncommon, an aortoduodenal fistula is usually due to pressure erosion of an abdominal aneurysm into the duodenum or complex atherosclerotic disease of the abdominal aorta, with a chronic inflammation and foreign body reaction. Symptoms include abdominal pain, gastrointestinal bleeding, and sepsis in 30% of patients. The preferred imaging modality for this type of fistula is also an MDCTA (34).

Contraindications

Contrast allergy

All iodinated contrast media are known to cause hypersensitivity reactions. It is thought that severe immediate reactions may be IgE-mediated, while most non-immediate skin reactions are T-cell mediated. The severity of the allergic response to the contrast determines the preparation for a CTA.

Please refer to the "Patient preparation" section earlier in this chapter for more details.

Renal dysfunction

As previously discussed, contrast material–induced renal failure is possible, especially in individuals with preexisting conditions such as diabetes mellitus or renal insufficiency (9). Medical centers have a cutoff value of creatinine levels above which a contrast study cannot be performed.

Pregnancy and breastfeeding

The physical and chemical effects of ionizing radiation results in cell death and DNA changes. With women who are pregnant, this can lead to growth retardation, congenital malformations, mental retardation, and even still birth. The effects of the radiation are dose dependent. These defects have been most detectable in high doses at weeks 3–4 and weeks 18–27 of menstrual age (35). Continued controversy and uncertainty regarding the preferred diagnostic imaging examination for acute distress in a pregnant patient still exists. The risks and benefits should be discussed with a pregnant woman before any imaging occurs (36). For a breastfeeding mother, pumping milk before a study for the use afterward is appropriate. Females younger than 35 years old should not undergo CTA unless comparable diagnostic imaging procedures that do not involve exposure to radiation have been considered.

Limitations and risks

Artifact

It is recommended that a negative oral contrast agent such as water be used, as a positive contrast agent can hinder the quality and lead to higher incidences of artifact. This appears as an area of active extravasation of contrast (23). Vessels adjacent to metal prostheses, such as joint replacements, are also not well visualized due to artifact.

Radiation exposure

The increased exposure to ionizing radiation during MDCT imaging should not go overlooked. Evidence has linked exposure to low-level ionizing radiation at doses used in medical imaging to the development of cancer. CT as a whole produces nearly half of the population's medical radiation exposure (37). MDCTA exposes a patient to more radiation than a patient undergoing a traditional CT. Care in using size-dependent protocols, enabling scanner dose-reduction tools, reducing the number of passes, and reducing duplicate coverage should be taken when the choice has been made to use this imaging modality (38). Radiation exposure standards still do not exist for pediatric cases, and this has put them at risk for excess exposure (39).

Dye infiltration

Contrast extravasation out of a catheter and vessel and into surrounding soft tissue can cause pain and swelling. For more information on risks and complications, please see Chapter 28.

Clinical images

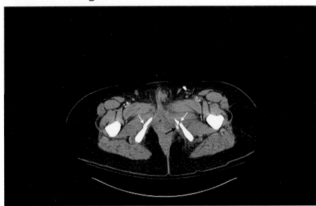

Figure 35.1. Axial CTA of the pelvis in a 29-year-old patient posttrauma/MVA showing bilateral pelvic fractures (*white arrows*). Note a focal round area (*black arrow*) of contrast accumulation adjacent to the left pelvic fracture consistent with a pseudoaneurysm or active arterial extravasation.

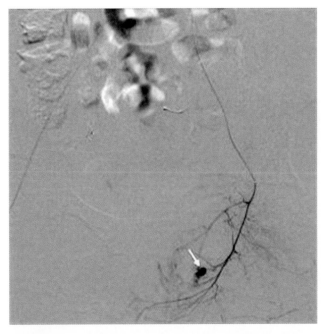

Figure 35.2. Superselective angiogram of the anterior subdivision of the left internal iliac artery demonstrating an area of pseudoaneurysm or active arterial extravasation (*white arrow*).

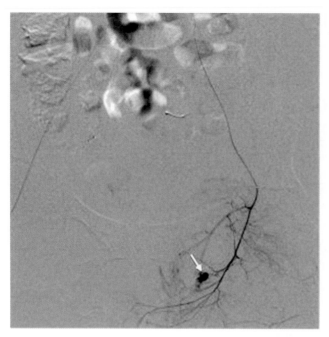

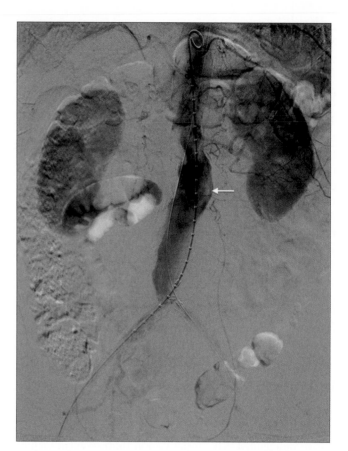

Figure 35.3. Angiogram status postcoil embolization of the anterior subdivision of the left anterior iliac artery demonstrating total occlusion of the target artery (*white arrow*) without opacification of the previously described pseudoaneurysm.

Figure 35.4. Abdominal aortic angiogram demonstrating a fusiform dilatation of the midabdominal aorta, consistent with AAA (*white arrow*).

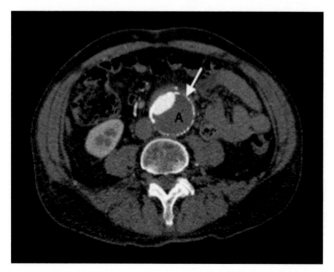

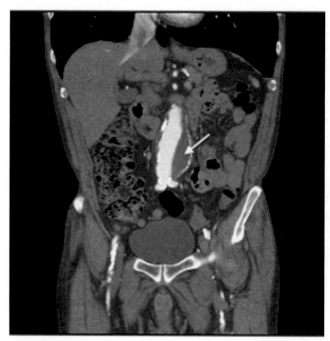

Figure 35.5. Axial arterial phase CT scan at level of midabdomen demonstrating a large abdominal aortic aneurysm measuring 5.6 cm in diameter (*white arrow*). Note the large eccentric mural thrombus within the lumen (A).

Figure 35.6. Coronal arterial phase postcontrast CT of the abdomen of the same patient (as in Fig. 35.5) demonstrates a large aneurysm, with eccentric mural thrombus (*white arrow*).

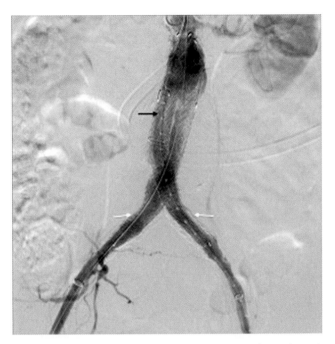

Figure 35.7. Abdominal aortic angiogram status post-endovascular aortic repair (EVAR) shows satisfactory placement of the main body (*black arrow*) stent graft with bilateral iliac limbs (*white arrows*).

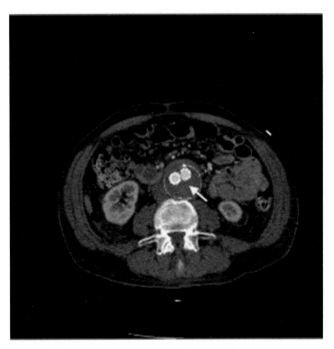

Figure 35.8. Axial arterial phase CT scan post-EVAR of the same patient (as in Fig. 35.7) shows satisfactory exclusion of the aneurysm sac (*white arrow*), with no contrast filling within the aneurysm sac to suggest endoleak.

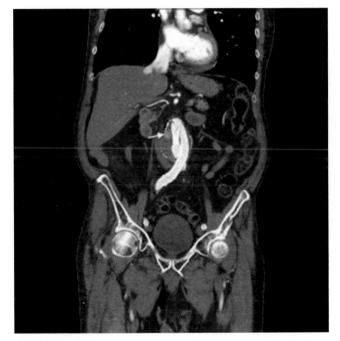

Figure 35.9. Coronal CTA of the abdomen status post-EVAR with endoleak. Note the dense contrast material within the aneurysm sac is consistent with endoleak (*white arrow*).

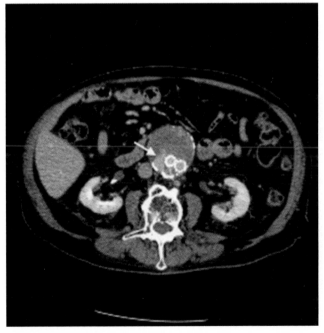

Figure 35.10. Axial venous phase CTA of the abdomen of the same patient (as in Fig. 35.9) demonstrating pooling of contrast within the aneurysm sac (*white arrow*) consistent with endoleak.

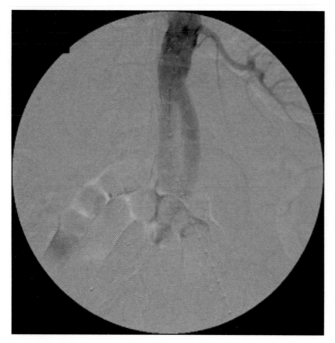

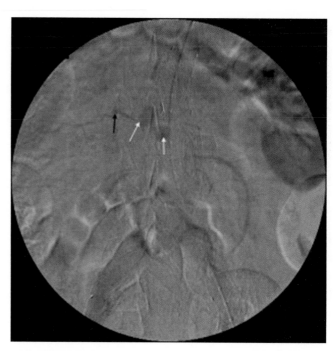

Figure 35.11. Early phase of abdominal aortic angiogram status post-EVAR of the same patient (as in Figs. 35.9 and 35.10), showing normal contrast enhancement of the abdominal aorta/main body of the stent graft and the bilateral iliac limbs.

Figure 35.12. Delayed phase of the abdominal aortic angiogram of the same patient (as in Fig. 35.11) status post-EVAR showing retrograde filling of the right lumbar artery (*black arrow*) contributing to the endoleak within the aneurysm sac (*white arrows*).

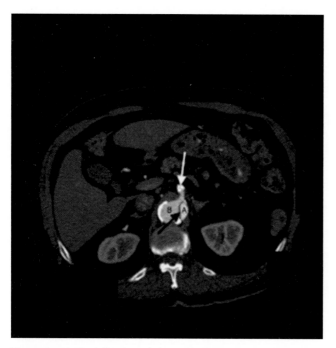

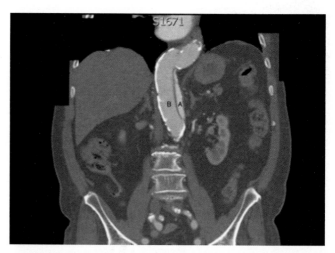

Figure 35.14. Coronal CTA of the abdomen of the same patient (as in Fig. 35.13) demonstrating the intimal flap consistent with aortic dissection. Again note the larger lumen with lower density of contrast representing the false lumen (B) and the smaller lumen with higher density of contrast representing the true lumen (A).

Figure 35.13. Axial CTA through the midabdomen demonstrates an abdominal aortic dissection (*black arrow*) causing two lumens within the abdominal aorta. The true lumen (A) is commonly of smaller size and with higher density of contrast. The false lumen (B), which is usually larger, is typically less dense relative to the true lumen. Note also that the false lumen is supplying the celiac trunk (*white arrow*).

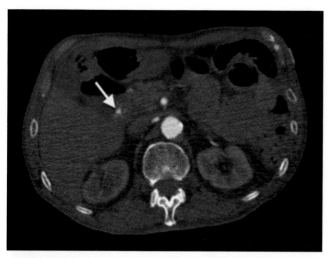

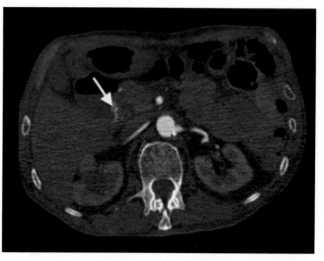

Figure 35.15. Axial CTA of the abdomen in a 76-year-old patient with a gastrointestinal bleed showing a rounded focus of contrast within the wall of the proximal duodenum (*white arrow*). This is consistent with a pseudoaneurysm as also confirmed during upper GI endoscopy to be located at the base of a duodenal ulcer.

Figure 35.16. Axial CTA of the same patient (as in Fig. 35.15) through the more distal aspect of the duodenum showing spillage and pooling of contrast leaking from the above-mentioned pseudoaneurysm within the duodenum (*white arrow*).

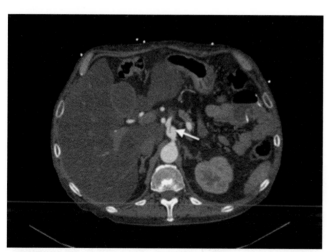

Figure 35.17. Axial arterial phase CT scan of the abdomen demonstrating a saccular aneurysm of the celiac trunk measuring 1.6 cm in diameter (*white arrow*). This is an incidental finding. Note also diffuse low-density appearance of the liver consistent with hepatic steatosis or diffuse fatty infiltration.

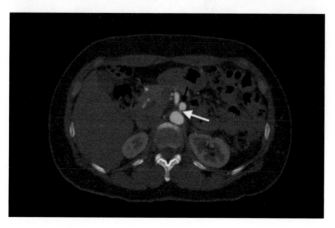

Figure 35.18. Axial CTA image of the abdomen showing severe stenosis of the proximal celiac artery (*white arrow*) with prominent post-stenotic dilatation (*black arrow*) in a patient with median arcuate ligament syndrome.

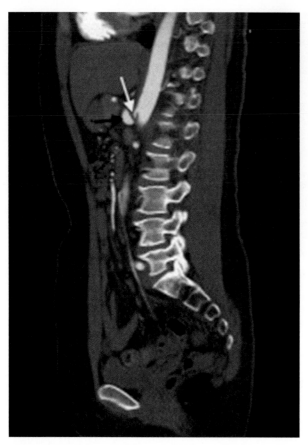

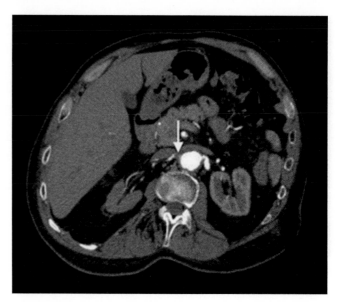

Figure 35.20. Axial CTA of the abdomen at the level of the renal arteries showing severe stenosis of the right renal artery at the ostial level (*white arrow*). Note the prominent chronic atrophy of the right kidney compared with the left kidney related to underlying hypoperfusion secondary to stenosis of the right renal artery as described.

Figure 35.19. Sagittal CTA image of the same patient (as in Fig. 35.18) at the level of the celiac artery origin showing severe stenosis (*white arrow*) of the proximal celiac artery with post-stenotic dilatation (*black arrow*). This is the classic appearance for median arcuate ligament syndrome.

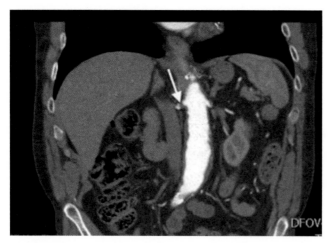

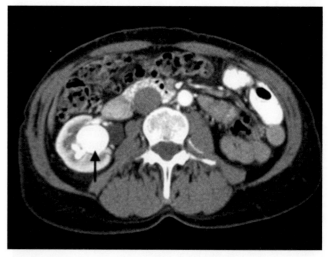

Figure 35.21. Coronal CTA of the abdomen of the same patient (as in Fig. 35.20) at the level of the renal arteries showing severe stenosis/occlusion of the right renal artery (*white arrow*).

Figure 35.22. Axial CTA of the abdomen through the level of the right kidney in a patient post–right kidney biopsy showing an area of arteriovenous fistula associated with a nidus in the region of the right renal hilum (*black arrow*). The patient had a kidney biopsy about 4 months earlier.

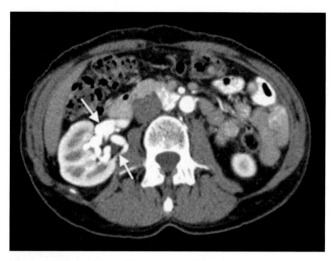

Figure 35.23. Axial CTA of the abdomen of the same patient (as in Fig. 35.22) showing early filling of the right renal veins (*white arrows*) due to direct communication between the artery and vein in the setting of underlying arteriovenous fistula.

Works Cited

1. Regine G, Stasolla A, Miele V: Multidetector computed tomography of the renal arteries in vascular emergencies. *Eur J Radiol* 2007;**64**(**1**):83–91.

2. Ptak T, Rhea JT, Novelline RA: Experience with a continuous, single-pass whole-body multidetector CT protocol for trauma: the three-minute multiple trauma CT scan. *Emergen Radiol* 2001;**8**(**5**):250–6.

3. Güven K, Acunaş B: Multidetector computed tomography angiography of the abdomen. *Eur J Radiol* 2004;**52**(**1**):44–55.

4. Feller I, Woodburne RT: Surgical anatomy of the abdominal aorta. *Ann Surg* 1961;**154**(**6**):239–52.

5. Lin PH, Chaikof EL: Embryology, anatomy, and surgical exposure of the great abdominal vessels. *Surg Clin N Am* 2000;**80**(**1**):417–33.

6. Moore KL: *Essential clinical anatomy*, 4th ed. Philadelphia: Lippincott Williams and Wilkins, 2010.

7. Ozkan U, Oğuzkurt L, Tercan F, et al.: Renal artery origins and variations: angiographic evaluation of 855 consecutive patients. *Diagn Interv Radiol* 2006;**12**(**4**):183–6.

8. Thomsen HS: Guidelines for contrast media from the European Society of Urogenital Radiology. *Am J Roen* 2003;**181**(**6**):1462–71.

9. Parfrey PS, Griffiths SM, Barrett BJ, et al.: Contrast material-induced renal failure in patients with diabetes mellitus, renal insufficiency, or both. *N Engl J Med* 1989;**320**:143–9.

10. Brockow K, Romano A, Aberer W, et al.: Skin testing in patients with hypersensitivity reactions to iodinated contrast media – a European multicenter study. *Allergy* 2009;**64**(**2**):234–41.

11. Brockow K, Christiansen C, Kanny G, et al. Management of hypersensitivity reactions to iodinated contrast media. *Allergy* 2005;**60**(**2**):150–8.

12. Budovec JJ, Pollema M, Grogan M: Update on multidetector computed tomography angiography of the abdominal aorta. *Radiol Clin N Am* 2010;**48**(**2**):283–309.

13. Maruyama T, Yoshizumi T, Tamura R, et al.: Comparison of eight- versus 16-slice multidetector-row computed tomography for visibility and image quality of coronary segments. *Am J Cardiol* 2004;**94**(**12**):1539–43.

14. Uyeda JW, Anderson SW, Sakai O, Soto JA: CT angiography in trauma. *Radiol Clin N Am* 2010;**48**(**2**):423–38.

15. Coll AR: Ultrasound surveillance of ectatic abdominal aortas. *Surg Engl* 2008;**90**(**6**):477–82.

16. Erbel R, Eggebrecht H: Aortic dimensions and the risk of dissection. *Heart* 2006;**92**(**1**):137–42.

17. Jeffrey RB Jr.: CT angiography of the abdominal and thoracic aorta. *Semin Ultrasound CT* 1998;**19**(**5**):405–12.

18. Borioni R, Garofalo M, De Paulis R, et al.: Abdominal aortic dissections: anatomic and clinical features and therapeutic options. *Tex Heart Inst J* 2005;**32**:70–3.

19. Nienaber CA, Eagle KA: Aortic dissection: new frontiers in diagnosis and management: part I: from etiology to diagnostic strategies. *Circulation* 2003;**108**:628–35.

20. Jonker FHW, Schlösser FJ, Moll FL, Muhs BE: Dissection of the abdominal aorta: current evidence and implications for treatment strategies: a review and meta-analysis of 92 patients. *J Endovasc Ther* 2009;**16**:71–80.

21. Horton KM, Fishman EK: CT angiography of the mesenteric circulation. *Radiol Clin N Am* 2012;**48**(**2**)331–45.

22. Lee EW, Laberge JM: Differential diagnosis of gastrointestinal bleeding. *Tech Vasc Interv Radiol* 2005;**7**(**3**):112–22.

23. McKinsey JF, Gewertz BL: Acute mesenteric ischemia. *Surg Clin North Am* 1997;**77**(**2**):307.

24. Wyers MC: Acute mesenteric ischemia: diagnostic approach and surgical treatment. *Semin Vasc Surg* 2010;**23**(**1**):9–20.

25. Fleischmann D: Multiple detector-row CT angiography of the renal and mesenteric vessels. *Eur J Radiol* 2003;**45**(**1**):S79–S87.

26. Scovell S, Hamdan A: *Celiac artery compression syndrome.* Waltham, MA: UpToDate, 2014.

27. Baldassarre E, Torino G, Siani A, et al.: The laparoscopic approach in the median arcuate ligament syndrome: a case report. *Swiss Med Wkly* 2007;**137**(**23–24**):353–4.

28. Gümüş H, Gümüş M, Tekbaş G, et al.: Clinical and multidetector computed tomography findings of patients with median arcuate ligament syndrome. *Clin Imag* 2012;**36**(**5**):522–5.

29. Pellerin O, Sapoval M, Trinquart L, et al.: Accuracy of multi-detector computed tomographic angiography assisted by post-processing software for diagnosis atheromatous renal artery stenosis. *Diagn Interv Imag* 2013;**94**(**11**):1123–31.

30. Sabharwal R, Vladica P, Coleman P: Multidetector spiral CT renal angiography in the diagnosis of renal artery fibromuscular dysplasia. *Eur J Radiol* 2007;**61**(**3**):520–7.

31. Litmanovich DE, Yildirim A, Bankier AA: Insights into imaging of aortitis. *Insights Imaging* 2012;**3**(**6**):545–60.

32. Cura M: Vascular malformations and arteriovenous fistulas of the kidney. *Acta Radiologica* 2009;**51**(**2**):144–9.

33. Wajid H, Herts BR: Renal arteriovenous malformation. *J Urol* 2014;**191**(4):1128–9.

34. Lemos AA, Sternberg JM, Tognini L, et al.: Nontraumatic abdominal hemorrhage: MDCTA. *Abdom Imaging* 2006;**31**(1):17–24.

35. Shetty MK: Abdominal computed tomography during pregnancy: a review of indications and fetal radiation exposure issues. *Semin Ultrasound CT* 2010;**31**(1):3–7.

36. Katz DS, Klein MA, Ganson G, Hines JJ: Imaging of abdominal pain in pregnancy. *Radiol Clin N Am* 2012;**50**(1):149–71.

37. Mettler FA, Bhargavan M, Faulkner K, et al.: Radiologic and nuclear medicine studies in the United States and worldwide: frequency, radiation dose, and comparison with other radiation sources – 1950–2007. *Radiology* 2009;**253**(2):520–31.

38. Sodickson A: Strategies for reducing radiation exposure in multi-detector row CT. *Radiol Clin N Am* 2012;**50**(1):1–14.

39. Naumann DN, Raven D, Pallan A, Bowley DM: Radiation exposure during paediatric emergency CT: time we took notice? *J Pediatr Surg* 2014;**49**(2):305–7.

Chapter 36

CT Angiography of the Head and Neck

Saud Siddiqui and Monica Wattana

Noninvasive imaging techniques are playing an ever-increasing role in the diagnosis and management of patients with lesions of the vascular structures of the head and neck. In addition to identifying the site and severity of stenosis, occlusion, or trauma, imaging of the vasculature of the head and neck can provide vital information regarding tissue injury and perfusion (location, size, and degree of reversibility or hypoperfusion). The choice of the imaging test depends on patient characteristics, the disease condition, the availability of technique and equipment, and the preference of the interpreting physician.

Increasingly, CT angiography (CTA) and magnetic resonance angiography (MRA) are replacing digital subtraction angiography (DSA) in the evaluation of cervicocranial vascular disorders. Evaluation of many vascular disorders is easily accomplished by either MRA or CTA, and the choice between the two may well rest on the availability of equipment or the preference of the interpreter. In many instances, DSA may be reserved for occasions when CTA and MRA findings are equivocal or not consistent with clinical symptoms. In the case of CTA, the rapid availability of information allows the astute physician to triage patients to appropriate therapies quickly, when the opportunity to treat patients with salvageable tissue who may benefit most from acute therapies is greatest. In one scanning session, CTA can provide information regarding early ischemic changes, demonstrate hypoperfusion/ischemic penumbra, and locate vascular lesions. In addition, because most CTA studies follow established technical parameters for acquisition of data, the level of ability or experience of the operator has a relatively small effect on the quality of the clinical information provided by such studies.

In comparison with catheter angiography, what CTA gives up in resolution and dynamic properties, it makes up for with rapid acquisition of a 3D dataset and the potential for assessment of whole-brain perfusion. Moreover, CTA illustrates not only arterial stenosis or occlusion but also the vessel wall. This factor is most pertinent in the assessment of intramural dissection and thrombosed aneurysms, both of which may complicate evaluation of stroke patients. Most important, CTA is minimally invasive when compared with conventional angiography, and because CTA uses a peripheral venous contrast injection, there is a reduced risk of local hematoma, pseudoaneurysm, spasm, thrombosis, dissection, and distal embolization when compared with the arterial puncture required for conventional angiography.

The 3D reconstructions produced by CTA are similar to those obtained with MRA, and the short imaging time of CTA may improve patient compliance when compared with MRA (especially in the claustrophobic patient). Unlike MRA, CTA can provide information about the presence of calcifications within atherosclerotic plaques, a feature that may be valuable to the physician performing angioplasty. Another area in which CTA is superior to MRA is in depiction of the relationship of intracranial aneurysms to adjacent bony structures. Of course, CT remains indispensable where there are contraindications to MRI, such as pacemakers and patient intolerance due to anxiety or motion.

Multimodal CT techniques – that is, scans that employ noncontrast CT, CT perfusion (CTP) imaging, and CTA – can rapidly provide data regarding the state of vascular anatomy and tissues in the head and neck and thereby allow physicians to streamline the care of the hyperacute patient. CTA and CTP can be performed immediately after conventional CT scanning, while the patient is still in the scanner, requiring only 5 to 10 minutes of additional time. Although detailed quantitative assessment of tissue perfusion is still evolving, CTP offers the advantages of assessing both reversible and irreversible ischemia through the generation of maps of cerebral blood volume, cerebral blood flow, and contrast mean transit time.

In addition to providing information about the severity of ischemia, CTP can be used to differentiate the core infarcted area from ischemic penumbra and to predict tissue outcome (1). Thus, CTA and CTP may aid the physician in identifying those regions of salvageable brain tissue, which may be amenable to reperfusion therapy. An alternative method involves the use of source images of CTA (CTA-SI) to produce whole-brain perfused cerebral blood volume-weighted images. This is attractive in that it provides some crude perfusion data and predicts final infarct volume better than noncontrast CT (NCCT) (2). It has been shown that CTA-SI rapid protocol for acute stroke overestimates infarct size compared with diffuse weighted imaging (DWI) on MR (3), obviating the need for further studies. Compared with CTA-SI, perfusion-weighted map (PWM) and perfused blood volume (PBV) have been shown to have similar performance, with PBV showing higher sensitivity for detecting infarct (4).

Indications

CTA of the head and neck is perhaps most useful in the management of patients who present with signs and symptoms of acute stroke; where the use of IV recombinant tissue plasminogen activator must be considered; in patients with suspected rupture of intracranial aneurysms or subarachnoid hemorrhage; and in patients who present posttrauma with penetrating neck injuries, where the decision must be made between managing the patient medically or surgically. In addition, conditions that can mimic stroke such as seizures, metabolic abnormalities, and nonorganic conditions may be difficult to distinguish from acute brain ischemia on purely clinical grounds. CTA is thus valuable as a diagnostic study that is widely available, rapid, and easily interpretable and therefore is of great value in triaging patients to appropriate therapies.

Ischemic and hemorrhagic stroke

Stroke is now the fourth most common cause of death and the most common cause of disability in the United States. Suspected stroke is triaged with the same importance of severe trauma or acute myocardial infarction (5). The time-critical nature of this disease has been shown in many studies, with dexterous management having been shown to significantly improve outcome and lower the chances of the hemorrhagic complications (6–16). Timely and accurate imaging is necessary in guiding admission, anticoagulation, thrombolysis, and other forms of treatment.

Risk factors for stroke include age older than 45 years, hypertension, previous stroke or transient ischemic attack, diabetes mellitus, high cholesterol, cigarette smoking, atrial fibrillation, migraine with aura, and thrombophilia. Key components of a history include the time course of the onset of symptoms; seizure activity; any recent events (stroke, myocardial infarction, trauma, surgery, bleeding); comorbid diseases (most importantly, hypertension and diabetes mellitus); and the use of anticoagulants, insulin, or antihypertensives. Physical exam of the head and neck may reveal signs of trauma or seizure (contusions or lacerations), carotid bruits, or jugular venous distention. If there is clinical suspicion of acute stroke, a thorough neurological exam should be performed immediately. Exam of other systems is most likely to reveal comorbid conditions such as myocardial ischemia, valvular conditions, jaundice, purpura, and petechia.

The presentations of stroke are manifold, and the initial evaluation of suspected ischemic or hemorrhagic stroke requires a rapid, but broad, assessment. The most common cause of hemorrhagic stroke is subarachnoid hemorrhage, the classic presentation of which is sudden onset of a severe headache, often described as "the worst headache of my life" or a "thunder-clap" headache, in the absence of focal neurological deficit. The onset of the headache may be associated with a brief loss of consciousness, seizure, nausea, vomiting, buckling of the knees, or stiff neck. In distinction, intracerebral hemorrhage typically presents with the abrupt onset of focal neurological deficit that worsens steadily over 30 to 90 minutes. Altered level of consciousness, stupor, coma, seizure, headache, vomiting, and signs of increased intracranial

pressure are also common. Although these presentations are familiar to most physicians, it is also clear that the constellation of symptoms with which hemorrhagic stroke may present are many and varied, can be quite vague, and thus require a keen eye on the part of the diagnostician.

The most common cause of ischemic stroke is atherosclerosis, with or without superimposed thrombosis; an embolic cause of ischemic stroke is much less common. The most relevant historical item in distinguishing between embolic and atherosclerotic ischemic stroke subtypes is the time course of neurological symptoms. The neurological deficits of stroke related to atherosclerosis and thrombosis often occur in a progressive but fluctuating manner, with symptoms occurring and remitting sporadically. The central feature of acute embolic stroke is one of sudden focal neurological deficit, with the severity of symptoms being maximal at onset. Rapid recovery from symptoms also points to an embolic cause. The patient with either type of ischemic stroke classically awakens from sleep with the neurological deficit (which may make determination of time of onset difficult), but symptoms may appear at any time. The clinical features of the presentation of ischemic stroke depend on the artery that is occluded, with the middle cerebral artery (MCA) being most common. Neurological deficits seen with involvement of the MCA include, but are not limited to, contralateral hemiplegia and hemisensory loss, aphasia (if the dominant hemisphere is involved) or dysarthria, apraxia, and contralateral body neglect.

The mean arterial pressure of patients with acute stroke is usually elevated, which may represent chronic hypertension or a physiological response to hypoperfusion of the central nervous system. The latter of these two etiologies must be considered when making treatment decisions, which is to say that one must be wary of a decline in neurological function when blood pressure is lowered. Patients with acute stroke may also present with hypoventilation and resultant hypercapnia, which can produce a deleterious increase in intracranial pressure and may require artificial ventilation.

CTA is of particular use in identifying subtle, early potential sources of embolism or low flow in ischemic stroke, as well as in detecting possible aneurysms or vessel malformations in hemorrhagic stroke, all of which may affect decisions about treatment. Signs of large or evolved infarction are correlated with a higher risk of hemorrhagic transformation after treatment with thrombolytic agents and are thus contraindications to such treatment. Neuroimaging with CTA or CTP may improve the selection of patients to be treated with reperfusion therapies by identifying regions of salvageable brain tissue, a low risk for hemorrhagic transformation, or occlusions of large arteries that may or may not be amenable to therapy. The information provided by CTA regarding the precise site of vascular occlusion and the patency of major sources of collateral flow may in fact make it possible to immediately target the vessel of interest and, thereby, avoid the need for other tests that may further delay thrombolytic administration. If perfusion imaging is unable to demonstrate territories at risk for infarction, it may be that the risk of hemorrhage outweighs the potential for benefit from thrombolysis. Imaging done prior to the administration of thrombolytic agents should address this question. Also, by detecting persistent occlusion after thrombolytic treatment, CTA may expedite patient triage to catheter-based interventions.

The American Heart Association and American Stroke Association's 2013 guidelines regarding the use of CT in the evaluation of patients with acute stroke state that, for patients who are candidates for reperfusion therapy, the goal is to complete the CT (noncontrast CT or multimodal CT) examination within 25 minutes of arrival at the ED, with study interpretation occurring within an additional 20 minutes (5). For patients with symptoms of ischemic stroke that occurred or have persisted for several days to weeks, CTA of the head and neck without perfusion imaging, followed by conventional brain MRI, may be most useful. CTP is not generally needed because most available treatments for patients in this clinical scenario do not involve perfusion data input (e.g., carotid endarterectomy), but individual cases may vary.

Trauma

For patients who suffer traumatic injuries to the head or neck, there is little controversy regarding the management of those who are hemodynamically unstable or those who present with direct evidence of vascular injury – surgical exploration or intervention is generally agreed on. However, controversy remains with regard to the management of patients with stable vital signs where the low yield of both surgical exploration and conventional angiography, as well as the morbidity associated with each, begs for a more conservative approach (17–20).

CTA is accurate, more rapid, less expensive, and requires less staffing than surgical exploration or conventional angiography. In other words, CTA is a cost- and time-effective method for the acquisition of angiographic data that are easy to integrate into rapid trauma workup. Often, patients with signs of vascular injury on CTA may be taken directly to surgery without further imaging or conventional angiography. In addition, postprocessing techniques available with CTA allow for 3D reconstructions that may be useful in surgical planning, especially those reconstructions that resemble the conventional angiogram images familiar to many surgeons. The caveat to CTA in this setting is that, although CTA has been shown to be useful in the evaluation of penetrating trauma of the head and neck, the utility of CTA in the management of blunt trauma is more equivocal.

Carotid or vertebral artery dissection is most commonly caused by blunt (severe hyperextension) or penetrating (stab or gunshot wound) trauma, but it may also be spontaneous and has been associated with certain risk factors, including hypertension, diabetes mellitus, smoking, hyperlipidemia, and prolonged hyperextension or lateral rotation of the cervical spine. The pathogenesis of spontaneous dissections is frequently unknown but may be related to certain connective diseases, including fibromuscular dysplasia, Ehlers–Danlos type IV, Marfan syndrome, autosomal dominant polycystic kidney disease, osteogenesis imperfecta type I, and cystic medial necrosis. Patients with arterial dissection typically present with headache (usually preceding a cerebral ischemic event, unlike the headache of stroke, which accompanies or follows the ischemic event), episodic blindness (amaurosis fugax), ptosis with miosis and pain (i.e., a painful partial Horners syndrome), neck swelling, or pulsatile tinnitus. Conventional arteriography remains the gold standard for diagnosis of dissection, but, for the reasons already given, a less invasive study is desirable when appropriate. In the hemodynamically stable patient, MRI and MRA usually show superior soft tissue contrast and have a higher sensitivity for detection of ischemia (21) and thus may be the preferable noninvasive study for arterial dissection. When a more rapid workup is needed, or when there is a contraindication to MRI or a lack of availability of equipment, CTA is indicated.

Diagnostic capabilities

Ischemic and hemorrhagic stroke

It is important to have a triage mechanism that can quickly distinguish patients who are truly experiencing cerebral ischemia or hemorrhage from patients who present with similar symptoms but are not experiencing a stroke. Initial noncontrast-enhanced CT (NECT) followed immediately by CTA and CTP provides a rapid yet thorough assessment of potential intracranial hemorrhage, large evolved infarct, arterial clot and stenosis, infarct size and location, and penumbra. The traditional reason for performing noncontrast CT initially is to exclude hemorrhage and obvious non-infarct disorders (e.g., tumor). Although useful in this regard, noncontrast CT may also yield signs leading directly to a diagnosis of infarct. Note that initial NECT is also helpful to rule out stroke mimics. A recent study showed at least 3% of patients with stroke mimics have been treated by mistake with intravenous tPA (22). This percentage should be lower with the use of NECT alone (5).

Rapid availability of MRI may tempt the physician to use MRI in lieu of CT scanning in the evaluation of acute stroke, but in most situations, multimodal CT scanning can be performed before the patient is cleared and prepared for MRI. CT methods may, in fact, provide more useful data, such as increased vessel detail, as described previously. Nevertheless, a recent study has shown that MRI is superior in detecting acute ischemia and chronic hemorrhage in emergency situations when compared with CTA. MRI had a sensitivity of 83% and CT of 26% for any acute stroke (22). This suggests possible increased use of MRI as an initial imaging modality in evaluating cases of suspected acute cerebral ischemia even in emergencies.

Various studies have shown that CTA, when compared with DSA, has sensitivities between 92% and 100% and specificities of 82% to 100% in identifying stenosis or occlusion of large intracerebral vessels (23). In addition, systematic reviews of the literature have concluded that CTA compared with conventional angiography is an accurate method for diagnosis of 70% to 99% carotid artery stenosis (24, 25). Sensitivity and specificity have ranged from 77% to 97% and 95% to 99%, respectively. This is an important conclusion given the implication that CTA, used cautiously, may replace the more invasive conventional angiography and that certain authors recommend surgery for asymptomatic patients with 60% to 99% stenosis and for symptomatic patients with 50% to 99% stenosis. CTA has also been found to have a superior sensitivity of 97% when compared with MRA (92%–95%) and color Doppler ultrasonography (76%) in evaluating degree of carotid artery stenosis (26). Compared with DSA, CTA has shown a sensitivity of at least 89% for detecting flow abnormalities in the circle of Willis (27). In addition, CTA has shown to have a sensitivity of 100% in identifying vertebral artery dissection, when compared with MRA at 77% and Doppler ultrasonography at 71%, when using DSA as the reference (28).

CTA, in combination with either CTP or CTA-SI, has been shown to be accurate in the detection of cerebral ischemia, with a sensitivity and specificity of at least 78% and 93%, respectively, when compared with follow-up CT or MRI (29–31). These tests have also demonstrated a high sensitivity and specificity (>0.90) in the evaluation of stroke extent as estimated by ASPECTS score. In addition, it seems that these techniques are equivalent to diffusion- and perfusion-weighted MRI in the assessment of acute cerebral perfusion deficit (30–33), but they are free of the logistical considerations inherent to MRI.

Rupture of an intracranial aneurysm is a leading cause of nontraumatic subarachnoid hemorrhage (SAH), which carries a very poor prognosis – a case fatality rate between 27% and 44% within 30 days of initial bleed (34). Surgical intervention is directed at minimizing the occurrence of rebleeding, the risk of which is highest in the 24 hours after initial hemorrhage; thus, if indicated, surgical intervention should be performed as soon as possible. Although neither achieves the resolution of conventional angiography, CTA and MRA are both noninvasive tests that are useful for screening and presurgical planning after diagnosis of SAH by noncontrast CT. In the acute stages of SAH, MRA is less appropriate than CTA due to constraints that MRA may place on patient monitoring, motion artifacts from patient movement, and the need to move the patient to an MR suite after performance of a noncontrast CT. As one might ascertain, while the patient is still in the scanner, CTA can immediately follow the initial noncontrast CT with which the diagnosis of SAH has been made. Additional scan time is minimal, and CTA has been shown to reliably detect aneurysms 3 to 5 mm or larger (35–37), which often obviates the need for conventional angiography and the associated complications and costs.

In addition, CTA has been shown to provide more information than conventional angiography regarding the shape of an aneurysm, its relationship to surrounding bony and vasculature structures, and the characteristics of the neck of the aneurysm (particularly the presence of calcifications and its relationship to the skull). This 3D information can be very useful in surgical planning. For these reasons, CTA is increasingly used in lieu of conventional angiography in patients with suspected or known SAH. The sensitivity and specificity of CTA for the detection of aneurysms 3 mm or larger, with conventional angiography as the standard, are greater than 93% and 88%, respectively, with numerous reports, including unity in their estimation of both (35, 37, 38). The accuracy of CTA in the detection of aneurysms smaller than 3 mm is less established, and although transcranial Doppler ultrasound may improve diagnostic performance, aneurysms of this size may not be reliably detected. A more recent meta-analysis that included data from newer generation CT scanners found CTA to have a pooled sensitivity of 98% and specificity of 100% when identifying cerebral aneurysms in patients presenting with SAH, using findings at treatment and autopsy as the reference standard (39).

Trauma

Many patients who present with signs of trauma to the head, neck, or great vessels receive noncontrast CT imaging as part of the initial diagnostic workup, making the utility of CTA in patients with suspected vascular injury due to trauma potentially quite large. As discussed previously, CTA can be performed after initial noncontrast CT while the patient is still in the scanner. In addition, CTA provides diagnostic information about adjacent structures, such as the cervical spine and aerodigestive tract, which one cannot expect from conventional angiography. CTA may be preferable to ultrasound in many instances because of greater emergent availability of equipment and operator skill, while concerns over metallic foreign bodies as well as the logistic feasibility of performing MRI in acutely injured patients may preclude the use of MRI or MRA in some cases.

In comparison with the gold standard of conventional arteriography, CTA has been shown to be both highly sensitive and specific (values range from 90% to 100%) in the diagnosis of all vascular and aerodigestive tract injuries caused by penetrating trauma (40–42). As noted previously, the utility of CTA in blunt trauma is more equivocal; CTA has not yet been shown to be a viable substitute for cerebral angiography. Previous studies with 16- and 32-channel CTA have shown poor and variable sensitivities when detecting blunt cerebrovascular injury (BCVI). Nevertheless, a recent study showed that 64-multichannel CTA showed a sensitivity of 68%, a marked improvement from previous studies. This suggests that CTA may play a larger role as a screening tool for BCVI (43). The discrepancy in the diagnostic capability of CTA for injuries caused by penetrating and blunt trauma might be because injuries caused by penetrating trauma are usually close to the visualized injury tract, whereas vascular injuries related to blunt trauma may occur anywhere along the course of the carotid or vertebral arteries.

498

Imaging pitfalls and limitations

Technical factors such as slice thickness, length of coverage, kilovolt and milliampere settings, and bolus delay time can influence the accuracy and speed with which a CTA is obtained. For example, studies may be less than optimal if the bolus delay time is not adjusted such that the time of scanning coincides with the time of peak intraarterial contrast concentration. Technical specifications are especially important in the use of perfusion maps generated using CT, where motion artifact may not only make the maps uninterpretable but may also lead to erroneous interpretation. Although scanners from different manufacturers may vary slightly in the combination of technical specifications that produce optimum studies, many of these specifications are provided or known, and CTA alone usually represents a relatively low technical burden on both operator and patient.

Because CTA requires an iodinated contrast bolus, known or suspected renal failure is a relative contraindication for its use. This is especially true in patients with diabetes or congestive heart failure. Allergy to the contrast material may also preclude the use of CTA. If either factor emerges as a contraindication to CTA, triage of the patient to MRI, gadolinium-based CT imaging, or catheter angiography may be indicated.

The radiation dose administered during CTA is comparable to that of conventional angiography and is within the safe limits for diagnostic radiological assessments for adults. Concern may arise with multiple repeat scans, where the most likely adverse effect of radiation exposure is cataract formation or thyroid malignancy. Care should also be exercised in children and pregnant women, where the risks of radiation exposure from CT scanning are, to a large extent, unknown, but certain studies have shown an increased risk for malignancy or retardation (44).

Stroke

As discussed previously, CTA can be very useful in the emergent imaging and diagnosis of stroke. However, conventional angiography may still be required after CTA in certain cases. These include dissecting aneurysms where information about true and false lumens is desired; aneurysms where CTA is unable to demonstrate the nature of certain small arteries (conventional angiography has higher spatial resolution, and CTA does not always delineate arteries less than 1 mm in diameter); and aneurysms located in close proximity to the skull base, where it may be difficult to distinguish them amidst

bony structures. The performance of DSA after a questionable CTA requires the administration of greater amounts of potentially nephrotoxic contrast. However, this may be well tolerated in the setting of good renal function, adequate hydration, and possible pre- and postimaging diuretic treatment.

In the case of aneurysms that are directed inferiorly and are located close to the skull base, it may be necessary to carefully remove the bone from image reconstructions, which is a time-consuming process. This could potentially delay treatment in a setting where such a delay could have far-reaching implications. As mentioned in the "Diagnostic capabilities" section earlier in this chapter, it should also be kept in mind that CTA is relatively insensitive for the detection of aneurysms less than 3 mm.

Trauma

Artifacts produced by bullet or other metallic fragments may limit the utility of CTA in the setting of penetrating trauma of the neck. Lack of visualization of an arterial segment because of an artifact should be considered an indication for conventional angiogram. Conventional angiography also has the advantage of allowing for therapeutic interventions immediately following diagnosis, whereas CTA only provides information for triage to endovascular therapy.

Clinical images

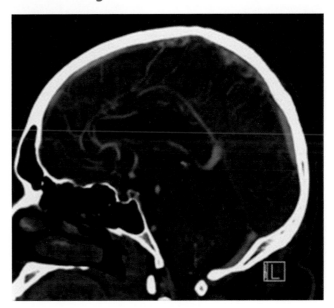

Figure 36.1. Normal CT angiogram of the head.

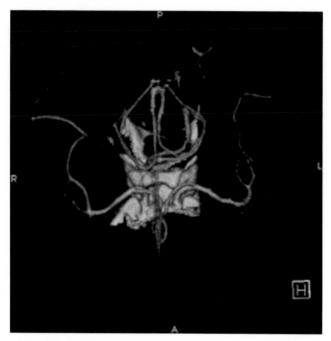

Figure 36.2. Normal 3D reconstruction done from CT angiogram of the head.

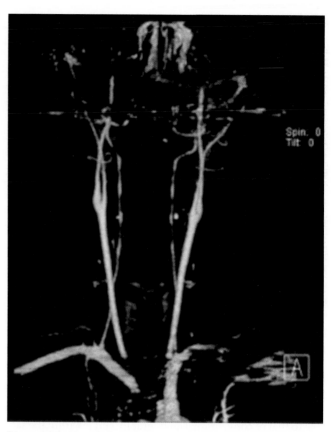

Figure 36.3. Normal 3D reconstruction done from CT angiogram of the neck.

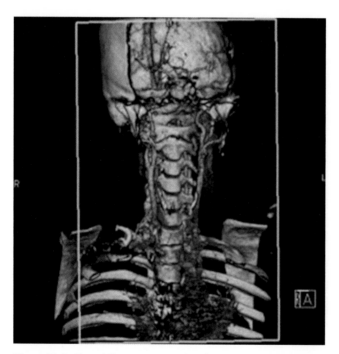

Figure 36.4. Normal 3D reconstruction done from CT angiogram of the neck with bony structures.

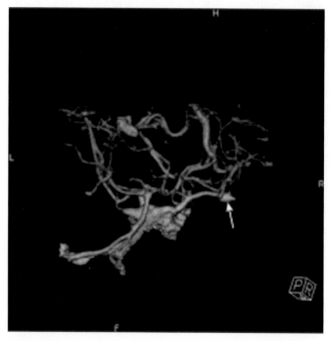

Figure 36.5. Aneurysm of the right middle cerebral artery bifurcation measuring approximately 3 × 7 mm. A nipple that extends into the apparent right temporal lobe hematoma suggestive of dissecting aneurysm.

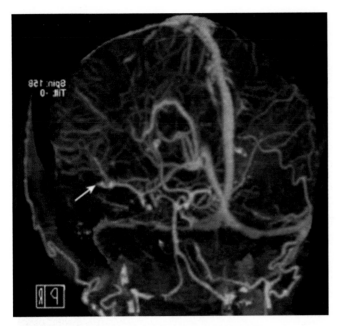

Figure 36.6. Slice view of the same aneurysm in Figure 36.5.

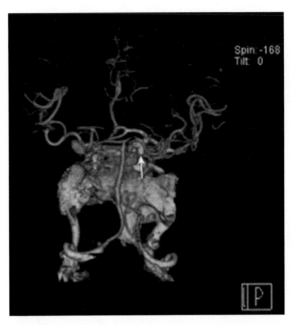

Figure 36.7. An aneurysm of the right internal carotid artery at the level of the right posterior communicating artery projecting posteriorly and inferiorly measuring 6 mm. The neck measures 4 mm.

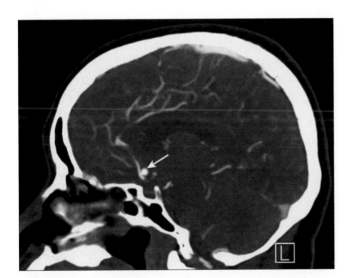

Figure 36.8. Sagittal section of a 0.6 cm aneurysm in the anterior communicating artery.

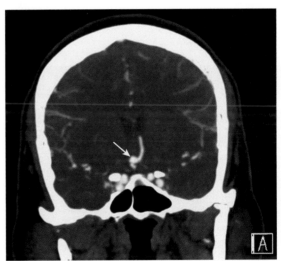

Figure 36.9. Coronal section of same aneurysm in Figure 36.8.

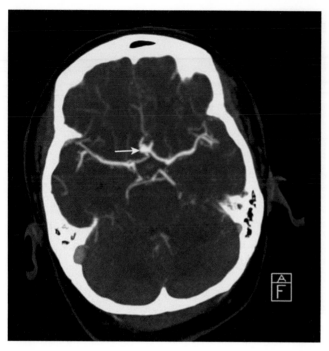

Figure 36.10. Transverse section of same aneurysm in Figs. 36.8 and 36.9.

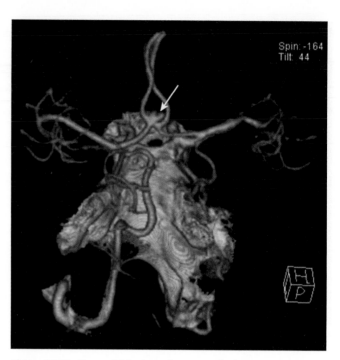

Figure 36.11. Six mm bilobed anterior communicating artery aneurysm.

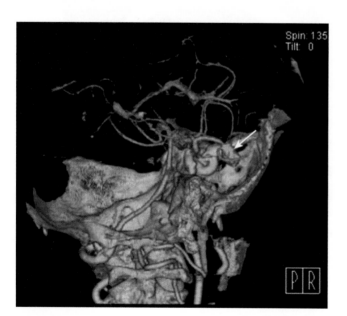

Figure 36.12. 3D view of large right middle cerebral artery bifurcation aneurysm measuring 1.1 cm by 0.7 cm and surrounding structures.

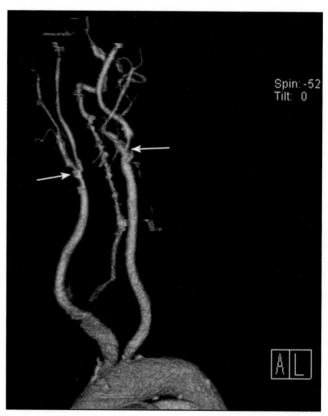

Figure 36.13. Eighty-five percent stenosis at the bifurcation of the left carotid artery. Seventy-five percent stenosis at the bifurcation of the right carotid artery. There is a large amount of vascular calcification.

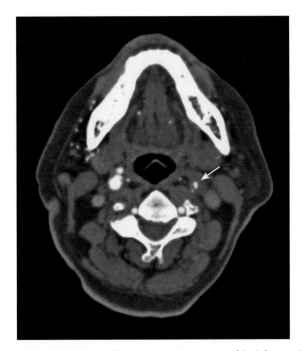

Figure 36.14. Eighty-five percent to 90% stenosis of the left carotid artery at the bifurcation.

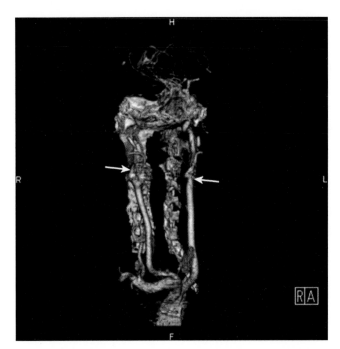

Figure 36.15. Eighty-five percent stenosis of the right internal carotid artery – of the proximal, mid, and distal portions. Tubular narrowing extends to the cavernous portion of the right internal carotid artery.

References

1. Parsons MW, Pepper EM, Chan V, et al.: Perfusion computed tomography: prediction of final infarct extent and stroke outcome. *Ann Neurol* 2005;**58**(5):672–9.

2. Bhatia R, Bal S, Shobha N, et al.: CT angiographic source images predict outcome and final infarct volume better than noncontrast CT in proximal vascular occlusions. *Stroke* 2011;**42**(6):1575–80.

3. Yoo A, Hu R, Hakimelahi R, et al.: CT Angiography source images acquired with a fast-acquisition protocol overestimate infarct core on diffusion weighted images in acute ischemic stroke. *J Neuroimaging* 2012;**22**(4):329–35.

4. Buerke B, Wittkamp G, Dziewas R, et al.: Perfusion-weighted map and perfused blood volume in comparison with CT angiography source imaging in acute ischemic stroke: different sides of the same coin? *Acad Radiol* 2011;**18**(3):347–52.

5. Jauch E, Saver J, Adams H, et al.: Guidelines for the early management of patients with acute ischemic stroke: a guideline for healthcare professionals from the American Heart Association/ American Stroke Association. *Stroke* 2013;**44**(3):870–947.

6. Albers GW, Amarenco P, Easton JD, et al.: Antithrombotic and thrombolytic therapy for ischemic stroke. *Chest* 2004;**126**(3):483S–512S.

7. Vo KD, Lin WL, Lee JM: Evidence-based neuroimaging in acute ischemic stroke. *Neuroimaging Clin N Am* 2003;**13**(2):167.

8. Grunwald I, Reith W: Non-traumatic neurological emergencies: imaging of cerebral ischemia. *Eur Radiol* 2002;**12**(7):1632–47.

9. Rother J: CT and MRI in the diagnosis of acute stroke and their role in thrombolysis. *Thromb Res* 2001;**103**:S125–33.

10. Lev MH, Segal AZ, Farkas J, et al.: Utility of perfusion-weighted CT imaging in acute middle cerebral artery stroke treated with intra-arterial thrombolysis – prediction of final infarct volume and clinical outcome. *Stroke* 2001;**32**(9):2021–7.

11. Lev MH, Farkas J, Rodriguez VR, et al.: CT angiography in the rapid triage of patients with hyperacute stroke to intraarterial thrombolysis: accuracy in the detection of large vessel thrombus. *J Comput Assist Tomogr* 2001;**25**(4):520–8.

12. Adams HP, del Zoppo G, Alberts MJ, et al.: Guidelines for the early management of adults with ischemic stroke – a guideline from the American Heart Association/American Stroke Association Stroke Council, Clinical Cardiology Council, Cardiovascular Radiology and Intervention Council, and the Atherosclerotic Peripheral Vascular Disease and Quality of Care Outcomes in Research Interdisciplinary Working Groups. *Circulation* 2007;**115**(20):E478–534. (Reprinted from *Stroke* 2007;38:1655–711.)

13. Laloux P: Intravenous rtPA thrombolysis in acute ischemic stroke. *Acta Neurol Belg* 2001;**101**(2):88–95.

14. Warach S: New imaging strategies for patient selection for thrombolytic and neuroprotective therapies. *Neurology* 2001;**57**(5):S48–52.

15. Wildermuth S, Knauth M, Brandt T, et al.: Role of CT angiography in patient selection for thrombolytic therapy in acute hemispheric stroke. *Stroke* 1998;**29**(5):935–8.

16. Suwanwela N, Koroshetz WJ: Acute ischemic stroke: overview of recent therapeutic developments. *Ann Rev Med* 2007;**58**:89–106.

17. Mittal VK, Paulson TJ, Colaiuta E, et al.: Carotid artery injuries and their management. *J Cardiovasc Surg* 2000;**41**(3):423–31.

18. Azuaje RE, Jacobson LE, Glover J, et al.: Reliability of physical examination as a predictor of vascular injury after penetrating neck trauma. *Am Surg* 2003;**69**(9):804–7.

19. Asensio JA, Valenziano CP, Falcone RE, Grosh JD: Management of penetrating neck injuries – the controversy surrounding zone-injuries. *Surg Clin North Am* 1991;**71**(2): 267–96.

20. Willinsky RA, Taylor SM, TerBrugge K, et al.: Neurologic complications of cerebral angiography: prospective analysis of 2,899 procedures and review of the literature. *Radiology* 2003;**227**(2):522–8.

21. Stringaris K: Three-dimensional time-of-flight MR angiography and MR imaging versus conventional angiography in carotid artery dissections. *Int Angiol* 1996;**15**(1):20–5.

22. Spokoyny I, Raman R, Ernstrom K, et al.: Imaging negative stroke: diagnoses and outcomes in IV t-PA treated patients. *J Stroke Cerebrovasc Dis* 2014;**23**(5):1046–50.

23. Chalela J, Kidwell C, Nentwich L, et al.: Magnetic resonance imaging and computed tomography in emergency assessment of patients with suspected acute stroke: a prospective comparison. *Lancet* 2007;**369**(9558):293–8.

24. Latchaw R, Alberts M, Lev M, et al. Recommendations for imaging of acute ischemic stroke a scientific statement from the American Heart Association. *Stroke* 2009;**40**(11):3646–78.

25. Wardlaw JM, Chappell FM, Best JJ, et al.: Noninvasive imaging compared with intra-arterial angiography in the diagnosis of symptomatic carotid stenosis: a meta-analysis. *Lancet* 2006;**367** (9521):1503–12.

26. Koelemay MJW, Nederkoorn PJ, Reitsma JB, Majoie CB: Systematic review of computed tomographic angiography for assessment of carotid artery disease. *Stroke* 2004;**35**(10): 2306–12.

27. Anzidei M, Napoli A, Zaccagna F, et al.: Diagnostic accuracy of colour Doppler ultrasonography, CT angiography and blood-pool-enhanced MR angiography in assessing carotid stenosis: a comparative study with DSA in 170 patients. *La Radiologia Medica* 2012;**117**(1):54–71.

28. Katz DA, Marks MP, Napel SA, et al.: Circle of Willis – evaluation with spiral CT angiography, MR-angiography, and conventional angiography. *Radiology* 1995;**195**(2):445–9.

29. Gottesman R, Sharma P, Robinson K, et al.: Imaging characteristics of symptomatic vertebral artery dissection: a systematic review. *Neurologist* 2012;**18**(5):255–60.

30. Kloska SP, Nabavi DG, Gaus C, et al.: Acute stroke assessment with CT: do we need multimodal evaluation? *Radiology* 2004;**233**(1):79–86.

31. Schramm P, Schellinger PD, Klotz E, et al.: Comparison of perfusion computed tomography and computed tomography angiography source images with perfusion-weighted imaging and diffusion-weighted imaging in patients with acute stroke of less than 6 hours' duration. *Stroke* 2004;**35**(7):1652–7.

32. Wintermark M, Fischbein NJ, Smith WS, et al.: Accuracy of dynamic perfusion CT with deconvolution in detecting acute hemispheric stroke. *Am J Neuroradiol* 2005;**26**(1):104–12.

33. Schramm P, Schellinger PD, Fiebach JB, et al.: Comparison of CT and CT angiography source images with diffusion-weighted imaging in patients with acute stroke within 6 hours after onset. *Stroke* 2002;**33**(10):2426–32.

34. Wintermark M, Reichhart M, Cuisenaire O, et al.: Comparison of admission perfusion computed tomography and qualitative diffusion- and perfusion-weighted magnetic resonance imaging in acute stroke patients. *Stroke* 2002;**33**(8):2025–31.

35. Nieuwkamp D, Setz L, Algra A, et al.: Changes in case fatality of aneurysmal subarachnoid haemorrhage over time, according to age, sex, and region: a meta-analysis. *Lancet Neurol* 2009;**8**(7): 635–42.

36. White PM, Wardlaw JM, Easton V: Can noninvasive imaging accurately depict intracranial aneurysms? A systematic review. *Radiology* 2000;**217**(2):361–70.

37. Kangasniemi M, Mäkelä T, Koskinen S, et al.: Detection of intracranial aneurysms with two-dimensional and three-dimensional multislice helical computed tomographic angiography. *Neurosurgery* 2004;**54**(2):336–40.

38. Chappell ET, Moure FC, Good MC: Comparison of computed tomographic angiography with digital subtraction angiography in the diagnosis of cerebral aneurysms: a meta-analysis. *Neurosurgery* 2003;**52**(3):624–30.

39. Wintermark M, Uske A, Chalaron M, et al.: Multislice computerized tomography angiography in the evaluation of intracranial aneurysms: a comparison with intraarterial digital subtraction angiography. *J Neurosurg* 2003;**98**(4):828–36.

40. Westerlaan H, Van Dijk J, Jansen-Van Der Weide M, et al.: Intracranial aneurysms in patients with subarachnoid hemorrhage: CT angiography as a primary examination tool for diagnosis – systematic review and meta-analysis. *Radiology* 2011;**258**(1):134–45.

41. Munera F, Soto JA, Palacio DM, et al.: Penetrating neck injuries: helical CT angiography for initial evaluation. *Radiology* 2002;**224**(2):366–72.

42. Soto JA, Soto JA, Palacio DM, et al.: Focal arterial injuries of the proximal extremities: helical CT arteriography as the initial method of diagnosis. *Radiology* 2001;**218**(1):188–94.

43. Inaba K, Munera F, McKenney M, et al.: Prospective evaluation of screening multislice helical computed tomographic angiography in the initial evaluation of penetrating neck injuries. *J Trauma-Injury Infect Crit Care* 2006;**61**(1):144–9.

44. Paulus E, Fabian T, Savage S, et al.: Blunt cerebrovascular injury screening with 64-channel multidetector computed tomography: more slices finally cut it. *J Trauma Acute Care Surg* 2014;**76**(2):279–85.

45. Etzel RA: Risk of ionizing radiation exposure to children: a subject review. *Pediatrics* 1998;**101**(4):717–19.

Chapter 37

CT Angiography of the Extremities

Nilasha Ghosh, Chanel Fischetti, Andrew Berg, and Bharath Chakravarthy

While contrast angiography has been known as the gold standard for documenting blood vessels of the extremities, CT angiography (CTA) is more commonly used (1). The latest CT equipment, called 64-slice detector scanners, can produce excellent images of arteries without the invasiveness of conventional angiography. By eliminating the invasive component of angiography, the possibility of causing iatrogenic arteriovenous fistulas, pseudoaneurysms, hematomas, and arterial dissections is eliminated (2). These thinner slices provide higher spatial resolution (3) and reduced motion and respiration artifact (1). The use of these scanners has also shortened examination time, and thus radiation exposure, as compared with older angiography techniques (1). CTA is often more convenient for emergent evaluation because it does not require mobilization of the interventional radiography team. Lastly, CTA has also been found to be considerably more cost-effective (4). This chapter discusses the indications, diagnostic capabilities, and limitations of CTA of the upper and lower extremities, followed by images of important pathological findings.

Indications

CTA should be performed after traumatic injuries in patients whose injured extremity is pulseless, has a neurological deficit, has an expanding hematoma, or has a bruit or thrill (5). It may also be required in penetrating trauma where the path of injury lies near an important vessel, with limb color or temperature change, or in blunt trauma with a suspicious mechanism, such as knee dislocations. Conventional angiography can also be used in these cases. However, Wallin and colleagues conducted a study evaluating the initial treatment of penetrating trauma in the lower extremity and concluded that CTA should supplant the use of conventional angiography due to proven accuracy, cost-effectiveness, and rapidity of administration and interpretation of results (6).

Nontraumatic indications include patients who present with a cool, painful extremity suggestive of acute arterial insufficiency (7) or in suspected arteriovenous fistulas or aneurysms. Other indications more appropriate to the outpatient setting include evaluation of the extent of peripheral vascular disease for operative planning and evaluation of existing vascular grafts for patency (8).

Diagnostic capabilities

CTA can characterize a vessel in several planes creating a 3D image to allow thorough evaluation of its walls, course, and continuity (2). Thus, it can be used to detect most vascular lesions, including thrombus, aneurysm, arteriovenous fistulas, and injury to the vessel wall. Furthermore, it provides 3D reconstructions of adjacent bones and soft tissue (9), which can be helpful in the complete evaluation of an extremity. All nonvascular images can be removed, and the resulting model can be rotated to view vessels from different angles and to remove overlapping vessels from the field of view. These capabilities allow for great accuracy, thus leading to sensitivity and specificity rates around 98% for detecting peripheral arterial disease (PAD) (3).

CTA is useful in detecting traumatic injuries, as well, with a sensitivity of 95% and specificities from 87% to 98% (10, 11). While some trauma cases require prompt surgical exploration, most will allow time for evaluation to define a specific treatment strategy (12). Because these images can often be composed and assessed more rapidly than other modalities, CTA can provide important lifesaving information in the workup of a trauma (13). CTA should also be considered for cases of microvascular reconstruction to accurately assess vascular anatomy prior to the procedure (4).

The 3D reconstruction of CTA allows for the creation and manipulation of images of the arterial system of the involved extremity. Often these images show disease not detected by other modalities (14), which include magnetic resonance angiography (MRA) and duplex ultrasonography. Each modality has its advantages and disadvantages. For example, duplex ultrasonography is easily accessible and not as harmful to the patient, but it has a lower sensitivity than MRA and CTA. MRA, with a specificity and sensitivity comparable to CTA (14), has higher diagnostic costs and several restrictions for use, such as in those patients with pacemakers and metal implants (13). The limitations of CTA are discussed next.

Imaging pitfalls and limitations

Suitable images require multidetector scanners and appropriate reconstruction software. Scanners with a smaller number of detectors, such as 8 or 16, will offer lower-quality images than newer 64-detector scanners. Furthermore, a narrow viewing window can make high-attenuation objects, such as calcified plaques and stents, appear larger than they really are, a phenomenon known as "blooming." This can lead to an overestimation of a supposed stenosis or occlusion (9). In general, full evaluation requires acquisition and manipulation of large amounts of data without a visual lag, which requires speed and significant computational resources (15).

Incorrect patient positioning and patient movement can decrease the image quality and produce artifacts suggestive of stenosis when none actually exist (8). In addition, it is important to coordinate the timing of the injection with scanning. The contrast material is rapidly injected into a peripheral vein and followed with a bolus dose of saline. The material then enters the arterial circulation, and scanning must be timed to coincide with filling of the vessels. This can be difficult in low-flow states such as poor cardiac output and significant stenosis, with incomplete opacification resulting in poor-quality images (16).

Furthermore, because most CTA is not performed in real time but rather is a compilation of static images, it may be difficult to delineate vascular occlusion and other vascular injuries from vasospasm. However, real-time CTA is starting to be used more frequently. Its use is well documented in dynamic testing of popliteal arterial entrapment syndrome (17).

CTA is not recommended for screening purposes due to the high doses of radiation and potential contrast nephrotoxicity (1). Frequent use of the multidetector CT scanner exposes the patient to large amounts of potentially carcinogenic ionizing radiation (18), so it is advised to limit a patient's exposure. The amount of contrast medium is reduced compared with conventional angiography (2), but it is still a substantial amount that could lead to nephrotoxicity (3). CTA uses iodinated contrast agents, whose adverse effects may be reduced by adequate hydration and possibly acetylcysteine; however, that measure is still debatable (19, 20). Patients with dye allergies may not tolerate the contrast either.

Clinical images

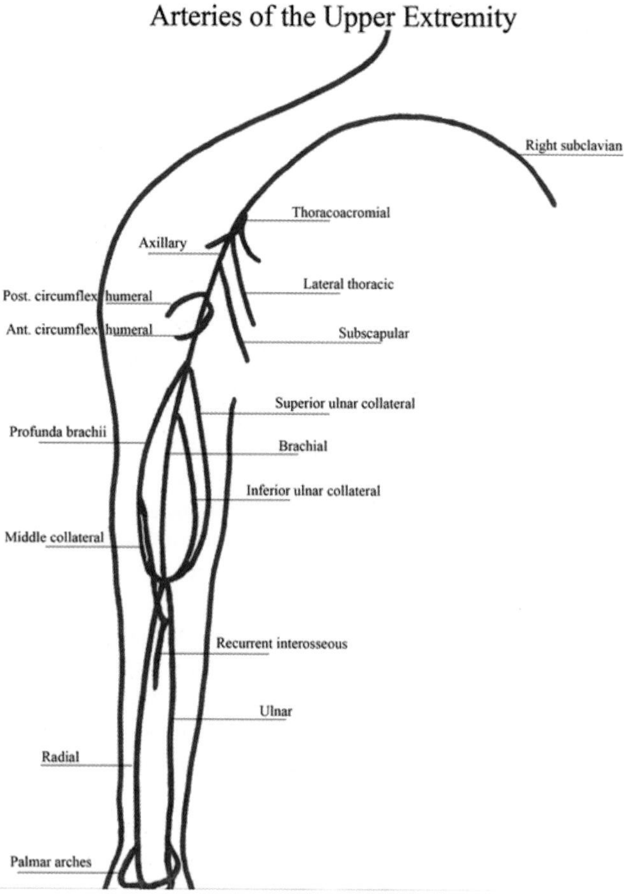

Arteries of the Upper Extremity

Right subclavian

Thoracoacromial

Axillary

Lateral thoracic

Post. circumflex humeral

Ant. circumflex humeral

Subscapular

Superior ulnar collateral

Profunda brachii

Brachial

Inferior ulnar collateral

Middle collateral

Recurrent interosseous

Ulnar

Radial

Palmar arches

Figure 37.1. Major arteries of the upper extremity.

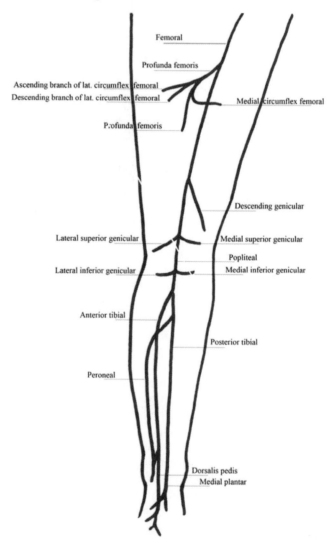

Femoral

Profunda femoris

Ascending branch of lat. circumflex femoral
Descending branch of lat. circumflex femoral

Medial circumflex femoral

Profunda femoris

Descending genicular

Lateral superior genicular

Medial superior genicular

Popliteal

Lateral inferior genicular

Medial inferior genicular

Anterior tibial

Posterior tibial

Peroneal

Dorsalis pedis
Medial plantar

Arteries of the Lower Extremity

Figure 37.2. Major arteries of the lower extremity.

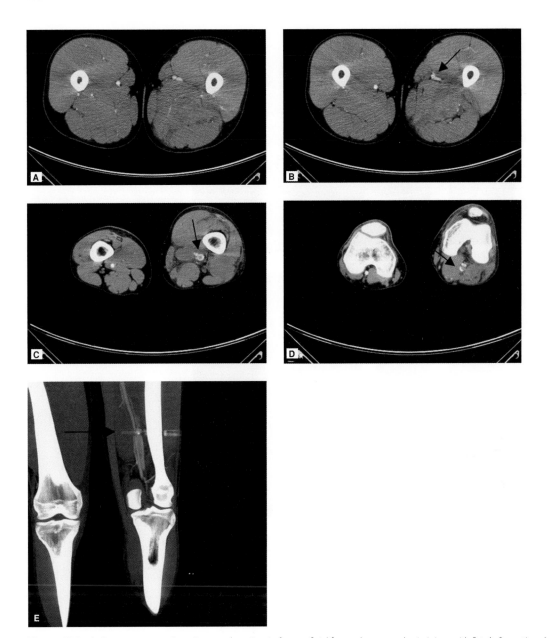

Figure 37.3. A–D, transverse sections; E, coronal section. Left superficial femoral artery and vein injury with fistula formation. A thrombus is also noted in the left popliteal vein. The patient suffered a gunshot wound to the distal left femur.

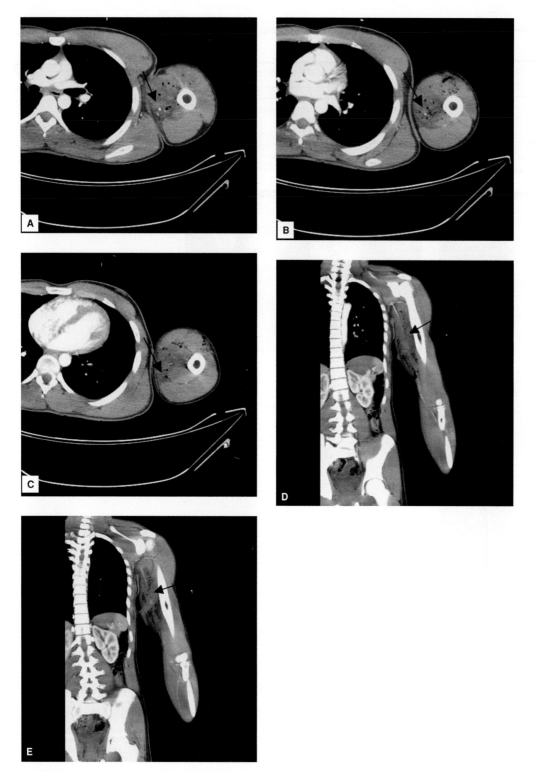

Figure 37.4. A–C, transverse sections; D–E, coronal sections. Disruption of the left brachial artery. The patient sustained a gunshot wound to the left arm.

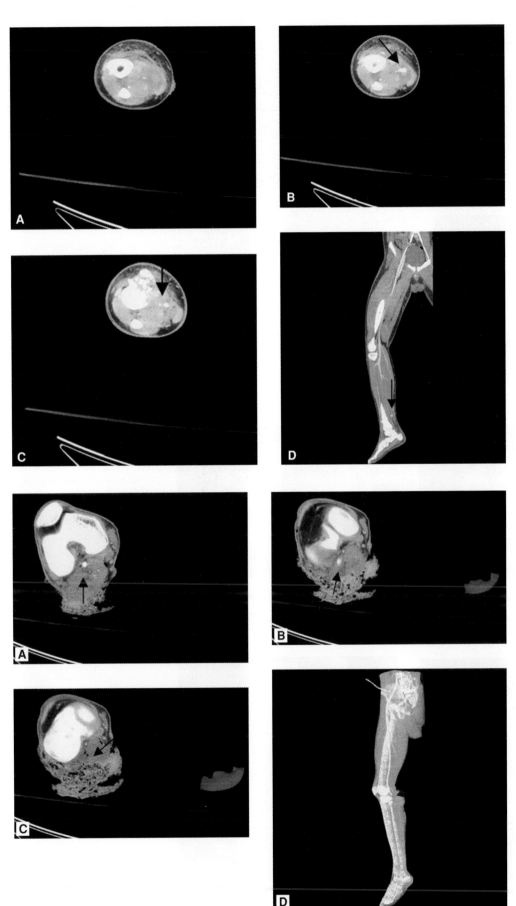

Figure 37.5. A–C, transverse sections; D, coronal section. Right posterior tibial artery pseudoaneurysm. The patient suffered a gunshot wound to the right leg with associated right tibial and fibular fractures.

Figure 37.6. A–C, transverse sections; D, coronal sections. Right distal popliteal artery occlusion. The patient sustained a deep laceration to his right calf after being injured by a circular saw.

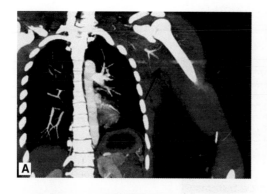

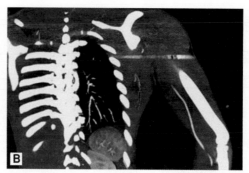

Figure 37.7. A–B, coronal sections; C, 3D reconstruction. Left axillary artery transection. The patient suffered a gunshot wound to the left axilla.

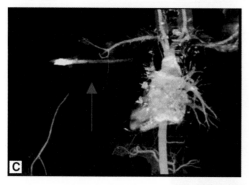

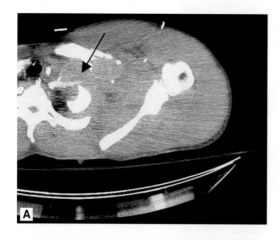

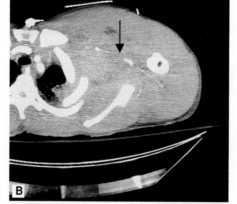

Figure 37.8. A–C, transverse sections; D, coronal section. Left subclavian artery transection. The patient sustained multiple gunshot wounds to the left chest and distal right forearm.

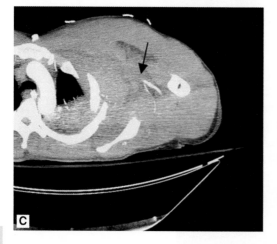

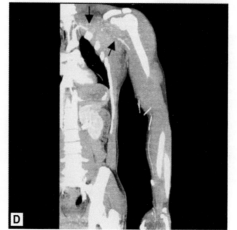

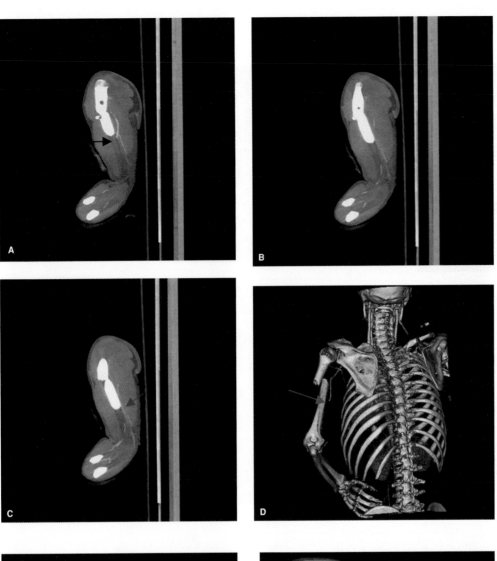

Figure 37.9. A–C, coronal sections; D, 3D reconstruction. Left brachial artery transection. The patient was trapped between a forklift and a piece of machinery. He also suffered an open humerus fracture to the left arm.

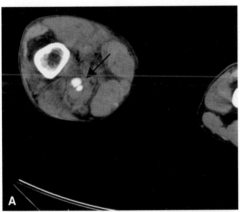

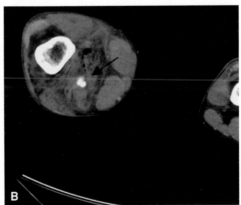

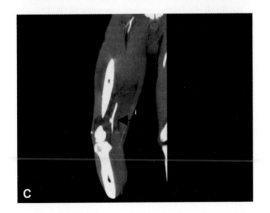

Figure 37.10. A–B, transverse sections; C, coronal sections. Right popliteal artery pseudoaneurysm. The patient sustained a gunshot wound to the right medial thigh.

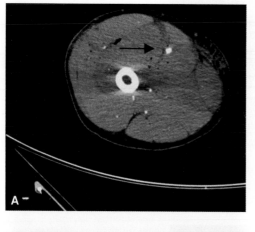

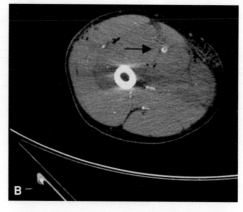

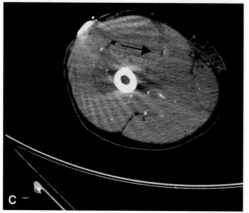

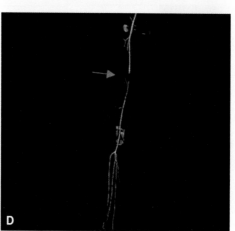

Figure 37.11. A–C, transverse sections; D, 3D reconstruction. Right superficial femoral artery occlusion. The patient suffered multiple gunshot wounds to his bilateral thighs and the right scapular region.

References

1. Norgren L, Hiatt WR, Dormandy JA, et al.: Inter-society consensus for the management of peripheral arterial disease (TASC II). *J Vasc Surg* 2007;**45**(1, Suppl):S5–S67.

2. Chan D, Anderson ME, Domatch BL: Imaging evaluation of lower extremity infrainguinal disease: role of the noninvasive vascular laboratory, computed tomography angiography, and magnetic resonance angiography. *Tech Vasc Interv Radiol* 2010;**13**(1):11–22.

3. Schernthaner R, Stadler A, Lomoschitz F, et al.: Multidetector CT angiography in the assessment of peripheral arterial occlusive disease: accuracy in detecting the severity, number, and length of stenoses. *Eur Radiol* 2008;**18**(4):665–71.

4. Lee GK, Fox PM, Riboh J, et al.: Computed tomography angiography in microsurgery: indications, clinical utility, and pitfalls. *Eplasty* 2013;13:e42.

5. McCorkell SJ, Harley JD, Morishima MS, Cummings DK: Indications for angiography in extremity trauma. *AJR Am J Roentgenol* 1985;**145**(6):1245–7.

6. Wallin, D, Yaghoubian A, Rosing D, et al.: Computed tomographic angiography as the primary diagnostic modality in penetrating lower extremity vascular injuries: a level I trauma experience. *Ann Vasc Surg* 2011;**25**(5):620–3.

7. Bell KW, Heng RC, Atallah J, Chaitowitz I: Use of intra-arterial multi-detector row CT angiography for the evaluation of an ischaemic limb in a patient with renal impairment. *Australas Radiol* 2006;**50**(4):377–80.

8. Willmann JK, Wildermuth S: Multidetector-row CT angiography of upper- and lower-extremity peripheral arteries. *Eur Radiol* 2005;**15**(Suppl 4):D3–9.

9. Fleischmann, D: Lower-extremity CTA. In Reiser MF, Becker CR, Nikolaou K, Glazer G (eds), *Multislice CT*. Springer, 2009:321–30.

10. Soto JA, Múnera F, Morales C, et al.: Focal arterial injuries of the proximal extremities: helical CT arteriography as the initial method of diagnosis. *Radiology* 2001;**218**(1):188–94.

11. Rieger M, Mallouhi A, Tauscher T, et al.: Traumatic arterial injuries of the extremities: initial evaluation with MDCT angiography. *AJR Am J Roentgenol* 2006;**186**(3):656–64.

12. Jens S, Kerstens MK, Legemate DA, et al. Diagnostic performance of computed tomography angiography in peripheral arterial injury due to trauma: a systematic review and meta-analysis. *Eur J Vasc Endovasc Surg* 2013;**46**(3):329–37.

13. Jakobs T, Wintersperger B, Becker C: MDCT-imaging of peripheral arterial disease. *Semin Ultrasound CT MR* 2004;**25**(2):145–55.

14. Met, R, Bipat S, Legemate DA, et al.: Diagnostic performance of computed tomography angiography in peripheral arterial disease. *JAMA* 2009;**301**(4):415–24.

15. Anderson SW, Lucey BC, Varghese JC, Soto JA: Sixty-four multi-detector row computed tomography in multitrauma patient imaging: early experience. *Curr Probl Diagn Radiol* 2006;**35**(5):188–98.

16. Miller-Thomas MM, West OC, Cohen AM: Diagnosing traumatic arterial injury in the extremities with CT angiography: pearls and pitfalls. *Radiographics* 2005;**25**(Suppl 1):S133–42.

17. Anil G, Tay K-H, Howe TC, Tan BS: Dynamic computed tomography angiography: role in the evaluation of popliteal artery entrapment syndrome. *Cardiovasc Intervent Radiol* 2011;**34**(2):259–70.

18. Brenner DJ, Hall EJ: Computed tomography: an increasing source of radiation exposure. *N Engl J Med* 2007;**357**(22): 2277–84.

19. European Stroke Organisation, Tendera M, Aboyans V, et al.: ESC guidelines on the diagnosis and treatment of peripheral artery diseases: document covering atherosclerotic disease of extracranial carotid and vertebral, mesenteric, renal, upper and lower extremity arteries: the Task Force on the Diagnosis and Treatment of Peripheral Artery Diseases of the European Society of Cardiology (ESC). *Eur Heart J* 2011;**32**(22): 2851–906.

20. Kelly AM, Dwamena B, Cronin P, et al.: Meta-analysis: effectiveness of drugs for preventing contrast-induced nephropathy. *Ann Intern Med* 2008;**148**(4):284–94.

The Physics of MRI

38

Joseph L. Dinglasan, Jr., and J. Christian Fox

Although CT continues to be the diagnostic imaging modality of choice for many clinical situations facing the emergency physician, MRI is quickly becoming the preferred alternative for evaluating certain complaints. Not only does MRI spare the patient from exposure to the ionizing radiation of CT, but it also has a well-deserved reputation of producing superior images of soft tissue structures, such as tumors, abscesses, the brain, and the spinal cord. This chapter elucidates how these amazing images are derived, in the simplest of terms and without any of the anxiety-inducing equations for which physics is famous.

Essential physical principles

Before one can understand the physics of MRI, it is important to review some of the essential physical principles that make MRI possible. Recall from your high school physics class that the hydrogen atom consists of a proton nucleus, which carries a unit of positive electrical charge, and a single electron, which carries a negative charge equal in magnitude to that of the proton. These hydrogen atoms are the simplest and most abundant elements in the human body, serving as the basic building blocks of everything from water molecules to lipids to proteins. The atomic nuclei of these hydrogen atoms, in addition to many others, act as small magnets due to the small magnetic dipole moments that they carry. These "moments" refer to the tendency of the object to move, as in "momentum."

These protons also carry an angular momentum in addition to their magnetic moment, which can be visualized in real time by the same spinning tops that continue to amuse children today. Angular momentum is the tendency for a spinning object to continue to spin about the same axis. When the axis of rotation is altered by an applied force, the angular momentum results in *precession*, such that these objects or particles rotate around such forces (Fig. 38.1).

The rate at which an object precesses is directly proportional to both its angular momentum and the strength of the forces that tend to change it.

Another important principle to understand is the reciprocal relationship between magnetism and electricity. Not only does a current of moving electrical charges generate a magnetic field, but time-varying magnetic fields in turn create electrical fields that promote the flow of electrical charges. In these magnetic fields, magnets experience an aligning force, whereby the "north" pole of one magnet tends to be attracted to the "south" pole of another, driven by the goal of achieving a lower energy state in which the entire system is in equilibrium.

MRI instruments take advantage of these fundamental principles. In fact, all MRI instruments contain a homogeneous magnetic field that is required to establish longitudinal magnetization of the protons within it. Many instruments achieve this by using permanent magnets that directly create magnetic fields, which are oriented along an axis extending between the two poles of a magnet. This is illustrated in Figure 38.2A, in which the magnetic field generated by the permanent magnet is

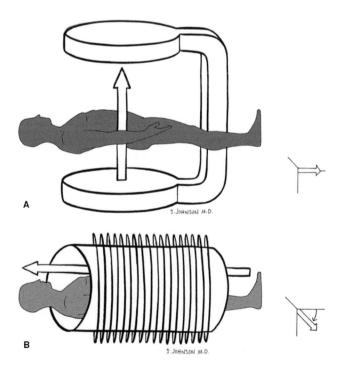

Figure 38.2. The magnetic field, BO, may run either (A) perpendicular to the axis of the body in an "open" configuration or (B) parallel to the body in a "closed" configuration.

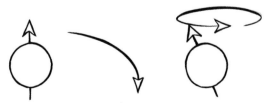

Figure 38.1. When an external force is applied to change the axis of rotation of an atom, angular momentum results in these particles rotating around such forces. This is known as *precession*.

perpendicular to the scanner table in an "open" configuration. In contrast, a magnetic field can also be generated perpendicular to an electrical current flowing along a cylindrical coiled wire, resulting in a "closed" configuration, in which the subject is enclosed in the magnet. The strength of the magnetic field generated by most standard MRI machines is 0.5 tesla (T), which is approximately 5,000 gauss, or equivalent to 10,000 times the strength of the Earth's magnetic field. Newer MRI machines used for research applications generate even stronger magnetic fields of 1.0 T and higher. This is done using superconducting magnets that take advantage of special materials and cooler temperatures to minimize the resistance to the flow of electrical current.

Formation of the MRI

The secret of MRI lies in nuclear magnetic resonance (NMR) technology first pioneered by Felix Bloch and Edward Purcell in 1946. Typically, at any given moment, the proton spins of atomic nuclei are randomly oriented in space, dictated by the intrinsic magnetic moments mentioned previously that are derived from the angular momentum of revolving electrons. Bloch and Purcell independently discovered that placing hydrogen atoms in a powerful magnetic field aligns the intrinsic spins of these protons almost in parallel or antiparallel with the applied field (Fig. 38.3).

Radio waves generated from an electrical coil can then be used to excite these protons so they flip their spins away from the direction of the magnetic field. The longer the frequency of this radio pulse, the larger the net magnetization vector M will deviate from the direction of this field. Once the pulse stops, the proton spins relax back to their lower energy state, releasing energy as electromagnetic waves at frequencies that can be detected by the same emission-reception coil. A different set of coils can then be used to apply magnetic gradients that alter these frequencies in such a way that their location can be determined in three dimensions.

Initially, a wide range of frequencies corresponding to the various locations along the imaging gradients comprise a continuously varying, or analog, waveform. Before these data can directly indicate the spatial location of the protons from which they originated, the MR signals must first undergo analog-to-digital conversion, such that the initial waveform is now in the form of a set of numbers that represent distinct time points along the waves. An MR acquisition computer then processes this information and arranges it into a 2D map of digital space known as *k-space*.

Each point in k-space contains data from all portions of an MRI. For example, the data point forming the dark center of the k-space image contains information about the intensity and contrast of the entire image. The data points in the periphery, however, encode information about the fine details of the image. This 2D image of k-space then undergoes a process known as Fourier transform analysis, which yields pixel data that represent the MR signal amplitude from that spatial location, generating the 3D MRI that we have all come to appreciate.

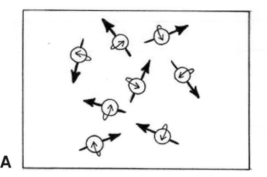

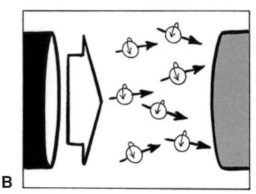

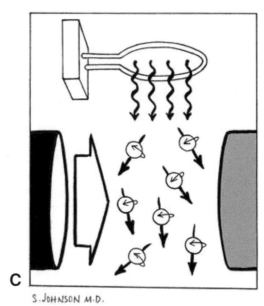

S. JOHNSON M.D.

Figure 38.3. Electron excitation. A: Proton spins normally orient randomly in the absence of an external magnetic field so the net magnetization vector M is 0. B: When an external field is applied, the intrinsic proton spins align either in parallel or in antiparallel with the magnetic field so M is parallel with the *Z-axis*. C: A radiofrequency pulse applied to the magnetic field causes the protons to flip their spins away from the field so M approaches the *x-y plane*.

Image characteristics

The intensity of MRI signals traditionally correlates to three characteristics of the tissue being imaged: proton density, T1 relaxation time, and T2 relaxation time. As the proton spins return to their relaxed state following radiofrequency excitation, they travel in both the *Z-axis* (which corresponds to the

Table 38.1: Ranges of NMR relaxation times for several biological tissues

Tissue Type	T1 (ms)	T2 (ms)
Bone	0.001–1	0.001–1
Muscle	460–650	26–34
Fat	180–300	47–63
Body fluid	1,000–2,000	150–480
White matter	220–350	80–120
Gray matter	340–610	90–130

T1 *longitudinal* relaxation time in parallel with the magnetic field) and the *x-y plane* (which corresponds to the T2 *transverse* relaxation time perpendicular to the magnetic field).

Properties of the tissue's molecular environment directly influence the T1 and T2 relaxation values. Proton–proton interactions, the efficiency of energy absorption, and inhomogeneities in the magnetic field may all play a role. Depending on the tissue involved, T1 values may range from roughly 300 to 2,000 ms, whereas T2 values can be found significantly lower from about 30 to 150 ms. MRI studies using different radio wave pulse sequences can be tailored to accentuate either of these T1 or T2 values, depending on what characteristic of the tissue would like to be emphasized on the image. Most studies currently employ the spin echo (SE) pulse sequence by modifying the repetition time (TR) and echo time (TE) intervals to accentuate either value.

TR is a direct reflection of image acquisition time during T1 relaxation, whereas TE corresponds with the image formulated during T2 relaxation time. Image contrast is maximized in either short TR intervals (<600 ms) or long TE intervals. Therefore, when the image is captured so that both TR and TE intervals are short, the T1 relaxation is emphasized, and the image is said to be *T1 weighted*. Likewise, when longer TR and TE intervals are used during image acquisition, the T2 relaxation time is emphasized, and the image is said to be *T2 weighted*. When a mix of both is achieved, using a long TR and short TE, the image depends mainly on *proton density* and is neither T1 nor T2 weighted. Table 38.1 lists representative relaxation times for several biological tissues.

T1 times are generally longer than T2 times. The greater proportion of free water molecules in low-viscous compounds such as body fluids and muscle account for the longer relaxation times not seen in rigid compounds such as bone.

T1, T2, and proton density depend largely on the state of matter of the biological tissue, ranging from free water to solid bone. There is a dynamic equilibrium in soft tissue between the water molecules bound to proteins and the water molecules that are essentially free (Fig. 38.4). Because the free water component has intrinsically longer T1 and T2 value times, it comprises the largest percentage of the MRI signal. The bound component of water and the dynamic division between free and bound water alter the relaxation processes between different tissues, thus contributing to the three contrast mechanisms.

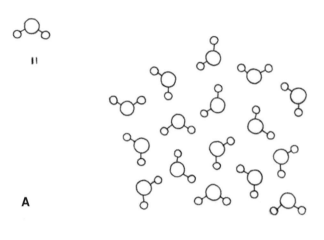

A

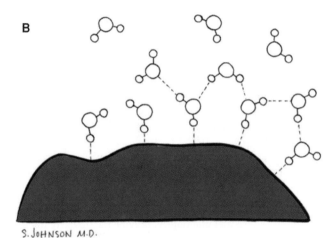

B

S. JOHNSON M.D.

Figure 38.4. Free water versus bound water. A: Biological water that is considered "free" is not in immediate proximity to macromolecules such as phospholipids, proteins, or DNA, making it highly disorganized and mobile. B: "Bound" water, in contrast, is restricted in its movement primarily by hydrogen macromolecules.

How do these three different contrast mechanisms translate to images with different visual characteristics? Here is an oversimplified rule of thumb: T1-weighted images look similar to gross specimens. This is because water appears dark while fatty tissues appear bright on T1-weighted images. In other words, cerebrospinal fluid (consisting predominantly of water molecules) looks black, gray matter (which has a high water content) is gray, and white matter (which has a high lipid content due to the myelin sheaths) appears white.

Contrast this with another key rule to remember: T2-weighted images look somewhat like the film negatives of T1-weighted images. Therefore, cerebrospinal fluid will be white, gray matter will still be gray, and epidural fat will be black. If you ever forget which one is which, just remember the mnemonic WW2, in which *water* is *white* in T2-weighted images.

Proton density–weighted images are different from T1- and T2-weighted images in that the contrast between predominantly water-based mediums and lipid-based mediums is minimized. This is best exemplified in brain tissue, in which the transition between white matter and gray matter is less pronounced, enabling the viewer to pick up on subtle abnormalities in the parenchyma that may represent serious pathology, such as edema or infarction.

Safety considerations

In addition to understanding the distinctions among T1-, T2-, and proton density–weighted images, the emergency physician must also consider the safety implications when ordering an MRI. The contraindications for MRI include the presence of a cardiac pacemaker; implanted cardiac defibrillator; aneurysm clip; carotid artery vascular clamp; neurostimulator; insulin or infusion pump; any implanted drug-infusion device; bone growth or fusion stimulator; or a cochlear, otologic, or ear implant. Not only may these devices serve as "missiles" under the control of powerful magnetic forces, but they may also dissipate heat, induce electrical current, and cause artifact that may be misread as an abnormality. With that said, newer devices composed of materials that are less ferromagnetic and therefore less responsive to magnetic fields are already on the market with an even larger number currently in development. When in doubt, contact the manufacturer of the device for MRI compatibility before proceeding.

Also, keep in mind that patients with any history of injury by a metal object such as a bullet or shrapnel (i.e., veterans or metal workers) should undergo a thorough evaluation prior to imaging. These metallic objects may be particularly harmful if they are lodged in a loose medium such as the eye, which would harbor very little resistance to magnetic forces. It is also worth mentioning that MRI machines produce a substantial amount of noise that may produce anxiety, distress, and even temporary hearing loss. Luckily, the advent of active noise-cancellation techniques and the utility of simple ear plugs decrease this noise by at least 50% to 70%.

The issue of using MRI in pregnancy often arises as well, particularly when the safety of CT is called into question due to the risk of exposing a growing fetus to ionizing radiation. To date, there have been no demonstrated deleterious effects linked to the use of MRI in pregnancy. However, it will be years before this can be said with certainty. For now, the MR Safety Committee of the Society for Magnetic Resonance Imaging recommends the use of MRI in pregnant women only if other nonionizing modalities such as ultrasound are inadequate or if the study provides valuable information that would otherwise require exposure to ionizing radiation.

Suggested Readings

Ahmed S, Shellock FG: Magnetic resonance imaging safety: implications for cardiovascular patients. *J Cardiovasc Magn Reson* 2007;3(3):171–82.

Blumenfeld H: *Neuroanatomy through clinical cases*. Sunderland, MA: Sinauer Associates, 2002.

Chakeres DW, Schmalbrock P: *Fundamentals of magnetic resonance imaging*. Baltimore, MD: Williams & Wilkins, 1992.

Feast R, Gledhill M, Hurrell M, Tremewan R: *Magnetic resonance imaging safety guidelines*. Available at: www.nrl.moh.govt.nz/publications/1996-5.pdf

Guy C, Ffytche D: *An introduction to the principles of medical imaging*, revised ed. London: Imperial College Press, 2005.

Mitchell DG, Cohen MS: *MRI principles*, 2nd ed. Philadelphia: Saunders, 2004.

Mugler JP III: Basic principles. In: Edelman RR, Hesselink JR, Zlatkin, MB, Crues JV III (eds), *Clinical magnetic resonance imaging*, 3rd ed. Philadelphia: Saunders, 2006.

Nitz W: Principles of magnetic resonance imaging and magnetic resonance angiography. In: Reimer P, Parizel PM, Stichnoth FA (eds), *Clinical MR imaging*, 2nd ed. Berlin: Springer-Verlag, 2003.

Shellock FG, Kanal E, Society for Magnetic Resonance Imaging (SMRI) Safety Committee: SMRI report: policies, guidelines, and recommendations for MR imaging safety and patient management. *J Magn Reson Imaging* 1991;1:97–101.

Chapter 39

MRI of the Brain

Asmita Patel, Colleen Crowe, and Brian Sayger

In recent years, there have been tremendous advances in the field of radiology, specifically in radioimaging. The development of an accurate way to visualize structures in the body has improved the diagnosis of patients and has allowed for less invasive methods in their evaluation. MRI represents a breakthrough in medical diagnostics and research, and it is becoming especially valuable in the evaluation of neurological and musculoskeletal pathology.

The field of MRI is still evolving and continually improving. Although its role as the modality of choice in the ED remains limited, MRI remains indispensable in the evaluation of brain tumors, strokes, and chronic demyelinating disorders, including multiple sclerosis.

In 1946, two scientists working independently on nuclear magnetic resonance (NMR) research laid the groundwork for the future development of MRI. Dr. Felix Bloch, working at Stanford University, and Dr. Edward Purcell from Harvard University simultaneously accomplished the first successful NMR experiment. In 1952, they were both awarded the Nobel Prize in Physics for their work in the study of the composition of chemical compounds.

Principles of MRI

The fundamental concept of MRI is based on resonance – specifically, nuclei of certain atoms, most commonly hydrogen atoms, resonate when placed in powerful magnetic fields. When radiofrequency energy (or radio waves) is projected toward the atoms, the nuclei absorb some of the energy, thus becoming "excited." Subsequently, the nuclei "relax" and return to their previous energy level, thereby emitting their own radio signals. These nuclear magnetic signals are then computer processed to form an image.

Protons, or the nuclei of hydrogen atoms, are found abundantly in the human body in the form of water. MRI scanning uses the difference in water content and its distribution in various body tissues to provide contrast resolution and tissue differentiation. To better understand how the images of MRI are generated, certain parameters must first be discussed.

As mentioned, when excited protons return from the high-energy to the low-energy state, they emit energy to the protons in their immediate environment, or lattice. T1 and T2, fundamental concepts of MRI, are based on this relaxation time. T1, known as the longitudinal relaxation time, is determined by interactions between the excited and surrounding protons, known as the "spin–lattice interaction."

T2, in contrast, does not involve a *loss* of energy, but the *exchange* of energy between the high- and low-energy protons, known as the "spin–spin interaction." In other words, it measures the duration of time protons remain in the excited phase prior to returning to their previous low-energy state.

T1 and T2 relaxation times are dependent on the environment of the resonating protons, and, therefore, each method derives characteristic images based on the various tissue scanned. Still, to understand MRI generation, two more parameters, repetition time (TR) and echo time (TE), should also be discussed. In generating an image, a sequence of repetition produces a nuclear resonance signal. TR stands for the time between repetitions. TE represents the time between the application of this radiofrequency pulse and the generation and detection of the nuclear signal, or spin echo. These parameters are paramount to the difference in T1- and T2-generated images. Short TRs and short TEs enhance tissues with short T1 relaxation times, thus generating T1-weighted images. Alternatively, long TR and long TE pulse sequences enhance tissues with long T2 times; therefore, such sequences generate T2-weighted images. As a consequence of these properties, T1-weighted images are more valuable in defining anatomy, whereas T2-weighted images are often used in identifying pathology of tissue.

Applying these concepts to the human body, cerebrospinal fluid has a long T1 relaxation time; it appears dark in T1-weighted images and bright in T2-weighted images. Fat has a relatively short T1, thus appearing bright on T1-weighted images and dark on T2-weighted images. Certain material such as air and bone that have similar T1 and T2 times appear dark on both images. In fact, understanding these imaging parameters and manipulating the TR and TE accordingly can improve differentiation of normal tissue from pathological lesions.

The fluid-attenuated inversion recovery (FLAIR) sequence is similar in appearance to T2 but with the CSF nulled-out (dark), allowing subtle areas of T2 signal abnormality to be visualized more easily. With FLAIR, vasogenic and cytotoxic edema is differentiated from the CSF signal (see Figs. 39.41, 39.56). This is also a useful sequence for detecting multiple sclerosis (MS) lesions (see Figs. 39.47 and 39.48), which also appear bright on FLAIR. FLAIR is the best MR sequence for detecting subarachnoid hemorrhage (SAH), though CT remains the preferred initial imaging for SAH.

Diffusion weighted imaging (DWI) characterizes the ease of water diffusion between cells, which is restricted by cellular edema. Restriction of water proton diffusion causes a high-intensity (bright) signal on DWI sequences. DWI utilizes the apparent diffusion coefficient (ADC) of water, which is automatically calculated by the software and displayed on an ADC map. The ADC map helps differentiate new from old infarcts and cytotoxic from vasogenic edema when compared to DWI sequences. ADC also helps differentiate true DWI signal from "T2 shine-through" – apparent brightness on DWI caused by a very hyperintense signal on T2. DWI is primarily used for early detection of acute stroke and hypoperfusion, differentiating old versus new MS plaques and detecting cerebral abscesses.

Indications

Currently, the use of MRI in the emergency setting is limited to the diagnosis and evaluation of spinal cord compression. It also has a role in the evaluation of certain orthopedic injuries, including the evaluation of radiographically occult femoral neck fractures. Other nonemergent indications for conventional MRI include study of musculoskeletal joints, including the knee, shoulder, and several smaller joints, such as the temporomandibular joint.

A growing area in the emergent setting that uses MRI involves aortic dissection. MRI has been found to be equal in utility, if not superior, to contrast-enhanced CT for diagnosing aortic dissection. MRI may also be equivalent to transesophageal echocardiogram; however, the inability of unstable patients to undergo the procedure limits the use of MRI for this indication.

Neuroimaging provides timely and crucial information in the assessment and management of stroke. It helps delineate the extent of infarction, the degree of hemorrhage, and the amount of tissue injury. At present, CT scanning for the evaluation of stroke remains the most cost-effective and practical imaging modality used in the ED. The advent of helical CTs and CT angiograms obviate the use of MRIs in the initial evaluation of most central nervous system disorders. Nevertheless, the most valuable use of MRI remains in the field of acute ischemic stroke.

Diagnostic capabilities

In general, MRI is superior to CT in detecting injuries to soft tissues such as the brain and spinal cord. It is highly sensitive in diagnosing small intercerebral and brainstem lesions; small cerebral contusions; and injuries to muscles, ligaments, and tendons. It is also more sensitive in detecting changes that occur after ischemic strokes.

One appealing aspect of MRI is the lack of radiation exposure, which makes it ideal for pregnant patients and for patients who need repeat imaging throughout their lives due to their disease process. The high resolution of MRI provides better quality images and allows for visualization of otherwise difficult-to-visualize structures, including the posterior fossa. It has multiplanar-imaging capabilities and provides excellent soft tissue contrast and gray–white matter differentiation. The patency of blood vessels in the body can also be easily determined.

Imaging pitfalls and limitations

The lack of widespread availability of MRI and the high cost compared with CT scanning make its use limited in the ED. In addition, MRI requires long scanning durations, sometimes as long as 30 to 60 minutes. Patients are required to hold still because movement degrades the quality of the images. This becomes a significant obstacle in agitated trauma patients and in pediatric patients who require sedation. Also, acutely ill patients who need close monitoring may not tolerate such long scanning times. Certain patients who are overweight (heavier than 300 pounds) or have a fear of enclosed spaces may also have difficulty undergoing MRI. With the advent of open MRI, more patients are able to tolerate the procedure.

Patients who have metallic implants or foreign bodies such as pacemakers, cochlear implants, nerve stimulators, and certain metallic brain aneurysm clips are unable to undergo imaging. There have been reports of welders with implanted metal in their eyes who have gone blind after MRI. In the diagnosis of subarachnoid hemorrhage, MRI has decreased sensitivity. Although safer than the contrast used for CT scanning but not as commonly seen, there still remains a risk of allergic reaction to the contrast agent (gadolinium) used for MRI. These are all factors that should be taken into consideration when deciding which imaging modality is best for a particular patient.

Clinical images

MRI images of the normal anatomy of the brain are included first, along with detailed diagrams to explain the images. Then, pathological images are shown in various cuts and sequences.

Normal anatomy of the brain

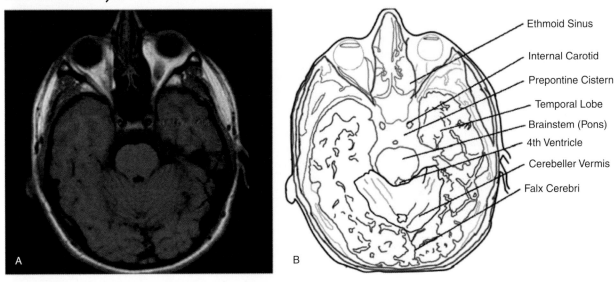

Figure 39.1. Axial view T1 without contrast.

Labels in diagram (B):
- Ethmoid Sinus
- Internal Carotid
- Prepontine Cistern
- Temporal Lobe
- Brainstem (Pons)
- 4th Ventricle
- Cerebeller Vermis
- Falx Cerebri

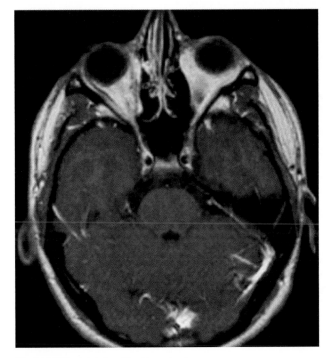

Figure 39.2. Axial view T1 with contrast.

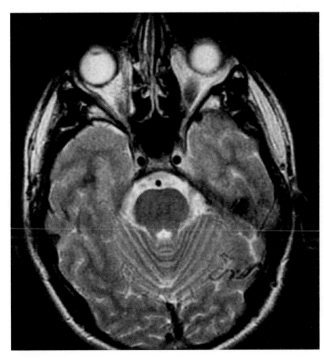

Figure 39.3. Axial view T2.

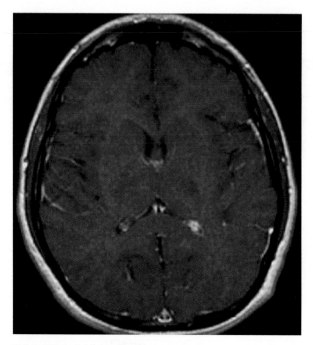

Figure 39.4. Axial view T1 without contrast.

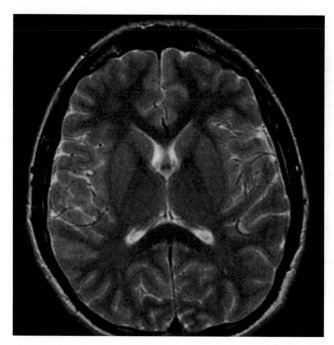

Figure 39.5. Axial view T1 with contrast.

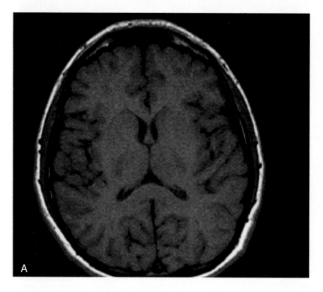

A

Figure 39.6. Axial view T2.

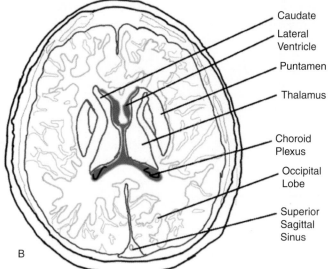

B

Caudate

Lateral Ventricle

Puntamen

Thalamus

Choroid Plexus

Occipital Lobe

Superior Sagittal Sinus

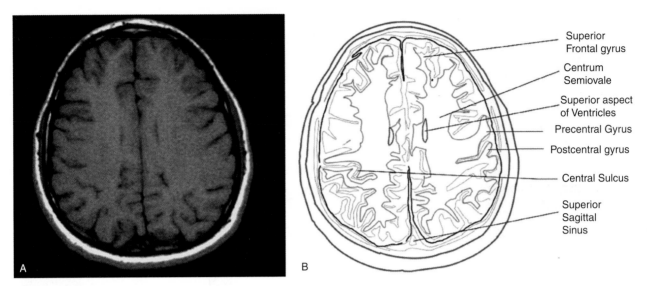

Superior Frontal gyrus

Centrum Semiovale

Superior aspect of Ventricles

Precentral Gyrus

Postcentral gyrus

Central Sulcus

Superior Sagittal Sinus

A

B

Figure 39.7. Axial view T1 without contrast, upper.

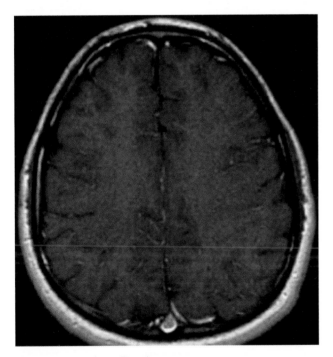

Figure 39.8. Axial view T1 with contrast, upper.

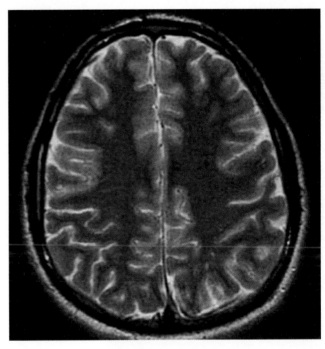

Figure 39.9. Axial view T2, upper.

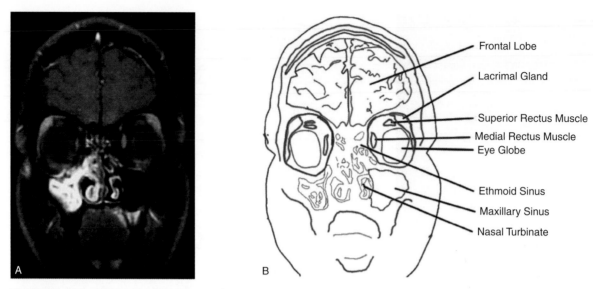

Figure 39.10. Coronal view T1 without contrast, frontal view.

Figure 39.11. Coronal view T2, frontal view.

Frontal Lobe

Lacrimal Gland

Superior Rectus Muscle
Medial Rectus Muscle
Eye Globe

Ethmoid Sinus

Maxillary Sinus

Nasal Turbinate

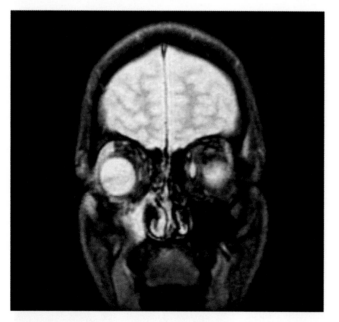

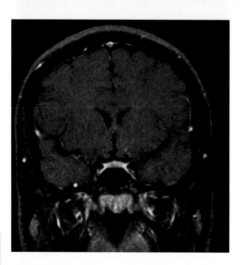

Figure 39.12. Coronal view T1 without contrast.

Lateral Ventricles

3rd Ventricle

Optic chiasm

Internal Carotid Artery

Sphenoidal sinus

Nasopharnyx

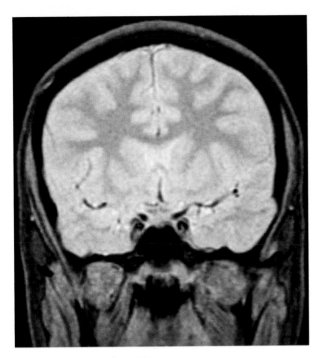

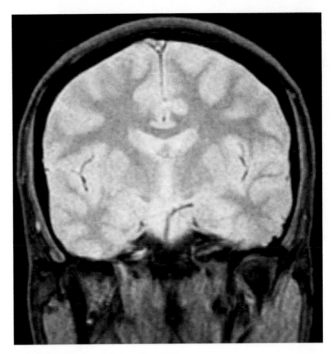

Figure 39.13. Coronal view T2.

Figure 39.15. Coronal view T2, middle.

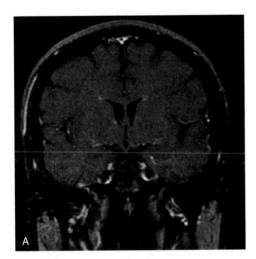

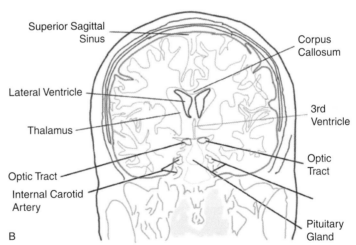

Figure 39.14. Coronal view T1.

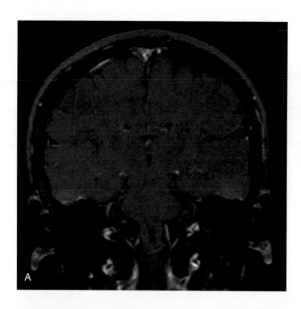

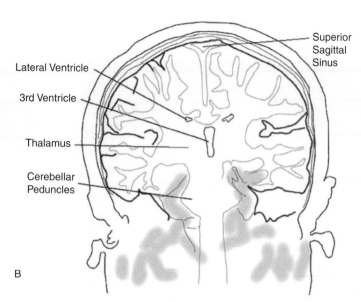

Figure 39.16. Coronal view T1, middle.

Figure 39.17. Coronal view T2.

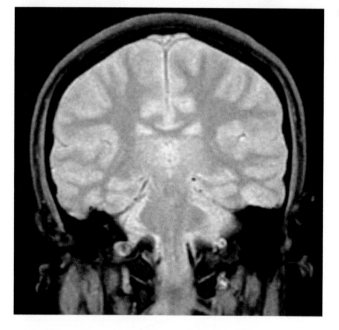

Figure 39.18. Coronal view T1 without contrast, posterior view.

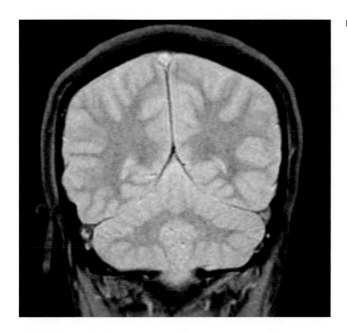

Figure 39.19. Coronal view T2.

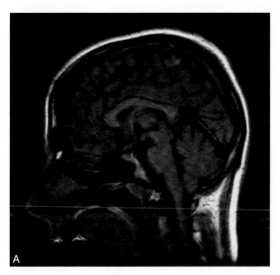

A

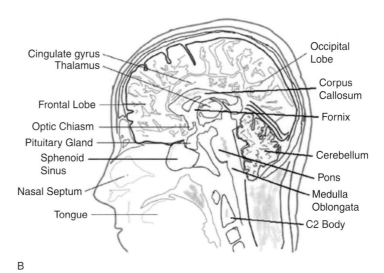

B

Cingulate gyrus
Thalamus
Frontal Lobe
Optic Chiasm
Pituitary Gland
Sphenoid Sinus
Nasal Septum
Tongue

Occipital Lobe
Corpus Callosum
Fornix
Cerebellum
Pons
Medulla Oblongata
C2 Body

Figure 39.20. Sagittal view T1.

Abnormal brain MRI images

Ischemia

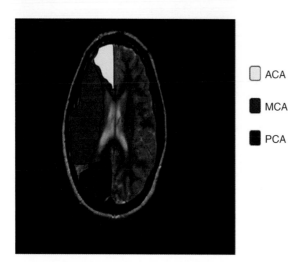

Figure 39.21. Distribution of strokes based on vascular territory. ACA = anterior cerebral artery; MCA = middle cerebral artery; PCA = posterior cerebral artery.

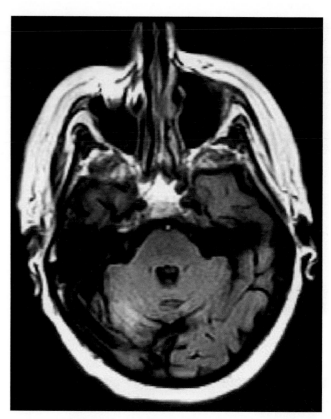

Figure 39.22. Right cerebellar infarct, wedge shaped, T2 axial FLAIR. Note the hyperintense signal of the infarct on T2WI.

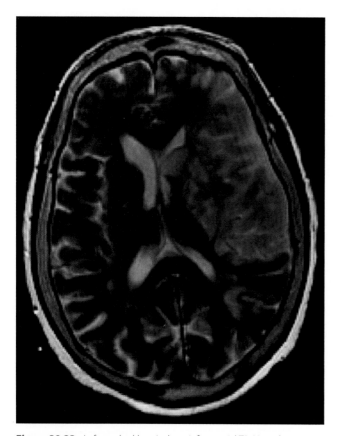

Figure 39.23. Left cerebral hemisphere infarct, axial T2. Note the hyperintense signal of the infarct on T2WI.

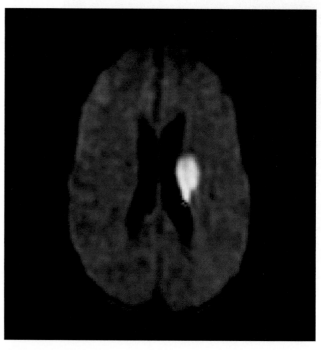

Figure 39.24. Left basal ganglia, left thalamus infarcts, bright on T2 DWI.

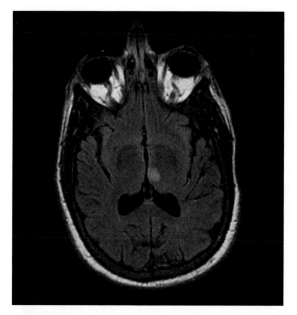

Figure 39.25. Left thalamus infarct, bright on T2 FLAIR.

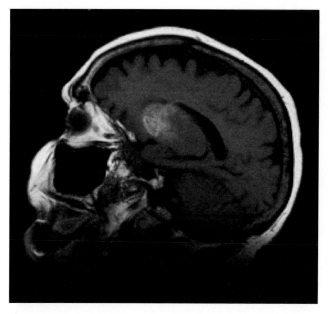

Figure 39.26. Left cerebral hemisphere infarct with right basal ganglia bleed, emphasis on right basal ganglia bleed, bright on T1 sagittal.

Intracranial hemorrhage

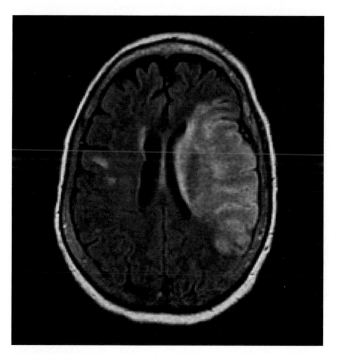

Figure 39.27. Left cerebral hemisphere infarct in the left MCA territory with right basal ganglia bleed (bright), emphasis on left cerebral infarct, bright on axial FLAIR.

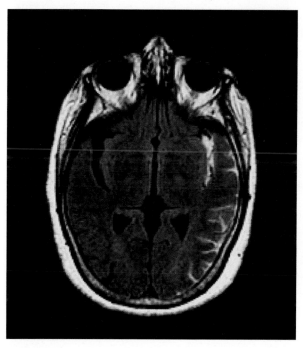

Figure 39.28. Left subarachnoid hemorrhage in the left temporal, parietal, and occipital lobes, bright on axial FLAIR.

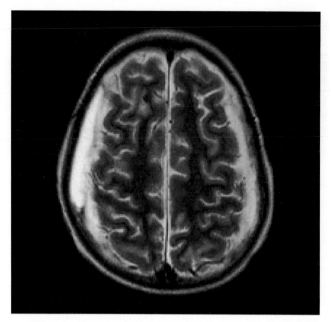

Figure 39.29. Right subdural hematoma, hyperintense (bright) on axial T2.

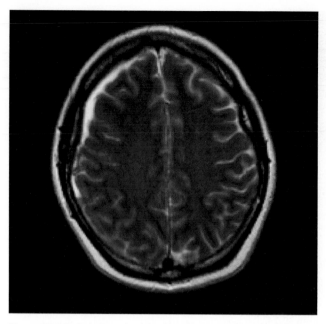

Figure 39.30. Right frontal subdural hematoma, bright on DWI.

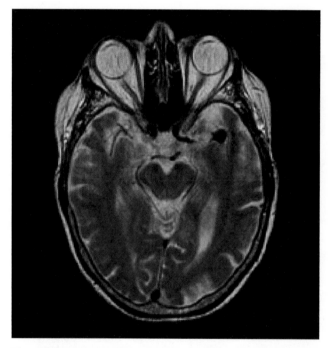

Figure 39.31. Berry aneurysm, located in the left temporal lobe, dark on axial T2.

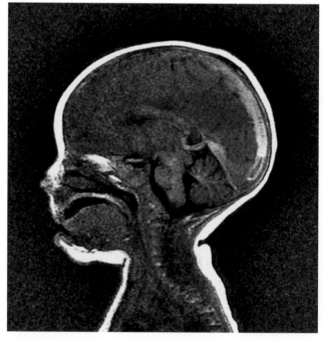

Figure 39.32. Dural sinus thrombosis (pediatric), bright on T1 flair sagittal.

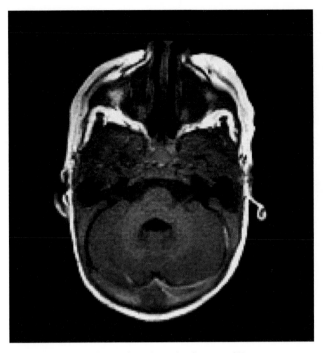

Figure 39.33. Dural sinus thrombosis, bright on axial T1.

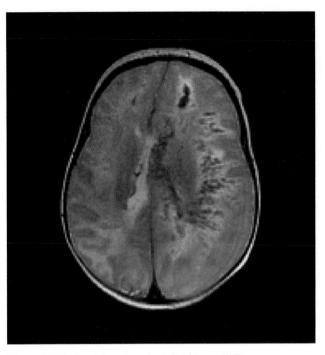

Figure 39.34. Dural sinus thrombosis, bright on axial T2.

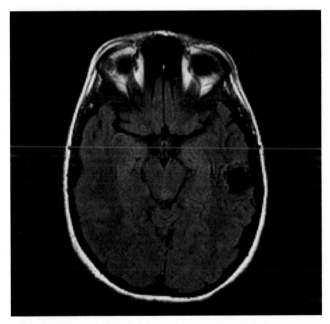

Figure 39.35. AVM, left temporal lobe, dark on axial T2 FLAIR.

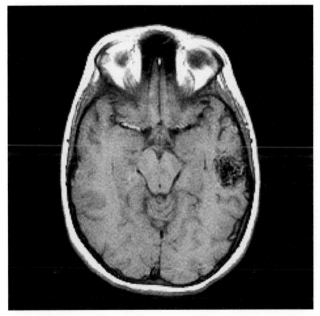

Figure 39.36. AVM, left temporal lobe, dark on axial T1.

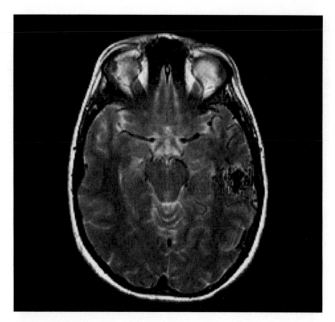

Figure 39.37. AVM, left temporal lobe, dark on axial T2.

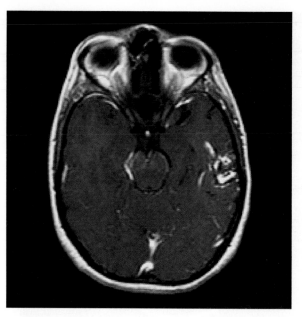

Figure 39.38. AVM, left temporal lobe, enhancing on axial T1 + contrast.

Infectious diseases of the brain

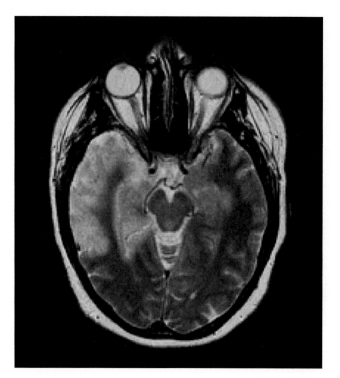

Figure 39.39. Right temporal lobe, acute herpes encephalitis, bright on axial T2. Herpes simplex encephalitis favors the medial temporal lobe, insula, and cingulum and acutely (<5d) appears bright (hyperintense) on FLAIR and T2 (as seen in this image).

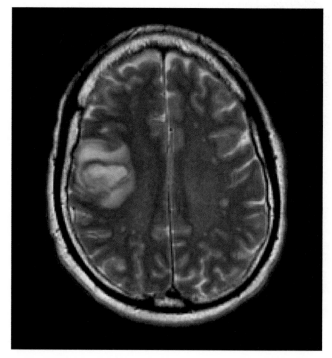

Figure 39.40. Brain abscess, axial T2.

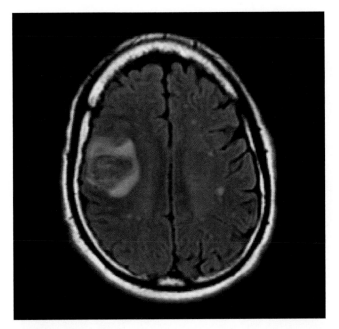

Figure 39.41. Brain abscess in right frontal lobe with surrounding vasogenic edema bright on axial T2 FLAIR.

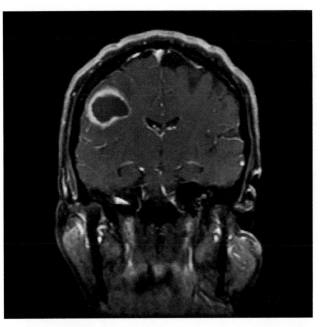

Figure 39.42. Brain abscess in the right parietal lobe demonstrating post-contrast ring-enhancement on coronal T1.

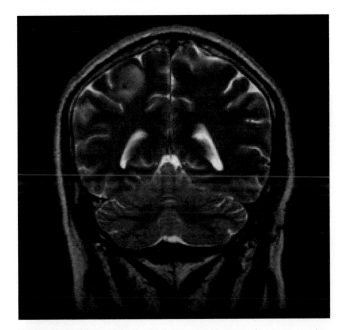

Figure 39.43. Neurocystericosis, right parietal lesion with vasogenic edema, bright on coronal T2.

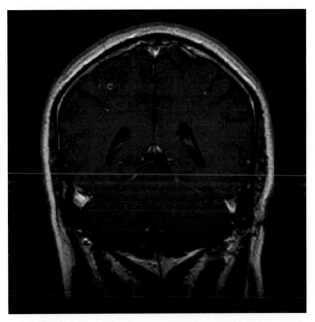

Figure 39.44. Neurocystericosis, right parietal post-contrast ring-enhancing lesion, coronal T1 + contrast.

Non-infectious diseases of the brain

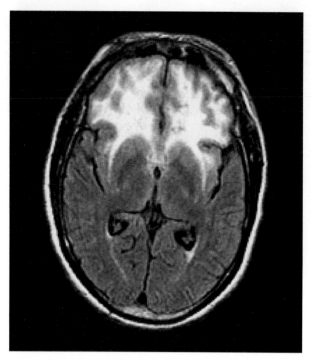

Figure 39.45. Neurosarcoidosis with encephalitis, bilateral frontal horn involvement, bright on axial FLAIR.

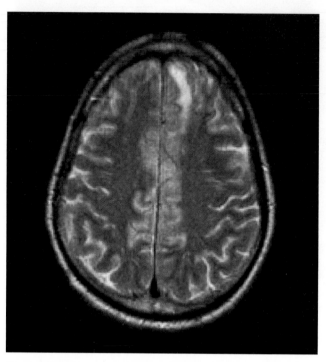

Figure 39.46. Neurosarcoidosis with encephalitis, paramedian posterior frontal lobe involvement, bright on DWI.

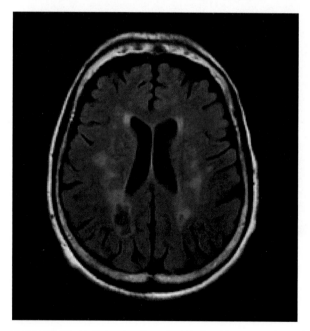

Figure 39.47. Multiple sclerosis, periventricular white matter plaques bright on T2 FLAIR.

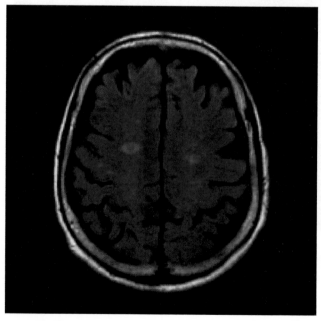

Figure 39.48. Multiple sclerosis, donut-shaped periventricular white matter plaques bright on axial T2 FLAIR.

Brain neoplasms

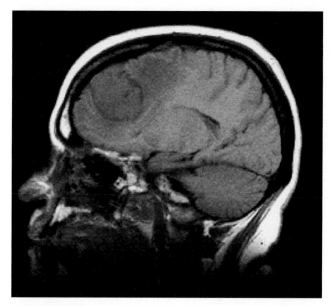

Figure 39.49. Left frontal meningioma, isointense to gray matter on sagittal T1. Meningiomas are characteristically isointense to slightly hypointense (dark) when compared to gray matter on T1 and enhance with contrast.

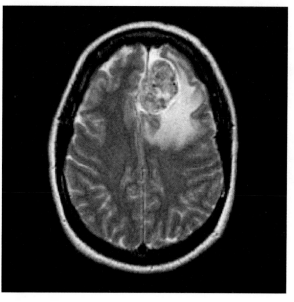

Figure 39.50. Left frontal meningioma (isointense to gray matter) with bright (hyperintense) vasogenic edema on T2 axial.

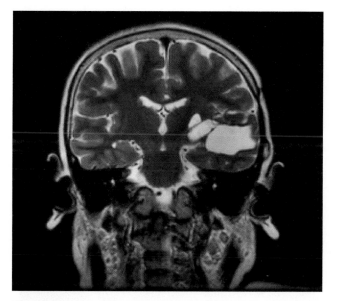

Figure 39.51. Cystic left temporal lobe mass, bright on coronal T2.

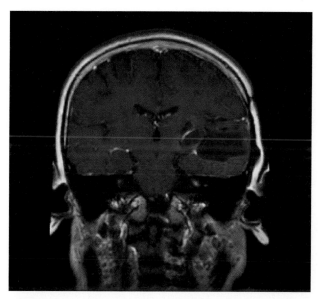

Figure 39.52. Cystic left temporal lobe mass, dark on coronal T1 (compare with Fig. 39.51).

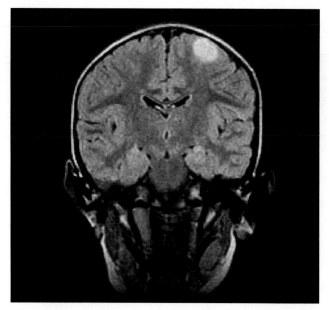

Figure 39.53. Left parietal glioma, coronal FLAIR. Gliomas are typically bright on FLAIR and may or may not enhance with contrast.

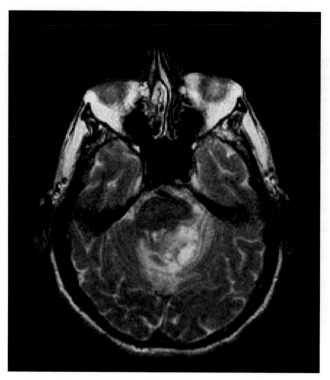

Figure 39.54. Left cerebellar mass with necrosis and hemorrhage, bright on axial T2.

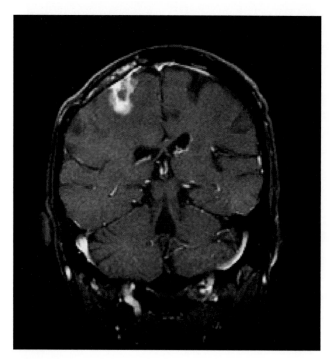

Figure 39.55. Right frontoparietal lobe metastasis showing contrast enhancement, T1 + contrast. Metastatic tumors are the most common intracranial neoplasm, typically located at the gray–white junction and often with significant vasogenic edema. The most common primary tumors are lung, breast, melanoma, renal cell, and thyroid carcinoma.

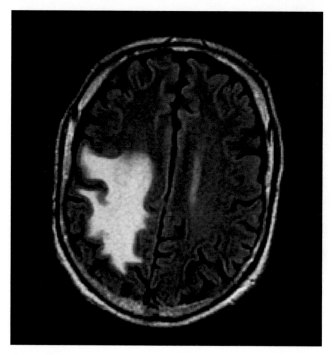

Figure 39.56. Right frontoparietal lobe metastasis with vasogenic edema, bright on axial FLAIR.

Orbital pathology

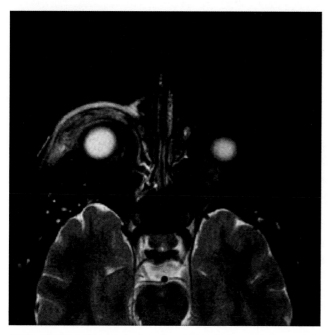

Figure 39.57. Right periorbital swelling, foreign body to soft tissue, axial T2.

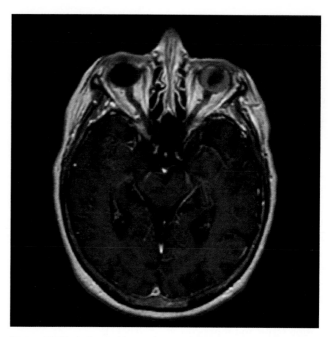

Figure 39.58. Left retinal hemorrhage and detachment, bright on axial T1.

Suggested Readings

Allen LM, Hasso AN, Handwerker J, Farid H: Sequence-specific MR imaging findings that are useful in dating ischemic stroke. *Radiographics* 2012;**32**(5):1285–97; discussion 97–9.

Avci E, Fossett D, Aslan M, et al.: Branches of the anterior cerebral artery near the anterior communicating artery complex: an anatomic study and surgical perspective. *Neurol Med Chir (Tokyo)* 2003;**43**(7):329–33; discussion 333.

Bloch F, Hansen WW, Packard M: Nuclear induction. *Phys Rev* 1946;**69**(3–4):127.

Bradley WG Jr.: MR appearance of hemorrhage in the brain. *Radiology* 1993;**189**(1):15–26.

Fleetwood IG, Marcellus ML, Levy RP, et al.: Deep arteriovenous malformations of the basal ganglia and thalamus: natural history. *J Neurosurg* 2003;**98**(4):747–50.

Fox RJ, Rudick RA: Multiple sclerosis: disease markers accelerate progress. *Lancet Neurol* 2004;**3**:10.

Jackson EF, Ginsberg LE, Schomer DF, Leeds NE: A review of MRI pulse sequences and techniques in neuroimaging. *Surg Neurol* 1997;**47**(2):185–99.

Kuker W, Nägele T, Schmidt F, et al.: Diffusion-weighted MRI in herpes simplex encephalitis. *Neuroradiology* 2004;**46**(2):122–5.

Osborn A, Blaser S, Salzman K: *Diagnostic imaging: Brain.* Salt Lake City, UT: Amirsys, 2004.

Purcell EM, Torrey HC, Pound RV: Resonance absorption by nuclear magnetic moments in a solid. *Phys Rev* 1946;**69**(1–2):37–8.

Schaefer PW, Grant PE, Gonzalez RG: Diffusion-weighted MR imaging of the brain. *Radiology* 2000;**217**(2):331–45.

Schellinger PD, Fiebach JB, Hoffmann K, et al.: Stroke MRI in intracerebral hemorrhage: is there a perihemorrhagic penumbra? *Stroke* 2003;**34**(7):1674–9.

Tintinalli J: *Emergency medicine: a comprehensive study guide*, 6th ed. New York: McGraw-Hill, 2004.

Tsuchiya K, Katase S, Yoshino A, Hachiya J: Diffusion-weighted MR imaging of encephalitis. *AJR Am J Roentgenol* 1999;**173**:1097–9.

Yousem DM, Grossman RI: *Neuroradiology: the requisites.* Philadelphia, PA: Mosby/Elsevier, 2010.

Chapter 40

MRI of the Spine

Aaron J. Harries, Andrew V. Bokarius, Armando S. Garza, and J. Christian Fox

Clinical indications

MRI has become accepted as the most appropriate imaging modality for the study of spine pathology in many cases. Specifically, in the examination of spinal cord trauma, soft tissue injury, and acute intervertebral disc injury, MRI has a higher soft tissue resolution than any other modality. However, despite optimal visualization of MRIs, it is often not the most appropriate initial imaging study because plain film radiographs and CT scans can provide diagnostic information faster and more cost-effectively (1).

MRI is indicated in blunt spinal trauma patients with neurological findings suggestive of spinal cord injury without a clear explanation following radiographs or CT (2). Emergent MRI of the spine is also generally indicated in the evaluation of spinal cord pathology with signs of myelopathy, radiculopathy, and progressive neurological deficit. Despite these seemingly clear indications, the risk of missing a spinal cord injury makes this decision a major dilemma for physicians. The medical and legal ramifications of restricting diagnostic MRI and failing to diagnose a patient with an unstable spine injury are clearly evident. In contrast, the ubiquitous use of expensive and time-consuming imaging equipment can inappropriately drive up the cost of medical care and possibly render emergency resources unavailable to other patients. Therefore, it is important to gain as much information as possible from the history, physical exam, and preliminary imaging studies to aid the physician's decision for selecting MRI for potential spinal cord pathology (3).

Spinal injuries are one of the most devastating and life-altering of all trauma-related injuries. Every year in the United States, there are approximately 12,000 new cases of spinal cord injuries, which are predominately seen in young men (4, 5). The majority of spinal cord injuries are caused by blunt trauma, with approximately 50% due to motor vehicle accidents, followed by falls, gunshot wounds, and sports injuries (6). Cervical cord injury is the most common and devastating of the spinal cord injuries, which is seen in 65% of patients with isolated spinal cord injury. In patients with isolated upper cervical fracture with associated neurological deficit, MRI resulted in treatment modification in 25% of patients (7). However, in patients with an upper cervical spine fracture without neurological findings, MRI did not change treatment. Thus, MRI has not been shown to be a useful or cost-effective screening tool in upper cervical fractures without neurological deficit (7).

After a trauma patient has been stabilized and immobilized, a history and physical examination must be performed to assess the possibility of a spinal cord injury. Important information to be included in the history is the presence or absence of neck or back pain, mechanism of injury (MOI), and any loss of consciousness. The MOI is of vital importance because the type of vertebral fracture has been shown to be unique to the vector forces placed upon it. This is particularly seen in acute cervical spine fractures being classified by MOI based on the primary spinal movements of flexion, extension, compression, lateral flexion, rotation, or a combination of these forces (8).

A thorough history is also important in nontraumatic patients who present with back pain. It is one of the most common medical complaints, often related to disc herniations, muscle strains, or osteoarthritis or degenerative joint disease (DJD). MRI may be beneficial for patients suffering from severe or persistent pain, sciatica (shooting pain down the leg), muscle weakness, and numbness or tingling. In a stable patient, follow up can be safely performed in a nonemergent setting. In addition, a history of back pain, fever, and laboratory evidence of infection may suggest discitis, osteomyelitis, or an epidural abscess requiring further evaluation with MRI. Past medical history questioning can also be important for diagnosing more cryptic etiologies of spinal disease. For example, previous history of cancer may suggest new vertebral metastasis, history of tuberculosis may manifest as Pott disease, or a patient with multiple sclerosis (MS) history with may present with neuropathic pain.

Important components of the history – such as the presence of radiculopathic pain, urinary or fecal incontinence, or muscle weakness – can help guide a physician's physical exam. The physical exam, in particular, the neurological exam, is vital to diagnosing potential spinal pathology. Findings of motor or sensory loss or abnormal reflexes can delineate the level of spinal cord injury and determine the region of the spine to be imaged. For example, a trauma patient with lower extremity paralysis and decreased sensation up to the xiphoid process will need MR imaging of the thoracic spine as the sensory deficit corresponds to T6 (thoracic spinal nerve level 6), which could have been missed if only a lumbar spine MRI were performed. In contrast, cauda equina syndrome affecting the lumbar spine would show signs of decreased sensation only to the lower extremities with saddle anesthesia and decreased rectal sphincter tone. In addition, noting the specific area of spine tenderness on palpation can also help identify underlying structural abnormalities. These physical findings can help localize the suspected level of spinal cord injury and assist in identifying the area of pathology on MRI.

It is important to complete an initial neurological exam at the time of presentation because the patient may later deteriorate, and a comparison may then be needed. A patient without symptoms in the field or at the time of presentation who neurologically deteriorates in the ED requires emergent treatment.

When requesting any radiological study, it is important to include relevant clinical history and diagnostic information to assist the radiologist in determining the most appropriate imaging study to perform. Specifically, include the patient's clinical history, neurologic deficits, any history of neoplasm or immunosuppression, and previous imaging studies on the request form.

Diagnostic capabilities

MRI has several major advantages over other imaging modalities that often make it the most appropriate diagnostic tool for common spine pathology. Unlike CT and plain radiographs, MRI does not use ionizing radiation, which are associated with long-term cancer risks. Due to the inherent physics underlying the principles of MRI, it has a higher contrast resolution, allowing for better soft tissue discrimination. MRI is sensitive for detecting spinal cord pathology associated with traumatic spinal cord injuries, disc herniations, neoplastic lesions, degenerative joint disease, and infections. In addition, MRI can effectively visualize spinal cord inflammatory conditions, such as MS and myelitis (9).

According to the ACR Appropriateness Criteria, traumatic spine injury would most commonly be imaged by CT, with sagittal and coronal reconstruction images. MRI imaging is useful for evaluating patients with neurological abnormalities, looking for cord abnormalities, or evaluating ligamentous injury and edema (10). While plain radiographs were standard in the past, now they are mainly used as tools for follow-up in patients with a known fracture.

Complex spine fractures and retropulsed fracture fragments are best characterized by CT (11). Spine trauma associated with neurological dysfunction suggesting possible spinal cord injury requires emergent MRI. MRI is the only imaging modality that directly visualizes the spinal cord; thus, its high contrast resolution is used to diagnose suspected spinal cord compression, hemorrhage, edema, purulent, or transection within the spinal canal (12). MRI has been shown to be useful in establishing a prognosis and for planning treatment associated with spinal cord injuries, with the degree of cord compression being the most important factor (13). Plain films or CT may be able to visualize bone fractures or dislocations in trauma patients, but they may be unable to detect associated traumatic disc herniations and occult ligamentous injuries, which may later be picked up by MRI (14).

Traumatic injury to cervical soft tissues and ligaments may occur in the absence of fractures or subluxations as evaluated by radiography or CT. If the injuries are significant, the resulting instability could lead to further injury or deformity, requiring surgical stabilization (15). These patients may report persistent neck pain or neurological deficits after violent cervical acceleration-deceleration, such as those seen in motor vehicle accidents. Alternatively, ligamentous injury may occur in severely obtunded patients, whose neurological status cannot be reliably evaluated. High clinical suspicion for ligamentous injury should prompt further evaluation with MRI, even in the setting of an unremarkable CT, as these tests provide complementary information (16). Flexion and extension radiographs are considered significantly less helpful, as they are relatively insensitive to soft tissue injury and may be confounded by muscle spasm in the acute setting.

Spinal stenosis resulting in compression of the spinal cord or nerve roots is often caused by impinging osteophytes and intervertebral disc herniations. Furthermore, disc herniations are one of the most common causes of severe, nontraumatic back pain presenting in the ED. Often radiographs may be obtained because they are fast and inexpensive and may detect any unsuspecting lesions, such as compression fractures or degenerative changes. MRI is considered the most sensitive imaging study for detecting disc herniations and determining degree of associated spinal canal or neural foraminal stenosis (17, 18). Depending on the presenting nature and severity of the disc protrusion, MRI may be performed safely in a nonemergent setting if the patient is stable. When MRI is contraindicated, CT myelography is a slightly less sensitive secondary modality for imaging disc herniations and is associated with higher risk due to invasive insertion of intrathecal contrast (19). Osteophytes or calcific components of other lesions causing compression on the spinal cord or roots can occasionally be missed on MRI. In these occult cases, CT can be used as an adjunct imaging study because of its fine depiction of osseous detail (20).

MRI is very sensitive in its visualization of bone marrow abnormalities. Abnormal bone marrow appearance in vertebral bodies can suggest a variety of disorders, such as anemia, infection, and metastatic disease. With the suspicion of osseous metastasis, plain radiographs provide an adequate first stage of screening; however, bone destruction abnormalities may not be appreciated until at least 50% of trabecular bone has been destroyed. With the use of MRI, early visualization of tumor replacement of normal bone marrow can be appreciated. Previous studies have shown that MRI has a higher sensitivity and earlier detection of vertebral metastasis than plain films, CT, and radionuclide bone scans; it also has >90% sensitivity for detecting early hematogenous dissemination of the tumor to the skeletal system (20, 21).

MRI is often used to detect early infection and to evaluate the full extent of potentially life-threatening lesions affecting the spine, such as osteomyelitis, discitis, and epidural abscess. For example, the earliest sign of vertebral osteomyelitis can be detected by MRI, due to its high sensitivity to bone marrow edema (22, 23). Also, sagittal images can directly assess early disc space and endplate abnormalities associated with discitis, which can evolve into osteomyelitis (24).

In the diagnosis of spinal tuberculosis (Pott disease), MRI has been shown to be more sensitive than radiography and more specific than scintigraphy due to the specific anatomical pattern of involvement, often demonstrating disc sparing. MRI provides early detection of spinal tuberculosis, up to 4 to 6 months earlier than other techniques, which could reduce destruction and diminish the need for surgery (25).

MRI has high sensitivity for visualization of inflammatory myelopathies, such as MS. Unfortunately, it exhibits a low specificity for differentiating from the variety of intramedullary lesions (26). Therefore, the diagnosis of MS is based on clinical criteria, with MRI playing an important supportive role due to its limited specificity (27). MRI of the cervical spine is recommended in patients with suspected MS with symptoms of spinal cord involvement because 10% to 15% of patients with spinal cord lesions have no intracranial disease (28, 29).

The sensitivity of MRI can be improved with the use of gadolinium IV contrast agents to diagnose spinal disease in the intramedullary, intradural extramedullary, and extradural compartments. Gadolinium-enhanced MRI of intramedullary disease is sensitive for detecting primary tumors (ependymomas and astrocytomas), metastasis, inflammation, and demyelination. In intradural extramedullary disease, enhancement is useful for diagnosing drop metastases, meningiomas, and nerve-sheath tumors (30).

Imaging pitfalls and limitations

MR safety continues to evolve with the proliferation of more sophisticated MRI-compatible implants and monitoring devices. MRI is contraindicated in patients with implanted cardiac pacemakers, defibrillators, ferromagnetic aneurysm clips, other ferromagnetic implants (cochlear electronic devices), and intraocular metallic foreign bodies from occupational exposure. The strong magnetic fields used in MRI can displace small metallic structures and cause electronic device malfunction. In general, orthopedic metallic hardware is not contraindicated; however, metallic prosthesis can induce susceptibility artifacts in MRI, limiting the evaluation of nearby structures. Therefore, it is important to provide appropriate information on any internal metallic objects so the radiologist can properly protocol the scan to minimize metallic artifact (31).

Traditionally, CT has been the imaging modality of choice for unstable patients requiring life-support equipment, which normally contains ferromagnetic components or sensitive electronic devices that will not tolerate large magnetic fields. MRI scans usually take longer than CT scans, which is unfavorable in emergent settings. Therefore, MRI is typically used once a patient has been stabilized. However, MRI-compatible respirators and physiological monitoring equipment are available, allowing patients requiring supportive care to be safely monitored during MRI (32).

The use of MRI has further limitations based on the constricted physical confines of the scanner. Morbidly obese patients may not be able to fit in the scanner because most MRI scanners have an approximate weight limit of 400 pounds and a maximum bore diameter of 70 cm; in addition, receiver coils may have specific restrictions. MRI in the pediatric population, especially those younger than 6 years, may be difficult to perform because they have to remain still for an extended period of time. Movement can produce motion artifact. Claustrophobic patients may also have difficulty with the tight confines of the MRI scanner. Both pediatric and claustrophobic patients may easily be treated with mild sedation.

With pregnant patients, ultrasound or MRI are usually preferable to CT or radiographs that use ionizing radiation. It is important to determine pregnancy status in females of reproductive age prior to requesting a study, because this may decide the appropriate imaging modality.

Gadolinium MRI contrast agents have been associated with much less toxicity and adverse reactions, including decreased incidence of renal failure, as compared with IV CT contrast agents (33). However, it is important to know a patient's renal function prior to MRI because gadolinium contrast agent is contraindicated in patients with preexisting renal failure due to associations of nephrogenic systemic fibrosis (NSF) (34, 35). According to the ACR contrast guidelines, the use of gadolinium-based contrast agents is generally contraindicated in patients with a GFR under 30 or in acute kidney injury (36). Certain precautions are advised in patients with asthma, allergy history, and prior iodinated or gadolinium-based contrast reactions. For example, corticosteroids and antihistamines may be given to patients prophylactically, prior to an MRI study.

The use of gadolinium-based MR contrast agent in pregnant patients is not routinely performed; however, in a case-by-case basis, it requires a well-documented risk–benefit analysis. Previous studies have shown that gadolinium ions pass through the placental barrier and enter the fetal circulation, causing possible side effects to the fetus. Therefore, an in-depth analysis of the potential benefits to the patient and fetus, outweighing the potential risks of gadolinium ion exposure to the developing fetus, is required (37).

Clinical images

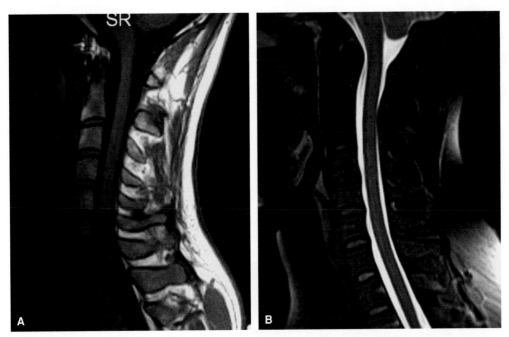

Figure 40.1. Normal cervical spine. A: Sagittal T1 image through the normal cervical spine demonstrates vertebral body bone marrow as hyperintense, or high signal (bright), compared with the intervertebral discs that appear as isointense, or intermediate signal. Cerebrospinal fluid (CSF) is hypointense, or low signal (dark), with the spinal cord appearing as an intermediate signal. The vertebral cortical margins are well demarcated with low signal and blend anterior and posteriorly with the respective longitudinal ligaments. B: Sagittal T2 image demonstrates vertebral body bone marrow as low signal with the intervertebral discs as high signal. CSF appears as a high signal surrounding the spinal cord, which is a lower signal.

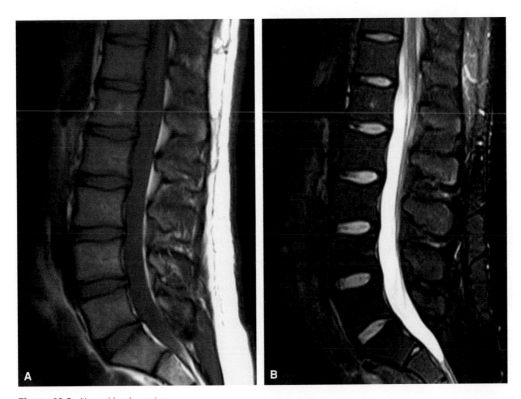

Figure 40.2. Normal lumbar spine.
   A: Sagittal T1 image through the normal lumbar spine demonstrates bone marrow as hyperintense signal (bright), intervertebral discs as isointense signal, CSF as hypointense signal (dark), and spinal cord as isointense signal. B: Sagittal T2 image shows bone marrow as hypointense signal, intervertebral discs as hyperintense signal, CSF as hyperintense signal, and spinal cord as hypointense signal.

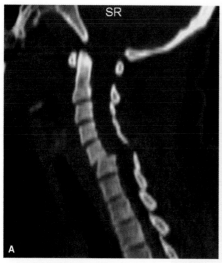
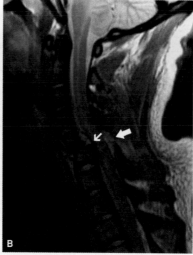

Figure 40.3. A: CT of the cervical spine with posttraumatic grade 2 (50%) vertebral body anterolisthesis at C5–6. There is disruption of the posterior elements and ligamentous structures, making this an unstable fracture.

B: Sagittal T2 image also demonstrates anterolisthesis at C5–6 with associated posterior longitudinal disruption and evidence of cord compression (*small white arrow*). There is also disruption of the anterior longitudinal ligament with associated edema marked by high signal (*black arrow*). Also shown is widening of the posterior elements with disrupted interspinous ligaments marked by increased edema (*large white arrow*) due to flexion injury.

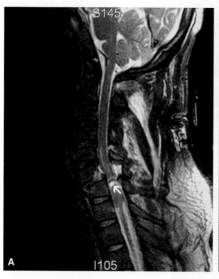
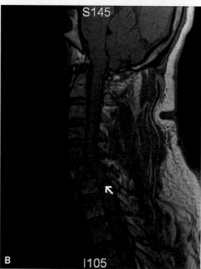

Figure 40.4. Cervical cord transection. This type of cervical fracture-dislocation is a classic extension injury. A: Sagittal T2 image through the cervical spine demonstrates subluxation of C6 on C7, with a fracture through the posterior inferior endplate of C6 and anterior superior endplate of C7. The hyperintense transverse signal (*arrow*) in the spinal cord indicates cord transection. B: Sagittal T1 image shows similar features with hypointense transverse signal (*arrow*) at the cord transection.

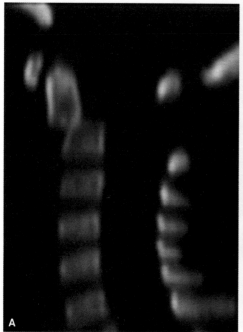
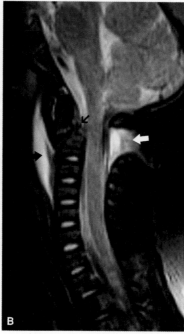

Figure 40.5. Odontoid fracture. A: CT of the cervical spine shows a type II odontoid fracture (fracture line through the base of the odontoid at its attachment to the body of C2). B: Sagittal T2 image also shows evidence of fracture, with the odontoid base being offset approximately 1 cm from the body of C2 (*small black arrow*). The fracture fragment is displaced anteriorly with no apparent signal abnormality in the spinal cord. There is also wide separation of posterior elements of C1–2, with complete ligamentous disruption shown by hyperintense signal (*large white arrow*). In addition, there is evidence of significant prevertebral soft tissue edema, also marked by hyperintense signal (*large black arrow*).

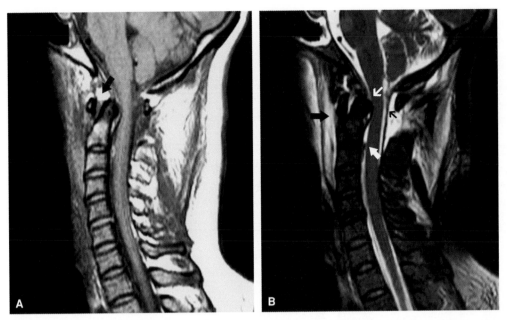

Figure 40.6. C1-C2 subluxation. This 33-year-old female suffered a craniocervical separation injury as a pedestrian when she was hit by a car. A: Sagittal T1 image shows widening of the pre-dens space, indicating anterior subluxation of C1 on C2 (*black arrow*) and compromise of the transverse ligament causing impingement of the dens on the anterior surface of the spinal cord. B: Sagittal T2 image also shows C1–2 subluxation with better appreciation of cord compression (*small white arrow*). There are also multiple ruptured ligaments involving the upper cervical spine evidenced by increased space between the basion and the dens, indicating injury to the apical ligament, tectorial membrane and alar ligaments. There is disruption of the anterior longitudinal ligament with prevertebral swelling at the C1 and C2 levels (*large black arrow*). A small epidural hematoma marked by low T2 signal (*small black arrow*) is seen at the posterior epidural space of C1. There is also a small area of low T2 signal posterior to the C2–3 interspace likely representing hemorrhage and injury to the posterior longitudinal ligament (*large white arrow*).

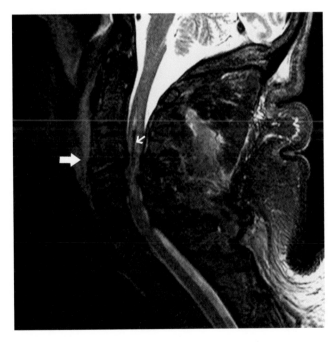

Figure 40.7. Cervical fracture with hemorrhagic cord contusion. This 64-year-old male suffered a severe spinal cord injury, resulting in quadriplegia below C4 after falling off a horse. Sagittal T2 image shows evidence of subtle C3 and C4 fractures with underlying chronic degenerative changes resulting in marked narrowing of the spinal canal to 5 mm, leading to linear hemorrhagic contusion marked by hypointense signal (*small arrow*) of the spinal cord from C2 to the lower body of C4. There is a likely tear of the anterior spinal ligament at the point of a teardrop fracture of the anterior inferior border of C3 (*large arrow*). There is also soft tissue abnormality with prevertebral edema associated with fracturing of C3–4.

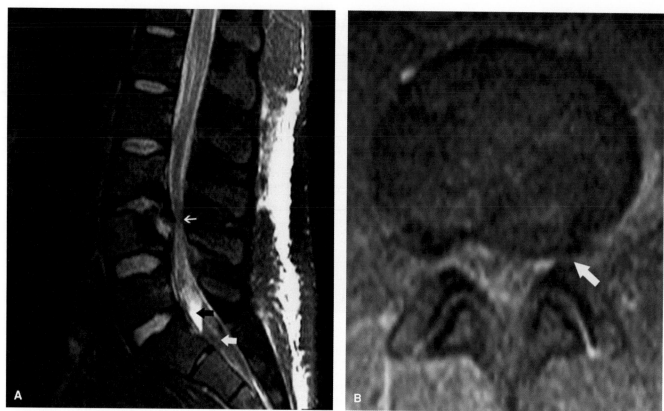

Figure 40.8. Lumbar fractures with spinal stenosis status post gunshot wound. This 20-year-old male presented with traumatic back pain secondary to a gunshot wound, with decreased sensory and motor functions in the lower extremities bilaterally. A: Sagittal T2 image shows fractures of the L3–4 vertebra with retropulsion of bony fragments (*small white arrow*) into the spinal canal. The combination of bone fragments and associated hemorrhagic products result in focal spinal stenosis at L4 narrowed down to 4 mm. There is also presumed injury to the posterior longitudinal ligament at this level. In addition, there is a hematocrit level (*large white arrow*) in the caudal thecal sac, indicating hemorrhage with serum supernatant as high signal (*black arrow*). B: Axial T1 postcontrast image shows retropulsed vertebral body fragments causing left neural foraminal and spinal canal stenosis (*white arrow*).

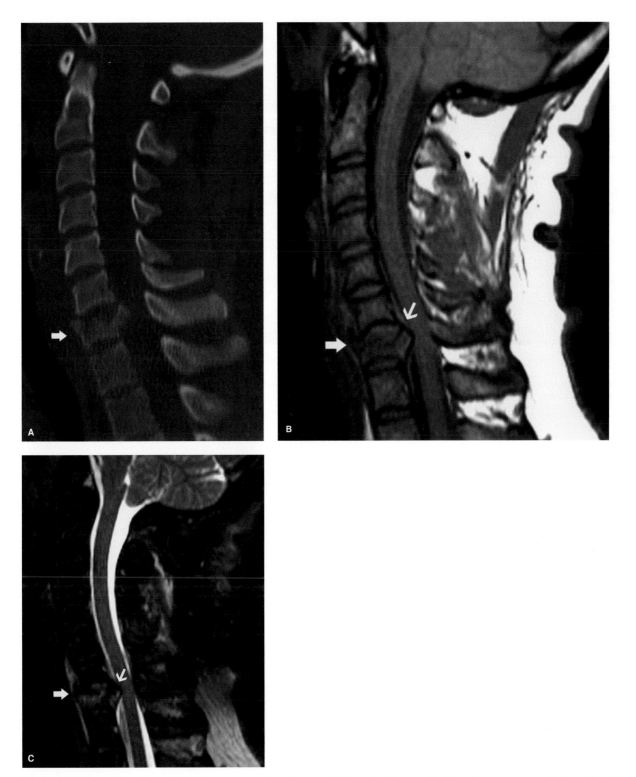

Figure 40.9. Cervical burst fracture. A: CT demonstrates a burst fracture of C7 (*arrow*) with retropulsed bone fragments in the spinal canal. Sagittal T1 (B) and T2 (C) images further characterize this traumatic injury by confirming the C7 burst fracture and visualizing the associated rupture of the anterior (*large arrow*) and posterior (*small arrow*) longitudinal ligaments. The retropulsed bone fragments cause narrowing of the spinal canal with resultant cord compression. There is associated pre-vertebral soft tissue edema.

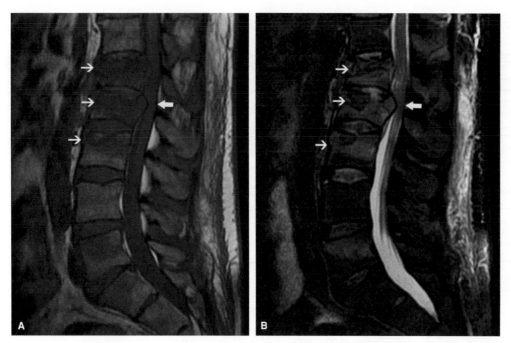

Figure 40.10. Traumatic compression fracture with spinal stenosis. Sagittal T1 (A) and short tau inversion recovery (STIR) (B) images show posttraumatic multilevel lumbar spine fractures (*small arrows*), most severe at L1. Note the disruption of the superior endplates and anterior cortex. STIR image shows evidence of edema as high signal within the vertebral bodies. There is severe canal stenosis (*large arrow*) due to posterior displacement of fracture fragments and increased signal in the adjacent spinal nerve roots with imaging confirming a clinical diagnosis of cauda equina syndrome.

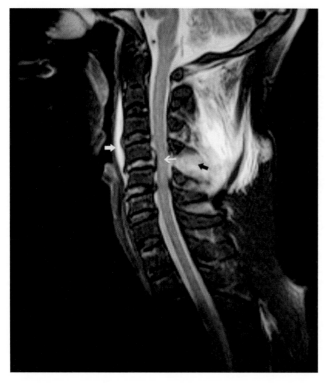

Figure 40.11. Traumatic cervical disc extrusion with cord compression. Sagittal STIR T2 image of cervical spine demonstrates multilevel disc osteophyte complexes and a disc extrusion at C4–5 (*small white arrow*), which effaces the anterior thecal sac, causing mild compression and edema of the anterior cord marked by abnormal signal. Evidence of edema with high signal in the intervertebral discs, combined with disruption of both the anterior longitudinal ligament and the interspinous ligaments (*black arrow*), indicates that an acute flexion injury has resulted in traumatic disc extrusion. There is also prevertebral edema marked by hyperintense signal (*large white arrow*). Mild cord contusion without hemorrhage can improve, whereas a cord hematoma is less likely to regress.

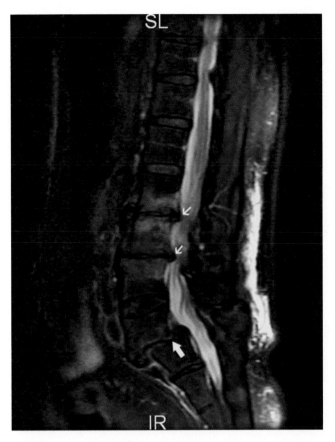

Figure 40.12. Chronic degenerative changes resulting in spinal stenosis. Sagittal STIR image through the lumbar spine with multifactorial spinal canal stenosis. There are degenerative changes at L2–3, L3–4, L4–5, L5-S1 with loss of intervertebral disk height, disc desiccation (loss of normal signal in disk), and Modic type I degenerative endplate changes at L2–3 and L3–4 marked by T2 high signal. Disc bulges (*small arrows*) at these levels combined with endplate and facet hypertrophy and grade I-II anterior spondylolysthesis at L5-S1 (*large arrow*) result in moderate spinal canal stenosis.

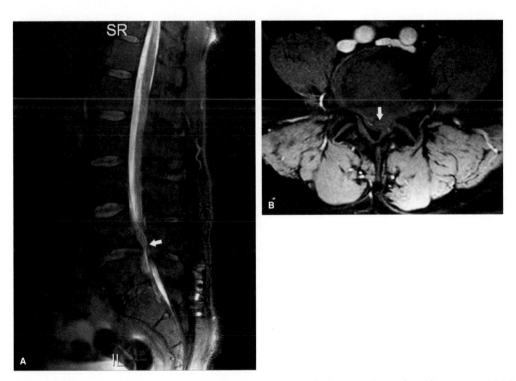

Figure 40.13. Lumbar disc herniation. A: Sagittal T2 image through the lumbar spine shows a large disc extrusion at L4–5 with cranial migration posterior to the vertebral body of L4, resulting in severe spinal stenosis (*arrow*). B: Axial T1 postcontrast image through L4/5 interspace also shows severe stenosis as the disc extends into the spinal canal (*arrow*).

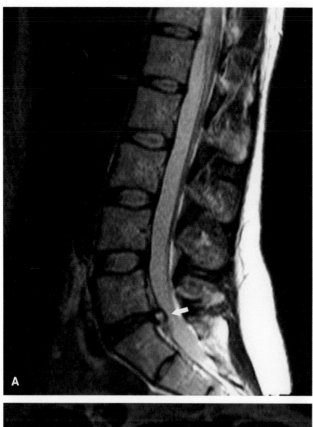

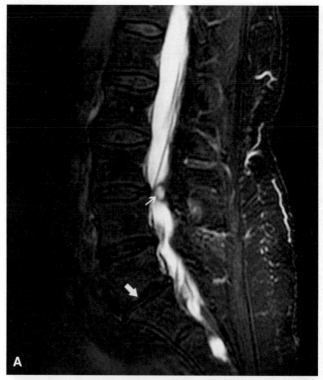

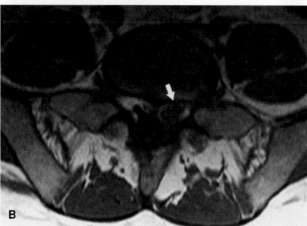

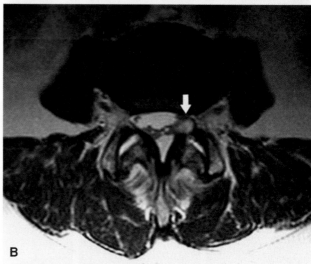

Figure 40.14. Lumbar disc extrusion with sequestration. This 28-year-old female presented with left leg numbness. A: Sagittal proton density image of the lumbar spine shows a 9 mm left posterolateral disc extrusion at the L5-S1 level. The axial view better demonstrates 1.4 cm sequestered disc fragment. There is also desiccation of the L5-S1 disc evidenced by decreased signal. B: Axial T1 image shows the disc extrusion (*arrow*) extending laterally into the left L5-S1 neural foramen and left lateral recess.

Figure 40.15. Synovial cyst with neural foraminal stenosis. A: Sagittal T2 image through the lumbar spine shows evidence of a synovial cyst (*small arrow*) marked by a round fluid signal indenting the thecal sac at the L3–4 interspace level. B: Axial T2 image through the L3–4 interspace shows the synovial cyst marked by a round fluid signal with a hypointense peripheral rim (*arrow*) in the left posterolateral spinal canal adjacent to the facet joint, causing severe neural foraminal stenosis and compression of adjacent nerve root. On axial T2 image, synovial cysts can be differentiated from herniated discs as they are normally found next to the facet joints.

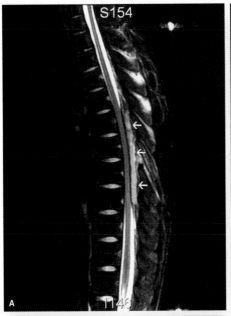
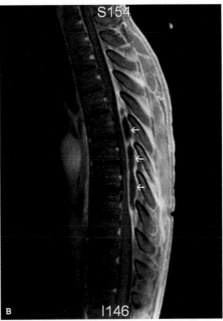
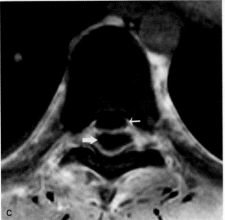

Figure 40.16. Epidural abscess. This patient presented with severe back pain with sensory and motor deficits. A: Sagittal T2 image through the thoracic spine shows evidence of a large posterior epidural fluid collection, likely abscess (*arrows*), extending from approximately T8 to T12. The epidural collection demonstrates increased signal and effaces the posterior thecal sac compressing the cord. B: Sagittal T1 postcontrast image shows peripheral enhancement around the collection. The internal contents do not enhance, thus making neoplasm very unlikely. C: Axial T1 postcontrast image shows the posterior epidural abscess (*large arrow*) compressing the spinal cord, which is anterior (*small arrow*).

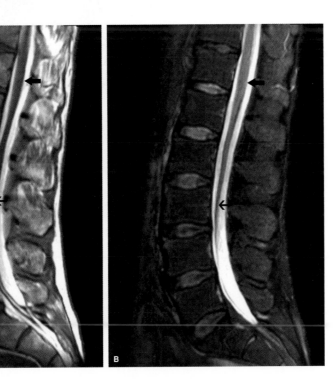

Figure 40.17. Subdural hematoma. This 49-year-old male with seizure disorder status post fall injury presented with lower back pain, bilateral lower extremity numbness, and muscle weakness. A: Sagittal T1 image shows extensive high signal surrounding the spinal cord throughout the subdural space, most consistent with blood product/protein. B: Sagittal T2 fat saturated image also shows failure of suppression, suggesting an alternate etiology such as hemorrhage. There is associated mass effect with compression of the conus medullaris (*large black arrow*) and spinal nerve roots (*small black arrow*). This mass effect would be less likely in subarachnoid space, and the diffuse involvement is less likely an epidural process. This subdural process extends all the way to the thoracic spine.

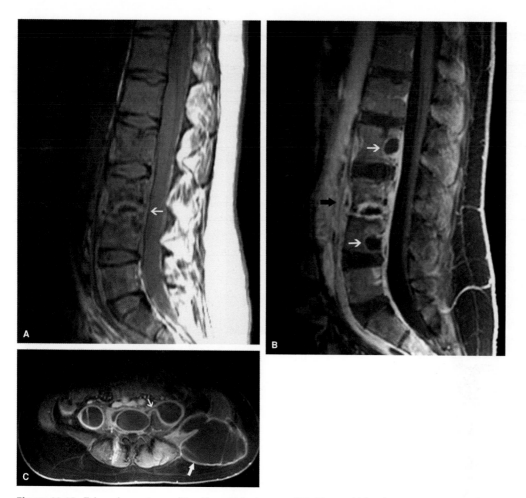

Figure 40.18. Tuberculous osteomyelitis with multiple abscesses. This 22-year-old female presented with left flank mass and severe back pain with a history of tuberculosis exposure. A: Sagittal proton density image of the lumbar spine shows abnormal signal principally in the L2, L3, and L4 vertebral bodies and at the L3–4 disc (*white arrow*). B: Sagittal T1 postcontrast image tuberculous granulomas. Enhancement at L3–4 disc is compatible with discitis, which is a late finding. There is also a large prevertebral phlegmon anterior to L2, L3, and L4 (*large black arrow*). C: The axial T1 postgadolinium image shows paraspinal, pelvic, left psoas (*small white arrow*) and a 10 cm left gluteal abscesses (*large white arrow*).

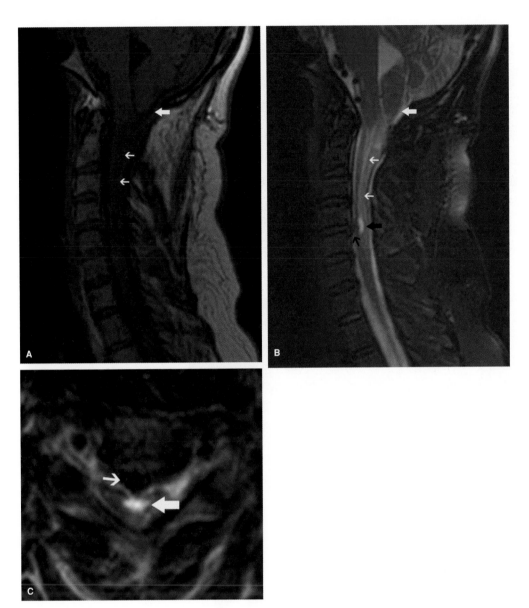

Figure 40.19. Tuberculosis with syrinx and Chiari I malformation. Sagittal proton density T1 (A) and T2 (B) images show gross tuberculous myelopathic changes of the cord from C1 through C5 (*small white arrows*). There is evidence of a syrinx (i) at the C4–5 interspace level, low signal on T1, and high signal on T2. At this same level, there is mild cord compression and associated disc osteophyte complex (*small black arrow*). There is also evidence of Chiari I malformation with 9 mm pointed tonsillar herniation (*large white arrow*). C: Axial T2 image clearly shows the syrinx (*large white arrow*) and the osteophyte complex (*small white arrow*).

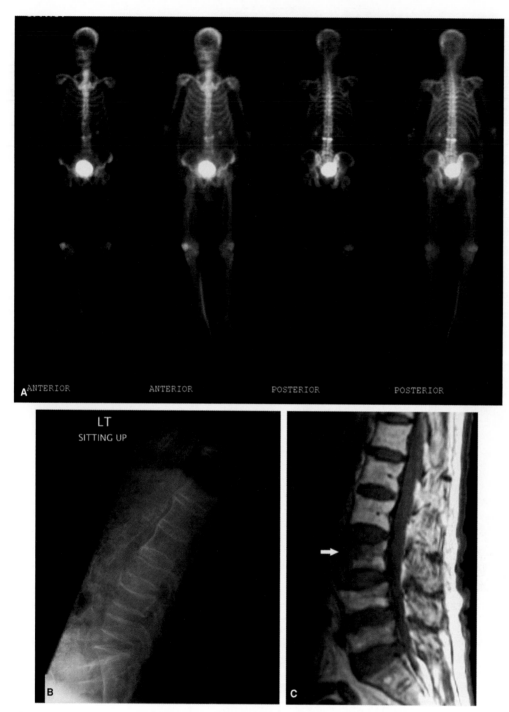

Figure 40.20. Gastric cancer metastasis to lumbar spine. This patient with known gastric cancer presented with lower back pain. A: Tc-99 MDP bone scan shows evidence of focal uptake in L3 vertebral body. B: Lateral plain film demonstrates diffuse osteopenia, loss of the normal lordotic curve, and compression deformities at L3–5. C: Sagittal T1 image demonstrates a hypointense focus in the anterior L3 vertebral body (*arrow*), compatible with a metastatic lesion.

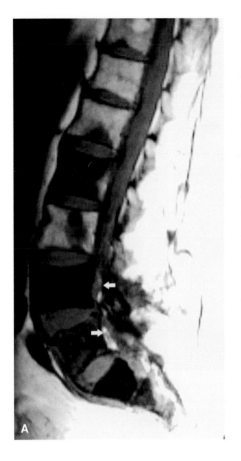
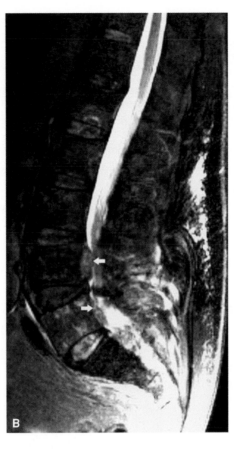

Figure 40.21. Prostate cancer metastasis to lumbar spine. Sagittal T1 (A) and T2 (B) images through the lumbar spine show diffuse signal abnormalities in the lumbar vertebral bodies, indicating replacement of normal marrow with metastatic disease. This patient demonstrates the diffuse metastatic pattern typical of prostate cancer. Lesions that demonstrate hypointensity on both T1 and T2 are compatible with sclerotic metastases. There is also evidence of epidural tumor extension behind the vertebral bodies of L4 and L5 (*arrows*). The aggressive nature of the metastatic tumor rarely confines itself to the borders of the bone and often extends into the epidural space.

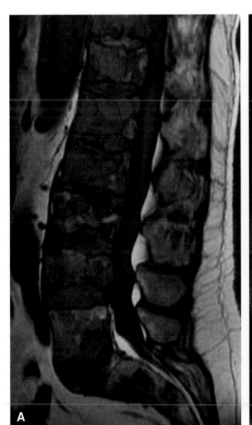
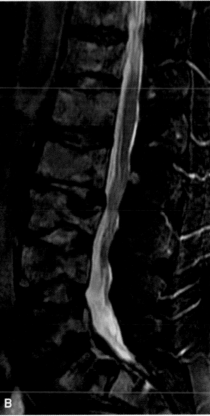

Figure 40.22. Multiple myeloma with compression fractures. Sagittal T1 (A) and T2 (B) images through the lumbar spine show extensive signal abnormality with focal lytic lesions of bone destruction typical of multiple myeloma. Multiple myeloma is the most common primary bone tumor, typically occurring between ages 45 and 80 years.

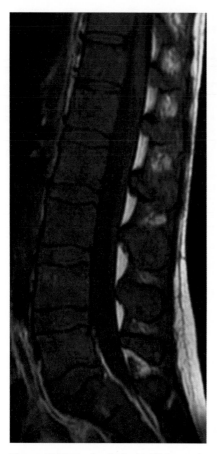

Figure 40.23. Leukemia. Sagittal T1 image through the lumbar spine of a patient with leukemia evidenced by diffuse, homogenous replacement of normal fat signal in vertebral bodies secondary to leukemia. The tumor bone marrow signal is isointense in signal to the intervertebral discs as compared with normal T1 marrow signal being brighter than adjacent discs.

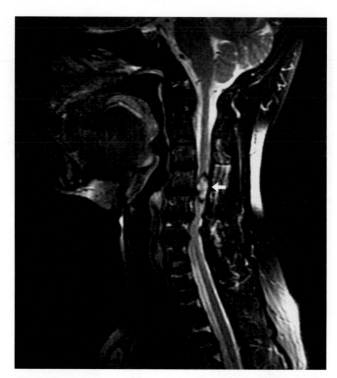

Figure 40.24. Cavernous hemangioma. Sagittal T2 through the cervical spine demonstrates an intramedullary lesion (*arrow*) with expansion of the cord at level C4–5. The lesion has a heterogeneous signal with a peripheral rim of hypointense signal representing blood products in multiple stages of evolution. The "popcorn" appearance is commonly seen with cavernous hemangiomas.

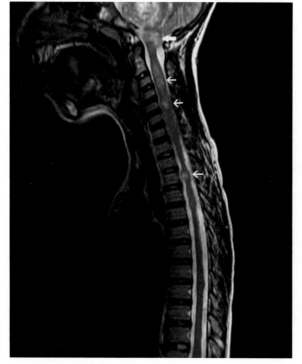

Figure 40.25. Multiple ependymomas. This young patient with neurofibromatosis type 1 presented with progressive weakness of the extremities. Sagittal T2 image of the cervical and thoracic spine demonstrates multiple intramedullary lesions (*small arrows*) with beaded expansion of the spinal cord marked by heterogeneous signal. There is also a mass in the posterior fossa, indicating a brainstem tumor (*large arrow*).

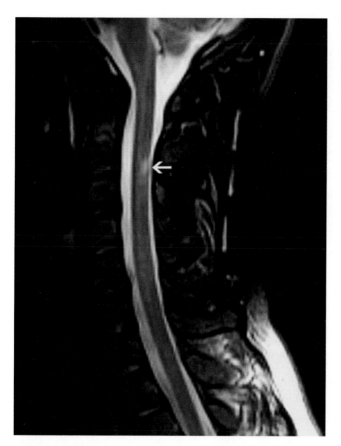

Figure 40.26. A classic MS case with fluctuating neurological deficits in space and time. Sagittal T2 image of the cervical spine demonstrates an MS plaque as a focal hyperintense intramedullary lesion (*arrow*) in the cervical spinal cord at C2–3 level without cord expansion. MS can mimic a spinal cord neoplasm; however, this is less likely if there is no mass effect in the cord. Most MS lesions occupy less than half the diameter of the cord, are less than two vertebral body lengths in size, and are normally located peripherally. Focal plaques are typically found twice as often in the cervical cord as compared with the lower cord levels.

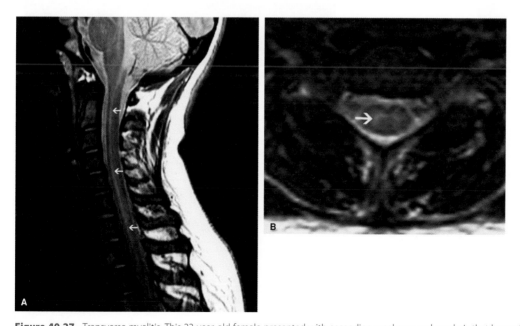

Figure 40.27. Transverse myelitis. This 23-year-old female presented with ascending weakness and paralysis that began in the lower extremities and rapidly progressed to the upper extremities. A: Sagittal proton density T2 image shows hyperintense signal (*arrows*) in the cervical cord from the craniocervical junction to the upper thoracic region. There is no evidence of cord expansion. B: Axial T2 image also shows a hyperintense signal (*arrow*) in the center of the spinal cord. These findings of transverse myelitis in this patient were associated with Guillain–Barré syndrome, and the patients' symptoms improved within a few months, with subsequent MRI showing decreased signal intensity.

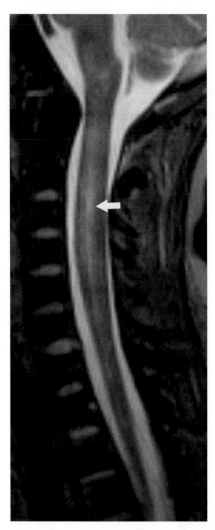

Figure 40.28. Postviral transverse myelitis. This child presented with headache, neck stiffness, and progressive extremity weakness. Sagittal T2 image shows diffuse swelling of the cervical cord with increased signal (*arrow*) associated with postviral transverse myelitis. The inflammatory process of transverse myelitis is typically a monophasic illness that usually resolves in weeks to months.

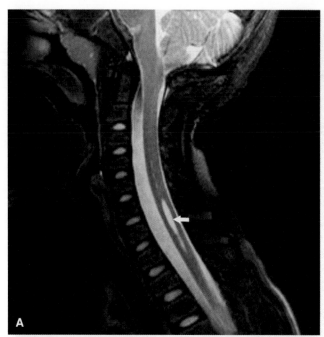

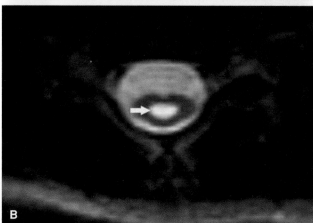

Figure 40.29. Syringomyelia. A: Sagittal T2 image through the cervical spine shows a homogeneous signal, isointense with CSF, and smooth, well-defined borders of a syrinx (*arrow*). B: Axial T2 image through the cervical cord demonstrates the high signal of the syrinx (*arrow*). The combination of defined margins, homogeneity, and isointensity with CSF helps differentiate syrinx from tumor. Clinical symptoms associated with syringomyelia are progressive dissociated sensory loss of pain and temperature of the upper extremities, without motor and proprioceptive deficits.

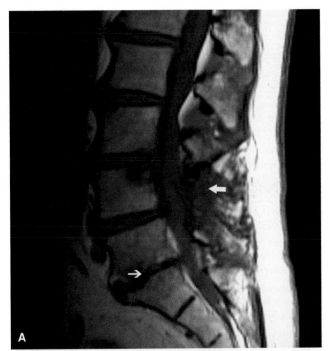

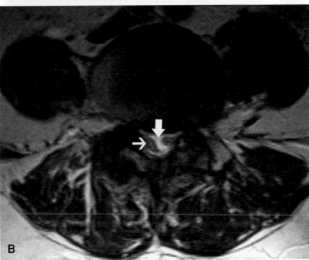

Figure 40.30. Postlaminectomy arachnoiditis. A: Sagittal T1 image through the lumbar spine shows evidence of postsurgical defect with the absence of posterior elements at L4–5 and associated hypointense signal indicating scar formation (*large arrow*). There is also evidence of degenerative disc disease at L5-S1 (*small arrow*). B: Axial T2 image shows the spinal nerve roots clumping (*small white arrow*) on the periphery of the spinal canal, with the appearance of a bright empty thecal sac known as the "empty sac" sign (*large white arrow*) characteristic of arachnoiditis.

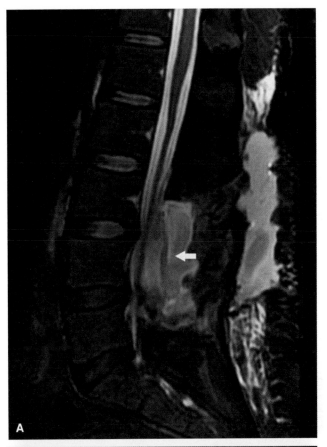

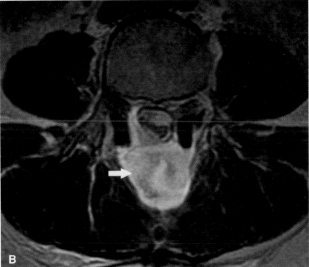

Figure 40.31. Postlaminectomy pseudomeningocele. A: Sagittal T2 image through the lumbar spine demonstrates postsurgical defects with absent posterior elements at L3–5 and a posterior fluid signal collection contiguous with the lumbar dural sac (*arrow*). B: Axial T2 image shows evidence of postlaminectomy pseudomeningocele demonstrated by a large CSF collection marked by hyperintense signal (*arrow*).

References

1. Chin CT: Spine imaging. *Semin Neurol* 2002;**22**(2):205–20.

2. Tintinalli J, Stapczynski J, Ma OJ, et al. (eds): *Tintinalli's emergency medicine: a comprehensive study guide*, 6th ed. New York, NY: McGraw-Hill, 2004.

3. Van Goethem JW, Maes M, Ozsarlak O, et al.: Imaging in spinal trauma. *Eur Radiol* 2005;**15**(3):582–90.

4. Burney RE, Maio RF, Maynard F, Karunas R: Incidence, characteristics, and outcome of spinal cord injury at trauma centers in North America. *Arch Surg* 1993;**128**(5):596–9.

5. National Spinal Cord Injury Statistical Center (NSCIS): Spinal cord injury: facts and figures at a glance. *J Spinal Cord Med* 2011 Nov;**34**(6):620–1.

6. Farmer JC, Vaccaro AR, Balderston RA, et al.: The changing nature of admissions to a spinal cord injury center: violence on the rise. *J Spinal Disord* 1998;**11**(5):400–3.

7. Vaccaro AR, Kreidl KO, Pan W, et al.: Usefulness of MRI in isolated upper cervical spine fractures in adults. *J Spinal Disord* 1998;**11**(4):289–93.

8. Sances A Jr, Myklebust JB, Maiman DJ, et al.: The biomechanics of spinal injuries. *Crit Rev Biomed Eng* 1984;**11**(1):1–76.

9. Bates D, Ruggieri P: Imaging modalities for evaluation of the spine. *Radiol Clin North Am* 1991;**29**(4):675–90.

10. Daffner RH, Hackney DB: ACR appropriateness criteria on suspected spine trauma. *J Am Coll Radiol* 2007 Nov;**4**(11):762–75.

11. Orrison WW Jr, Benzel EC, Willis BK, et al.: Magnetic resonance imaging evaluation of acute spine trauma. *Emerg Radiol* 1995;**2**(3):120–8.

12. Slucky AV, Potter HG: Use of magnetic resonance imaging in spinal trauma: indications, techniques, and utility. *J Am Acad Orthop Surg* 1998;**6**(3):134–45.

13. Yamashita Y, Takakoshi M, Malosuno Y, et al.: Acute spinal cord injury: magnetic resonance imaging correlated with myelopathy. *Br J Radiol* 1991;**64**:201–9.

14. Mhuircheartaigh NN, Kerr JM, Murray JG: MR imaging of traumatic spinal injuries. *SeminMusculoskelet Radiol* 2006;**10**(4):293–307.

15. Benedetti PF, Fahr LM, Kuhns LR, et al.: MR imaging findings in spinal ligamentous injury. *AJR Am J Roentgenol* 2000;**175**(3):661–5.

16. Daffner, RH, Hackney DB: ACR appropriateness criteria on suspected spine trauma. *J Am Coll Radiol* 2007;**4**(11):762–75.

17. Kim KY, Kim YT, Lee CS, et al.: Magnetic resonance imaging in the evaluation of the lumbar herniated intervertebral disc. *Int Orthop* 1993;**17**(4):241–4.

18. Forristall RM, Marsh HO, Pay NT: Magnetic resonance imaging and contrast CT of the lumbar spine: comparison of diagnostic methods and correlation with surgical findings. *Spine* 1988;**13**(9):1049–54.

19. Janssen ME, Bertrand SL, Joe C, Levine MI: Lumbar herniated disk disease: comparison of MRI, myelography, and post-myelographic CT scan with surgical findings. *Orthopedics* 1994;**17**(2):121–7.

20. Yousem DM, Atlas SW, Goldberg HI, Grossman RI: Degenerative narrowing of the cervical spine neural foramina: evaluation with high-resolution 3DFT gradient-echo MR imaging. *Am J Neuroradiol* 1991;**12**(2):229–36.

21. Steinborn MM, Heuck AF, Tiling R, et al.: Whole-body bone marrow MRI in patients with metastatic disease to the skeletal system. *J Comput Assist Tomogr* Jan-Feb 1999;**23**(1):123–9.

22. Avrahami E, Tadmor R, Dally O, Hadar H: Early MR demonstration of spinal metastasis in patients with normal radiographs and CT and radionuclide bone scans. *JCAT* 1989;**13**(4):598–602.

23. Baleriaux DL, Neugroschl C: Spinal and spinal cord infection. *Eur Radiol* 2004;**14**(Suppl 3):E72–83.

24. Erdman WA, Tamburo F, Jayson HT, et al.: Osteomyelitis: characteristics and pitfalls of diagnosis with MR imaging. *Radiology* 1991;**180**(2):533–9.

25. Unger E, Moldofsky P, Gatenby R, et al.: Diagnosis of osteomyelitis by MR imaging. *AJR Am J Roentgenol* 1988;**150**(3):605–10.

26. Agosta F, Absinta M, Sormani MP, et al.: In vivo assessment of cervical cord damage in MS patients: a longitudinal diffusion tensor MRI study. *Brain* Aug 2007;**130**:2211–9.

27. Traboulsee AL, Li DK: The role of MRI in the diagnosis of multiple sclerosis. *Adv Neurol* 2006;**98**:125–46.

28. Poser CM, Brinar VV: Diagnostic criteria for multiple sclerosis. *Clin Neurol Neurosurg* 2001;**103**(1):1–11.

29. Kidd D, Thorpe JW, Kendall BE, et al.: MRI dynamics of brain and spinal cord in progressive multiple sclerosis. *Ann Neurol* 1992;**32**:643–50.

30. Bradley WG: Use of gadolinium chelates in MR imaging of the spine. *J Magn Reson Imaging* 1997;**7**(1):38–46.

31. Kanal E, Borgstede JP, Barkovich AJ, et al.: American College of Radiology white paper on MR safety. *AJR Am J Roentgenol* 2002;**178**(6):1335–47.

32. Kanal E, Shellock FG: Patient monitoring during clinical MR imaging. *Radiology* 1992;**185**(3):623–9.

33. Schrader R: Contrast material-induced renal failure: an overview. *J Interv Cardiol* 2005;**18**(6):417–23.

34. Pedersen M: Safety update on the possible causal relationship between gadolinium-containing MRI agents and nephrogenic systemic fibrosis. *J Magn Reson Imaging* 2007;**25**(5):881–3.

35. Aydingoz U: The need for radiologists' awareness of nephrogenic systemic fibrosis. *Diagn Interv Radiol* 2006;**12**(4):161–2.

36. American College of Radiology: *Manual on contrast media*, 7th ed. 2010.

37. Kanal E, Borgstede JP, Barkovich AJ, et al.: American College of Radiology white paper on MR safety: 2004 update and revisions. *AJR Am J Roentgenol* 2004;**182**(5):1111–4.

Chapter 41

MRI of the Heart and Chest

Jonathan Patane, Bryan Sloane, and Mark Langdorf

Clinical indications

The development and maturation of MRI has revolutionized the clinician's ability to noninvasively assess pathology with incredible detail and accuracy. Unfortunately, the limited availability and cost are major prohibitive factors in the prevalence of MRI as a first-line imaging modality in emergency medicine. Recent technological advances have decreased cardiac MRI studies to between 30 and 90 minutes, which must be taken into consideration in determining the role of cardiac MRI in patients with severe cardiac pathology (1). A growing body of research and technological advancement suggests that MRI of the chest and heart will play a prominent role in future screening and monitoring of appropriate patients. It has been suggested that MRI, specifically cardiac MRI, has a role in patients presenting with acute chest pain and normal EKG findings without ST elevation or depression (2). Cardiac MRI may be helpful in these patients to rule out non-ST segment elevation myocardial infarction (NSTEMI) or other cardiac pathologies such as myocarditis without subjecting the patient to invasive coronary angiography and potential complications (2).

Even though MRI of the heart has matured to accurately assess cardiac structure, function, perfusion, and myocardial viability with a capacity unmatched by any other imaging modality, it comprises only 0.1% of all noninvasive cardiac studies ordered (3). The sensitivities and specificities for MRI detection of chest (some cardiovascular) pathologies are demonstrated in Table 41.1. Although current clinical guidelines limit the use of MRI of the chest and heart, it should be used more frequently in acute care as logistical concerns regarding the technology are overcome, most notably the cost and time required for MRI examinations.

A careful history, physical exam, and relevant diagnostic studies are fundamental to the assessment of a patient before choosing the appropriate imaging modality. It is important to document a patient's presenting complaint and symptoms, along with results from prior investigations, when requesting the study. The stability of the patient's condition will steer the physician's management of the patient. An unstable patient may not be able to tolerate diagnostic tests of extended length such as MRI. However, with recent technological advances, the rise time (time needed to achieve maximum gradient strength) and number of channels available for signal detection have increased, leading to faster acquisition of high-quality images (1).

Pregnant patients may want to avoid the increased risk of fetal malformation or cancer from CT irradiation or multiple radiographs. Research on the long-term risk of MRI to the fetus has not found evidence for or against its use; however, research articles have stated that pediatric patients who were exposed to MRI between 20 weeks and term in utero have shown normal pediatric exams through 9 months of age (4). Even though small prospective studies on pregnant patients and surveys of pregnant healthcare workers exposed to MRI devices to date have not identified increased risks, caution is still recommended in the first trimester (5).

Patients with renal insufficiency or CT contrast allergies may be better candidates for higher-resolution MRI studies. However, the gadolinium contrast in patients with renal insufficiency or on dialysis should be avoided. Gadolinium is not recommended due to the increased risk of nephrogenic fibrotic dermopathy (NFD)/nephrogenic systemic fibrosis (NSF), a rare condition of unclear etiology.

The strongest indication for MRI of the heart in the emergent setting is to diagnose suspected aortic dissection. The American College of Radiology (ACR) Appropriateness Criteria rate MRI of the heart as 8 out of 9 for aortic dissections, with limitations related to cost and study time (6). Patients presenting with acute thoracic aortic dissections (TADs) commonly complain of tearing or sharp chest pain. Anterior chest pain is associated with aneurysms of the ascending aorta, neck and jaw pain are associated with the aortic arch, and pain in the intrascapular area is associated with descending aortic dissections.

Thoracic vascular catastrophes may present additionally as diaphoresis, nausea, vomiting, lightheadedness, and severe apprehension, as well as focal neurologic deficits. The mortality for aortic dissection is 1 to 5 per 100,000 - per year. Risk factors for aortic dissection include uncontrolled hypertension, prior cardiac surgery, bicuspid aortic valve, increased age, male gender, connective tissue disorders such as Marfan and Ehlers–Danlos syndrome, and pregnancy. Although trauma secondary to high-speed decelerations commonly results in aortic rupture, this is a distinct injury from aortic dissection (7).

Pulmonary embolism (PE) is one of the most common, missed fatal events. More than 400,000 cases of PE are missed annually in the United States, resulting in the death of more than 100,000 patients. Approximately 10% of the PE deaths occur within 60 minutes of the initial onset of symptoms. Patients presenting with PE classically have pleuritic chest pain, acute dyspnea, tachypnea, hemoptysis, leg swelling, tachycardia, syncope, and discomfort in the legs (7).

However, atypical presentations are common and include nonpleuritic chest pain, fever, absent leg symptoms and normal exam, and thoracic back pain. Although much consideration is given toward PE arising from lower extremity deep venous thrombosis (DVT), it is important to recognize the risk factors for upper extremity DVT as well, such as central venous catheters, malignancy, and coagulopathy (8). Embolism is the leading cause of maternal mortality in pregnancy, accounting for up to 20% of all maternal deaths due to the estrogen-induced hypercoaguable state. (9). The chest radiograph is normal in more than 50% of pregnant patients who are subsequently proven to have PE (10). Radiation exposure during helical CT pulmonary angiography (CTPA) is viewed as a negligible risk to the fetus and less than that of ventilation-perfusion scans (11). Magnetic resonance angiography (MRA) of the lungs is rated 4 out of 9 on the ACR Appropriateness Criteria. For those patients without contraindications, x-ray and CTPA are recommended. The ACR comments that MRA of the chest may be an alternative modality for those unable to tolerate CT contrast (12).

Cardiac MRI (cMRI) has a number of advantages. The inherent high contrast of spin echo's dark blood and gradient echo's bright blood enable exceptional visualization of internal cardiac structures (13). This has led to cMRI being the gold standard for cardiac function tests. Transthoracic ultrasound continues to be the dominant imaging modality due to lower cost and convenience to patients; however, it lacks the sensitivity and specificity of cMRI. In fact, it has been argued that the increased sensitivity of cardiac MRI for detecting myocardial infarctions can lead to decreased cost of hospitalization in patients who present to the emergency department with emergent chest pain through the use of cardiac observation units (14).

The American Heart Association/American College of Cardiology (AHA/ACC) guidelines recognize cMRI's higher spatial resolution and ability to recognize both the transmural and circumferential extent of myocardial infarction (MI), but the AHA/ACC task force report stated that more experience and comparison to other methods for predicting infarct size is required before they make clinical recommendations (15). The remarkable potential of cMRI for accurately defining myocardial infarcts should lead to promising clinical research in acute care.

Diagnostic capabilities

MRI obtains high-resolution 3D images noninvasively without contrast. Using spin echo techniques, rapidly moving blood is void of signal and appears black, whereas slow-moving blood has an increased signal. These MRI characteristics make it easier to identify true and false lumens and intimal flaps. Cine MRI is used to reference obtained images to ECG recording, providing reconstructed, real-time cardiac imaging (16). Adding a cine MRI protocol to spin echo techniques adds 15 to 31 minutes to the procedure and provides detailed information regarding valvular disease, regurgitant flow, and turbulent flow

(17). A complete cardiac MRI exam can be completed in under 30 minutes and gives information on ventricular function, identifies edema suggestive of acute injury, and can evaluate myocardial perfusion (18).

The use of MRI for aortic dissection was first described in 1983 (19). For the diagnosis of thoracic aortic dissection (TAD), MRI of the great vessels has proven efficacy. A 1993 prospective study of 110 patients compared MRI to the sensitivities for detecting TAD for MRI, transesophageal echocardiography (TEE), x-ray CT, and transthoracic echocardiography (TTE); they were 98.3%, 97.7%, 93.8%, and 59.3%, respectively. Specificities were 97.8%, 76.9%, 87.1%, and 83%, respectively (Table 41.1). The authors of the study recognized the superiority of MRI in accurately diagnosing and detailing the extent of dissection. They recommended initial TTE for rapid assessment with a follow-up TEE or MRI and advised against the less accurate, contrast-based CT and more invasive, costly angiography. A more recent meta-analysis of 16 studies involving helical CT, MRI, and TEE demonstrated similar sensitivities and specificities among all imaging modalities with MRI having a slightly higher pooled positive predictive value, suggesting that all modalities yield equally reliable diagnostic information (20). The diagnostic information provided with TEE is less comprehensive than the higher-resolution 3D views from MRI, but both tests provide all the diagnostic information a surgeon requires to properly treat the patient.

In their 2010 practice guidelines, the American College of Cardiology Foundation (ACCF) and AHA recommend selecting an imaging modality that best suits the patient based on patient condition and intuitional limitations (21).

For patients presenting with acute nonspecific chest pain and low probability of coronary artery disease (CAD), the ACR rates MRI and MRA of the aorta as 5 out of 9 on its appropriateness scale after chest x-ray, nuclear myocardial perfusion scan, CT, ultrasound, and V/Q scan. The ACR highlights the ability of MRI to identify vascular pathology and encourages its use in patients who have contraindications to CT contrast (22). For suspected aortic dissection and nontraumatic aortic disease, the ACR rates MRA of the chest and abdomen as 8 out of 9 after chest x-ray and CTA due to limited accessibility and expertise causing delay in diagnosis, but the ACR promote its use in patients who cannot tolerate CT contrast (6, 23). However, the ACR rates MRI of the heart above all other modalities to assess for non-ischemic cardiomyopathy and highlights its ability to assess anatomy, local and total function, and overall viability (24).

The AHA does not recommend any specific noninvasive imaging modality over another to detect ischemic change due to low sample sizes in existing studies. The ACR also notes that large-scale studies on cardiac MRI are lacking and does not definitively recommend it at this time (22, 25).

The diagnostic capabilities of MRA in detecting pulmonary embolus are currently limited to larger emboli in the main pulmonary artery through the segmental branches. The strengths of MRA are its ability to acquire volumetric data of the lung vasculature with reconstruction and

Table 41.1: Relative sensitivity, specificity, accuracy, positive predictive value (PPV), and negative predictive value (NPV) among TTE, TEE, CT, and MRI

Findings (%)	Sensitivity	Specificity	Accuracy	PPV	NPV
All dissections					
TTE	59.3	83.0	69.8	81.4	61.9
TEE	97.7	76.9	90.0	87.7	95.2
CT	93.8	87.1	91.1	91.8	90.0
MRI	98.3	97.8	98.0	98.3	97.8
Type A dissections					
TTE	78.1	86.7	84.1	71.4	90.3
TEE	96.4	85.7	90.0	81.8	97.3
CT	82.6	100	94.9	100	93.3
MRI	100	98.6	99.0	96.8	100
Type B dissections					
TTE	10.0	100	80.4	100	80.0
TEE	100	96.4	97.1	88.2	100
CT	96.0	88.9	91.1	80.0	98.0
MRI	96.5	100	99.0	100	98.7
Site of entry					
TTE	26.2	100	71.0	100	67.7
TEE	72.7	100	86.8	100	79.5
CT	–	–	–	–	–
MRI	88.0	100	95.2	100	92.6
Thrombus formation					
TTE	11.8	100	72.7	100	71.7
TEE	68.4	100	91.3	100	89.3
CT	92.0	95.6	94.4	92.0	95.6
MRI	98.2	98.5	95.2	97.0	94.4
Aortic regurgitation					
TTE	96.9	94.7	95.4	88.6	98.6
TEE	100	95.3	97.1	92.9	100
CT	–	–	–	–	–
MRI	83.2	100	96.6	100	96.8
Pericardial effusion					
TTE	75.0	100	98.2	100	98.1
TEE	100	100	100	100	100
CT	100	100	100	100	100
MRI	100	100	100	100	100

From Nienaber CA, von Kodolitsch Y, Nicolas V, Siglow V, Piepho A, Brockhoff C, Koschyk DH, Spielmann RP: The diagnosis of thoracic aortic dissection by noninvasive imaging procedures. *N Engl J Med* 1993;328(1):1–9.

visualization in various spatial planes. The ability to detect subsegmental PE is limited, but the technology continues to advance with faster gradients, parallel imaging, motion control, and shorter acquisition times (26).

Prospective investigation of pulmonary embolism diagnosis (PIOPED) evaluated the accuracy of computed tomography pulmonary angiography (CTPA) with venous-phase imaging for DVT in diagnosing acute PE. The results reinforced the superior accuracy of CTPA in diagnosing PE. However, a significant portion of patients presenting with a suspected PE may have contraindications to CTPA. The PIOPED study evaluated 7,284 patients suspected of having a PE. Of those,

25% were not eligible due to concerns regarding the contrast agent, 1,350 had elevated creatinine or were on dialysis, 184 were pregnant, and 272 were allergic to contrast agents (27).

The PIOPED study was followed by a multicenter MRA targeted study (PIOPED III). This study showed a sensitivity of 78%, with specificity of 99% for MRA alone, and a sensitivity of 92% and specificity of 96% for MRA combined with MR venography. However, there was a high rate of technically inadequate studies across all centers (11% to 52%), and the authors concluded that MRA for the diagnosis of PE should be performed only at centers with experience and only on patients with specific contraindications to other modalities (28).

Patients ineligible for CTPA or angiography due to irradiation or contrast concerns may be good candidates for MRA with gadolinium-based contrast agents. Ersoy and colleagues demonstrated a 94% to 95% detection of emboli from the main pulmonary artery, although the segmental branches using time-resolved 3D MRA in 27 patients who had contraindications for CTPA (29). Delayed-enhancement cardiac MRI (DE-cMRI) has shown significant promise in assessing myocardial ischemia and damage. Patients receive gadolinium-based contrast agents 10 to 30 minutes before imaging. Cine MRI is then ECG gated, and a reconstruction of cardiac function is provided at increased spatial resolution. The longer study times of standard imaging protocols have made this impractical for patients presenting with suspected myocardial infarction. Research published from the Duke Cardiovascular Magnetic Resonance Center described new techniques for rapid detection of MI using subsecond, free-breathing DE-cMRI. Sensitivity, specificity, and accuracy for their rapid method was 87%, 96%, and 91%, respectively, compared with the standard technique, which was 98%, 100%, and 99%, respectively. The subsecond techniques required less than 30 seconds to complete imaging, only 5% to 10% of the time required for standard techniques (30).

Existing noninvasive imaging techniques have high negative predictive values but lack the ability to positively identify ACS. New cardiac MRI protocols can detect acute coronary syndrome and differentiate it from old infarct and other myocardial damage through the inclusion of T2-weighted imaging. It may also be able to differentiate unstable angina from NSTEMI. A protocol including T2-weighted imaging, FP-MRI, cine left ventricle function, and DE-MRI was able to detect ACS with a sensitivity of 85%, specificity of 96%, PPV of 85%, and NPV of 96%. Imaging was completed within 32 ± 8 minutes (31). When compared with single positron emission CT (SPECT), a commonly utilized modality of cardiac stress testing, cardiac MRI had improved sensitivity and negative predictive values (86.5% and 90.5% vs. 66.5% and 79.1%) in a study of 752 patients (32). The use of cardiac MRI for detection of cardiac pathology will likely increase in the future.

A single-center study of 110 patients showed that utilization of cardiac stress MRI in an ED cardiac observation unit did not miss any cases of acute coronary syndrome and reduced costs associated with hospitalization of intermediate- to high-risk patients who would otherwise have been admitted (14). The use of cardiac MRI in emergency departments will likely increase as technology becomes faster and more available.

MRI of the chest and heart, with its high spatial resolution and tissue-blood contrast, may identify incidental structures such as cardiac masses, congenital malformations, or pulmonary tumors. Recent technologies are even making gains in visualizing coronary artery disease with some notable results (33). Studies suggest MRI of the lungs may be helpful in diagnosing and monitoring pulmonary hypertension, COPD, chronic thromboembolic pulmonary hypertension, vasculitis, and arteriovenous malformations (34, 35).

Imaging pitfalls and limitations

Cost and on-call availability are the major limitations for routine use of MRI of the chest and heart. Plain films, ultrasound, and CT have benefited from drastic reductions in cost and easy accessibility in EDs. As the availability of MRI improves, we may expect similar changes in cost.

The second significant limitation is the time required to image patients using MRI. The alternation of powerful magnetic fields, directed radiofrequencies, and data acquisition are technologically and computationally intensive processes. Attempting to image the only significantly moving targets within the body, the heart and lungs, is a remarkable challenge for medical technology. To limit motion blurring, patients may be required to perform 10- to 30-second breath-holds. Gating data acquisition to ECGs has been successful, but the technology for synchronizing to a patient's respiration rate is not as promising. Another limitation is that patients presenting in an emergency setting may not be able to physically perform breath-holds or slow-breathing techniques for quality images.

Medical equipment for intubation, ECG leads, and patient lines have been engineered to be MRI compatible. Patients may be monitored acutely during imaging protocols. For example, there is no evidence that patients receiving MRI for suspected aortic dissections are at increased morbidity or mortality risks by having extended MRI studies (16). New techniques for rapid MRI of the thoracic aorta using half-Fourier rapid acquisition have reduced mean imaging times to 48 seconds for ECG gated and 30 seconds for nontriggered acquisition (36).

Patients with cardiac pacemakers and cardioverter defibrillators are currently contraindicated to receive MRI due to the effect of strong magnetic fields on the devices. Research is being done to assess the safety of pacemakers in MRI. Studies sampling the current generation of pacemakers have found no device malfunctions or heating effect (37). Most prosthetic valves and coronary stents are safe for cMRI but may lead to artifacts that degrade images. The safety profile depends on each specific device and manufacturer. The MRI precautions from most stent package inserts recommend avoiding MRI 8 weeks post-stenting for proper endothelialization, minimizing the stent-migration risk. Retrospective studies on patients receiving stents and cMRI post-MI found no increased risks or adverse effects (38).

Gadolinium-based contrast agents are considerably safer than CT contrast and dyes. Patients with renal insufficiency are contraindicated to receive CT-based contrast agents. However, a recent association between gadolinium-based MRA contrast in dialysis patients and NFD/NSF, a rare systemic condition of fibroblastic proliferation, is cause for some concern. There were no known cases of NFD before 1997, yet the Centers for Disease Control and Prevention (CDC) database of cases was in the hundreds as of 2007. The CDC recommends that gadolinium-containing contrast agents be avoided in patients with advanced renal failure, particularly in patients who are undergoing peritoneal dialysis (39).

Clinical images

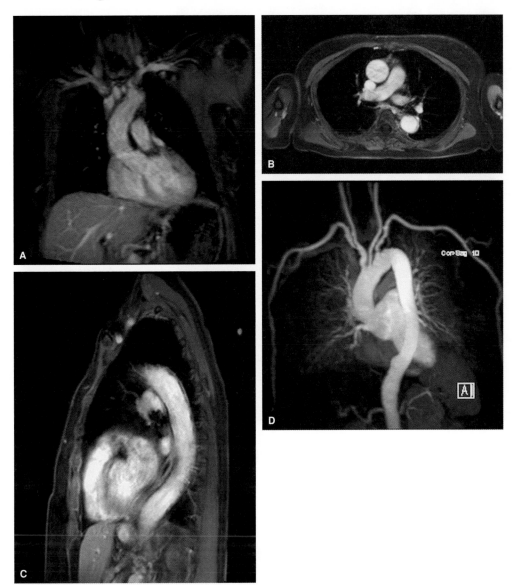

Figure 41.1. A: Normal thoracic aorta coronal T1-weighted fat suppressed postgadolinium image through the normal thorax demonstrates hyperintense blood flow within the cardiac and arterial structures. The aortic root and outlet are nicely displayed. Soft tissue fat signal is suppressed for improved contrast. The pulmonary alveolar air contributes a hypointense, black signal surrounding the cardiac silhouette. Hepatic arterial blood flow is also contrasted well against the isointense hepatic tissue. B: Axial FLASH postgadolinium delayed image of the thorax demonstrates the hyperintense signal of the great vessels superior to the heart. The aorta and superior vena cava are noted anteriorly. Beneath the aortic arch, we see the right and left pulmonary arteries. Posteriorly is the hyperintense descending aorta. C: Sagittal T1-weighted fat suppressed postgadolinium image displays the hyperintense curved descending aorta entering below the level of the diaphragm distally. The heart structures anteriorly are blurred secondary to cardiac motion. D: MRA 3D arterial reconstruction of thoracic vasculature demonstrates the hyperintense signal of the left and right ventricle, aorta, pulmonary arterial vasculature, origin of the brachiocephalic trunk, common carotid, and left subclavian artery. Bilateral common carotids in the neck and abdominal celiac blood flow are noteworthy.

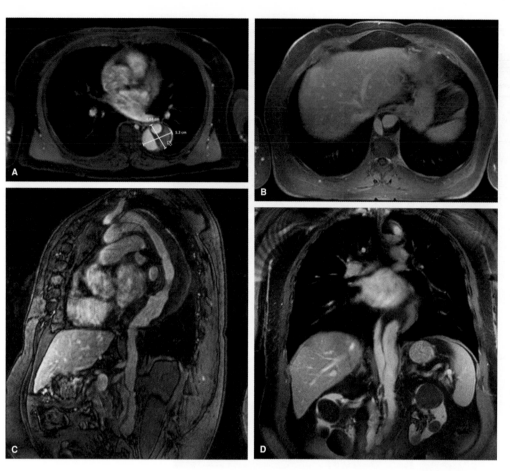

Figure 41.2. Aortic dissection. A 65-year-old male with Stanford type B aneurysm and dissection involving the descending aorta. A: Axial T1 FLASH postgadolinium image displays a dual hyperintense lumen in the descending aorta with isointense intraluminal thrombus (*arrow*). The descending aorta measures 5.3 × 4.64 cm in diameter. The hyperintense true lumen anteriorly measures 1.81 cm in diameter, and the false lumen medial and posteriorly measures 3.63 × 2.28 cm. B: Axial T1 FLASH postgadolinium image at the level of the diaphragm demonstrates continuation of the dual aortic lumens and thrombus. C: Sagittal T1 3D postgadolinium image demonstrates the dissection flap originating near the origin of the left subclavian artery and progression of the aortic dissection well below the level of the diaphragm with significant thrombus in the posterior aspect of the aortic lumen. D: Coronal T1 FLASH postgadolinium image demonstrates the hyperintense true and false lumen entering the diaphragm distally and terminating near the level of the celiac trunk.

Concordant Hyperenhancement Patterns

Patient example 1: nearly transmural MI

Patient example 2: subendocardial MI

Patient example 3: partly transmural and subendocardial MI

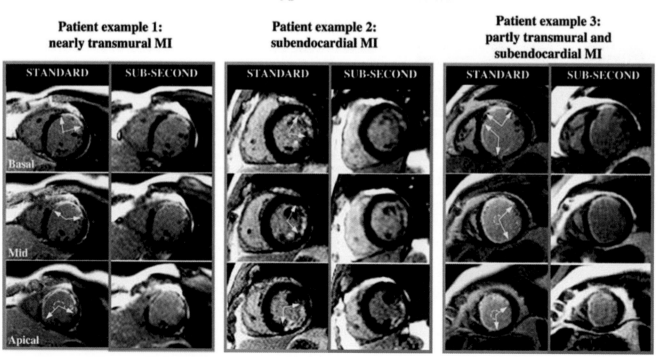

Figure 41.3. MI. Study compares routine breath-hold delayed contrast enhancement cardiovascular magnetic resonance to subsecond (<30 s) for the detection of MI. Representative images in three patients showing concordant hyperenhancement patterns between standard and subsecond imaging. Courtesy of Raymond J. Kim, MD, Duke Cardiovascular Magnetic Resonance Center, Durham, NC.

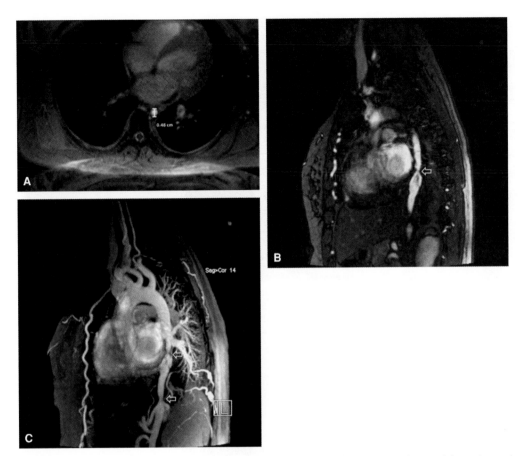

Figure 41.4. Coarctation. A: A 30-year-old female with aortic coarctation, axial iPAT acquired postgadolinium image demonstrates hyperintense signal of the descending aorta with significant stenosis to 0.48 cm. B: Sagittal FLASH 3D postgadolinium image demonstrates a point of stenosis (*arrow*) posterior to the heart with aortic dilation distally. C: Sagittal MIP 3D reconstruction image demonstrates coarctation of the aorta posterior to the heart and stenosis at the level of the diaphragm.

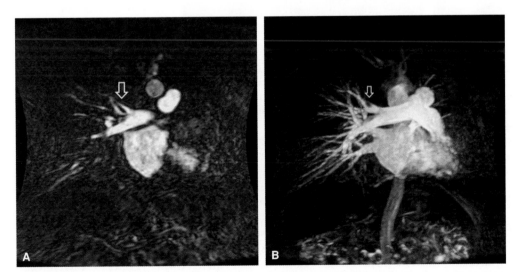

Figure 41.5. PE. A 56-year-old man with a history of heart transplant in 1999 and lung cancer who is experiencing shortness of breath, lower extremity edema, and left popliteal DVT. 3D TRICKS MRA with the IV administration of 40 mL gadolinium contrast. Coronal thin MIP (A) and 3D volume (B) demonstrate acute thrombus (*arrows*) within the right upper lobe artery. Courtesy of Hale Ersoy, MD, Cardiovascular Imaging Section, Department of Radiology, Brigham and Women's Hospital and Harvard Medical School, Boston.

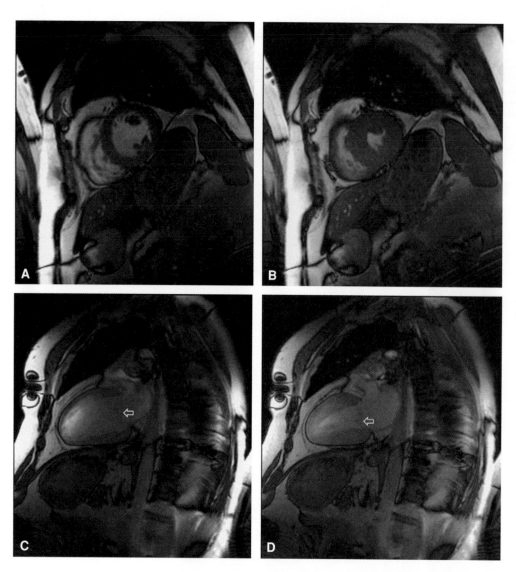

Figure 41.6. Restrictive cardiomyopathy/cardiac function. A 61-year-old male with history of amyloidosis; heart function evaluated with cardiac gated postgadolinium sequential magnetic imaging. A: Oblique sagittal IR/turbo FLASH short-axis image demonstrates a cross-section of the right and left ventricle in diastole. Note the detail of the hypointense left ventricular papillary muscles in the hyperintense blood-filled chamber. B: The systolic image from the same sequence demonstrates maximal cardiac contraction and mild left ventricular hypertrophy in this patient. C: Oblique sagittal IR/turbo FLASH long-axis image demonstrates the left ventricle and left atrium during diastole. Note the thin hypointense line demonstrating the mitral valve leaflets (*arrows*). D: The systolic image from the same sequence demonstrates the left ventricle in maximal contraction.

References

1. Atalay MK: Establishing a cardiac MRI program: problems, pitfalls, and limitations. *J Am Coll Radiology* 2005;**2**(9):740–8.

2. Smulders MW, Kietselaer BL, Das M, et al.: The role of cardiovascular magnetic resonance imaging and computed tomography angiography in suspected non-ST-elevation myocardial infarction patients: design and rationale of the cardiovascular magnetic resonance imaging and computed tomography angiography (CARMENTA) trial. *Am Heart J* 2013; **a66**(6):968–75.

3. Earls JP, Ho VB, Foo TK, et al.: Cardiac MRI: recent progress and continued challenges. *J Magn Reson Imaging* 2002;**16**:111–27.

4. Clements H, Duncan KR, Fielding K, et al.: Infants exposed to MRI in utero have a normal paediatric assessment at 9 months of age. *Br J Radiol* 2000;**73**:190–4.

5. De Wilde JP, Rivers AW, Price DL: A review of the current use of magnetic resonance imaging in pregnancy and safety implications for the fetus. *Progr Biophys Molec Biol* 2005;**87**: 335–53.

6. American College of Radiology (ACR): ACR appropriateness criteria: acute chest pain – suspected aortic dissection. 2011. Available at: www.acr.org/~/media/ACR/Documents/AppCriteria/Diagnostic/AcuteChestPainSuspectedAorticDissection.pdf

7. Marx JA: *Rosen's emergency medicine: concepts and clinical practice*, 8th ed. St. Louis, MO: Mosby, 2014.

8. Schleyer AM, Jarman KM, Calver P, et al.: Upper extremity deep vein thrombosis in hospitalized patients: a descriptive study. *J Hosp Med* 2014;**9**(1):48–53.

9. Chang J, Elam-Evans LD, Berg CJ, et al.: Pregnancy-related mortality surveillance – United States, 1991–99. *MMWR Morb Mortal Wkly Rep* 2003;**52**(SS-2):1–8.

10. Scarsbrook AF, Evans AL, Owen AR, Glees FV: Diagnosis of suspected venous thromboembolic disease in pregnancy. *Clin Radiol* 2006;**61**:1–12.

11. Winer-Muram HT, Boone JM, Brown HL, et al.: Pulmonary embolism in pregnant patients: fetal radiation dose with helical CT. *Radiology* 2002;**224**:487–92.

12. American College of Radiology (ACR): ACR appropriateness criteria: acute chest pain – suspected pulmonary embolism. 2011. Available at: www.acr.org/~/media/ACR/Documents/App Criteria/Diagnostic/AcuteChestPainSuspectedPulmonaryEmboli sm.pdf

13 Raizner AE: *Indications for diagnostic procedures: topics in clinical cardiology*. New York: Igaku-Shoin Medical, 1997.

14. Miller CD, Hwang W, Hoekstra JW, et al.: Stress cardiac magnetic resonance imaging with observation unit care reduces cost for patients with emergent chest pain: a randomized trial. *Ann Emerg Med* 2009;**56**(3):209–19.

15. American College of Cardiology/American Heart Association (ACC/AHA): ACC/AHA guidelines for the management of patients with ST-elevation myocardial infarction: a report of the American College of Cardiology/American Heart Association Task Force on Practice Guidelines. *Circulation* 2004;**110**:588–636.

16. Nienaber CA, von Kodolitsch Y, Nicolas V, et al.: The diagnosis of thoracic aortic dissection by noninvasive imaging procedures. *N Engl J Med* 1993;**328**(1):1–9.

17. Sechtem U, Pflugfelder PW, Cassidy MM: Mitral or aortic regurgitation: quantification of regurgitant volumes with cine MR imaging. *Radiology* 1988;**167**:425–30.

18. Shapiro MD, Guarraia DL, Moloo J, Cury RC: Evaluation of acute coronary syndromes by cardiac magnetic resonance imaging. *Top Magn Reson Imaging* 2008;**19**(1):25–32.

19. Herfkens RJ, Higgins CB, Hricak H, et al.: Nuclear magnetic resonance imaging of the cardiovascular system: normal and pathologic findings. *Radiology* 1983;**147**:749–59.

20. Shiga T, Wajima Z, Apfel CC, et al.: Diagnostic accuracy of transesophageal echocardiography, helical computed tomography, and magnetic resonance imaging for suspected thoracic aortic dissection: systematic review and meta-analysis. *Arch Intern Med* 2006;**166**(13):1350–6.

21. Hiratzka LF, Bakris GL, Beckman JA, et al.: 2010 ACCF/AHA/ AATS/ACR/ASA/SCA/SCAI/SIR/STS/SVM guidelines for the diagnosis and management of patients with thoracic aortic disease. *Circulation* 2010;**121**(13):e266–369.

22. American College of Radiology (ACR): ACR appropriateness criteria: acute chest pain – acute nonspecific chest pain – low probability of coronary artery disease. 2011. Available at: www .acr.org/~/media/ACR/Documents/AppCriteria/Diagnostic/A cuteNonspecficChestPainLowProbabilityCoronaryArteryDis ease.pdf

23. American College of Radiology (ACR): ACR appropriateness criteria: nontraumatic aortic disease. 2013. Available at: www .acr.org/~/media/ACR/Documents/AppCriteria/Diagnostic /NontraumaticAorticDisease.pdf

24. American College of Radiology (ACR): ACR appropriateness criteria: nonischemic myocardial disease with clinical manifestations. 2013. Available at: www.acr.org/~/media/ACR /Documents/AppCriteria/Diagnostic/NonischemicMyocardial DiseaseWithClinicalManifestations.pdf

25. Anderson JL, Adams CD, Antman EM, et al.: 2012 ACCF/AHA focused update incorporated into the ACCF/AHA 2007 guidelines for the management of patients with unstable angina/non-ST-elevation myocardial infarction: a report of the American College of Cardiology Foundation/American Heart Association Task Force on Practice Guidelines. *J Am Coll Cardiol* 2013;**61**(23):e179–347.

26. Kluetz PG, White CS: Acute pulmonary embolism: imaging in the emergency department. *Radiol Clin North Am* 2006;**44**: 259–71.

27. Stein PD, Fowler SE, Goodman LR, et al.: Multidetector computed tomography for acute pulmonary embolism. *N Engl J Med* 2006;**354**(22):2317–27.

28. Stein PD, Chenevert TL, Fowler SE, et al.: Gadolinium-enhanced magnetic resonance angiography for pulmonary embolism: a multicenter prospective study (PIOPED III). *Ann Intern Med* 2010;**152**(7):434–43, W142–3.

29. Ersoy H, Goldhaber SZ, Cai T, et al.: Time-resolved MR angiography: a primary screening examination of patients with suspected pulmonary embolism and contraindications to administration of iodinated contrast material. *AJR Am J Roentgenol* 2007;**188**:1246–54.

30. Sievers B, Elliott MD, Hurwitz LM, et al.: Rapid detection of myocardial infarction by subsecond, free-breathing delayed contrast-enhancement cardiovascular magnetic resonance. *Circulation* 2007;**115**:236–44.

31. Cury RC, Shash K, Nagurney JT, et al.: Cardiac magnetic resonance with T2-weighted imaging improves detection of patients with acute coronary syndrome in the emergency department. *Circulation* 2008;**118**(8):837–44.

32. Greenwood JP, Maredia N, Younger JF, et al.: Cardiovascular magnetic resonance and single-photon emission computed tomography for diagnosis of coronary heart disease (CE-MARC): a prospective trial. *Lancet* 2012;**379**(9814): 453–60.

33. Constantine G, Kesavan S, Flamm SD, Sivananthan MU: Role of MRI in clinical cardiology. *Lancet* 2004;**363**:2162–71.

34. Coulden R: State-of-the-art imaging techniques in chronic thromboembolic pulmonary hypertension. *Proc Am Thorac Soc* 2006;**3**:577–83.

35. Pedersen MR, Fisher MT, van Beek EJR: MR imaging of the pulmonary vasculature – an update. *Eur Radiol* 2006;**16**: 1374–86.

36. Stemerman DH, Krinsky GA, Lee VS, et al.: Thoracic aorta: rapid black-blood MR imaging with half-Fourier rapid acquisition with or without electrocardiographic triggering. *Radiology* 1999;**213**:185–91.

37. Shellock FG, Fischer L, Fieno DS: Cardiac pacemakers and implantable cardioverter defibrillators: in vitro magnetic resonance imaging evaluation at 1.5-tesla. *J Cardiovasc Magn Reson* 2007;**9**(1):21–31.

38. Patel MR, Albert TS, Kandzari DE, et al.: Acute myocardial infarction: safety of cardiac MR imaging after percutaneous revascularization with stents. *Radiology* 2006;**240**(3):674–80.

39. Centers for Disease Control and Prevention (CDC): Nephrogenic fibrosing dermopathy associated with exposure to gadolinium-containing contrast agents – St. Louis, Missouri, 2002–2006. *MMWR Morb Mortal Wkly Rep* 2007;**56** (7):137–41.

Chapter 42

MRI of the Abdomen

Lance Beier, Nilasha Ghosh, Andrew Berg, and Andrew Wong

Clinical indications

Despite its status as the least-used imaging modality of the ED, MRI is a continually evolving technology that may one day be indispensable to the ED physician. The combination of superior contrast and resolution frequently provides more sensitive and specific diagnoses of abdominal pathology, relative to CT (1–3). MRI also carries the additional, and perhaps more important, benefit of producing its images by measuring the effect of a radiofrequency pulse on tissue within a static magnetic field (4). The clinical relevance of this is that high-quality images can be obtained without the use of ionizing radiation. In May 2005, the U.S. Food and Drug Administration released a report stating that the amount of radiation exposure from a single CT scan of the abdomen may be enough to increase the lifetime probability of a fatal cancer by 1 chance in 2,000 (5). As MRI becomes faster and increasingly cost-effective, it is not unreasonable to predict that it may eventually supplant CT scanning as first-line imaging in many indications.

Today, however, the American College of Radiology (ACR) offers a very specific list of indications for MRI of the abdomen (Table 42.1). Although these are useful, they do not become compelling without the presence of a strong contraindication for CT scanning. In the ED, this scenario is most commonly encountered in the pregnant patient. There is debate as to how much ionizing radiation exposure is acceptable in a pregnant patient, but it is generally agreed that this exposure is not without risk and should be avoided if possible (6). While it is not ideal to use CT in pregnancy, it is not an absolute contraindication. CT use in certain emergent situations can produce favorable outcomes for both mother and baby and therefore should be used without delay when necessary (7). Table 42.2 lists common ionizing radiation imaging studies and the radiation exposure to the fetus. Even though no study to date has shown adverse effects of MRI on a fetus, its use must be chosen carefully. The ACR currently recommends the use of MRI during pregnancy if 1) the information requested from the MR study cannot be acquired via non-ionizing means (e.g., ultrasonography), 2) the data are needed to potentially affect the care of the patient or fetus during the pregnancy, and 3) the referring physician does not believe it is prudent to wait until the patient is no longer pregnant to obtain these data (8).

Use of CT in the pediatric population also deserves special consideration with regards to ionizing radiation exposure.

The risk of radiation-caused cancer in children is higher than it is in adults due the relative increased dose as well as their increased lifetime risk (9). Therefore, it would be in the pediatric patient's best interest to explore non-radiation-exposing modalities, such as MRI, when indicated.

Diagnostic capabilities

In general, MRI is known for its superior ability to diagnose pathology of the abdomen due to its intrinsically high contrast. This, along with its ability to provide images in any plane and its low susceptibility to artifacts, often combine to provide uniquely useful imaging of the abdomen. Specifically, MRI can often create the highest quality imaging of the liver, gallbladder, biliary system, pancreas, spleen, and kidneys. This becomes useful considering that acute abdominal pain accounts for more than 7.5 million annual visits to EDs in the United States (10). Of the causes of acute abdominal pain, there is particularly good evidence for the use of MRI in diagnoses of cholecystitis, cholangitis, pancreatitis, appendicitis, and renal artery stenosis.

In the diagnosis of acute cholecystitis, it remains unquestioned that first-line imaging should always be ultrasound. It has a relatively high sensitivity and specificity – 88% and 80%, respectively (11) – and is quick and cost-effective. Occasionally, however, ultrasound can be nondiagnostic secondary to patient obesity, obstructing bowel gas, failure to visualize, or when a single calculus is impacted in the cystic duct (ultrasound sensitivity = 14%). In these situations, magnetic resonance cholangiopancreatography (MRCP) has been shown to have a significantly better sensitivity and accuracy (12, 13). MRCP is the study of choice in pregnant women with known or suspected pancreaticobiliary disease (14). Additionally, recent evidence has supported a greater role for MRCP in the assessment of biliary disease in the non-pregnant population.

When acute cholangitis is clinically suspected, based on the presence of Charcot's triad of jaundice, abdominal pain, and fever, the initial imaging is most often accomplished by ultrasound, which is then followed by endoscopic retrograde cholangiopancreatography (ERCP) for both confirmation of the diagnosis and therapeutic stone extraction. MRCP, however, is becoming a useful alternative when ERCP is unsuccessful or contraindicated. Heavily T2-weighted sequences can very accurately assess biliary and pancreatic ducts, allowing for the detection of choledocholithiasis (15). In fact,

Table 42.1: Abbreviated ACR indications for MRI of the abdomen

Pancreas

1. Detection or preoperative assessment of pancreatic tumors

2. Characterization of indeterminate lesions detected with other imaging modalities

3. Evaluation of pancreatic duct anomalies, obstruction, or dilatation

4. Evaluation of pancreatic or peripancreatic fluid collections

5. Evaluation of chronic pancreatitis or complications of acute pancreatitis

Spleen

1. Characterization of indeterminate lesions detected with other imaging modalities

2. Detection and characterization of suspected diffuse abnormalities of the spleen

Kidneys

1. Detection or preoperative assessment of renal tumors

2. Characterization of indeterminate lesions detected with other imaging modalities

3. Evaluation of the urinary collecting system for abnormalities of anatomy or physiology (MR urography)

Adrenal glands

1. Detection of pheochromocytoma and functioning adrenal adenoma

2. Characterization of indeterminate lesions detected with other imaging modalities

Vascular

1. Diagnosis and/or assessment of the following vascular abnormalities:

  i. Aneurysm or dissection of the aorta and its branch vessels

  ii. Stenosis or occlusion of the aorta and major branch vessels

  iii. Arteriovenous fistula or malformation

  iv. Portal, mesenteric, splenic vein, inferior vena cava (IVC), renal vein, or hepatic vein thrombosis

2. Vascular evaluation in one of the following clinical scenarios:

  i. Lower extremity claudication

  ii. Suspected renovascular hypertension

  iii. Suspected chronic mesenteric ischemia

  iv. Hemorrhagic hereditary telangiectasia

  v. Suspected Budd-Chiari syndrome

  vi. Portal hypertension

  vii. Suspected gonadal vein reflux

  viii. Detection of suspected leak following abdominal aortic aneurysm surgery or MR-compatible aortic stent graft placement

Bile ducts and gallbladder

1. Detection and post-treatment follow-up of bile duct and gallbladder cancer

2. Detection of bile duct or gallbladder stones

3. Evaluation of dilated bile duct

4. Evaluation of suspected congenital abnormalities of the gallbladder or bile ducts

Liver

1. Detection of focal hepatic lesions

Table 42.1: (cont.)

2. Lesion characterization (i.e., cyst, hemangioma, hepatocellular carcinoma, metastasis, focal nodular hyperplasia, hepatic adenoma)

3. Evaluation of vascular patency, including Budd-Chiari

4. Evaluation of diffuse liver disease such as cirrhosis, hemochromatosis, hemosiderosis, fatty infiltration

5. Clarification of findings from other imaging studies or laboratory abnormalities

6. Evaluation of congenital abnormalities

Gastrointestinal tract and peritoneum

1. Assessment of inflammatory disorders of the small or large bowel and mesenteries

2. Assessment of acute abdominal pain (e.g., appendicitis) in pregnant patients

3. Detection and evaluation of primary and metastatic peritoneal or mesenteric neoplasms

4. Detection and characterization of intraabdominal fluid collections

Other

1. Evaluation of the abdomen as an alternative to CT when radiation exposure is an overriding concern in susceptible patients such as pregnant or pediatric patients, or in patients with a contraindication to iodinated contrast agents.

2. Detection and characterization of extraperitoneal neoplasms other than above

Adapted from ACR: ACR practice guideline for the performance of magnetic resonance imaging (MRI) of the abdomen (excluding the liver). 2005, October 1 (revised 2010) Available at: www.acr.org/~/media/ACR/Documents/PGTS/guidelines/MRI_Abdomen.pdf; ACR: ACR practice guideline for the performance of magnetic resonance imaging (MRI) of the liver. 2005, October 1 (revised 2010). Available at: www.acr.org/~/media/ACR/Documents/PGTS/guidelines/MRI_Liver.pdf; ACR: ACR practice guideline for the performance of pediatric and adult body magnetic resonance angiography (MRA). 2015. Available at: www.acr.org/~/media/D1BC4FB23D4B4005872FDDAE018E0CE7.pdf

Table 42.2: Estimated fetal exposure from some common radiologic procedures

Procedure	Fetal Exposure
Chest x-ray (2 views)	0.02–0.07 mrad
Abdominal film (single view)	100 mrad
Hip film (single view)	200 mrad
Mammography	7–20 mrad
Barium enema or small bowel series	2–4 rad
CT† scan of head or chest	<1 rad
CT scan of abdomen and lumbar spine	3.5 rad
CT pelvimetry	250 mrad

† Abbreviation: CT, computed tomography
Data from Cunningham FG, Gant NF, Leveno KJ, et al.: General considerations and maternal evaluation. In: *Williams obstetrics*, 21st ed. New York: McGraw-Hill, 2001:1143–58.

MRCP has been shown to be the most sensitive of the non-invasive techniques for evaluating bile ducts and detecting stones in the common bile duct (16). For this reason, MRCP is recommended as the preferred imaging in patients with a high likelihood of choledocholithiasis (17).

MRI is also increasingly used in the diagnosis of acute pancreatitis. There is now strong evidence that nonenhanced MRI is as effective as contrast-enhanced CT in assessing the severity of acute pancreatitis as well as outcome prediction (18). This could be especially useful in the patient where clinical suspicion of acute pancreatitis is high and CT imaging is negative. T2-weighted sequences provide an advantage for assessing the level of necrosis: high-signal fluid would suggest that there is necrosis in the pancreatic parenchyma (15). Because MRI is able to provide excellent visualization without using contrast agents, MRI would be a beneficial alternative when the use of nephrotoxic contrast is contraindicated.

MRCP is similarly emerging as a diagnostic modality for chronic pancreatitis. ERCP remains the gold standard, but innovations in MRCP, such as secretin-enhanced MRCP (19) and combination with endoscopic ultrasound, are yielding sensitivities and specificities up to 98% and 100%, respectively (20). MRCP alone shows 90% to 95% concordance with ERCP without the associated mortality rate of 0.07% or the associated morbidity (7.5% of patients will suffer pancreatitis, infections, bleeding, or perforations) (21–23). It can even reduce the number of ERCP examinations obtained before cholecystectomy (14, 24). With these benefits, it is not unexpected that utilization of MRCP continues to increase.

Appendicitis, in the properly selected patient, can be diagnosed with nonenhanced MRI with comparable sensitivity and specificity as contrast-enhanced CT (25). This is particularly attractive in pregnant patients because they have a higher incidence of appendicitis, and there are the special considerations for avoiding unnecessary surgery in a pregnant patient as well as sparing the fetus exposure to ionizing radiation. A recent study demonstrated the superior sensitivity of MRI, 100%, as well as the competitive specificity, 94% (26), relative to the sensitivity and specificity of CT, 94% and 95%, respectively (27), in diagnosing appendicitis in a pregnant patient. Use of MRI has also been effective in detecting other possible causes for acute abdominal and pelvic pain in the pregnant population such as adnexal lesions, fibroids, abscess, acute cholecystitis, cholelithiasis, and urinary pathology (28). The pediatric population is susceptible to a high incidence of acute appendicitis as well. In the pediatric population, MRI has been shown to have a sensitivity and specificity of 100% and 96%, respectively, and is therefore an appropriate imaging modality that limits the exposure of younger patients to ionizing radiation (29).

In patients presenting with malignant hypertension, MR angiography (MRA) has emerged as an exquisitely sensitive modality for the diagnosis of renal artery stenosis. Studies have shown that enhanced MRA has a comparable sensitivity and specificity to that of CTA when detecting renal artery stenosis, that being 90% and 94%, compared with 94% and 93%, respectively (30). Additionally, nonenhanced MRA sequences have been developed that can reliably detect renal artery disease without the nephrotoxic contrast used in CTA (31). This moderate improvement in diagnosis, along with the inherent advantages of MR scanning versus CT scanning, has advanced MRA to first-line screening for renovascular hypertension in many institutions.

Imaging pitfalls and limitations

Despite the wide range of possible applications of MRI, there are several limitations that prevent its use in a wide range of patients. First and foremost is that MRI scans take a significant amount of time, and the risk of an unstable patient decompensating during the scan far outweighs the possible benefits of the imaging. For this reason, MRI of the abdomen is rarely indicated emergently. If imaging is believed to be necessary in this situation, a CT scan or bedside ultrasound should be the modality of choice.

In addition to selecting only hemodynamically stable patients, a thorough history and physical needs to be performed to screen for several additional contraindications for MRI. MRI, as its name implies, functions with the aid of strong magnets, which have the ability to displace any ferromagnetic implants and interfere with electronic devices. In general, cardiac pacemakers, intracranial aneurysm clips, certain neurostimulators, certain cochlear implants, and other electronic devices are absolute contraindications (32). Most orthopedic hardware, however, is safe but may cause an increase in artifacts (33).

In addition to these absolute contraindications, there are several relative contraindications that should be taken into account. Most MRI scanners are unable to accommodate patients who weigh more than 350 pounds or are greater than 60 cm in diameter, making scanning of morbidly obese patients difficult, if not impossible (34). There are open MRI systems that can accommodate patients up to 550 pounds, but they are, unfortunately, not widely available.

Preliminary lab work to establish good renal function is recommended if gadolinium contrast is needed. Gadolinium lacks the nephrotoxicity of iodinated contrast agents commonly used in CT scanning, but recent warnings have been issued against its use in patients with renal failure due to a potential link with a scleroderma-like illness, nephrogenic systemic fibrosis (35, 36). Although this complication is rare, it is considered severe enough to warrant these new precautions.

Finally, patients selected for MRI must be able to lie still for the duration of the scan to prevent motion artifact. This is a particularly important point to address in pediatric patients and patients with pain, in which case analgesics should be administered prior to the scan. Additional use of a sedative is often warranted to minimize movement.

Clinical images

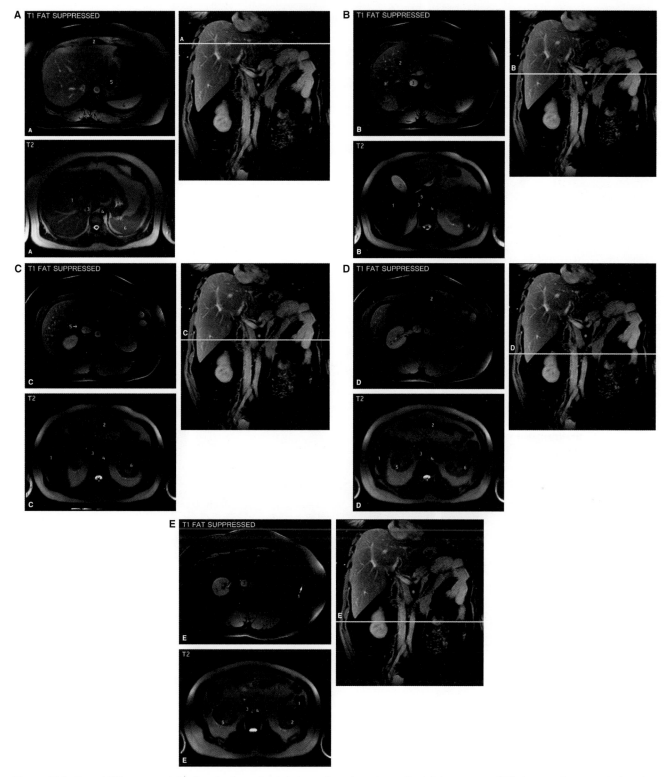

Figure 42.1. Normal MRI anatomy. A: 1 = liver, 2 = immediately below collapsed esophagus, 3 = inferior vena cava (IVC), 4 = aorta, 5 = stomach, 6 = spleen. B: 1 = liver, 2 = gallbladder, 3 = IVC, 4 = aorta, 5 = duodenum, 6 = spleen, 7 = body of pancreas. C: 1 = liver, 2 = transverse colon, 3 = IVC, 4 = aorta, 5 = duodenum, 6 = left kidney, 7 = pancreas. D: 1 = liver, 2 = transverse colon, 3 = IVC, 4 = aorta, 5 = right kidney, 6 = left kidney, 7 = pancreas. E: 1 = descending colon, 2 = left kidney, 3 = IVC, 4 = aorta, 5 = right kidney.

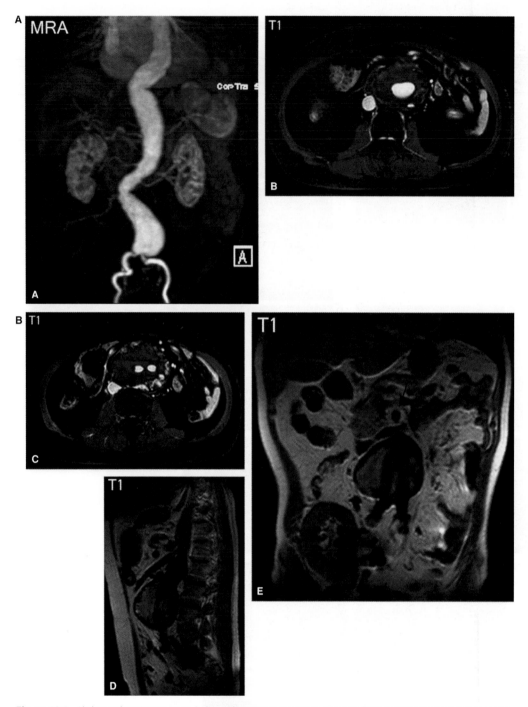

Figure 42.2. Abdominal aortic aneurysm. A: Coronal maximum intensity projection (MIP) reconstruction showing a large aneurysm measuring 4.8 × 4.7 cm in its largest diameter. This aneurysm does not extend into the common iliac arteries. B: Same patient in axial T1-weighted postgadolinium image showing high-intensity gadolinium in the lumen surrounded by low-intensity wall thrombus. C: Axial T1-weighted postgadolinium image in a second patient showing extension of an aneurysm into the common iliac arteries. Sagittal T1-weighted (D) and coronal T1-weighted (E) images of the same patient showing a very large 8.6 × 7 cm aortic aneurysm beginning just below the origin of the superior mesenteric artery (*arrows, e* and *f*).

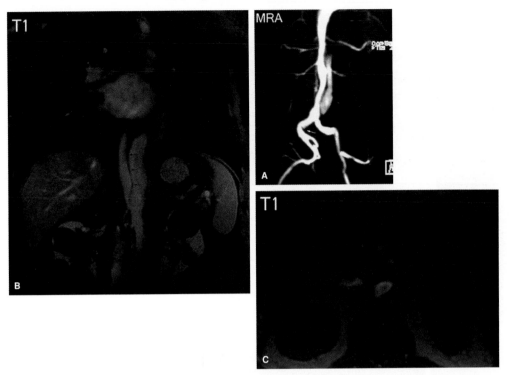

Figure 42.3. Aortic dissection. A: Coronal MIP reconstruction showing complex aortic dissection ending just proximal to the aortic bifurcation as well as 50% stenosis of the right common iliac artery (*arrow*). B: Coronal T1-weighted imaging with arrows indicating place of cleavage. C: Axial T1-weighted image showing an intimal flap separating the false and true lumens. The false lumen can be distinguished by its higher signal intensity in T1 due to its slower relative rate of flow.

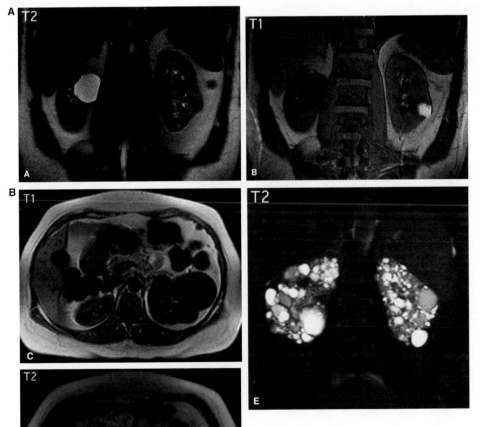

Figure 42.4. Simple and hemorrhagic renal cysts. Sagittal T2-weighted (A) and sagittal T1-weighted (B) images showing renal cysts. The cyst in the right kidney is hyperintense on T2 and hypointense on T1, indicating that it is a simple cyst. The opposite is true of the cyst in the left kidney, which is characteristic of a hemorrhagic cyst. Axial T1-weighted (C) and axial T2-weighted (D) images in a second patient demonstrating multiple simple cysts of the left kidney. E: Sagittal T2-weighted image of a patient with autosomal dominant polycystic kidney disease showing bilaterally enlarged kidneys with cysts involving nearly every part of the renal parenchyma.

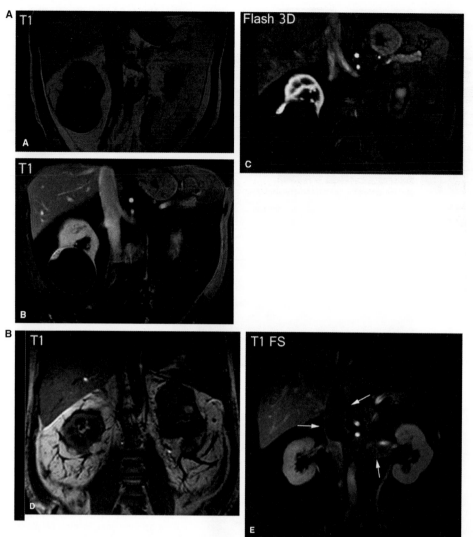

Figure 42.5. Renal cell carcinoma. Coronal T1-weighted (A) and coronal fat-suppressed T2-weighted (B) images showing an 8.5 × 7.6 cm cyst with 1.7 × 1.7 solid mass at its superior aspect. C: Coronal postgadolinium Flash 3D image showing stromal enhancement of the mass, an indication of malignancy. D: Coronal T1-weighted image from a second patient showing an advanced left 7.8-cm renal cell carcinoma. E: Coronal T1-weighted fat-suppressed image in the same patient showing the tumor's invasion into the left renal vein, through the inferior vena cava, and into the right atrium.

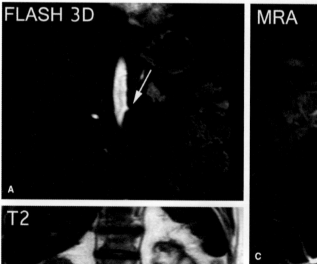

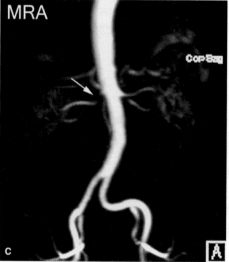

Figure 42.6. Renal artery stenosis. A: A coronal postgadolinium FLASH 3D image showing severe narrowing of the left renal artery (*arrow*). B: Coronal T2-weighted view of the same patient showing an atrophic left kidney with moderate hydronephrosis and cortical thinning, most likely secondary to arterial insufficiency. C: Coronal MIP reconstruction in a second patient showing greater than 50% origin stenosis of the right renal artery (*arrow*) and a duplicated left renal artery.

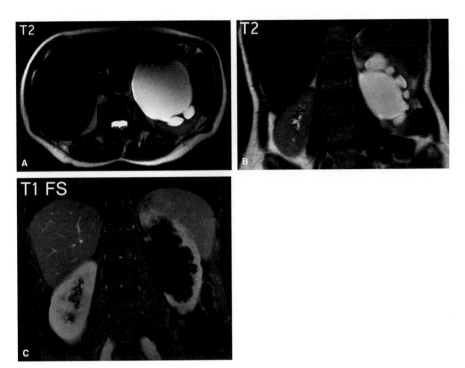

Figure 42.7. Hydronephrosis. Axial T2-weighted (A), coronal T2-weighted (B), and coronal fat-suppressed postgadolinium T1-weighted (C) views of severe left hydronephrosis in a patient with ureteropelvic junction obstruction.

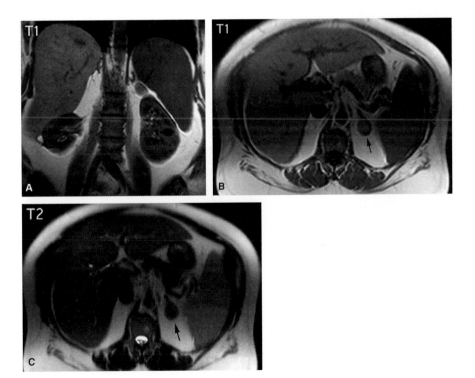

Figure 42.8. Adrenal adenoma. Coronal T1-weighted (A), axial T1-weighted (B), and axial T2-weighted (C) images showing a 3.1 × 2.4 × 2.7 cm left adrenal mass (*arrows*) in a patient with hepatosplenomegaly. Adrenal adenomas are usually solitary encapsulated lesions and are common incidental findings in imaging of the abdomen. Clinical workup is only recommended for adenomas greater than 2 cm in diameter.

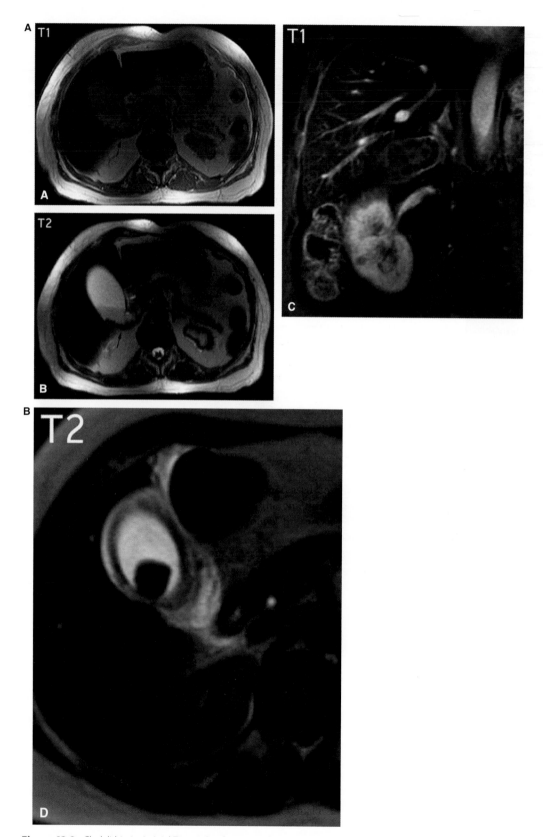

Figure 42.9. Cholelithiasis. A: Axial T1-weighted image with multiple round to faceted gallstones within the gallbladder. Axial T2-weighted (B) and coronal fat-suppressed postgadolinium T1-weighted (C) views in the same patient. D: Coronal T2-weighted image in a second patient showing cholelithiasis with pericholecystic fluid. Gallstones are most typically found incidentally and usually present as intraluminal, signal void, round, or faceted structures on both T1- and T2-weighted images.

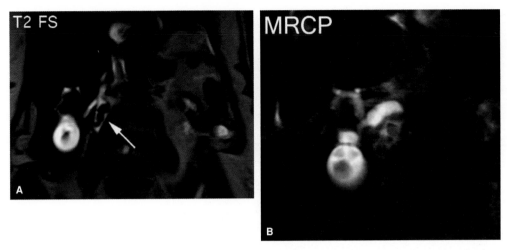

Figure 42.10. Choledocholithiasis. A: Coronal fat-suppressed T2-weighted image showing three faceted low-signal stones in a dilated common bile duct. Notice the meniscus of high-signal bile above the superior stone. B: Coronal T2-weighted MRCP image in the same patient.

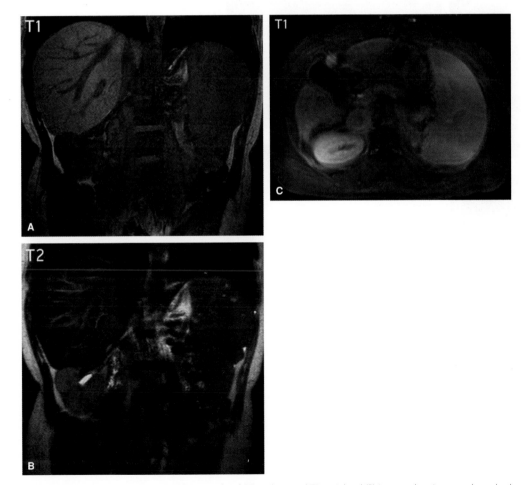

Figure 42.11. Splenomegaly. Coronal T1-weighted (A) and coronal T2-weighted (B) images showing an enlarged spleen, measuring 14.6 cm, with several hemangiomas. C: Axial T1-weighted view of a patient with cirrhosis and an enlarged spleen measuring 16.5 cm.

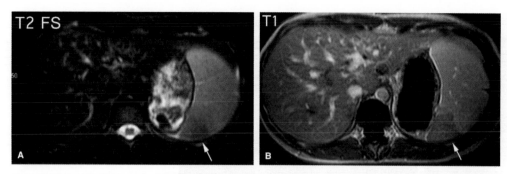

Figure 42.12. Splenic infarct. Axial fat-suppressed postgadolinium T2-weighted (A) and axial postgadolinium T1-weighted (B) images showing a wedge-shaped infarct that fails to enhance on postgadolinium images. Notice the peripherally enhancing splenic capsule around the defect.

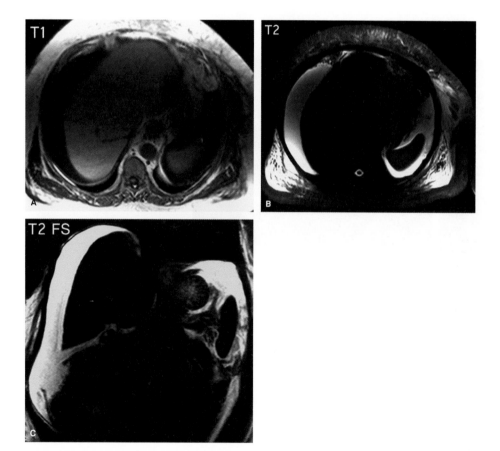

Figure 42.13. Ascites. Axial T1-weighted (A), axial T2-weighted (B), and coronal fat-suppressed T2-weighted (C) images of a cirrhotic patient showing excess fluid in the peritoneal cavity that has low signal intensity on T1-weighted and high signal intensity on T2-weighted images, consistent with a low-protein transudate. Exudative or hemorrhagic fluid collections would have the opposite presentation, giving the evaluator valuable clues to its pathogenesis.

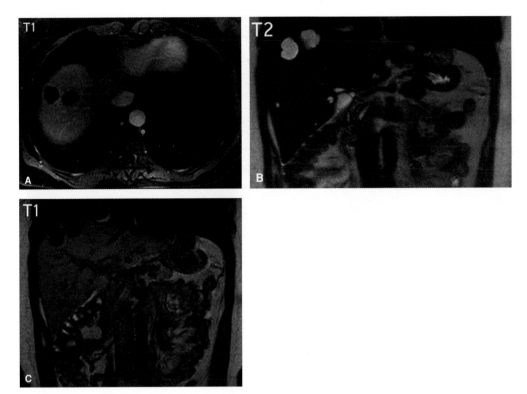

Figure 42.14. Simple hepatic cysts. Axial postgadolinium T1-weighted (A), coronal T2-weighted (B), and coronal T1-weighted (C) images of a patient with two simple hepatic cysts. They can be separated from potentially malignant lesions by their sharp borders, homogeneous interiors, and lack of enhancement on postgadolinium images.

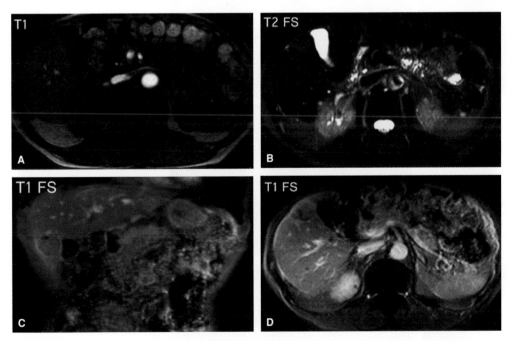

Figure 42.15. Hepatocellular carcinoma. A: Axial T1-weighted image showing 2.8-cm low-signal lesion adjacent to the gallbladder in liver segment V. Axial fat-suppressed T2-weighted (B), coronal fat-suppressed T2-weighted (C), and axial fat-suppressed postgadolinium T2-weighted (D) images from the same patient. Notice that postgadolinium, the lesion is heterogeneously enhancing with a clearly visible pseudocapsule.

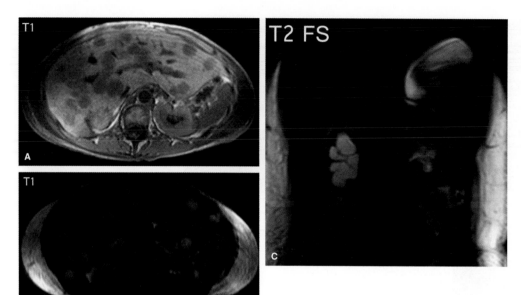

Figure 42.16. Metastatic liver disease. Axial T1-weighted (A) and axial postgadolinium T1-weighted (B) images showing an enlarged liver with extensive metastatic disease from a primary cervical cancer. C: Coronal fat-suppressed T2-weighted image in the same patient showing right hydronephrosis secondary to ureteral obstruction by the primary malignancy.

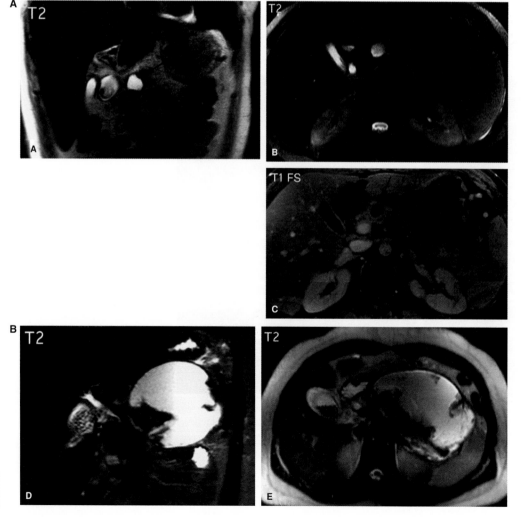

Figure 42.17. Pancreatic pseudocyst. Coronal T2-weighted (A) and axial fat-suppressed postgadolinium T1-weighted (B) image showing a small pseudocyst (*arrow*) of the pancreatic head in a patient with acute pancreatitis. C: Axial T2-weighted view showing communication of the pseudocyst with a prominent pancreatic duct. Coronal T2-weighted (D) and axial T2-weighted (E) images from a second patient showing a large hemorrhagic pseudocyst with very little normal residual tissue. Also seen is cholelithiasis with pericholecystic fluid.

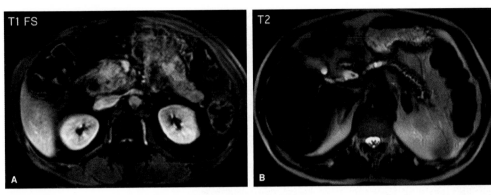

Figure 42.18. Pancreatic cancer. A: Axial fat-suppressed postgadolinium T1-weighted image of pancreatic cancer of the head of the pancreas. B: Axial T2-weighted image showing the pancreatic cancer as well as dilation of the pancreatic duct.

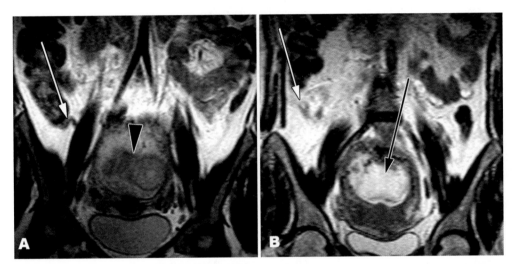

Figure 42.19. Appendicitis in pregnancy. A: Coronal T2-weighted image that shows a normal appendix (*white arrow*) and a gravid uterus (*black arrow*). B: Coronal T2-weighted image with an inflamed appendix (*white arrow*) and gravid uterus (*black arrow*).

References

1. Noone TC, Semelka RC, Chaney DM, Reinhold C: Abdominal imaging studies: comparison of diagnostic accuracies resulting from ultrasound, computed tomography, and magnetic resonance imaging in the same individual. *Magn Reson Imaging* 2004;**22**(1):19–24.

2. Lumachi F, Tregnaghi A, Zucchetta P, et al.: Sensitivity and positive predictive value of CT, MRI and ^{123}I-MIBG scintigraphy in localizing pheochromocytomas: a prospective study. *Nucl Med Commun* 2006;**27**(7):583–7.

3. Pedrosa I, Levine D, Eyvazzadeh AD, et al.: MR imaging evaluation of acute appendicitis in pregnancy. *Radiology* 2006;**238**(3):891–9.

4. Huk WJ, Gademann G: Magnetic resonance imaging (MRI): method and early clinical experiences in diseases of the central nervous system. *Neurosurg Rev* 1984;**7**(4):259–80.

5. U.S. Food and Drug Administration (FDA): Whole body scanning: what are the radiation risks from CT? 2007. Available at: www.fda.gov/cdrh/ct/risks.html

6. Hall EJ: Scientific view of low-level radiation risks. *Radiographics* 1991;**11**(3):509–18.

7. Wang PI, Chong ST, Kielar AZ, et al.: Imaging of pregnant and lactating patients: part 2, evidence-based review and recommendations. *AJR Am J Roentgenol* 2012 Apr;**198**(4):785–92.

8. Kanal E, Borgstede JP, Barkovich AJ: American College of Radiology white paper on MR safety. *AJR Am J Roentgenol* 2002;**178**(6):1335–48.

9. Brenner D, Elliston C, Hall E, Berdon W: Estimated risks of radiation-induced fatal cancer from pediatric CT. *AJR Am J Roentgenol* 2001;**176**(2):289–96.

10. McCaig LF, Nawar EW: *National hospital ambulatory medical care survey: 2004 emergency department summary.* Hyattsville, MD: National Center for Health Statistics, 2006:1–29.

11. Shea JA, Berlin JA, Escarce JJ, et al.: Revised estimates of diagnostic test sensitivity and specificity in suspected biliary tract disease. *Arch Intern Med* 1994;**154**(22): 2573–81.

12. Park MS, Yu JS, Kim YH, et al.: Acute cholecystitis: comparison of MR cholangiography and US. *Radiology* 1998;**3**:781–5.

13. Hkansson K, Leander P, Ekberg O, Hkansson H-O: MR imaging in clinically suspected acute cholecystitis: a comparison with ultrasonography. *Acta Radiol Choledocholithiasis* 2000;**41**(4):322–8.

14. Oto A, Ernst R, Ghulmiyyah L, et al.: The role of MR cholangiopancreatography in the evaluation of pregnant patients with acute pancreaticobilliary disease. *Br J Radiology* 2009;**82**:279–85.

15. ACR: ACR Appropriateness Criteria Acute Pancreatitis. 1998 (amended 2013). Available at: www.acr.org/qualitysafety /~/~/media/2712288FE06B48A4B87F20E9C4B7D652.pdf.

16. Maurea S, Caleo O, Mollica C, et al: Comparative diagnostic evaluation with MR cholangiopancreatography, ultrasonography and CT in patients with pancreatobiliary disease. *Radiol Med* 2009;**114**:390–402.

17. Lalani T, Couto CA, Rosen MP, et al.: ACR appropriateness criteria jaundice. *J Am Coll Radiol.* 2013 Jun;**10**(6):402–9.

18. Stimac D, Miletic D, Radic M, et al.: The role of nonenhanced magnetic resonance imaging in the early assessment of acute pancreatitis. *Am J Gastroenterol* 2007;**102**(5):997–1004.

19. Czakó L: Diagnosis of early-stage chronic pancreatitis by secretin-enhanced magnetic resonance cholangiopancreatography. *J Gastroenterol* 2007;**42**(Suppl 17): 113–17.

20. Pungpapong S, Wallace MB, Woodward TA, et al.: Accuracy of endoscopic ultrasonography and magnetic resonance cholangiopancreatography for the diagnosis of chronic pancreatitis: a prospective comparison study. *J Clin Gastroenterol* 2007;**41**(1):88–93.

21. Andriulli A, Loperfido S, Napolitano G, et al.: Incidence rates of post-ERCP complications: a systematic survey of prospective studies. *Am J Gastroenterol* 2007;**102**(8):1781–8.

22. Chan YL, Chan AC, Lam WW, et al.: Choledocholithiasis: comparison of MR cholangiography and endoscopic retrograde cholangiography. *Radiology* 1996;**200**(1):85–9.

23. Shanmugam V, Beattie GC, Yule SR, et al.: Is magnetic resonance cholangiopancreatography the new gold standard in biliary imaging? *Br J Radiol* 2005;**78**(934):888–93.

24. Williams EJ, Green J, Beckingham I, et al.: Guidelines on the management of common bile duct stones (CBDS). *Gut* 2008;**57**: 1004–21.

25. Leeuwenburgh MM, Wiarda BM, Wiezer MJ, et al.: Comparison of imaging strategies with conditional contrast-enhanced CT and unenhanced MR imaging in patients suspected of having appendicitis: a multicenter diagnostic performance study. *Radiology* 2013;**268**(1):135–43.

26. Pedrosa I, Beddy P, Pedrosa I: MR imaging evaluation of acute appendicitis in pregnancy. *Radiology* 2006;**238**(3):891–9.

27. Terasawa T, Blackmore CC, Bent S, Kohlwes RJ: Systematic review: computed tomography and ultrasonography to detect acute appendicitis in adults and adolescents. *Ann Intern Med* 2004;**141**(7):537–46.

28. Oto A, Ernst RD, Ghulmiyyah LM, et al.: MR imaging in the triage of pregnant patients with acute abdominal and pelvic pain. *Abdom Imaging* 2009;**34**(2):243–50.

29. Herliczek TW, Swenson DW, Mayo-Smith WW: Utility of MRI after inconclusive ultrasound in pediatric patients with suspected appendicitis: retrospective review of 60 consecutive patients. *AJR Am J Roentgenol* 2013;**200**(5):969–73.

30. Rountas C, Vlychou M, Vassiou K, et al.: Imaging modalities for renal artery stenosis in suspected renovascular hypertension: prospective intraindividual comparison of color Doppler US, CT angiography, GD-enhanced MR angiography, and digital substraction angiography. *Ren Fail* 2007;**29**(3):295–302.

31. Pei Y, Shen H, Li J, et al.: Evaluation of renal artery in hypertensive patients by unenhanced MR angiography using spatial labeling with multiple inversion pulses sequence and by CT angiography. *AJR Am J Roentgenol* 2012;**199**(5):1142–8.

32. ACR: ACR practice guideline for performing and interpreting magnetic resonance imaging (MRI). 2013, (amended 2014). Available at: www.acr.org/~/media/EB54F56780AC4C6994 B77078AA1D6612.pdf

33. Shellock FG: Biomedical implants and devices: assessment of magnetic field interactions with a 3.0-tesla MR system. *J Magn Reson Imaging* 2002;**16**(6):731–2.

34. Uppot RN, Sahani DV, Hahn PF, et al.: Impact of obesity on medical imaging and image-guided intervention. *AJR Am J Roentgenol* 2007;**188**(2):433–40.

35. Pederson M: Safety update on the possible causal relationship between gadolinium-containing MRI agents and nephrogenic systemic fibrosis. *J Magn Reson Imaging* 2007;**25**(5):881–3.

36. Grobner T: Gadolinium – a specific trigger for the development of nephrogenic fibrosing dermopathy and nephrogenic systemic fibrosis? *Nephrol Dial Transplant* 2006;**21**:1104–8.

Chapter 43

MRI of the Extremities

Kathryn J. Stevens and Shaun V. Mohan

Indications

Magnetic resonance imaging (MRI) is an excellent imaging modality for visualizing soft tissue and bony pathology. Although the majority of hospitals now have MRI scanners, they are still not widely available on call. MRI studies should be requested emergently only if the required diagnostic information cannot be adequately obtained from other imaging modalities such as radiographs, CT, or ultrasound. However, nonurgent MRI studies can be extremely helpful for the diagnostic workup of patients presenting to the ED, as long as quality of care is not compromised by the delay in imaging.

It is imperative to provide relevant clinical history and diagnostic information when requesting any radiologic study, as this will help determine the most appropriate imaging modality. Documentation of a patient's presenting symptoms or precipitating events on the request form is important, because a request that simply asks to "rule out" a particular diagnosis may cause insurance companies to deny subsequent reimbursement. It is also helpful to indicate pertinent laboratory work the patient has had prior to imaging and whether the results of these tests were abnormal.

In females of reproductive age, it is prudent to determine whether the patient is pregnant prior to requesting a study, as this will again alter the choice of imaging modality. During pregnancy, ultrasound or MRI are preferable to studies involving ionizing radiation such as CT or multiple radiographs, unless the risk to the mother from undiagnosed injuries outweighs the risk to the fetus from irradiation.

Knowledge of renal function is critical when considering which imaging modality to request. The radiologist must be informed about any potential renal compromise prior to booking any cross-sectional imaging study. Iodinated radiographic contrast agents are usually not given if renal function is compromised, particularly when associated with diabetes mellitus, as these patients are at increased risk of developing contrast-induced nephropathy (1–3). An MRI examination may provide more useful information than CT in these cases. However, the MRI contrast agent gadolinium is also contraindicated in patients with preexisting renal failure, particularly those with a glomerular filtration rate (GFR) of less than 30 mL/minute, as this has been linked to the development of nephrogenic systemic fibrosis, also known as nephrogenic fibrosing dermopathy. This entity was first described in 1997 and is characterized by skin thickening with inhibition of flexion and extension of joints due to contractures, eventually progressing to widespread fibrosis of other organs, which may be fatal. Gadolinium should be used with caution for patients with GFR between 30 mL/minute and 60 mL/minute, not exceeding doses of 0.1 mmol/kg. There are currently no contraindications to gadolinium administration in patients with GFR greater than 60 mL/minute (4).

MRI is exquisitely sensitive to bone marrow edema and can be used to evaluate for occult bony injuries that cannot be otherwise seen on radiography or even CT (5–8). MRI should still be considered for any patient with symptoms and physical findings highly suggestive of a fracture, even if the radiographs or CT are negative. An MRI scan should be requested emergently if the presence of a fracture may require surgical intervention, result in a patient's admission to hospital, or has the potential to displace if left untreated such as an occult fracture of the femoral neck. MRI can also be used to evaluate patients in whom an underlying soft tissue injury or internal joint derangement is suspected, to determine whether this injury requires surgical repair or would result in a significant change in the patient's subsequent management (9–18).

CT is more widely available and readily accessible, and it can be helpful in the initial evaluation of a septic patient. CT is useful to demonstrate subcutaneous edema, soft tissue abscesses, soft tissue gas, radiopaque foreign bodies, periosteal reaction, and bony destruction. However, if there is clinical or radiographic concern for soft tissue or bony infection, MRI can also be considered, both to confirm the diagnosis and define the extent of bony, soft tissue, or joint involvement (19, 20). MRI is more sensitive than CT for detection of early soft tissue edema or bone marrow edema and can elegantly demonstrate abscesses, interfascial fluid collections, skin defects, and bony destruction, particularly when intravenous gadolinium is given. Gradient echo sequences are also sensitive for picking up small bubbles of gas or metallic foreign bodies, manifesting as blooming areas of low-signal intensity or susceptibility artifact.

MRI can also be helpful to evaluate for inflammatory disorders and bony or soft tissue neoplasms. However, MRI may also detect incidental lesions or normal anatomic variants that simulate pathologic lesions. Therefore, it is important to correlate imaging findings with the clinical presentation and to have some knowledge of the normal anatomy of the musculoskeletal structures in the extremities to avoid over-diagnosing pathology.

Diagnostic capabilities

Trauma is one of the leading causes for a patient to present to the ED. Fractures and dislocations are common and are almost always associated with injuries to intra-articular structures and surrounding soft tissues. Although bony injuries are usually best demonstrated on radiographs or CT studies, the extent of associated soft tissue damage is often underestimated. Soft tissue swelling, joint effusions, and joint space asymmetry are signs for increased clinical suspicion for associated injuries. Fine detail of the adjacent soft tissues can also be appreciated relatively well with modern multidetector CT scanners, particularly with the ability to reformat images in multiple planes. Soft tissue injuries can also be evaluated with ultrasound, which can be used to accurately diagnose muscle tears, tendon injuries, and periarticular structures. Ultrasound has the unique advantage of dynamic scanning, as some abnormalities can be more easily detected when the affected limb is actively or passively moved, as in the case of tendon tears or muscle hernias. However, musculoskeletal ultrasound is very operator-dependent, and it can take considerable time to acquire the necessary skills. In addition, ultrasound may not be able to capture an entire anatomic structure in one frame, and in most joints it is not possible to interrogate deep intra-articular structures.

Trauma to ligaments, tendons, muscles, neurovascular bundles, and intra-articular structures is therefore best assessed with MRI. MRI scanners with higher field strength, new coil technology, fast pulse sequences, and increased use of contrast agents has expanded the use of MRI in musculoskeletal applications. The majority of radiology departments develop their own standard imaging protocols to ensure that studies are consistent and reproducible. However, the quality of the scan will vary with the strength of the MRI scanner and type of transmitter and receiver coils used, and it also depends to some extent on the training and skill of the MRI technologists and sequence selection chosen by radiologists. MRI is ideal for evaluating complex joint anatomy, given the multiplanar imaging capabilities. T1-weighted sequences are ideal for demonstrating fine anatomic detail, and fat-saturated fluid sensitive sequences such as T2 and proton density can demonstrate subtle pathology that may currently be overlooked with other imaging modalities.

Imaging pitfalls and limitations

MRI is noninvasive and does not involve irradiation; it is therefore ideal for younger patients. However, children under the age of 6 years may find it difficult to remain still for the duration of the scan, thereby resulting in motion artifact. Similarly, patients who are claustrophobic or are in significant pain may also be unable to tolerate lying in the scanner, but they can be premedicated with a mild sedative or pain killers if this is known ahead of time. It is not advisable to scan clinically unstable patients by MRI in an emergent situation, as sequence acquisition takes longer than a CT scan. However, monitoring equipment can now be made MR compatible, and patients requiring supportive care can be safely monitored while inside the MRI scanner (21, 22).

Most MRI scanners have a weight limit of approximately 400 pounds and a maximum bore diameter of 70 cm, thereby excluding morbidly obese patients. Even obese patients who can fit into the MRI scanner may still not fit into an appropriate extremity coil, which will yield poor image quality.

There are a number of absolute contraindications to obtaining an MRI, which include intracranial aneurysm clips, intraocular metallic foreign bodies, and cardiac pacemakers. Strong magnetic fields can cause displacement of small metallic structures and will cause malfunction of electronic devices. Orthopedic hardware is generally not ferromagnetic and therefore is not a contraindication to scanning. However, significant susceptibility artifact is created by metallic implants, particularly those containing stainless steel (23). It is important to provide appropriate information on any internal metallic hardware when requesting an MRI scan so that the radiologist can protocol the scan appropriately to minimize metallic artifact. This generally involves acquiring STIR images instead of T2-weighted images, using a lower strength magnet where available, and avoiding gradient echo sequences, in which metallic artifact is maximized. There are also a number of recently developed metal suppression sequences that can optimize imaging around metal implants (24).

Clinical images

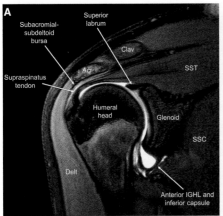

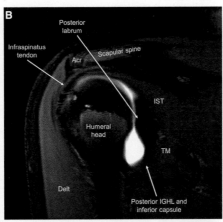

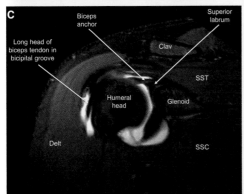

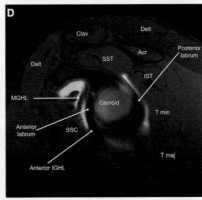

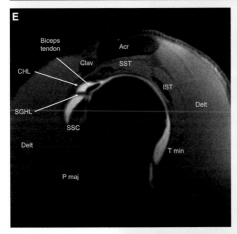

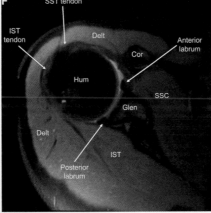

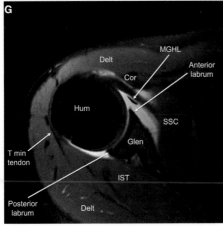

Figure 43.1. Normal anatomy of the shoulder. Patients are usually imaged with the arm at the side, either at neutral or externally rotated for optimal visualization of rotator cuff tendons.

Clav = clavicle, Acr = acromion, Cor = coracoid process, SSC = subscapularis, SST = supraspinatus, IST = infraspinatus, T min = teres minor, T maj = teres major, Delt = deltoid, P maj = pectoralis major, CHL = coracohumeral ligament, SGHL = superior glenohumeral ligament, MGHL = middle glenohumeral ligament, anterior IGHL = anterior band of the inferior glenohumeral ligament, posterior IGHL = posterior band of inferior glenohumeral ligament.

Coronal oblique fat-saturated T2- weighted (T2 FS) images (A, B) from an MR arthrogram prescribed in plane with the supraspinatus tendon, passing through the anterior humeral head and glenoid (A), and posterior humeral head and glenoid (B). Coronal oblique fat-saturated T1-weighted (T1 FS) MR arthrographic image (C) through the anterior humeral head in a different patient demonstrates the long head of biceps tendon inserting into the superior labrum, forming the bicipitolabral complex. Sagittal oblique fat-saturated T1-weighted (T1 FS) MR arthrographic image (D) at the level of the glenoid. Sagittal oblique fat-saturated T1-weighted (T1 FS) MR arthrographic image (E) at the level of the rotator interval (space between the supraspinatus and subscapularis tendons through which the biceps tendon passes to enter the glenohumeral joint). Axial fat-saturated proton density-weighted (PD FS) image (F) at the level of the superior glenoid. Axial T1 FS MR arthrographic image (G) at the level of the mid-glenoid.

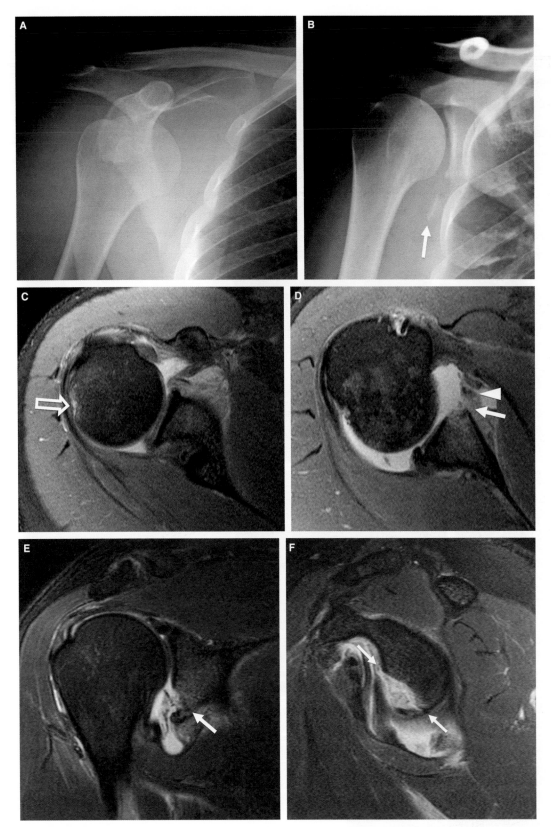

Figure 43.2. (A) Anteroposterior (AP) radiograph of the right shoulder in a 26-year-old male with acute anterior dislocation of the glenohumeral joint. (B) A subsequent Grashey view shows that the shoulder is relocated, but a bony fragment is now seen inferior to the glenohumeral joint (*arrow*). Axial PD FS images (C, D) demonstrate a small Hill–Sachs impaction fracture of the posterosuperior humeral head (open arrow), a fracture (bony Bankart lesion) of the anteroinferior glenoid (*arrow*), with detachment of the anterior labrum (labral Bankart) (*arrowhead*). Coronal oblique (E) and sagittal oblique T2 FS (F) images again demonstrates the fracture of the anteroinferior glenoid (*arrows*).

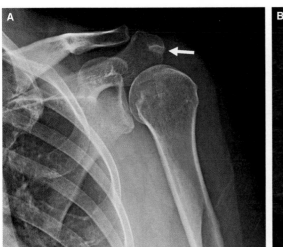

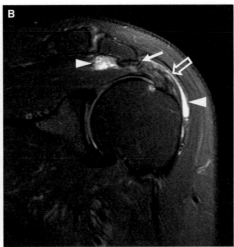

Figure 43.3. A 52-year-old female with severe shoulder pain. (A) A Grashey radiograph of the shoulder demonstrates a prominent subacromial spur (*arrow*). Coronal oblique T2 FS image (B) demonstrates the subacromial spur, with severe tendinopathy and bursal surface fraying of the supraspinatus tendon (*open arrow*) and subacromial/subdeltoid bursitis (*arrowhead*).

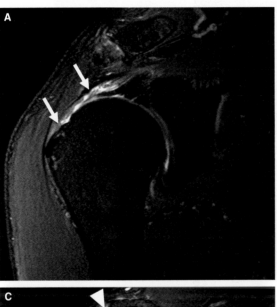

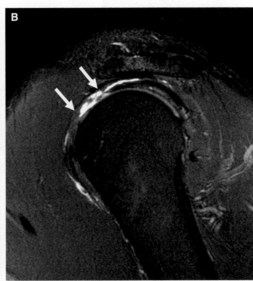

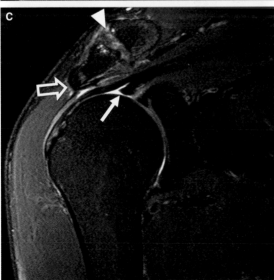

Figure 43.4. Coronal oblique PD FS (A) and sagittal oblique T2 FS (B) images of the right shoulder in a 51-year-old male with longstanding shoulder pain and recent fall. A full thickness tear of the supraspinatus tendon is visible (*arrows*). (C) A coronal oblique PD FS image more posteriorly shows an extensive undersurface delaminating cuff tear, with retraction of undersurface fibers (*arrow*). Severe degenerative change of the acromioclavicular joint is evident (*arrowhead*), with lateral down sloping of the acromion (*open arrow*), likely impinging on the supraspinatus tendon.

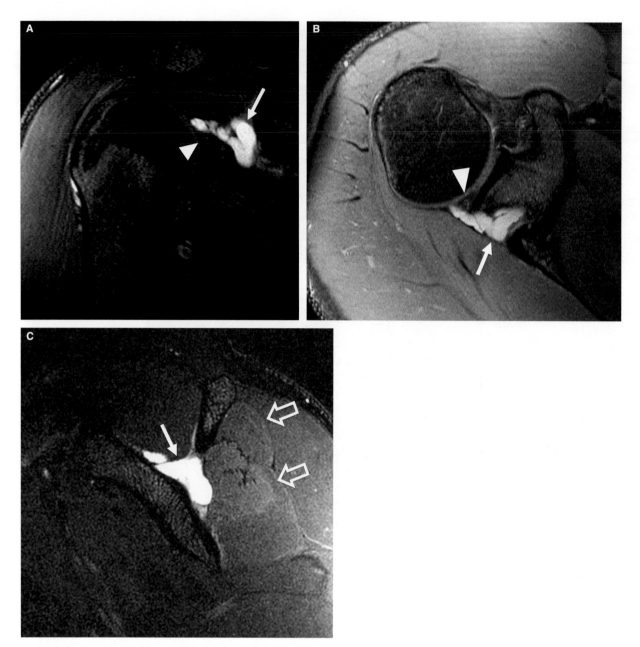

Figure 43.5. Coronal oblique T2 FS (A) and axial PD FS (B) images of the right shoulder in a 36-year-old male with shoulder pain and weakness demonstrate a tear of the posterosuperior labrum (*arrowhead*), with an associated paralabral cyst extending into the spinoglenoid notch (*arrow*). Sagittal T2 FS image (C) again demonstrates the paralabral cyst in the spinoglenoid notch (*arrow*). There is subtle edema within the infraspinatus muscle (*open arrows*), indicative of early denervation.

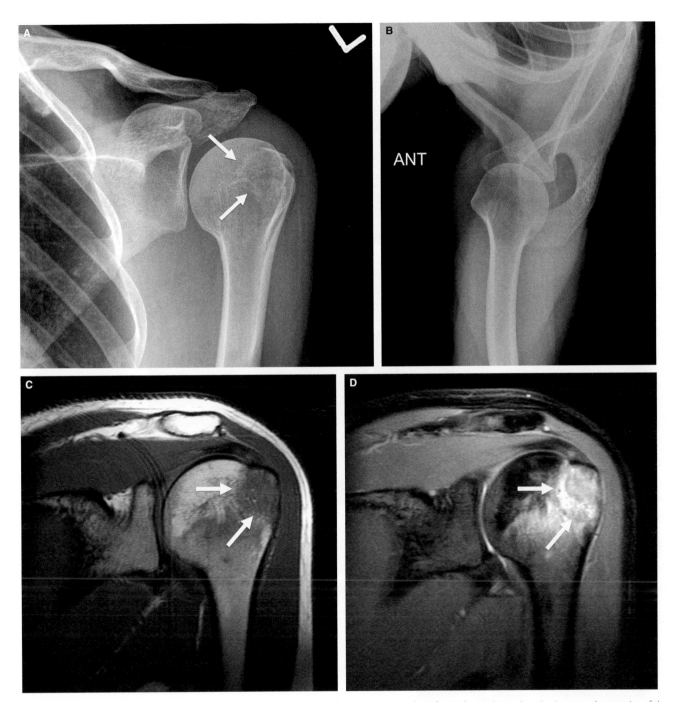

Figure 43.6. Grashey (A) and axillary (B) views of the left shoulder taken after a skiing injury show faint sclerosis (*arrows*) projecting over the margins of the greater tuberosity – but no obvious fracture line. Coronal oblique T1 (C) and T2 FS (D) images demonstrating a nondisplaced fracture of the greater tuberosity demarcated by a vague low-signal intensity fracture line (*arrows*), with extensive associated bone marrow edema.

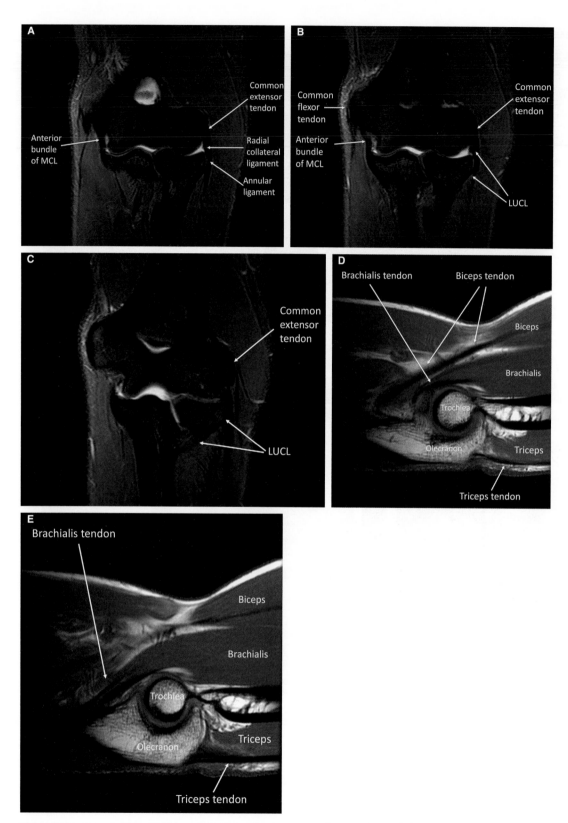

Figure 43.7. Coronal oblique T2 FS images (A–C) showing the common flexor tendon medially and common extensor tendon laterally. The ulnar collateral ligament is composed of three bands, of which the anterior bundle is the one best seen on coronal images. It is normal for the MCL to appear slightly attenuated proximally as in this example. There are also three components of the lateral collateral ligament, namely the radial collateral ligament (RCL), annular ligament, and lateral ulnar collateral ligament (LUCL). The LUCL acts as a supportive sling for the radial head and provides the primary restraint to varus stress. Sagittal T1 FS MR arthrographic images (D, E) show the biceps tendon inserting into the bicipital tuberosity of the radius (D) and the brachialis tendon inserting into the coronoid process of the ulna (D, E). The triceps tendon inserts into the olecranon and may have a wavy contour of the triceps tendon if the elbow is hyperextended.

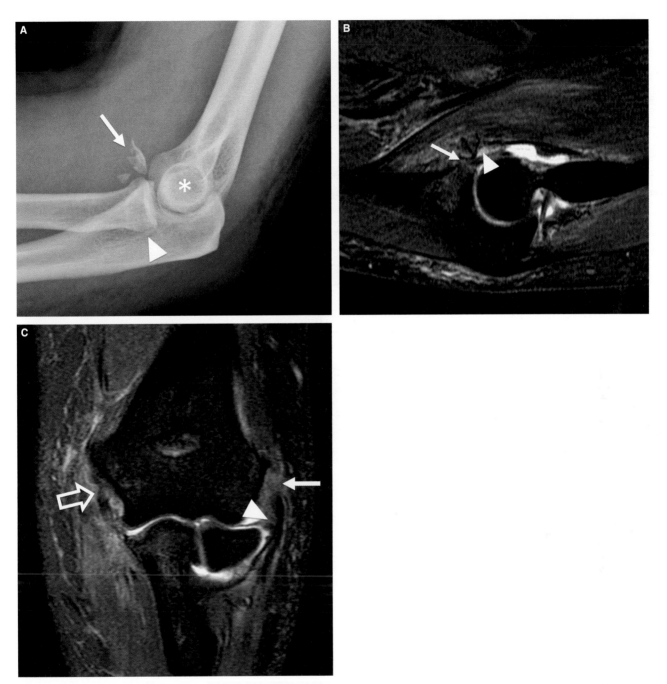

Figure 43.8. (A) Lateral radiograph of a 37-year-old male with recent elbow dislocation demonstrating a comminuted fracture of the coronoid process (*arrow*) and subtle posterior subluxation of the radial head (*arrowhead*) with respect to the center of the capitellum (*asterisk*). Sagittal T2 FS image (B) again demonstrates a fracture of the coronoid process (*arrow*), with a partial undersurface tear and reactive edema in the overlying brachialis muscle (*arrowhead*). Coronal T2 FS (C) image demonstrates complete tears of the common extensor tendon (*arrow*) and LUCL (*arrowhead*) from the lateral epicondyle, and there is a high-grade tear of the medial collateral ligament (*open arrow*).

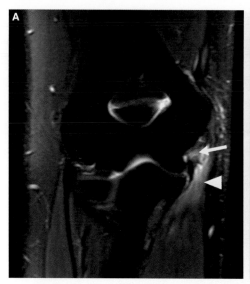

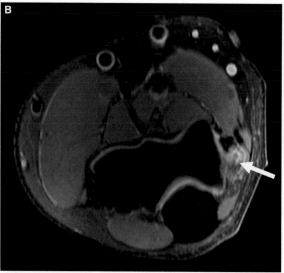

Figure 43.9. Coronal T2 FS (A) and axial PD FS (B) images of the elbow in a 22-year-old male following a valgus injury demonstrates a complete tear of the proximal fibers of the anterior bundle of the medial collateral ligament (*arrow*). Edema is seen in the adjacent flexor muscles (*arrowhead*).

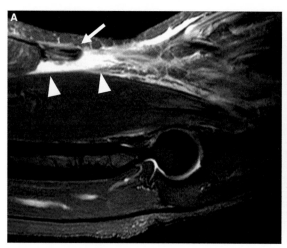

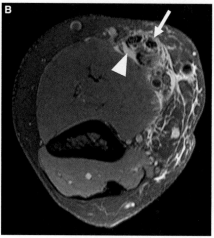

Figure 43.10. Sagittal T2 FS (A) and axial PD FS (B) images of the elbow in a 52-year-old man following a lifting injury resulting in rupture of the distal biceps tendon, with the tendon end retracted proximally (*arrow*) and adjacent hemorrhage and edema (*arrowheads*).

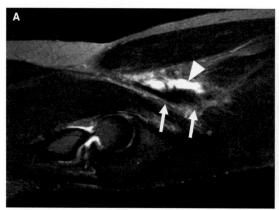

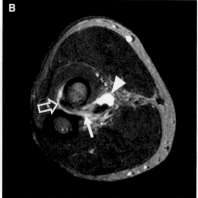

Figure 43.11. Sagittal T2 FS (A) of the elbow in a 46-year-old with elbow pain after working out in the gym. The distal biceps tendon appears thickened and irregular (*arrows*), with fluid in the adjacent bicipitoradial bursa (*arrowhead*). Axial PD FS image (B) demonstrates a high-grade tear of the distal biceps tendon (*arrow*). Excess fluid is seen in the bicipitoradial bursa (*arrowhead*), and there is mild bony hypertrophy of the bicipital tuberosity of the radius (*open arrow*).

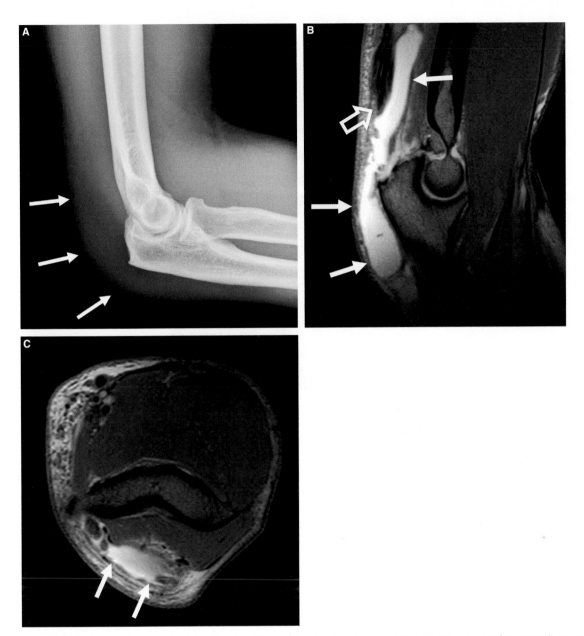

Figure 43.12. (A) Lateral radiograph of the elbow in a 22-year-old male with pain after a jujitsu fight. Prominent soft tissue swelling is seen posteriorly (*arrows*), but there is no obvious avulsion fracture. Sagittal T2 FS (B) and axial PD FS (C) images show a complete tear of the distal triceps tendon, with a retracted tendon end (*open arrow*). Extensive hemorrhage is seen in the olecranon bursa (*arrows*).

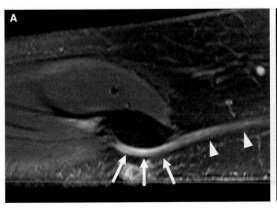
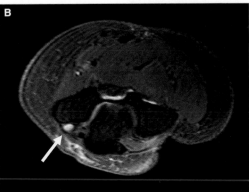

Figure 43.13. Sagittal (A) and axial T2 FS (B) images in a 40-year-old female with left elbow and forearm pain demonstrate increased T2 signal within the ulnar nerve as it runs along the posterior margin of the olecranon (*arrows*), compatible with ulnar neuritis. Normal signal intensity is seen in the ulnar nerve more proximally (*arrowheads*).

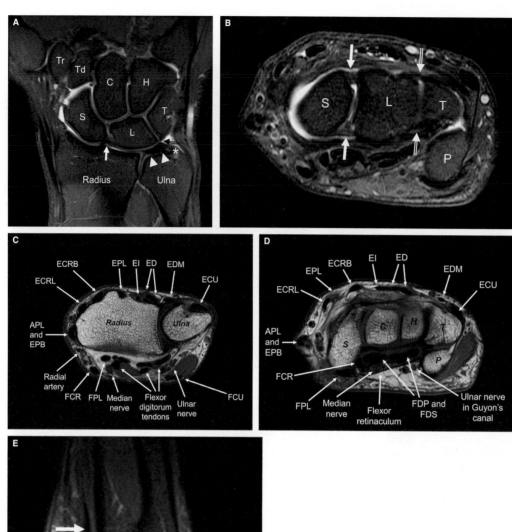

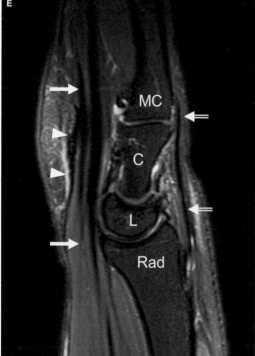

Figure 43.14. Normal anatomy of the wrist. The wrist can be imaged with the arm at the side, the arm overhead, or the arm flexed and the wrist placed over the abdomen. However, in the latter position, the arm must be separated from the abdominal wall, or there will be considerable artifact from respiration. High-resolution images can usually be obtained using a dedicated extremity coil and a small field of view.

Coronal T2 FS image (A) of the wrist showing normal anatomy. S = scaphoid, L = lunate, T = triquetrum, H = hamate, C = capitate, Tr = trapezoid, Td = trapezium. The central fibers of the scapholunate (*arrow*) and lunotriquetral (*black double line arrow*) ligaments are well seen, as well as the triangular fibrocartilage (*arrowheads*), which arises from the sigmoid notch of the radius and attaches to the ulna via the triangular ligament (*asterisk*). Axial T2 FS image (B) through the proximal carpal row demonstrates the dorsal and volar fibers of the scapholunate ligament (*arrows*) and lunotriquetral ligament (*double line arrow*). The dorsal fibers of the scapholunate ligament and volar fibers of the lunotriquetral ligament are the strongest and functionally important portions of the ligaments. S = scaphoid, L = lunate, T = triquetrum, P = pisiform. Axial T1 images (C, D) at the level of the distal radio-ulnar joint (C) and carpal tunnel (D) demonstrating normal anatomy. APL = abductor pollicis longus, EPB = extensor pollicis brevis, ECRL = extensor carpi radialis longus, ECRB = extensor carpi radialis longus brevis, EPL = extensor pollicis longus, EI = extensor indicis, ED = extensor digitorum tendons, EDM = extensor digiti minimi, ECU = extensor carpi ulnaris, FCR = flexor carpi radialis, FPL = flexor pollicis longus, FDP = flexor digitorum profundus, FDS = flexor digitorum superficialis, FCU = flexor carpi ulnaris. Sagittal T2 FS image (E) of the wrist demonstrating normal flexor tendons (*arrows*) in the carpal tunnel, with the overlying flexor retinaculum (*arrowheads*). Normal extensor tendons (*double line arrows*) are seen over the dorsal wrist. L = lunate, C = capitate, MC = metacarpal.

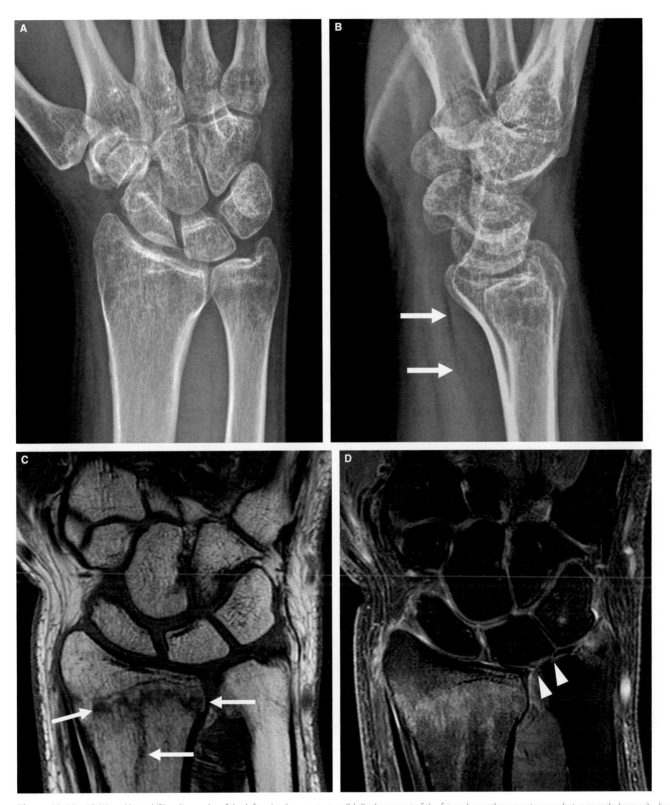

Figure 43.15. AP (A) and lateral (B) radiographs of the left wrist demonstrate mild displacement of the fat pad over the pronator quadratus muscle (*arrows*) – but no visible fracture. Coronal T1 (C) and T2 FS (D) images demonstrate a nondisplaced fracture of the distal radius (*arrows*), extending into the distal radioulnar joint, and a large tear of the triangular fibrocartilage (*arrowheads*).

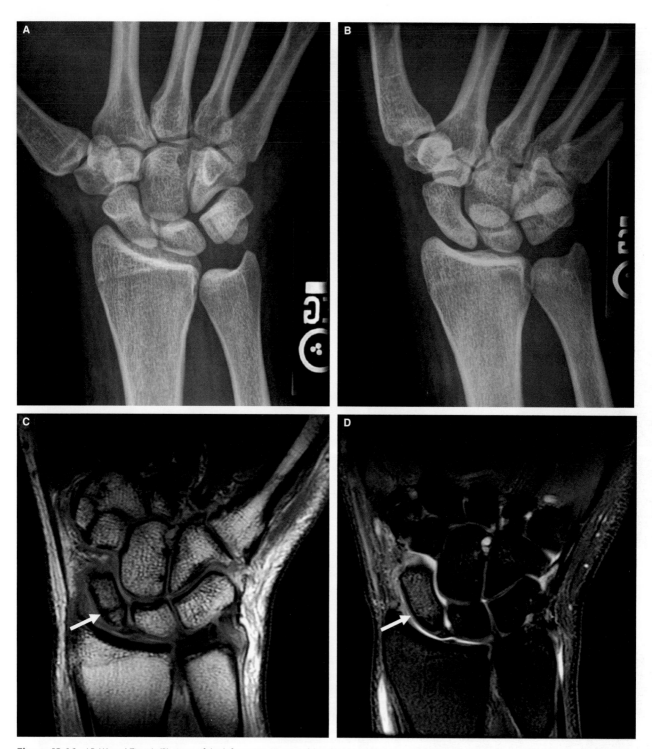

Figure 43.16. AP (A) and Zitter's (B) views of the left wrist in 20-year-old male with wrist injury. No fracture is visible. Coronal T1 (C) and T2 FS (D) one week later demonstrate a nondisplaced fracture of the scaphoid waist (*arrow*), with prominent bone marrow edema.

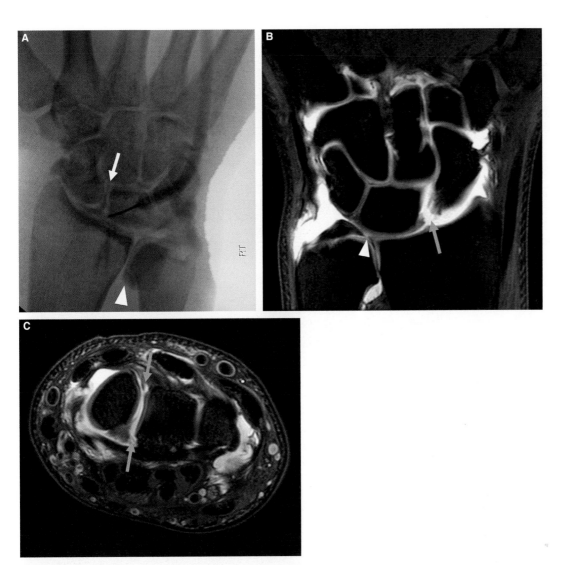

Figure 43.17. (A) AP fluoroscopic image taken during an injection of contrast into the radiocarpal joint demonstrating contrast extending into the distal radioulnar joint (*arrowhead*) and midcarpal joint (*arrowhead*), compatible with tears of the triangular fibrocartilage and scapholunate ligaments. Coronal T1 FS image (B) with intra-articular gadolinium demonstrates a large tear in the scapholunate ligament (*arrow*), as well as a small tear in the radial aspect of the triangular fibrocartilage (*arrowhead*). Axial T2 FS image (C) shows disruption of the dorsal and volar fibers of the scapholunate ligament (*arrows*).

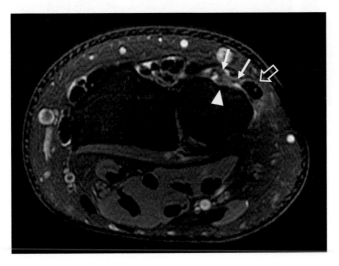

Figure 43.18. ECU tendon dislocation. Axial T2 FS image of the wrist demonstrates medial dislocation of the extensor carpi ulnaris tendon (*open arrow*) with a tear of the ulnar subsheath (*arrows*) that usually stabilizes the ECU tendon within the ulnar groove (*arrowhead*).

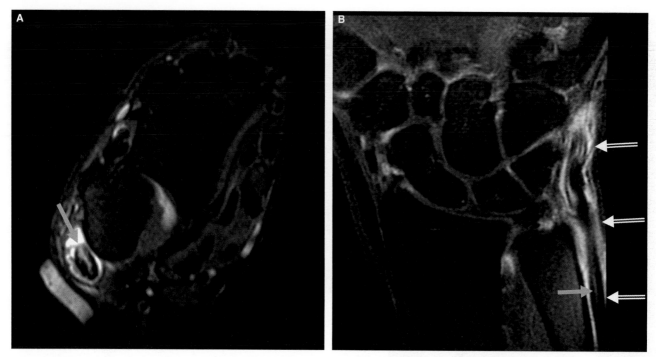

Figure 43.19. (A) Axial T2 FS image of the wrist demonstrates a split tear of the extensor carpi ulnaris tendon (*arrow*) with surrounding tenosynovial fluid and synovitis. Coronal T1 FS post-gadolinium (B) also shows the tendon tear (*arrow*), with marked peritendinous enhancement (*double line arrows*), compatible with tenosynovitis.

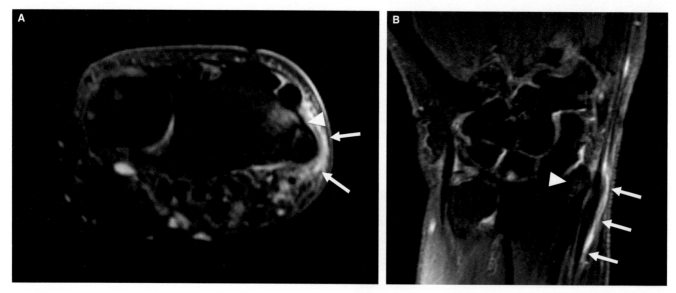

Figure 43.20. Axial (A) and coronal T2 FS (B) images in a 73-year-old woman with wrist pain demonstrates marked inflammatory changes around the first extensor compartment tendons (*arrows*), compatible with de Quervain's tenosynovitis. A bone spur and reactive bone marrow edema is seen along the radial styloid (*arrowhead*).

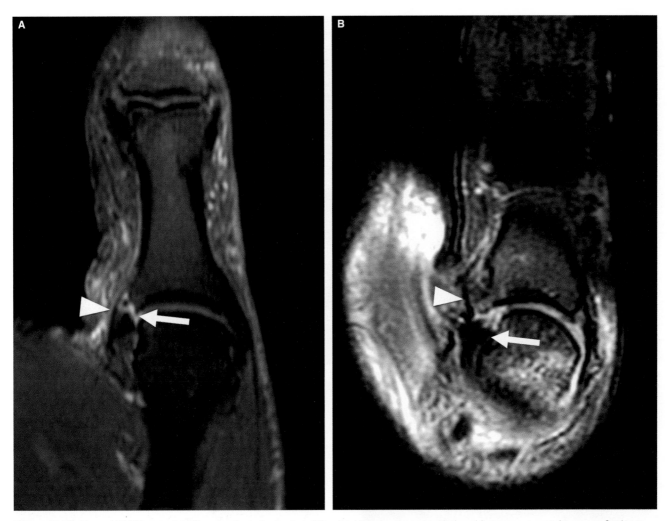

Figure 43.21. Coronal T2 FS images in different patients demonstrate (A) a distal UCL tear (*arrow*), with the adductor aponeurosis lying superficial to it (*arrowhead*), and (B) a Stener lesion, with the adductor aponeurosis (arrowhead) perched on the torn and retracted UCL (*arrow*), forming the so-called "yoyo on a string" appearance.

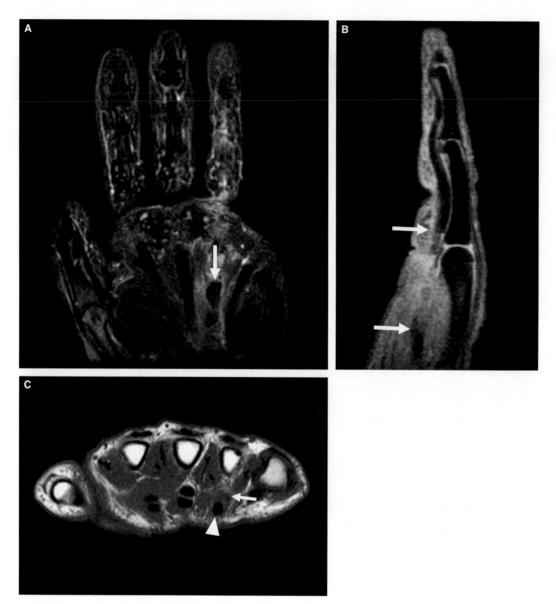

Figure 43.22. Coronal T2 FS (A), sagittal T2 FS (B), and axial T1-weighted (C) images in a patient with rheumatoid arthritis and sudden inability to flex the distal ring finger. The flexor digitorum profundus tendon is ruptured, with the disrupted tendon ends clearly identified (*arrows*). The overlying flexor digitorum superficialis tendon (*arrowhead*) appears intact.

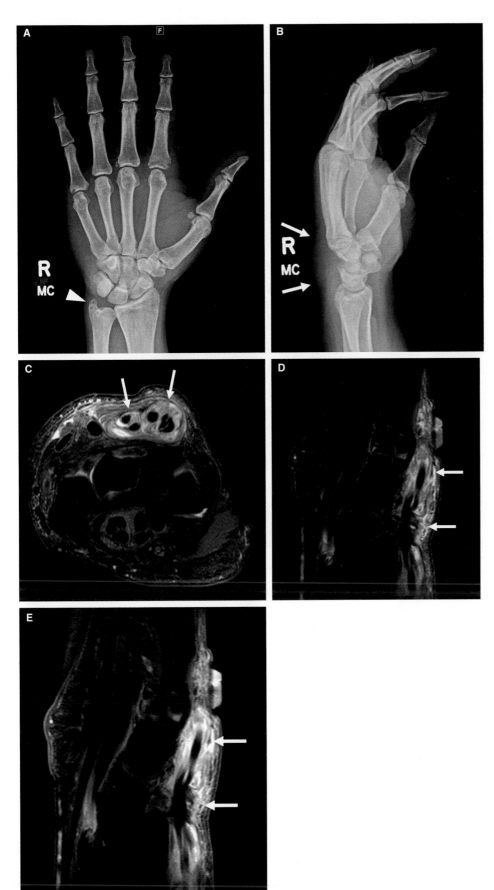

Figure 43.23. AP (A) and lateral (B) radiographs of the right hand in a 51-year-old diabetic man with pain and mass over dorsal wrist demonstrating well-defined erosions of the ulnar styloid (*arrowhead*), with no osteopenia or overlying soft tissue swelling, which would be atypical for rheumatoid arthritis. Marked soft tissue swelling is seen over the dorsal wrist (*arrows*). Axial T2 FS (C), sagittal T2 FS (D), and T1 FS post-contrast (E) images demonstrate severe enhancing tenosynovitis of the extensor digitorum tendons (*arrows*). The patient was subsequently found to have gout.

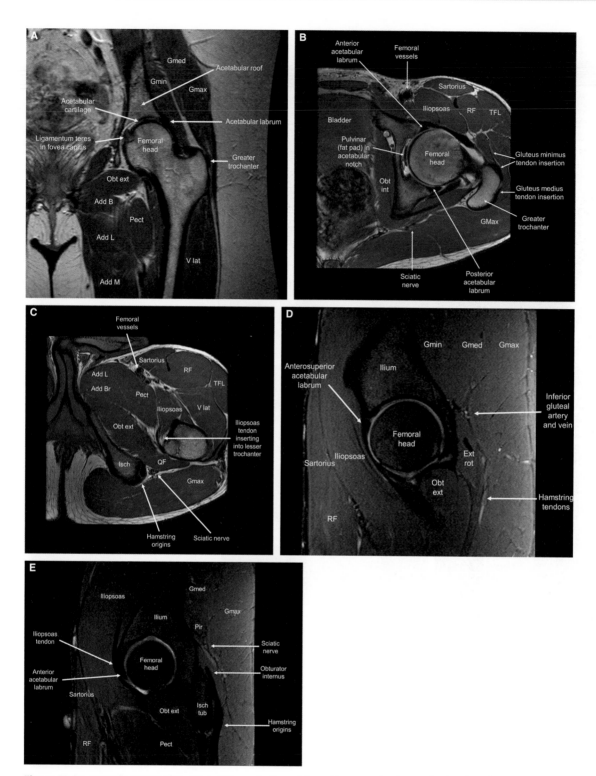

Figure 43.24. Normal anatomy of the hip. In MRI examinations of the pelvis or sacroiliac joints, a body coil can be used with a large field of view. This can be helpful when looking for multifocal pathology, or when the patient presents with vague or nonspecific symptoms that could be generated by a number of different anatomic structures within the pelvis. Some conditions such as osteonecrosis can occur bilaterally, and including both hips within the field of view may pick up occult disease on the asymptomatic side. If symptoms are localized to the hip, a surface coil and smaller field of view allows more detailed anatomic visualization. MR arthrography is commonly performed to look for intra-articular pathology, as the presence of fluid within the joint increases the sensitivity for diagnosis of labral tears or articular cartilage pathology.

Coronal T1 (A), axial T1 (B, C), and sagittal T2 FS (D, E) images through the left hip demonstrating normal anatomy. Gmin = gluteus minimus, Gmed = gluteus medius, Gmax = gluteus maximus, Obt ext = obturator externus, Obt int = obturator internus, RF = rectus femoris, TFL = tensor fascia late, V lat = vastus lateralis, Pir = piriformis, Pect = pectineus, Add L = adductor longus, Add B = adductor brevis, Add M = adductor magnus, QF = quadratus femoris.

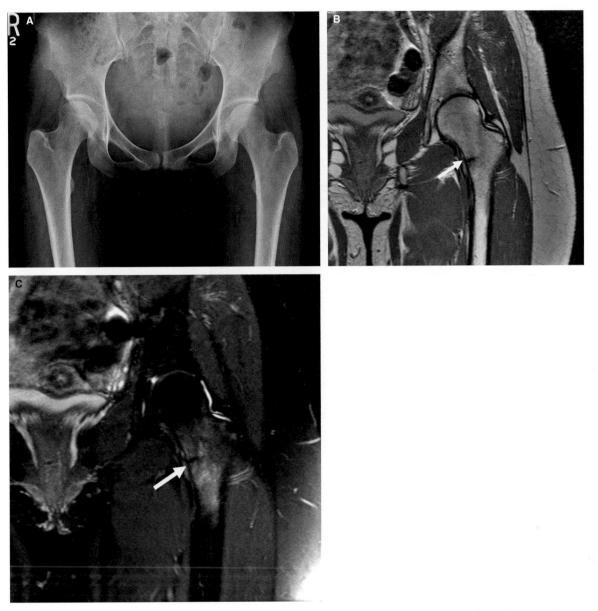

Figure 43.25. (A) AP radiograph of the pelvis in a 22-year-old college athlete with left hip pain demonstrates no bony abnormality. Coronal PD (B) and T2 FS (C) images of the left hip 9 days later demonstrate an incomplete stress fracture (*arrow*) across the medial aspect of the left femoral neck.

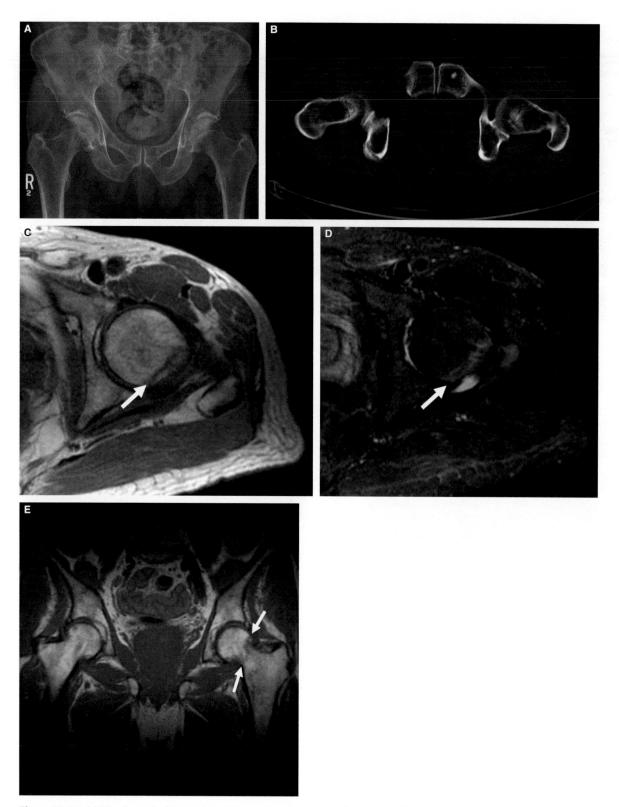

Figure 43.26. (A) AP radiograph of the pelvis in a 76-year-old male who tripped on a step and had severe left hip pain, but in whom no acute bony injury is seen. Axial CT image (B) of the left hip again demonstrates nonspecific lucencies in both femoral heads, but no obvious cortical disruption. Axial T1 (C), STIR (D), and coronal T1-weighted (E) images show linear signal traversing the subcapital portion of the femoral neck (*arrow*), with associated bone marrow edema, compatible with a nondisplaced fracture.

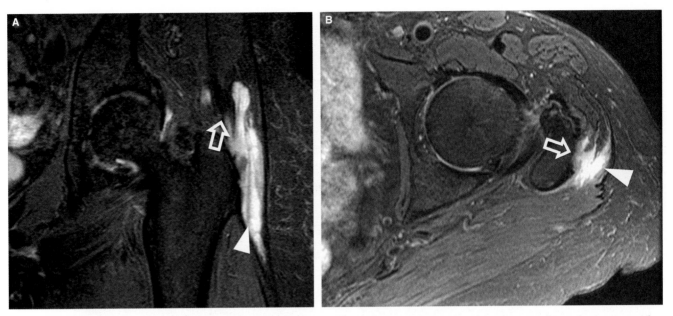

Figure 43.27. Coronal (A) and axial (B) T2 FS images in an 84-year-old woman after a fall demonstrate avulsion of the gluteus medius tendon (*open arrow*) from the middle facet of the greater trochanter, with an overlying bursal fluid collection (*arrowhead*).

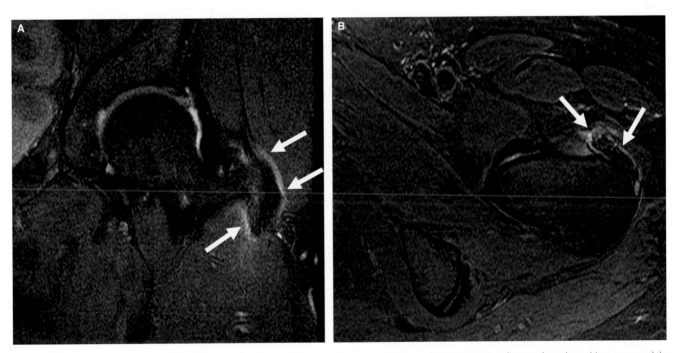

Figure 43.28. Coronal (A) and axial (B) T2 FS images of a 45-year-old female with recurrent hip pain. Prominent peritendinous edema (*arrow*) is seen around the gluteus minimus tendon insertion, compatible with peritendinitis.

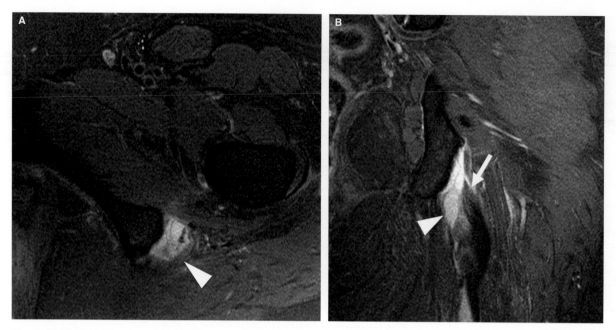

Figure 43.29. Axial (A) and coronal (B) T2 FS images of a 57-year-old man with acute posterior thigh pain. The proximal hamstring tendons have been completely avulsed, with retraction of the tendon ends (*arrow*) and focal fluid within the ischial bursa (*arrowheads*).

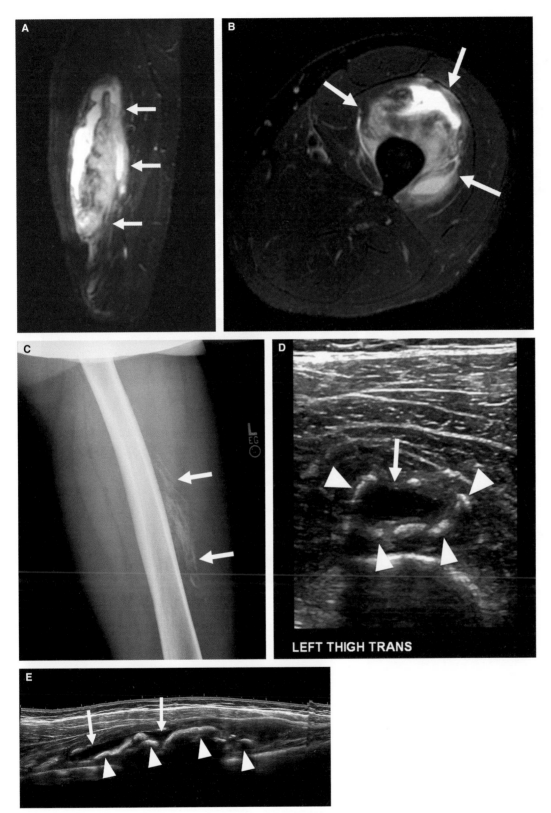

Figure 43.30. Sagittal (A) and coronal T2 FS (B) images in 20-year-old basketball player with a direct blow to his thigh demonstrates a large tear of the vastus intermedius muscle, with discontinuity of fibers and a large hematoma (*arrows*). Lateral x-ray (C) 3 weeks later demonstrates ill-defined calcification (*arrows*) in the anterior thigh, compatible with myositis ossificans. Axial (D) and sagittal (E) ultrasound images of the left anterior thigh demonstrate a hematoma in the anterior thigh (*arrow*), with peripheral areas of calcification (*arrowheads*).

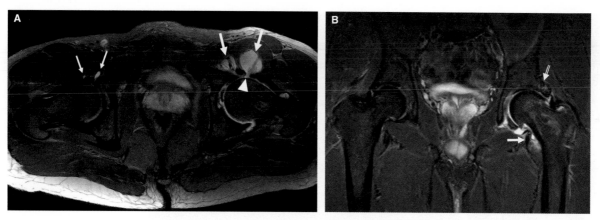

Figure 43.31. Axial T2 FS image (A) of a 49-year-old man with left hip pain demonstrates a bilobed fluid collection and synovitis adjacent to the left iliopsoas tendon (*arrow*), compatible with severe iliopsoas bursitis. The iliopsoas bursa communicates with the hip joint via a small defect in the anterior capsule (*arrowhead*). Mild iliopsoas bursitis is also present on the right (*small arrows*). Coronal STIR image (B) demonstrates edema around the distal iliopsoas tendon (*arrow*). Severe osteoarthritis is present in the left hip, with a joint effusion and synovitis. There is bony over-coverage of the femoral head, with a chronic stress fracture of the acetabular margin (*double line arrow*), suggesting that the patient has pincer-type femoral acetabular impingement.

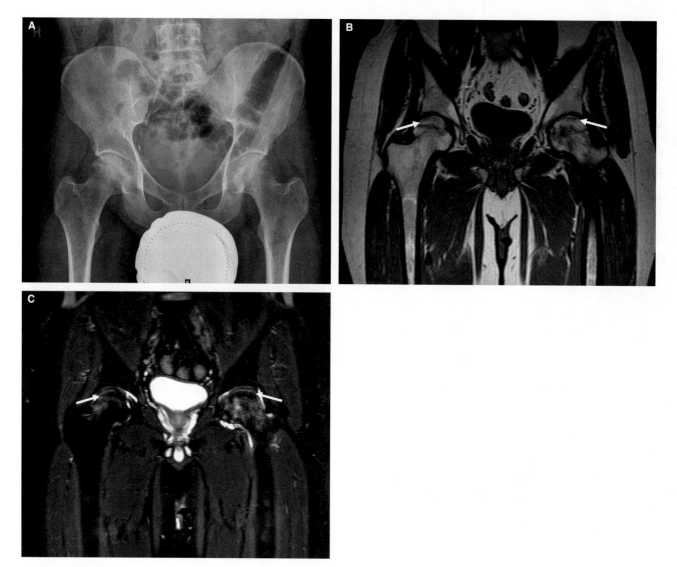

Figure 43.32. (A) AP radiograph of the pelvis in a 35-year-old renal transplant patient with bilateral hip pain. Surgical clips in the right hemipelvis are related to the transplant, but the hips look unremarkable. Coronal T1 (B) and T2 FS (C) demonstrate bilateral osteonecrosis of the femoral heads, with the characteristic double line sign. Necrotic bone retains the signal of normal bone marrow initially, although there would be no enhancement if gadolinium were given. Subtle subchondral linear signal is seen in both hips (*arrows*), compatible with subchondral fractures, but there is no evidence of articular surface collapse.

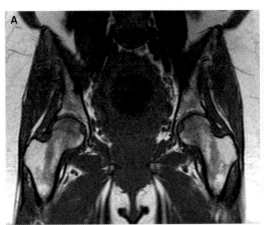

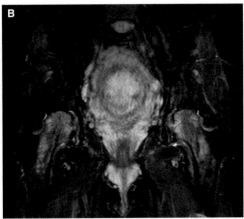

Figure 43.33. Coronal T1 (A) and T2 FS (B) images in a 38-year-old woman in the third trimester of pregnancy with hip pain, showing a pregnant uterus and symmetric bone marrow edema in the femoral necks bilaterally. The appearances are consistent with transient osteoporosis, which is usually self-limiting and resolves within 6 to 10 months.

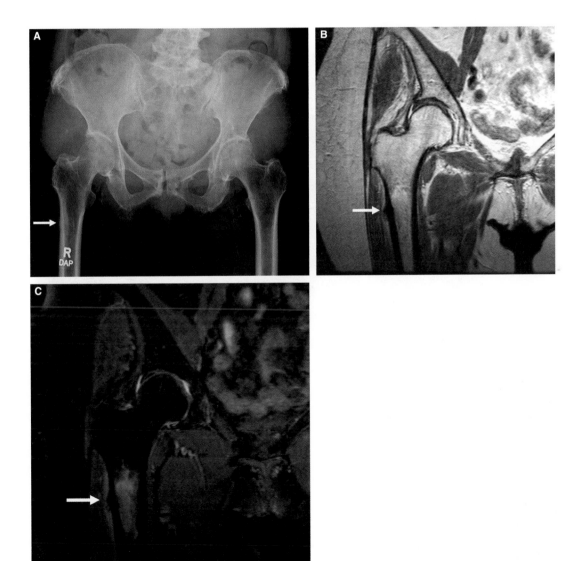

Figure 43.34. Patient with hepatocellular carcinoma and right hip pain. (A) AP radiograph demonstrates subtle periosteal reaction along the lateral aspect of the femoral shaft (*arrow*). Coronal T1 (B) and T2 FS (C) images demonstrate an early fracture with prominent bone marrow edema and periosteal edema (*arrow*). The appearances are typical of a bisphosphonate-induced subtrochanteric insufficiency fracture. The patient had been taking bisphosphonates for osteoporosis.

609

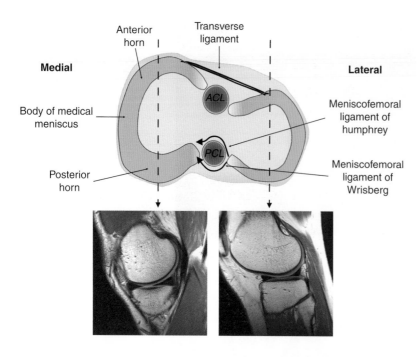

Figure 43.35. Diagrammatic representation of normal meniscal anatomy, with sagittal sections through the medial and lateral menisci. The medial meniscus shows that the posterior horn is twice as large as the anterior. The posterior horn of the lateral meniscus is the same size as the anterior horn.

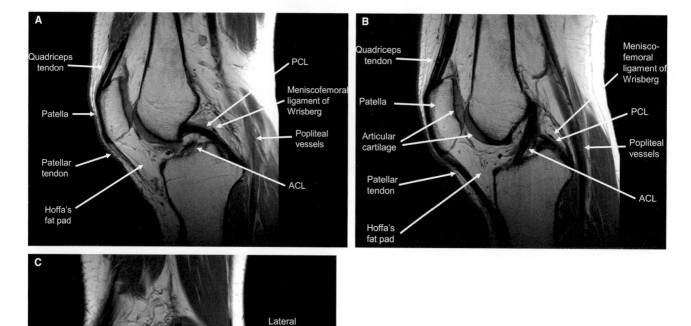

Figure 43.36. Normal anatomy. Sagittal PD images through the intercondylar notch (A, B). PCL = posterior cruciate ligament, ACL = anterior cruciate ligament. Sagittal PD image through the lateral knee (C) demonstrating normal anatomy.

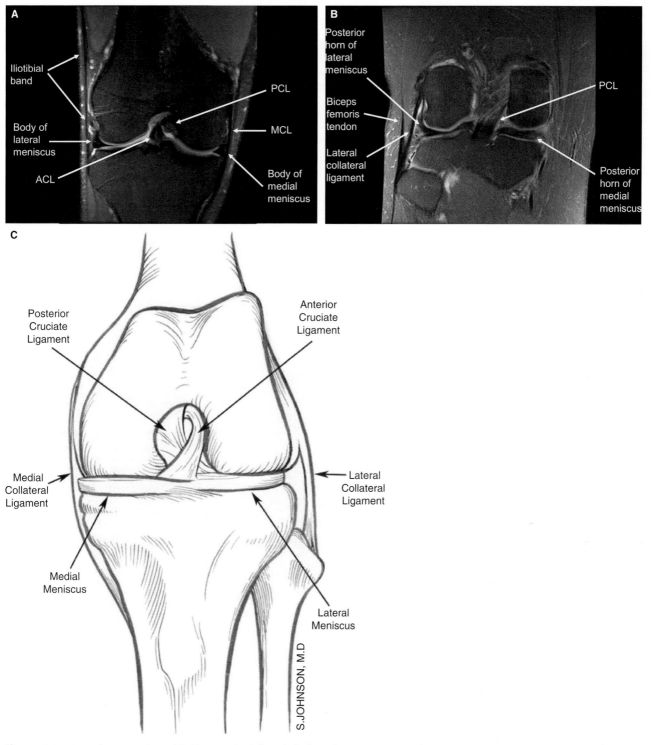

Figure 43.37. Normal anatomy. Coronal T2 FS images (A, B) through the knee demonstrating normal anatomy. ACL = anterior cruciate ligament, PCL = posterior cruciate ligament, MCL = medial collateral ligament. Diagrammatic representation of the normal anatomic structures (C).

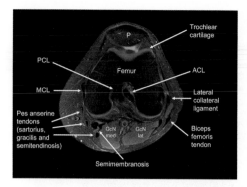

Figure 43.38. Normal anatomy. Axial PD FS image through the knee at the level of the intercondylar notch showing normal structures. P = patella, ACL = anterior cruciate ligament, PCL = posterior cruciate ligament, MCL = medial collateral ligament, GcN med = medial gastrocnemius, GcN lat = lateral gastrocnemius.

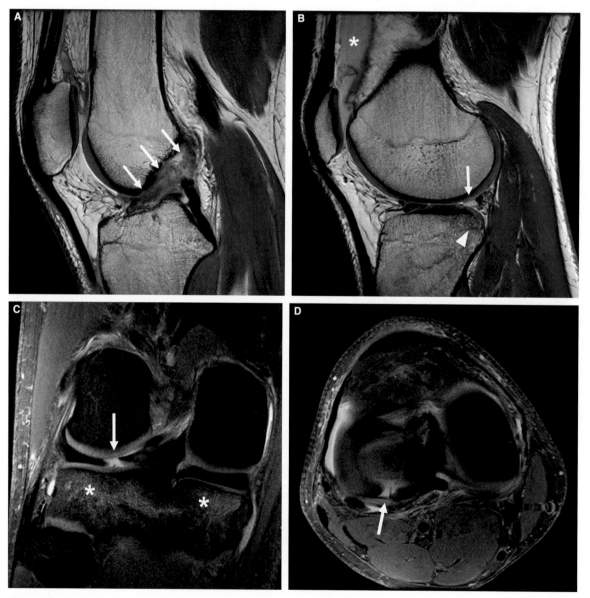

Figure 43.39. MR images of a 33-year-old patient who sustained a pivot injury to his right knee. Sagittal PD image (A) demonstrates diffuse disruption of ACL fibers compatible with a complete tear. Sagittal PD image (B) shows truncation of the posterior horn of the lateral meniscus (*arrow*), with a small underlying impaction fracture (*arrowhead*). A large joint effusion is evident in the suprapatellar bursa (*asterisk*). Coronal T2 FS (C) and axial PD FS (D) images demonstrate a large radial tear (*arrow*) in the posterior horn extending through the majority of the meniscal width. Bone marrow edema is seen within the proximal tibia posteriorly (*asterisks*).

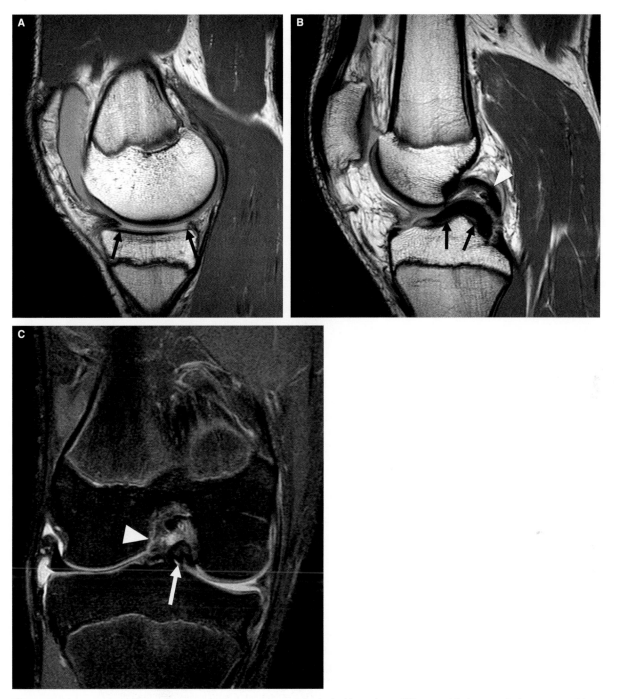

Figure 43.40. A 15-year-old boy with previous ACL tear presents with a locked knee. Sagittal PD image (A) shows marked truncation of the normal medial meniscus peripherally (*arrows*). Sagittal PD image (B) shows a large meniscal fragment (*arrows*) lying anterior to the PCL (*arrowhead*), resulting in a "double PCL" sign. Coronal PD FS (C) shows the large displaced bucket-handle tear (*arrow*). The ACL appears markedly irregular (*arrowhead*).

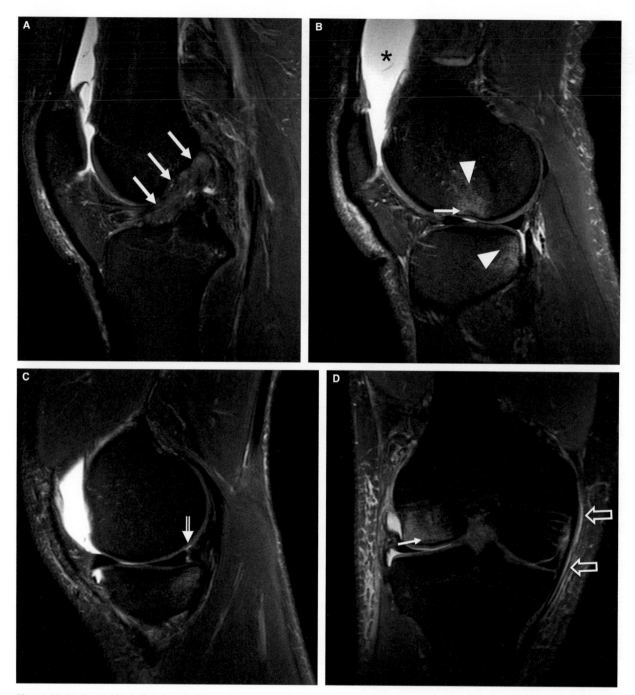

Figure 43.41. Sagittal (A, B, C) and coronal (D) T2 FS images in a 25-year-old soccer player with an acute twisting injury demonstrates diffuse disruption of the ACL (*arrows*), with "kissing contusions" on the lateral femoral condyle and lateral tibial plateau (*arrowheads*), where the two bones have impacted each other. A linear low-signal intensity line (*small arrow*) is visible in the lateral femoral condyle (*arrowhead*), compatible with a small impaction fracture. A large joint effusion is evident (*asterisk*). There is a vertical tear through the posterior horn of the medial meniscus (*double line arrow*), with subjacent bone marrow edema. The MCL is intact, but there is prominent periligamentous edema (*open arrow*), compatible with a low-grade sprain.

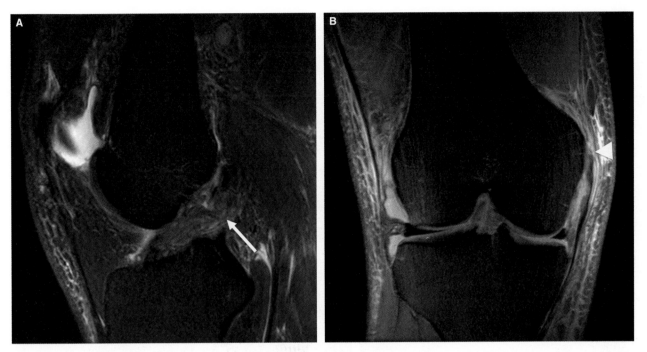

Figure 43.42. A 35-year-old male with skiing injury. Sagittal T2 FS image (A) demonstrates a complete tear of the proximal ACL (*arrow*). Coronal T2 FS image (B) shows a high-grade tear of the proximal MCL (*arrowhead*), with prominent periligamentous edema.

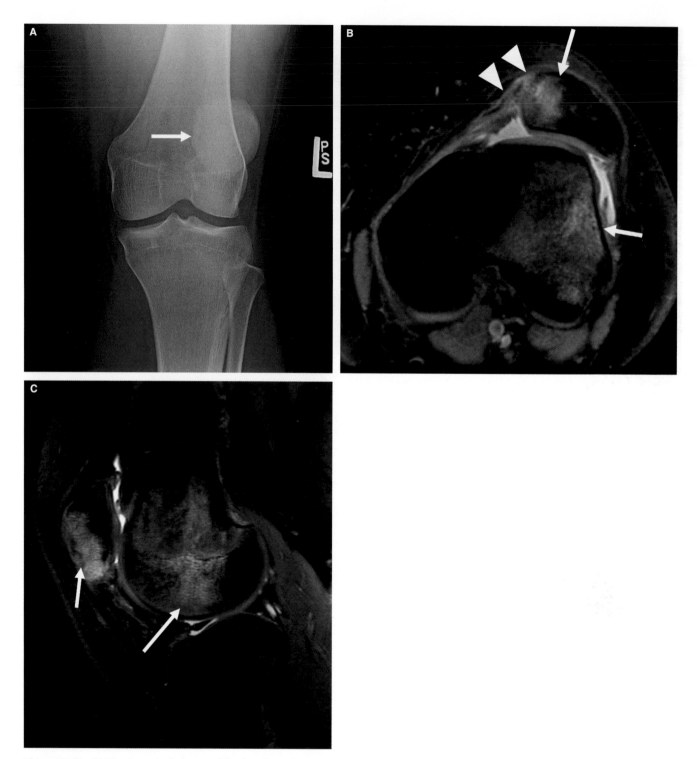

Figure 43.43. (A) AP radiograph of a 21-year-old hockey player after an acute knee injury demonstrating mild lateral displacement of the patella (*arrow*). Axial PD FS (B) and coronal T2 FS (C) images demonstrate "kissing contusions" on the medial patella and lateral femoral condyle (*arrows*), characteristic of recent lateral patellar dislocation, with high-grade sprain of the medial retinaculum (*arrowheads*).

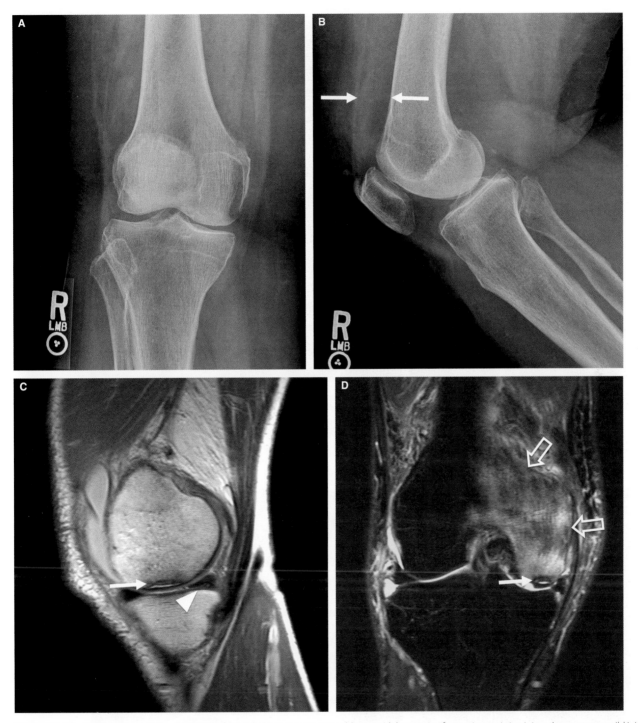

Figure 43.44. AP (A) and lateral (B) radiographs of the right knee in an 81-year-old man with knee pain after a minor twisting injury demonstrates mild joint space narrowing medially and a moderate joint effusion (*arrows*). Sagittal PD (C) and coronal T2 FS (D) images through the medial compartment demonstrate a curvilinear subchondral insufficiency fracture of the medial femoral condyle containing fluid (*arrow*), with extensive bone marrow edema (*open arrows*). There is a small undersurface tear of the posterior horn of the medial meniscus (*arrowhead*), with mild extrusion of the body. Subchondral insufficiency fractures are commonly associated with large tears of the posterior root of the medial meniscus, allowing extrusion of the meniscus, changing the weight-bearing stresses in the medial compartment.

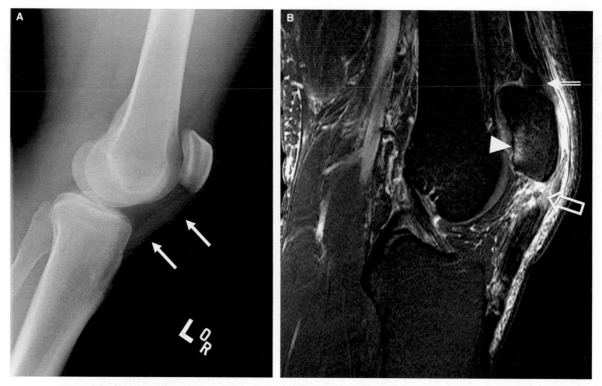

Figure 43.45. A 42-year-old male patient with sudden anterior knee pain after jumping off a high wall. The lateral x-ray (A) shows mild prepatellar soft tissue swelling (*arrows*) but no fracture. Sagittal T2 FS (B) image shows a complete tear of the proximal patellar tendon (*open arrow*) and low-grade tear of the distal quadriceps tendon (*double line arrow*). Minor subchondral edema is seen in the inferior patella (*arrowhead*).

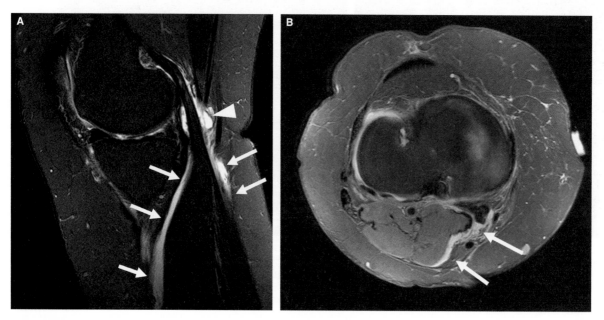

Figure 43.46. Sagittal (A) and axial PD FS (B) images in a patient with acute calf pain demonstrates a small fluid collection in the expected location of a Baker's cyst (*arrowhead*), with ill-defined fluid tracking distally around the medial gastrocnemius muscle (*arrows*), compatible with a ruptured Baker's cyst.

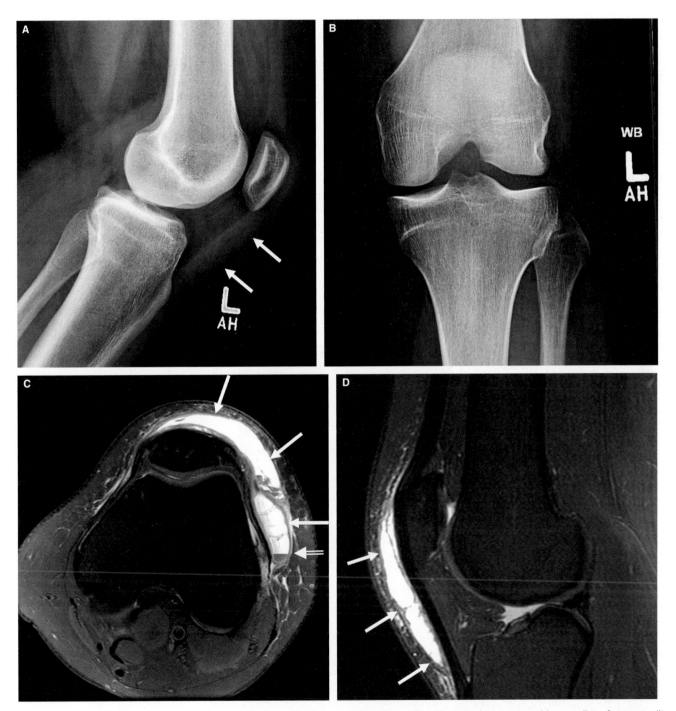

Figure 43.47. A 19-year-old female soccer player with a fall one month ago. AP (A) and lateral (B) radiographs demonstrate mild prepatellar soft tissue swelling (*arrows*) but are otherwise unremarkable. Axial PD FS (B) and sagittal T2 FS (C) images demonstrate a large hematoma (*arrows*) in the prepatellar soft tissues extending laterally. A fluid level is visible on the axial image (*double line arrow*). The appearances are compatible with a Morel-Lavallee lesion, resulting from a shearing injury between the subcutaneous fat and underlying fascia. These can develop a thick-walled capsule and may need percutaneous aspiration.

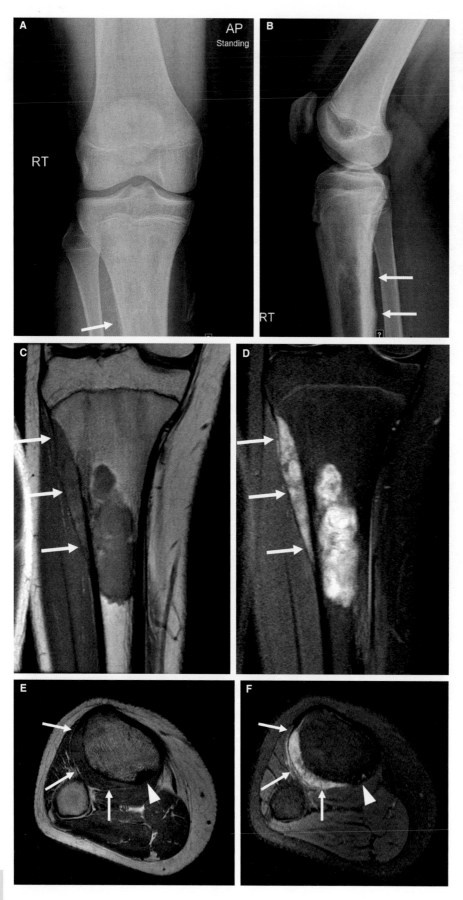

Figure 43.48. AP (A) and lateral (B) radiographs of the right knee in a 15-year-old patient with persistent knee pain after minor trauma 8 days ago demonstrates subtle periosteal reaction (*arrows*) along the posterolateral aspect of the proximal tibia. Coronal T1 (C) and T2 FS (D) images demonstrate a lobulated tumor in the proximal tibia, with subperiosteal tumor (*arrows*) extending superiorly along the lateral tibia. Axial T1 (E) and T2 FS (F) images showing extensive subperiosteal spread of tumor (*arrows*). An incidental small sclerotic fibrous cortical defect is seen posteriorly (*arrowhead*). Patients with osseous tumors can present to the emergency room with fairly nonspecific symptoms or may attribute their symptoms to a recent traumatic event. The findings can be extremely subtle on initial radiographic examinations, particularly if symptoms are poorly localized. MRI is very sensitive for tumor infiltration of bone marrow and extent of soft tissue involvement and is used both to diagnose and stage disease.

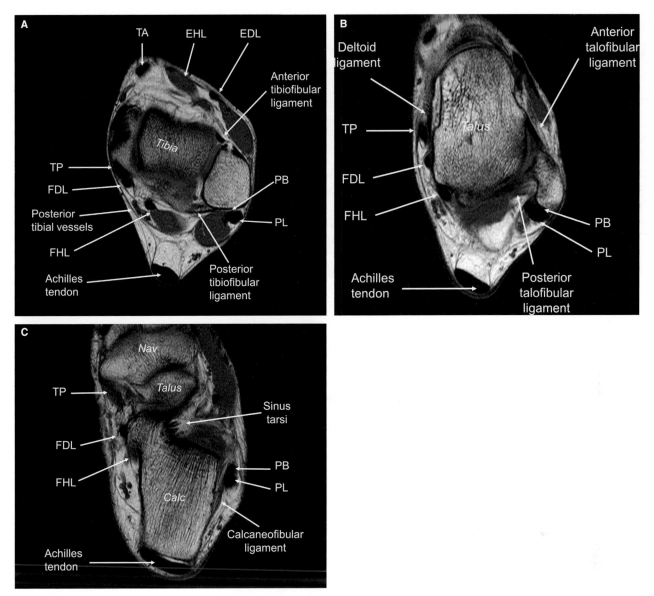

Figure 43.49. Normal anatomy of the ankle. (A) Axial T1 image through the ankle at the level of the inferior tibiofibular syndesmosis. TA = tibialis anterior, EHL = extensor hallucis longus, EDL = extensor digitorum longus, TP = tibialis posterior, FDL = flexor digitorum longus, FHL = flexor hallucis longus, PB = peroneus brevis, PL = peroneus longus tendons. (B) Axial T1 image at a slightly lower section through the talus. (C) Axial T1 image at a lower section through the calcaneus (Calc).

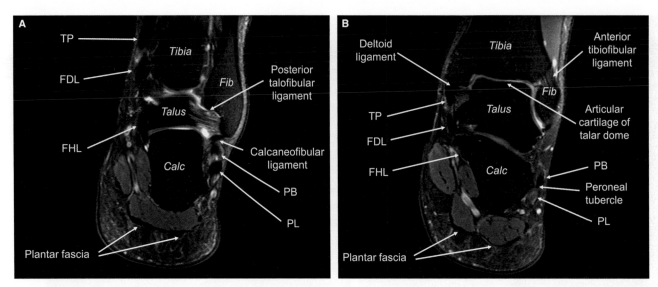

Figure 43.50. (A) Coronal T2-weighted image through the posterior ankle joint. Calc = calcaneus, Fib = fibula, TP = tibialis posterior, FDL = flexor digitorum longus, FHL = flexor hallucis longus, PB = peroneus brevis, PL = peroneus longus. (B) Coronal T2-weighted image through the mid portion of the ankle joint.

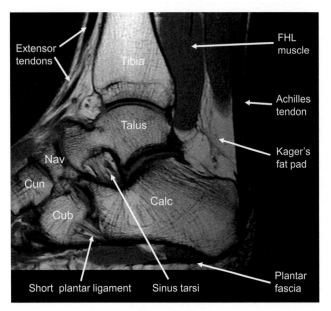

Figure 43.51. Sagittal PD image of the ankle showing normal anatomy. Calc = calcaneus, Cub = cuboid, Nav = navicular, Cun = cuneiform, FHL = flexor hallucis longus.

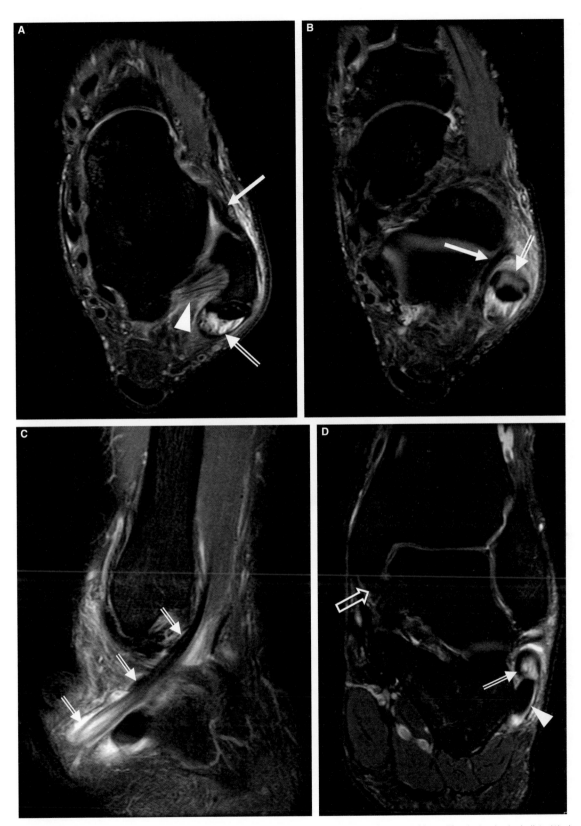

Figure 43.52. Axial PD FS images (A, B, C) through the ankle of a 23-year-old male who twisted his ankle playing basketball. In (A), the anterior talofibular ligament (*arrow*) is markedly thickened, compatible with grade 2 sprain. The posterior talofibular ligament appears intact, with mild interspersed edema (*arrowhead*). Tenosynovial fluid is seen in the peroneal tendon sheath (*double line arrow*). In (B), the calcaneofibular ligament (*arrow*) is thickened but intact. There is a split tear of the peroneus brevis tendon, manifesting as a C-shaped tendon (*double line arrow*), with marked surrounding inflammatory change. Sagittal PD FS (C) and coronal PD FS (D) images also demonstrate the longitudinal split tear (*double line arrows*) of peroneus brevis, with surrounding fluid and edema. Peroneus longus (*arrowhead*) appears intact. The deltoid ligament (*open arrow*) and articular cartilage of the talar dome are intact.

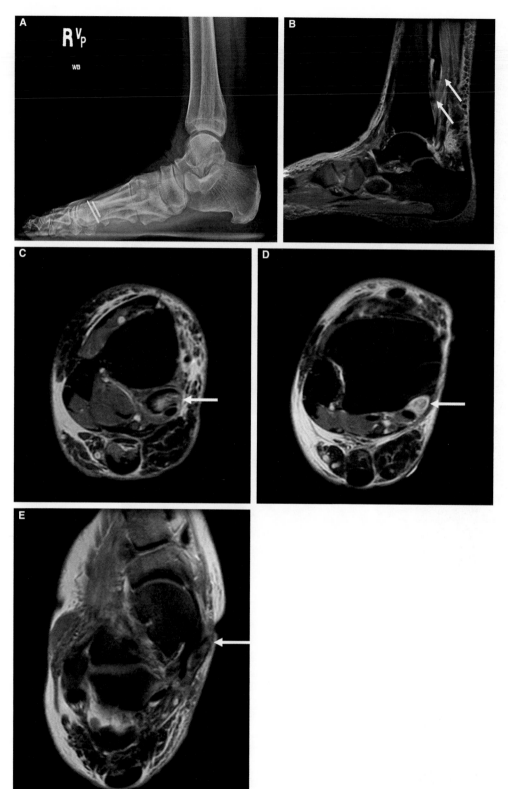

Figure 43.53. (A) Lateral radiograph of a 70-year-old woman with severe medial ankle pain after a stumble demonstrating mild pes planus (flat foot). Sagittal PD FS (B) image demonstrates a complete tear of the posterior tibial tendon (*arrow*), with the tendon end retracted proximally. Axial PD FS image above the tear (C) shows a thickened retracted tendon (*arrow*) with associated edema. Axial PD FS image at the level of the medial malleolus (D) demonstrates absence of the posterior tibial tendon in the tendon sheath, which contains hemorrhagic debris (*arrow*). Axial PD FS image more distally (E) demonstrates some retracted torn tendon fibers (*arrow*) at the level of the talar neck.

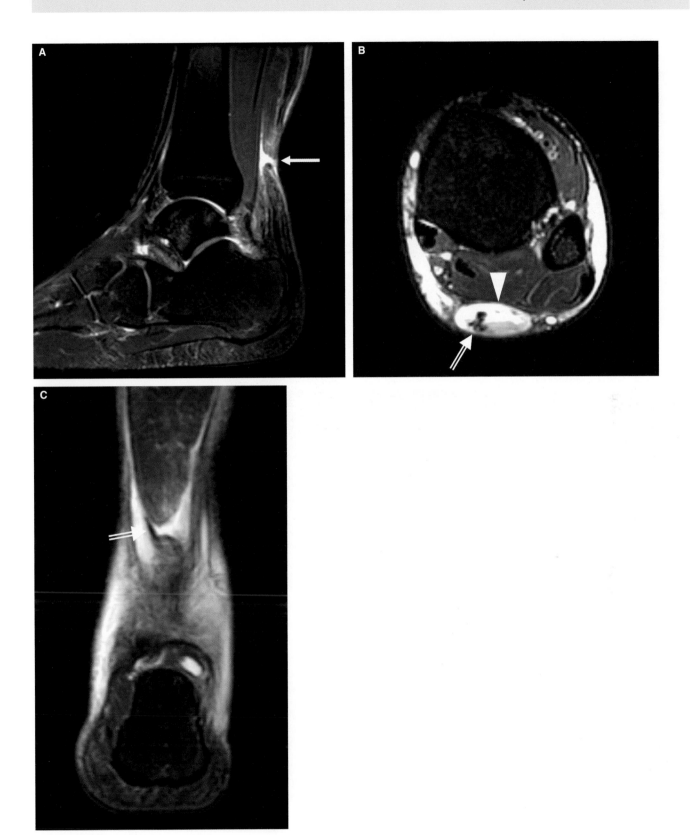

Figure 43.54. Sagittal T2 FS (A) of the left ankle in a 21-year-old athlete with sudden pain demonstrates a high-grade tear of the Achilles tendon at the myotendinous junction (*arrow*), with mild retraction of the tendon ends. On the axial T2 FS image (B) there appears to be a few tendon fibers remaining intact (*double line arrow*), with surrounding hematoma (*arrowheads*). However, on the coronal T2 FS image (C), the fibers are shown to be noncontiguous (*arrow*).

625

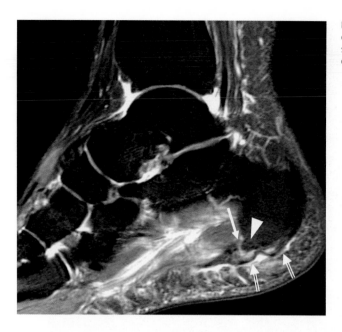

Figure 43.55. Sagittal T2 FS image in a football player with heel pain demonstrates detachment of the proximal plantar fascia (*arrow*), with periosteal stripping along the inferior calcaneus (*double line arrows*). A small plantar calcaneal spur is present (*arrowhead*).

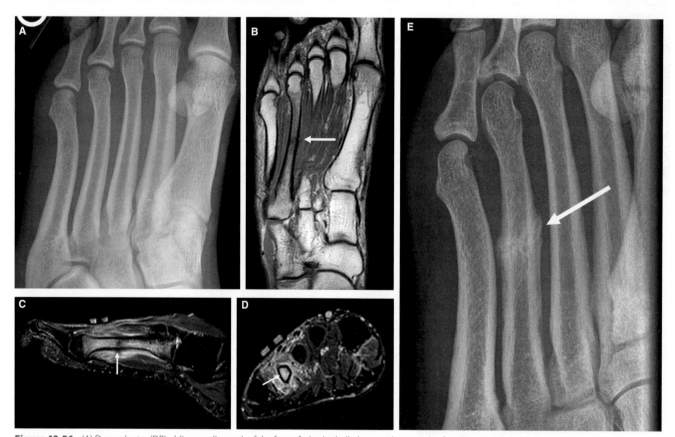

Figure 43.56. (A) Dorsoplantar (DP) oblique radiograph of the foot of a basketball player with pain in his fourth metatarsal. No abnormality can be seen, and an MRI was therefore requested. Axial T1 (B), sagittal T2 FS (C), and coronal T2 FS (D) images show severe edema in the 4th metatarsal shaft, with a low signal intensity line centrally, consistent with a stress fracture (*arrow*). Extensive edema is also seen within the surrounding soft tissues. A follow-up radiograph (E) 3 weeks later now clearly shows the stress fracture with surrounding callus formation.

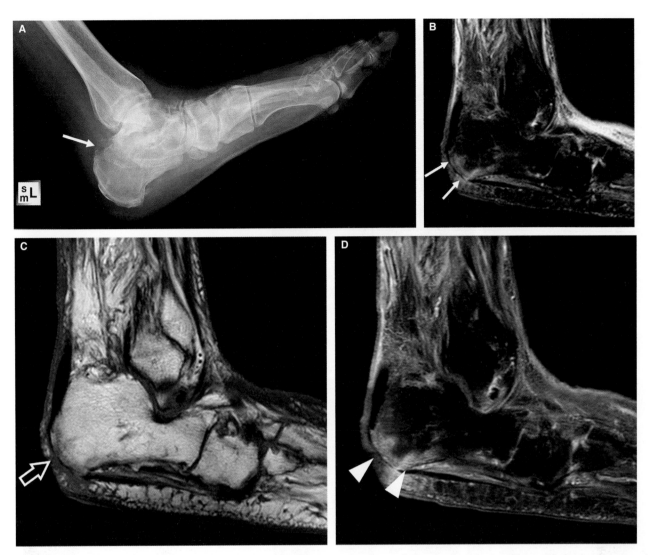

Figure 43.57. Lateral radiograph (A) of the left foot in an 81-year-old diabetic male with a small ulcer over the posterior calcaneus. The bones are osteopenic, and there is a pes planus deformity (flat foot), with prominent degenerative change of the mid foot. No obvious bony destruction is seen adjacent to the ulcer, although there is some irregularity of the posterior superior calcaneus (*arrow*). Sagittal T2 FS (B), T1 (C), and T1 FS post gadolinium (D) images of the foot demonstrate a large soft tissue defect over the posterior heel (*small arrows*), with underlying bone marrow edema. On T1, there is cortical irregularity of the calcaneus with subtle areas of low T1 signal intensity (*open arrow*) and enhancement following gadolinium (*arrowheads*) compatible with early osteomyelitis.

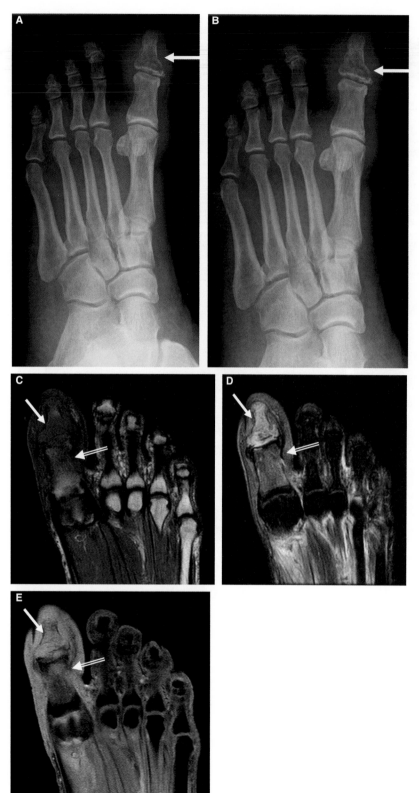

Figure 43.58. AP (A) and DP oblique (B) radiographs of a 55-year-old diabetic patient with a red swollen toe show soft tissue swelling and patchy lucency in the distal phalanx of the big toe (*arrow*). Coronal T1 image (C) shows that there is extensive osteomyelitis in the distal phalanx, with replacement of the normal fatty marrow (*arrow*), and poor visualization of the overlying cortex causing a "ghost sign." Coronal T2 FS (D) demonstrates with corresponding high T2 signal in the distal phalanx (*arrow*), but there is also mild bone marrow edema (*double line arrow*) in the proximal phalanx, with subtle areas of low signal on T1 (*double line arrow*), suggesting early spread of infection. Coronal T1 post gadolinium (E) shows diffuse enhancement in the distal phalanx (*arrow*) and mild enhancement in the proximal phalanx (*double line arrow*).

References

1. Schrader R: Contrast material-induced renal failure: an overview. *J Interv Cardiol* 2005;**18**:417–23.

2. Stacul F: Reducing the risks for contrast-induced nephropathy. *Cardiovasc Intervent Radiol* 2005;**28**(Suppl 2):S12–18.

3. Toprak O, Cirit M: Risk factors for contrast-induced nephropathy. *Kidney Blood Press Res* 2006;**29**:84–93.

4. Thomsen HS: How to avoid nephrogenic systemic fibrosis: current guidelines in Europe and the United States. *Radiol Clin North Am.* 2009 Sep;**47**(5):871–5.

5. Feldman F, Staron R, Zwass A, et al.: MR imaging: its role in detecting occult fractures. *Skeletal Radiol* 1994;**23**:439–44.

6. Frihagen F, Nordsletten L, Tariq R, et al.: MRI diagnosis of occult hip fractures. *Acta Orthop* 2005;**76**:524–30.

7. Memarsadeghi M, Breitenseher MJ, Schaefer-Prokop C, et al.: Occult scaphoid fractures: comparison of multidetector CT and MR imaging–initial experience. *Radiology* 2006;**240**:169–76.

8. Verbeeten KM, Hermann KL, Hasselqvist M, et al.: The advantages of MRI in the detection of occult hip fractures. *Eur Radiol* 2005;**15**:165–9.

9. Bencardino JT, Rosenberg ZS: Sports-related injuries of the wrist: an approach to MRI interpretation. *Clin Sports Med* 2006;**25**:409–32.

10. Campbell SE: MRI of sports injuries of the ankle. *Clin Sports Med* 2006;**25**:727–62.

11. Chaipat L, Palmer WE: Shoulder magnetic resonance imaging. *Clin Sports Med* 2006;**25**:371–86.

12. Gehrmann RM, Rajan S, Patel DV, et al.: Athletes' ankle injuries: diagnosis and management. *Am J Orthop* 2005;**34**: 551–61.

13. Hayes CW, Coggins CA: Sports-related injuries of the knee: an approach to MRI interpretation. *Clin Sports Med* 2006;**25**: 659–79.

14. Kaplan LJ, Potter HG: MR imaging of ligament injuries to the elbow. *Radiol Clin North Am* 2006;**44**:583–94.

15. Meislin R, Abeles A: Role of hip MR imaging in the management of sports-related injuries. *Magn Reson Imaging Clin N Am* 2005;**13**:635–40.

16. Morag Y, Jacobson JA, Miller B, et al.: MR imaging of rotator cuff injury: what the clinician needs to know. *Radiographics* 2006;**26**:1045–65.

17. Tuite MJ, Kijowski R: Sports-related injuries of the elbow: an approach to MRI interpretation. *Clin Sports Med* 2006;**25**:387–408.

18. Zlatkin MB, Rosner J: MR imaging of ligaments and triangular fibrocartilage complex of the wrist. *Radiol Clin North Am* 2006;**44**:595–623.

19. Pineda C, Vargas A, Rodriguez AV: Imaging of osteomyelitis: current concepts. *Infect Dis Clin North Am* 2006;**20**:789–825.

20. Struk DW, Munk PL, Lee MJ, et al.: Imaging of soft tissue infections. *Radiol Clin North Am* 2001;**39**:277–303.

21. Kanal E, Shellock FG: Patient monitoring during clinical MR imaging. *Radiology* 1992;**185**:623–9.

22. Kanal E, Shellock FG: MR imaging of patients with intracranial aneurysm clips. *Radiology* 1993;**187**:612–4.

23. White LM, Buckwalter KA: Technical considerations: CT and MR imaging in the postoperative orthopedic patient. *Semin Musculoskelet Radiol* 2002;**6**:5–17.

24. Hargreaves BA, Worters PW, Pauly KB, et al.: Metal-induced artifacts in MRI. *AJR.* 2011; **197**:547–55.

Index